EPIDEMIOLOGY OF
WORK RELATED DISEASES

EPIDEMIOLOGY OF
WORK RELATED DISEASES

Edited by
CORBETT McDONALD
Professor Emeritus in Occupational Medicine,
University of London,
Professor Emeritus in Epidemiology,
McGill University, Montreal

BMJ
Publishing
Group

© BMJ Publishing Group 1995

First published in 1995
by the BMJ Publishing Group, BMA House, Tavistock Square,
London WC1H 9JR

British Library Cataloguing in Publication Data

A catalogue record for this book is available
from the British Library

ISBN 0-7279-0856-1

Typeset in Great Britain by Apek Typesetters Ltd, Nailsea, Bristol
Printed and bound in Great Britain by Latimer Trend & Co. Ltd., Plymouth

Contents

METHODOLOGY

COMMENTARY

Contributors

Benjamin Amick
Department of Health and Social Behaviour
Harvard School of Public Health
Boston
Massachusetts
USA

Olav Axelson
Department of Occupational and Environmental Medicine
University of Linköping
Linköping
Sweden

Geoffrey Berry
Department of Public Health
University of Sydney
Sydney
Australia

Bruce Case
Department of Pathology
McGill University
Montreal
Canada

Nicola Cherry
Centre for Occupational Health
University of Manchester
Manchester
UK

CONTRIBUTORS

Pieter-Jan Coenraads
Department of Dermatology
University Hospital
Groningen
The Netherlands

Edward Emmett
National Occupational Health and Safety Commission
Worksafe Australia
Sydney
Australia

Yutaka Hosoda
Institute of Radiation Epidemiology
Radiation Effects Association
Tokyo
Japan

Stanislav Kasl
Department of Epidemiology and Public Health
Yale University School of Medicine
New Haven
Connecticut
USA

Alison McDonald
Department of Occupational Medicine
McGill University
Montreal
Canada

Corbett McDonald
Department of Occupational and Environmental Medicine
Royal Brompton National Heart and Lung Institute
London
UK

James Merchant
Institute of Agricultural Medicine and Environmental Health
University of Iowa
Iowa City
Iowa
USA

viii

Peter Pelmear
Department of Occupational and Environmental Health
St Michael's Hospital
Toronto
Ontario
Canada

Stephen Reynolds
Institute of Agricultural Medicine and Environmental Health
University of Iowa
Iowa City
Iowa
USA

Hilkka Riihimäki
Department of Epidemiology and Biostatistics
Finnish Institute of Occupational Health
Helsinki
Finland

Rodolfo Saracci
Unit of Analytical Epidemiology
International Agency for Research on Cancer
Lyon
France

Henriëtte Smit
Department of Chronic Disease and Environmental Epidemiology
National Institute of Public Health and Environmental Protection
Bilthoven
The Netherlands

Anthony Newman Taylor
Department of Occupational and Environmental Medicine
Royal Brompton National Heart and Lung Hospital
London
UK

Gilles Thériault
Department of Occupational Health
McGill University
Montreal
Canada

CONTRIBUTORS

H A Waldron
Department of Occupational Health
St Mary's Hospital
London
UK

Hans Weill
Section of Environmental Medicine
Tulane University Medical Center
New Orleans
Louisiana
USA

Peter Westerholm
Division of Occupational Medicine
National Institute of Occupational Health
Stockholm
Sweden

Craig Zwerling
Institute of Agricultural Medicine and Environmental Health
College of Medicine
University of Iowa
Iowa City
Iowa
USA

INTRODUCTION

1 Occupational epidemiology

CORBETT McDONALD

> This is the epidemiologist's main role, to test properly the ideas that he or a clinician, pathologist or laboratory investigator formulates.
>
> Sartwell (1974)[1]

To originate an idea is a matter of luck or inspired intuition, to test it requires skill and objectivity; if properly done, the result is a contribution to science. Thus epidemiology, together with the complementary disciplines of physiopathology and toxicology, provide the scientific basis for medicine, and occupational epidemiology for medical practice as related to the interface between health and work. The aim of this book is to provide a concise statement of what is currently known about the epidemiology of the main groups of work-related disease and, at the same time, to review methodological issues which the research has identified. It is not a comprehensive manual of epidemiology and each contributor has been asked to select only those topics that seemed most important, but with as detailed an evaluation as possible of the quality of studies on which conclusions are based. Sadly, it is the common experience of those with expert knowledge of any subject to be appalled when they read about it in a text. It would be quite an achievement if the contents of this book were not to evoke that reaction. In the final chapters some personal views are presented on the central question of whether all this scientific effort is fulfilling its theoretical purpose and, if not, we need to consider why.

Epidemiology is concerned with the causation of disease and by inference with its prevention. As it depends primarily on observation

1

and seldom on experiment it is not easy to define the point at which it became a science. Some, even in quite high places, would say it never has, perhaps without sufficient thought for whether there is any better alternative. It is hard to see that fully controlled experiments of the kind that are common in the laboratory will ever be more than occasionally feasible for assessing cause and effect in humans. Even in evaluating treatment the double blind randomised trial has its limitations and experimental results in one species cannot be confidently applied to another, especially to humans. We have therefore little choice but to rely on circumstantial evidence derived from observation in much the same way as guilt or innocence is determined in a court of law. The legal view is that "to prove a thing is to test it,"[2] perhaps less difficult with a suspected pathogen than a suspected criminal, in that the test can usually be repeated in differing circumstances. Moreover, as stated by Sartwell, it is for the epidemiologist to conduct the test properly, which is where the evolution of methods and designs of improved reliability has, particularly in the past 50 years or so, brought the unstructured observations of the past to something that justifies more respect as a scientific discipline. Just as cause and effect can never be proved beyond all possible doubt, even for cigarettes or asbestos, so the gradual development of epidemiology makes it difficult to specify the point in time when the transition took place. A useful milestone was the publication in 1959 of Witts' *Medical Surveys and Clinical Trials* in which Doll summarised the essential features of "prospective" and "retrospective" studies.[3] Examples were cited of studies conducted in the immediate post-war era which exemplified important features of longitudinal observations on a defined population cohort and of problems in the selection of cases and controls for retrospective inquiry.

For about 20 years this conceptual dichotomy prevailed in epidemiological research with the cross-sectional prevalence survey seen as a rather unsatisfactory though often necessary compromise of limited aetiological value. This primary concern for design structure was gradually invaded by a new and more unified concept introduced during the 1970s, which called for incident cases of disease always to be seen against a dynamic base population with specific characteristics. These ideas, for which Miettinen deserves much credit,[4] cut across the over-simplicity which until then influenced survey design strongly and at the same time provided logical principles for identifying the optimal study design and the potential seriousness of the inevitable trade-offs that might have to be made.

As shown in the chapters that follow, research achievements in occupational epidemiology during the past 40 years or so have been substantial. Although aimed at assessing the health effects of workplace conditions and exposures the findings have much wider implications, a point that I shall return to. What has been learned can be considered under three headings: identification of previously unforeseen hazards and risks; clarification of the essential nature of these and of already recognised risks; and quantification of exposure-effect relationships. In all three categories much research effort has been concerned with carcinogenicity. The capacity of mineral dusts, fibres, and metallic compounds to cause cancers of the respiratory tract, largely speculative until the 1950s, is now seen as having major health and industrial consequences. The role of physical and mineralogical factors has been considerably clarified and some progress made towards an understanding of exposure-response. The risks of cancer in several industries, such as those concerned with the production of coal gas, rubber, dyes, and mineral oils were generally known, but these have been better documented. Studies have confirmed the carcinogenic effects of other metallic compounds, several new industries (for example, furniture and leather), and some 20 or so specific chemicals. The risks from ionising radiation, long recognised, have been better quantified than most others, but to this problem must now be added suspicion about electromagnetic radiation.

It could be argued that malignant diseases have received a disproportionate amount of attention, perhaps because they reflect the preoccupations of an aging population, but also because deaths are easier to study than sickness. Certainly, such major causes of long-term disability as asthma, dermatoses, deafness, neurobehavioural toxicity, musculo-skeletal disease, and the effects of mental stress have not been investigated as fully as they deserve. Nevertheless, chapters in this book show that there are important findings in all of them. The increasing numbers of women in employment throughout the world, the falling birth rate, and consequent concern about the outcome of pregnancy have drawn attention to the need for epidemiological studies on work in pregnancy. Apart from confirming long held beliefs about adverse ergonomic effects and the possible toxicity of organic solvents the results have been mainly reassuring.

In the course of these substantial epidemiological efforts, methodological progress has also been made. Case-referent studies are more soundly based, tightly designed, and conducted than they were; cohorts are generally larger, better defined, and more assiduously followed; results are more appropriately analysed than in the past; cross-sectional studies are now conducted with greater insight into their limitations and attempts made to allow for them. Least evidence of progress is probably in the quantitative assessment of exposure-response, not because of any lack of concern, but because the measurement of exposure in any cumulative sense over long periods is the weakest link in the chain of cause and effect, whether in occupational or general epidemiology.

There is at present no solution in sight to this problem, which has both serious implications scientifically and important consequences socially.

3

With only the most approximate information on past levels of environmental exposure, let alone on effective human dose, all attempts to estimate risk in varied circumstances, particularly at low levels, are little better than guesswork. We are not even able to say with confidence, based on observation as opposed to assumption, whether a given relationship follows a straight or curved line and whether or not there is any identifiable "safe" level. At the workplace this is bad enough but traditionally at least there is some concept of acceptable risk that may allow this kind of ignorance to be glossed over. For our homes, public buildings, and general environment, however, it is another matter, especially when it is a question of cancer or other dire or dreaded consequence. If it is difficult to assess even approximately the level of risk in relation to a defined exposure in industry, how virtually impossible it is to do so by direct observation in the general population. Until this problem is overcome, occupational epidemiology will not be able to take its proper place as the cornerstone of environmental health.

Meanwhile, it will be evident to readers of the last two chapters of this book that all is not well even in the relation of occupational epidemiology to those who practice occupational health or to those who deal in public attitudes and policy. Waldron emphasises the apparent lack of relevance of epidemiological information to the occupational physician; he could probably have added, or to the hygienist or nurse. He makes the point that today's epidemiologists tend to have little direct knowledge of or contact with industry or indeed with medicine, which may explain a lack of interest in the daily concerns of occupational health professionals. Instead, their priorities may range from the abstractly scientific to the concerns of governmental agencies, the general public, and occasionally of the worker. The underlying problem may be that the occupational health professions, unlike those in public health, have not traditionally given much priority to epidemiology in their training requirements.

The views expressed by Hans Weill are also cause for concern, for where America is today the rest of us may be tomorrow. He contrasts the importance of epidemiological research in an industrial country with the forces that serve to obstruct and retard it. Free societies, unfortunately, do not necessarily promote responsibility in their journalists or discourage self interest in their lawyers. Indirectly, and no doubt unintentionally, the media and the courts have done much to retard epidemiological research, particularly of good quality, and to discredit the results. Partly this is the result of ignorance of the nature of epidemiological evidence and partly because of an almost paranoid preoccupation with research sponsorship rather than with quality. The fact is that good news and virtuous behaviour do not sell papers, and more money can be made from legal battles over past errors than from promoting better standards for the future. The net result is that industry has become wary about granting

4

facilities for epidemiological studies of their employees and quite reluctant to fund them. They have come to believe that if the research finds evidence of a health problem they will be the first to suffer and if it does not it will be said that they paid for it.

This is an unsatisfactory situation, which works against both workers' health and industrial prosperity. It will be corrected only by some change in the method of research funding and by ensuring access to the workplace for legitimate studies. It seems reasonable in a free enterprise society for employers to cover fair and necessary costs of protecting the health of those on whom they depend for their economic success. Good employers who make every effort to maintain safe conditions should clearly pay less than those in the same industrial sector who do not. Appropriately established research funds, which exist in some countries whether on a national or sector basis, could be the main source of support for occupational health studies. This framework might encourage competent investigators to remain in occupational epidemiology rather than abandon it for more tranquil areas where they are less subject to charges of bias and worse.

Fortunately, not all potential consumers of epidemiological data are part of this stormy confrontational media-distorted scenario. Apart from occupational physicians, hygienists, and nurses, we must also consider doctors in public health and clinical practice, and the general public, all with varied and legitimate concern for the effects of work on health. If occupational epidemiologists have failed to communicate effectively with these groups, for which there is some evidence, they have mainly themselves to blame. The problem may lie in the fact, as suggested by Waldron, that fewer and fewer occupational epidemiologists today have ever worked or been trained in these fields. Competent though the new breed of investigators may be in the design, conduct, and analysis of their studies, it is less evident that they have the needs or the interests of these people in mind. Occupational epidemiology is predominantly a multi-disciplinary science; it may suffer seriously if physicians and hygienists cease to participate fully.

What in the coming years should be the priority objectives for occupational epidemiology? There seems little doubt that the most serious failure in current research is to provide reliable quantification of exposure-response, particularly for diseases that are chronic or of long latency. It is unlikely that much can be done to improve environmental assessments, so every effort must be put into the development and validation of biological methods. The potential of this approach has been crudely demonstrated by lung burden analyses but the possibility of lasting effects of chemical exposures on human tissues should be intensively explored. Studies of exposure-response have also suffered from too frequent reliance on the prevalence of fully established disease as

5

against the incidence of early disease-related changes. Cohort studies will undoubtedly continue to command respect but they are usually expensive, time consuming, and dominated by mortality. It should be better appreciated that the case-referent approach based on complete ascertainment of incident disease within a well defined population can give as good or better results at lower cost.

The research objectives of recent years have been dominated by occupational cancer. Other work-related diseases of equal gravity (and which are responsible for more lengthy disability) have not received comparable attention. Seriously deficient also are any objective attempts to evaluate measures taken to prevent, control, or manage work-related diseases and accidents. This is one area in which occupational physicians and hygienists have both responsibility and opportunity. Finally, all research effort on work and health will have little impact if the general public and those whose job it is to inform them do not understand some fairly simple principles of causation, risk, and scientific evidence. This is going to take a long time so we had better start the education process as soon and as early in life as possible.

1 Sartwell PE. Retrospective studies. A review for the clinician. *Ann Intern Med* 1974; **81:** 381–6.
2 McDonald JC. Asbestos and lung cancer: has the case been proven? *Chest* 1980; **78:** 374s–6s.
3 Doll R. Retrospective and prospective studies. In: Witts LJ, ed. *Medical surveys and clinical trials.* London: Oxford University Press, 1959: 71–98.
4 Miettinen O. Design options in epidemiologic research. An update. *Scand J Work Environ Health* 1982; **8:** Suppl 1: 7–14.

2 Metals and chemicals

CORBETT McDONALD, RODOLFO SARACCI

Introduction (p 7). IARC assessment of agents encountered occupationally: Metals and metallic compounds (p 9); Non-metallic chemicals (p 9). Epidemiological studies of metals and their compounds: Group 1 carcinogens: Arsenic (p 13); Beryllium (p 16); Cadmium (p 17); Chromium (p 18); Nickel (p 18). Other metals: Cobalt (p 20); Lead (p 20); Mercury (p 20). Epidemiological studies of chemical compounds and industries: Group 1 carcinogens: Benzene (p 21); Chloromethyl methyl ether (CMME) (p 22); Ethylene oxide (p 22); Shale and mineral oils (p 23); Vinyl chloride (p 24). Group 2A carcinogens: Acrylonitrile (p 24); 1–3 butadiene (p 24); Creosote (p 26); Diethyl sulphate (p 26); Formaldehyde (p 27); Polychlorinated biphenyls (p 30). Conclusion (p 32).

Introduction

The potential carcinogenicity of chemical substances has been evident since various skin cancers associated with coal and tar were first identified at the end of the last century and, indeed, since 1795 when Percival Pott described scrotal cancer in chimney sweeps. Despite ore mining and smelting for at least 2000 years, metals came under suspicion only in the 1920s, perhaps because it is seldom metals themselves but certain of their compounds that are carcinogenic.

An appreciation of the magnitude of the threat posed by the manufacture of countless new products by the world's burgeoning chemical and metallurgical industries led the International Agency for Research on Cancer (IARC), a specialised research organisation within WHO, to establish an evaluation programme, which, from 1971 to date, has systematically assessed the carcinogenicity of more than 700 agents, mixtures, and occupational exposures. These evaluations, published in an extensive series of some 60 monographs, provide the basis and point of departure for this chapter.[1] The procedures used by the IARC should therefore be understood.

Each evaluation is made in Lyon by an invited international working group of scientific experts with special knowledge of the physical and chemical, epidemiological, toxicological, and environmental aspects of the materials under scrutiny. In preparation for each meeting of the working group a detailed review of published findings considered to be relevant is made by specialists selected by the Agency. After full discussion by the experts in groups and in plenary sessions a consensus is sought on the strength of the evidence of carcinogenicity (*a*) in humans and (*b*) in experimental animals, or short-term tests, classified as *sufficient* (S), *limited* (L), *inadequate* (I), *evidence suggesting lack* (ESL) or, often, *no data* (ND). For exact definition of these terms reference should be made to the preamble of one of the most recent volumes (for example, no 59 (1)) of the monographs series. In 1979 and again in 1982 and 1987, larger and differently constituted international groups of experts were assembled in Lyons to summarise, bring up to date, and, where appropriate to re-evaluate information relating to the carcinogenicity of all agents previously dealt with. The most recent supplement, resulting from the 1987 review, covers 631 agents or exposures (some complex).[2] Adding the subsequently considered agents and exposures brings the total at March 1994 to 775, classified in an overall evaluation of the human and experimental evidence of carcinogenicity (plus other relevant data—for example, on mechanisms of carcinogenicity) as follows:

Group 1: 63 agents considered to be human carcinogens
Group 2A: 50 agents considered to be probably carcinogenic to humans
Group 2B: 209 agents considered to be possibly carcinogenic to humans
Group 3: 452 agents not classifiable as to their carcinogenicity to humans
Group 4: 1 agent (caprolactan) considered probably not carcinogenic to humans

The lack of agents in Group 4 is explained by the fact that only agents for which some positive findings had been reported in the literature are generally selected for evaluation in the monograph series.

This chapter will be virtually limited to agents and exposures classified by the IARC as Group 1 or Group 2A carcinogens, giving rather greater attention to the epidemiological evidence (which by definition is less than conclusive) for those in Group 2A than Group 1. Dusts, fibres, ionizing radiation, electromagnetic fields, and pesticides are reviewed in chapters 3, 4, 5 and 12 and do not need further consideration here and, of the chemicals and metallic compounds that remain, only those in which occupational exposure is important will be discussed.

IARC assessment of agents encountered occupationally

Metals and metallic compounds

A summary is presented in table 2.1 of the evidence for carcinogenicity and the overall classification of nine metals or their compounds that have been assessed by the IARC. Arsenic, chromium, and nickel, at least in some form, have long been recognised as human carcinogens and beryllium and cadmium, for which the evidence in man has been more limited, only more recently. The evidence on iron was clear in that its carcinogenicity was evident in mining only with coincidental exposure to radon and in foundries where several other carcinogens are commonly present. Cobalt, mercury, and the inorganic compounds of lead were assessed but only as *possible* human carcinogens, mainly because of insufficient epidemiological evidence. In all these metallic agents, lung was the main organ affected, together with skin for arsenic and nasal sinuses for nickel. Four other metals: manganese, titanium, zinc, and platinum have shown evidence of carcinogenic potential in animal experiments but have not been reviewed formally by the IARC.[3]

With all nine metals shown in table 2.1 the main occupational exposures are in mining, smelting, and refining and less commonly in secondary industries. However, cadmium, chromium, and lead are also used widely in the manufacture of paints, pigments, and batteries, and arsenic in the production of pesticides.

Non-metallic chemicals

A similar but much longer list exists of almost 50 non-metallic compounds and exposures of occupational importance that have been classified by the IARC as Group 1 or Group 2A carcinogens (table 2.2). In addition, there are 20 or more therapeutic agents, mainly used in the treatment of malignant disease, which are themselves carcinogenic or probably so. These are also potential hazards during manufacture, but more importantly during administration by insufficiently protected health care workers. The remaining 40 or more agents can be considered in four main categories: (1) aromatic amines and n-nitroso chemicals; (2) alkylating agents; (3) polycyclic aromatic hydrocarbons (PAHs); and (4) a miscellaneous set of non-nitrogenous chemicals. This grouping is one of convenience and may not be entirely in line with the formal classification of agents used in authoritative chemical texts, such as that of Sontag.[4]

Table 2.1 IARC evaluation of carcinogenicity of metals and metallic compounds;[1,2] main industrial exposures and organs affected

Agent	IARC evaluation			Organs affected	Main industrial exposures
	Human*	Animal*	Overall**		
Arsenic	S	L	1	lung, skin	copper and other metal mining and smelting; production and use of pesticides and herbicides
Beryllium	S	S	1	lung	extraction, production, and fabrication
Cadmium	S	S	1	lung, prostate	smelting, alloying, welding, battery and paint manufacture
Chromium	S	S	1	lung	welding, stainless steel manufacture, plating, leather tanning, chromate and pigment manufacture
Nickel	S	S	1	lung, nasal sinuses	mining, smelting, refining
Iron					
haematite mining (with radon)	S	ND	1	lung	iron ore mining
iron and steel founding	S	ND	1	lung	iron and steel foundries
Cobalt	In	S	2B	lung	mining and metallurgy; hard metal production and use;
Mercury	In	S	2B	liver(?)	mining and processing; chloralkali industry
	(methyl mercury) L		–		
	(mercuric chloride) L		2B		
Lead					
inorganic	In	S	2B	digestive(?)	manufacture of paints, pigments, glass, batteries; smelting
organic	In	In	3	–	tetraethyl lead manufacture

*Degree of evidence: S = sufficient; L = limited; In = insufficient; ND = no data
**See text for definitions

Table 2.2 IARC evaluations of the carcinogenicity of non-metallic chemicals;[1,2] main industrial exposures and organs affected

Agent	IARC evaluation Human*	Animal*	Overall**	Organs affected	Main industrial exposures
Aromatic amines and other n-nitroso chemicals					
4 aminobiphenyl	S	S	1	bladder	
rubber industry	S	In	1	bladder	rubber and cable industries
2 naphthylamine	S	S	1	bladder	
benzidine	S	S	1	bladder	
benzidine-based dyes	In	S	2A	–	
auramine	S	S	1	bladder	dye industries
magenta	S	In	1	bladder	
4,4-methylene-bis-(2-chloroaniline) (MOCA)	In	S	2A	bladder	epoxy resin and polyurethane foam workers
n-nitrosodiethylamine	ND	S	2A	–	
n-nitrosodimethylamine	ND	S	2A	–	chemical and solvent workers
n-ethyl n-nitroso urea	ND	S	2A	–	
n-methyl n-nitroso urea	ND	S	2A	–	
Alkylating agents					
chloromethyl methylether (CMME)	S	S	1	lung	ion exchange resin production
ethylene oxide	L	S	1	leukaemia	
propylene oxide	In	S	2A	–	chemical manufacture
ethylene dibromide	In	S	2A	–	
epichlorhydrin	In	S	2A	not known	
diethyl sulphate	L	S	2A	not known	chemical industry and refinery workers
dimethyl sulphate	In	S	2A	many sites	formaldehyde production and use
formaldehyde	L	S	2A		
Polycyclic aromatic hydrocarbons (PAHs)					
benzo α-pyrene	ND	S	2A	skin	–
polychlorinated biphenyls (PCBs)	L	S	2A	skin, lung, bladder	chemicals and electrical industries
coal gasification	S	S	1	lung, bladder	coal gas production
coal tar pitch	S	S	1	skin, lung, bladder	highway maintenance; roofing
coke production	S	S	1	skin	coke oven workers
creosotes	L	S	2A	skin	timber treatment; brickmaking

11

Table 2.2—continued

Agent	IARC evaluation Human*	Animal*	Overall**	Organs affected	Main industrial exposures
soots	S	S	1	skin, lung	chimney sweeping; furnace maintenance
shale oils	S	S	1	skin	shale oil production
mineral oils	S	S	1	skin	metal machining
aluminium production (electrolytic)	S	In	1	skin, lung, bladder	aluminium smelting
petroleum refining	L	S	2A	various	
Miscellaneous non-nitrogenous chemicals					
benzene	S	S	1	leukaemia	petroleum and coking industries; shoe making
vinyl chloride	S	S	1	liver, brain, lung	PVC manufacture
vinyl bromide	ND	S	2A	–	?
acrylonitrile	L	S	2A	lung, prostate, stomach	rubber and textile industries
dimethyl carbamoyl chloride	In	S	2A	–	chemical industry
isopropyl alcohol	S	In	1	nasal sinuses	isopropyl alcohol manufacture
tris(2,3-dibromopropyl) phosphate	In	S	2A	–	chemical industry
styrene oxide	L	S	2A	?	?
boot and shoe manufacture and repair	S	ND	1	nasal sinuses	boot and shoe manufacture
furniture and cabinet making	S	In	1	nasal sinuses	hardwood furniture manufacture
hairdressers and barbers	S	ND	2A	bladder	
painters	S	ND	1	various	petroleum, rubber and plastics industries
1,3 butadiene	L	S	2A	?	many and various
strong inorganic acids	S	ND	1	larynx	

Therapeutic agents
Over 20 agents used mainly for cancer therapy but also for psoriasis (methoxalen) or for laboratory experimentation (n-methyl n-nitroguanidine) have been evaluated as grade 1 or grade 2A carcinogens

drug manufacture and administration; laboratory research

This table is limited to chemicals assessed as Group 1 or Group 2A carcinogens
*Degree of evidence: S = sufficient; L = limited; In = insufficient; ND = no data
**See text for definition

However, this grouping allows certain patterns to be seen. Thus the carcinogenicity of aromatic amines, encountered mainly in the rubber and dye industries, is strongly supported by both human and animal evidence; they cause bladder cancer. Much the same pattern is shown by the PAHs in a fairly well defined set of large industries; the main risks are cancer of the skin and in some, of the lung and bladder. In contrast, the evidence of carcinogenicity of the alkylating agents depends, with few exceptions, almost wholly on animal tests and so little on epidemiological evidence that the organs affected in man are often uncertain. Exposure to these agents is mainly in their manufacture. Finally, the miscellaneous group are intermediate both in the varied nature of the evidence, the organs affected, and in the range of industrial exposure.

Epidemiological studies of metals and their compounds

Group 1 carcinogens

Arsenic

The occupations most extensively studied have been copper miners and smelter workers mainly in the USA, but also in Sweden and Japan. Additional information has been obtained from workers employed in the manufacture and use of arsenical pesticides and herbicides, from general populations resident in the vicinity of smelters and a pesticide plant, and from communities in Taiwan exposed to high levels of arsenic in drinking water.

Findings from the main cohort studies in smelter workers are summarised in table 2.3. Six of the eight studies shown are based on the initial and updated observations on employees of copper smelters at Anaconda in Washington state and at Tacoma in Montana. The results in both were similar in showing a substantial risk of lung cancer closely related to estimates of cumulative exposure, probably to arsenic trioxide. Increased risk has not been confidently detected at concentrations below about 500 $\mu g/m^3$ and there is some indication that risk decreases with time since last exposure.[11] Findings in Swedish and Japanese smelters were similar.

Information on populations resident in the vicinity of smelters is not consistent. A study by Greaves et al. of patients with cancer of the lung (or of three other anatomical sites unassociated with smelter effluent) living within 20 km of one of 10 non-ferrous smelters in the western USA showed no evidence of a geographical association with lung cancer.[13] The same was true of a study by Rom et al. in the vicinity of a smelter of copper, lead, and zinc in El Paso, Texas.[14] On the other hand, a similar survey near a zinc smelter in eastern Pennsylvania, leading to high levels of

13

Table 2.3 Main cohort mortality studies of workers exposed to metals and metallic compounds classified by the IARC as human carcinogens

First author	Year	Country	Industry	Cohort	Lung cancer Obs	SMR	Comment
Arsenic							
Lee[5]	1969	USA	copper smelter (Anaconda)	8047	147	3·29	related to duration and intensity
Pinto[6]	1978	USA	copper smelter (Tacoma)	527	32	3·05	–
Tokudome[7]	1976	Japan	copper smelter	(case-control)	162	(RR12)	also colon and liver
Wall[8]	1980	Sweden	copper smelter	3919	79	2·88	stomach cancer (SMR 1·74)
Lubin[9]	1981	USA	copper smelter (Anaconda)	5403	139	1·66	related to cumulative index of exposure
Enterline[10]	1982	USA	copper smelter (Tacoma)	2802	100	1·95	effect within 10 yr and then diminished
Welch[11]	1982	USA	copper smelter (Anaconda)	1800	80	3·21	no evidence of risk <500 µg/m³, little effect of smoking
Lee-Feldstein[12]	1986	USA	copper smelter (Anaconda)	8045	302	2·85	linear increase with cumulative exposure
Beryllium							
Ward[23]	1992	USA	extraction and processing plants	9225	280	1·26	lung cancer SMR for men employed <1 yr:1·32
Cadmium							
Elinder[27]	1985	Sweden	nickel-cadmium battery	522	8	1·33	prostate observed 4 SMR 1·08
Sorahan[28]	1987	UK	nickel-cadmium battery	3025	110	1·30	prostate cancer observed 15 incident cases (RR 1·36)
Stayner[29]	1992	USA	cadmium recovery	576	24	1·49	possible exposure to arsenic
Kazantzis[30]	1992	UK	cadmium processing	6910	237	1·22	prostate observed 37 SMR 0·75, lung cancer risk related to exposure level
Chromium							
Hayes[31]	1979	USA	chromate production	1803	59	2·00	–

	Year	Country	Process	Number	Number	Ratio	Comments
Alderson[32]	1981	UK	chromate production	2715	116	2·40	two nasal cancers (SMR 7·1)
Satoh[33]	1981	Japan	chromium compounds	896	25	7·4	six nasal sinus cancers
Korallus[34]	1982	FRG	chromate production	1140	51	2·10	–
De Marco[35]	1988	Italy	chromate production	981	14	2·17	–
Frentzel-Beyme[36]	1983	FRG	pigment production	1396	19	2·04	–
Davies[37]	1984	UK	pigment production	1002	39	2·02	risk related to level of exposure
Hayes[38]	1989	USA	pigment production	1879	24	1·43	risk related to level of exposure
Sorahan[39]	1987	UK	chromium plating	2689	72	1·50	some exposure to nickel salts
Nickel							
ICNCM*[40]	1990	Canada (Sudbury, Ontario)	mining, refining, smelting	about 55 000	695	1·25	nasal cancer observed 31 SMR 7·38; lung and nasal cancer risks almost confined to 3769 sinter plant workers where buccal/pharyngeal cancers were also in excess (SMR 2·11)
		Canada (Falconbridge, Ontario)	mining, smelting	11 594	114	1·35	
		UK (Clydach, Wales)	refining	2521	216	2·73	nasal cancer observed 75 SMR 208·45; cancer risks almost confined to exposures before 1930
		Norway (Kristiansand)	refining	3250	77	2·62	nasal cancer observed 3 SMR 4·53
		USA (Oregon)	mining, smelting	1510	27	1·48	no nasal cancer
		USA (W Virginia)	nickel alloy, refining	3208	91	0·95	nasal cancer observed 2 SMR 2·20
		UK	nickel alloy	1907	30	0·98	
		USA	gaseous diffusion (metallic nickel)	814	9	0·54	no nasal cancer; limited power
Redmond[41]	1984	USA (Tennessee)	nickel alloy	28 261	332	1·09	nasal sinus cancer observed 2

*International Committee on Nickel Carcinogenesis in Man (ICNCM) arsenic and cadmium pollution, was not clearly negative[15] and another near a large copper smelter in northern Sweden found a two-fold increase in lung cancer risk in people living within 20 km of the plant.[16]

Studies of exposure to arsenical pesticides are limited. Surveys in and near a plant in Baltimore, Maryland where inorganic pesticides were manufactured showed an excess of respiratory tract cancer in employees (observed 24; expected 14·9)[17] and suggestive evidence of an excess among men but not women in selected adjoining areas over a limited number of years.[18] Several reports of chronic arsenical poisoning among wine growers in the Moselle region of Germany were published in the 1940s which led to a systematic analysis by Lüchtrath of autopsy reports (1960–1977) on 163 wine growers whose deaths had been attributed to contact with arsenical insecticide.[19] Lung cancers were observed in 66% of the series and skin cancers in 18%. Although striking, such data are difficult to interpret.

More impressive are the studies by Chien et al. in a village community in a circumscribed area of southwest Taiwan where the arsenic content of artesian well water ranged from 0·35–1·14 ppm (median 0·78 ppm).[20 21] Odds ratios for bladder, lung, and liver cancers in this population, as compared with those who used only water from shallow wells (median arsenic content 0·04 ppm) were 3·90, 3·39, and 2·67, respectively. The risk for all three cancer sites, after adjustment for age and sex, was related to years of exposure to water from the artesian wells.

Beryllium

Beryllium and its compounds have been suspected as possible carcinogens for many years but until the most recent review by the IARC in 1993[22] the epidemiological evidence in man was not considered *sufficient*. Animal studies, however, show the metal to be carcinogenic. The recent evaluation depended largely on a single major cohort study by Ward et al., published in 1992, based on mortality in 9225 male workers from seven processing plants in the USA (see table 2.3).[23] These plants had already been studied individually by Mancuso[24] and Wagoner et al.[25] and causes of death recorded until the mid 1970s had been analysed. These studies all provided limited evidence of excess lung cancer. The survey by Ward et al. included all plants studied previously and carried observations forward until the end of 1988, by which time there had been 3240 deaths from all causes (SMR 1·05) and 280 deaths from lung cancer (SMR 1·26; 95%CI: 1·12 to 1·42). Despite the narrow confidence interval an increase of this magnitude is quite capable of explanation by social and other confounding factors. The evidence was also weakened by lack of data on intensity of exposure and the fact that the SMR of men employed for less than one year (1·32) was slightly higher than that of men with longer employment. However, essentially the same estimate of risk was obtained compared with both national and local county mortality, SMRs in all plants increased with time since first employment, the excess was greatest in the plants with highest mortality from non-malignant respiratory disease, and in men in earlier decades when exposure was less controlled. An attempt to adjust for smoking habit, on the other hand, reduced the lung cancer SMR from 1·26 to 1·12.

Some additional evidence was obtained from studies of mortality in people listed in the American Beryllium Case Registry as having acute pneumonitis or chronic systemic disease. The most recent analysis of these data in 1991 by Steenland and Ward found significant excess mortality compared with United States death rates for all cancers (SMR 1·51), lung cancer (SMR 2·00), non-malignant respiratory disease (SMR 34·25) and all causes (SMR 2·19).[26] Interpretation of mortality in subjects on disease registers may be difficult because of the possibility of various types of selection.

Cadmium

Findings are set out in table 2.3 from two large cohorts in the UK and two smaller groups in the USA and Sweden of workers exposed to cadmium, two in the manufacture of nickel-cadmium batteries, and two in cadmium recovery or processing. The first pair of studies was subject inevitably to possible confounding from nickel and, in the recovery plant, there may have been some exposure to arsenic in the earlier years. Detailed analyses, however, did not suggest that either of these factors seriously affected the results.

The cohort of battery workers reported by Sorahan in 1987 had previously been studied in various ways by other investigators over a 20 year period but with smaller numbers and less significant results.[27] Even so, the SMR for lung cancer was only modestly raised (1·30; 95%CI: 1·07 to 1·57) and there was little evidence of a correlation with extent or duration of exposure. At various stages in the evolution of this cohort a possible excess of prostatic cancer was noted and in the final analysis 15 incident cases were identified in the regional cancer registry compared with 11 expected. The much smaller cohort of nickel-cadmium battery workers in Sweden was closely comparable for lung cancer (SMR 1·33) but no excess in deaths from prostatic cancer was observed.[28]

The results of the two studies in cadmium recovery and processing were similar. The large cohort of nearly 7000 employees in 17 British plants by Kazantzis et al.[29] had a modest but significantly increased SMR for lung cancer (1·22; 95%CI: 1·02 to 1·39), a finding with which the SMR of 1·49 observed in the much smaller American study by Stayner et al.[30] was again comparable. A tightly designed case-referent analysis based on 174 fatal cases of lung cancer from the larger study showed a 1·23-fold increase in risk for each mg/m^3 year of cumulative exposure.[29] The same type of analysis in the American study, though based on only 24 deaths from lung cancer, also showed a steady increase in risk with cumulative exposure of roughly the same gradient. In neither of the latter studies was any increase in prostatic cancer observed.

Chromium

The most informative epidemiological surveys on the carcinogenic effects of chromium and its compounds (see table 2.3) have been in three industries: chromate production,[31-35] chromate pigment manufacture,[36-38] and chromium plating.[39] In the first category, five well-designed cohort studies of substantial size have been published since 1979. Several earlier reports were for various reasons less easy to interpret. In four of the five later surveys from industries in Europe and North America, the SMRs for lung cancer ranged from 2·00 to 2·40, whereas in the fifth, from Japan, the ratio was appreciably higher (7·40). An apparent excess of nasal cancers was noted in two of these cohorts. In none was any quantitative analysis of exposure-response or the effect of smoking investigated.

In the manufacture of chromate pigments, three somewhat larger studies have been made with lung cancer SMRs of the same order (1·43 to 2·04). In one of these a significant trend was observed between risk and duration of exposure but, again, no information was given on smoking habits or on the incidence of nasal cancer.[38] Finally, in the chromium plating industry, a fairly large cohort of 1288 men and 1401 women was studied in the UK by Sorahan et al., although they noted the possibility of some exposure also to nickel salts.[39] A significant excess of lung cancer was observed in men (observed 63; SMR 1·58) but not in women (observed 9; SMR 1·11). Three deaths from nasal cancer were recorded, one in a man who had worked for 13 years plating nickel.

A number of other studies have been reported on cancer risks in people exposed to chromium in other forms; for example, in the production of ferrochromium alloys, zinc chromate, spray painting, nickel/chromium foundries, cement finishing, and chrome leather tanneries, but without conclusive results.

Nickel

The most recent and comprehensive data on the carcinogenic effects of nickel and its compounds are contained in a report of the International Committee on Nickel Carcinogenesis in Man (ICNCM) published in 1990.[40] The results of eight cohort studies included in that report are summarised in table 2.3; six of these were in mining, smelting, and refining industries in Canada, USA, UK, and Norway, one in a high-nickel alloy plant in the UK, and one in a uranium enrichment plant in the USA where exposure was to pure metallic nickel. Findings from a large cohort of 28 621 employees, 80% male, in 12 high-nickel alloy plants in the USA, reported by Redmond in 1984 are also shown.[41] The data indicate that there was little or no evidence of excess of lung or nasal cancer in workers exposed to metallic nickel (though this study had very limited power) or in those engaged in the manufacture of nickel alloys, in marked contrast to the findings from the other industries. Within the latter, however, the distribution of risk was far from homogeneous and apparently related to the nature of the industrial process and the predominating nickel species— metallic, oxidic, sulphidic or soluble nickel sulphate or chloride—in the airborne dust to which the workers were exposed. Thus, in the large cohort of employees in Sudbury, Ontario, the SMR for lung cancer among 3769 sinter plant workers was 2·61 and, for nasal cancer, 50·73 whereas among the 50 977 non-sinter workers the corresponding ratios were 1·10 and 1·42. Sinter plant workers were mainly exposed to high dust concentrations (up to 100 mg/m^3) predominantly of oxidic and sulphidic nickel. In the mines and smelter at Falconbridge, Ontario, where the lung cancer SMR was 1·35, and no significant excess at any other site, total exposures to nickel were below 1 mg/m^3.

At the Clydach refinery in South Wales where the association with lung and nasal cancers was first recognised 60 years ago there has been evidence of a substantial reduction in risk of both diseases. Whereas in men first employed before 1930 the SMRs for lung and nasal cancer were 3·93 and 211·20, respectively, the corresponding ratios for men first employed after that date were 1·25 and 5·26. In the earlier period, the highest risks attributable to nickel were in furnace and calcining areas where exposures were mainly to the oxidic, sulphidic, and metallic species at estimated airborne concentrations of perhaps 30 mg/m^3.

The pattern of mortality in the cohort from the Norwegian refinery at Kristiansand differed from that observed in Ontario in that the risk was higher in workers in the electrolysis plant than in roasting and smelting whereas in Sudbury it was the reverse. The main difference in exposure appears to have been an appreciably higher estimated airborne concentration of soluble nickel in the Norwegian electrolytic department. Earlier observations on a cohort of workers from the Kristiansand refinery suggested that the joint action of nickel and smoking was additive rather than synergistic.

The relatively high SMR for lung cancer (1·48) in men from the mining and smelting operations in Oregon is probably misleading in that the excess was mainly in men employed for less than one year. Overall, there was little evidence of malignant disease in this cohort, exposed on average to airborne nickel concentrations of less than 1 mg/m^3, with little soluble or sulphidic compounds. In summary, the available epidemiological data point to a risk of lung and nasal cancer related to duration and intensity of exposure to airborne nickel compounds mainly in roasting, sintering, and calcining and, in Norway, with electrolytic refining. In differing

19

circumstances, oxidic, sulphidic, and soluble nickel are all incriminated to varying degrees. On the other hand, increased risk from exposure to metallic nickel, pure or in alloy manufacture, or to nickel sulphide and oxides in ore mining has not been clearly shown in man.

Other metals

In addition to the five metals classified as Group 1 carcinogens, brief mention should be made of the other four—iron, cobalt, mercury, and lead—also included in table 2.1. As stated earlier, there is abundant evidence from epidemiological studies that foundry workers[42] and haematite miners,[43] who are also exposed to radon, are at excess risk from lung cancer, but in neither circumstance is it probable that iron or its compounds were responsible. The remaining three metals deserve more searching examination, however, if only because they have all been shown to be carcinogenic in experimental animals.

Cobalt[44]

Two fairly small cohorts, one in South Wales and one in France, were both seriously confounded by other potentially carcinogenic exposures, but a larger study from Sweden is less easily dismissed. In the latter cohort, 3163 men employed in three hard-metal production plants, and exposed to cobalt metal powder, had an SMR, all causes, of 0·96 and for lung cancer 1·34 (observed 17; 95%CI: 0·77 to 2·13). In men with 10 years' exposure and 20 or more years' latency, the lung cancer SMR was 2·78 (observed 7; 95%CI: 1·11 to 5·72).

Lead[45]

The results from six cohort studies—four in the USA and one each in the UK and Sweden—were reviewed by the IARC. One of these studies was of employees in the manufacture of tetraethyl-lead and the others were of workers in lead or copper smelters or in the manufacture of batteries. A significant excess of stomach or digestive tract cancer was observed in two battery plants and of respiratory cancer in one of them. There were suggestions of excess of renal and bladder cancers, based on small numbers, in two of the smelter cohorts. Overall, however, these findings were considered as *inadequate* evidence of human carcinogenicity.

Mercury[46]

Apart from the possibility that excess mortality from hepatic and oesophageal cancer in areas of high exposure to methyl mercury in Minamata, Japan, other studies of exposure to metallic mercury and its compounds have been inconclusive.

Epidemiological studies of chemical compounds and industries

In table 2.2 are listed chemical compounds and industrial exposures which at time of writing were classified by the IARC as carcinogenic (Group 1) or probably carcinogenic (Group 2A). Among these are about 10 exposures defined only in terms of industry, in all of which the epidemiological evidence was considered *sufficient* but the animal evidence was usually lacking; indeed, it would often have been difficult for the laboratory to know what material to test. In some of these industries known carcinogens would commonly have been present, for example, various aromatic amines in rubber and dye manufacture and in hairdressing, and polyaromatic hydrocarbons in aluminium production and processes related to the destructive distillation of coal. In other industries such as boot and shoe manufacture and furniture making the nature of the carcinogenic agent(s) remains unknown. In contrast, the apparent carcinogenicity of strong inorganic acid mists is a hazard in many industries, including, for example, the manufacture of isopropyl alcohol, which itself has been under suspicion.[47] These are extensive subjects and any brief attempt to review the epidemiological evidence would probably not be useful. We have chosen to concentrate instead on those Group 1 and Group 2A carcinogens that are more precisely defined, in particular, on the latter group where the uncertainties tend to lie with the epidemiological evidence. The discussion will be confined to agents for which there is at least *limited* epidemiological evidence of carcinogenicity in man.

Group 1 carcinogens

Benzene

For many years there have been reports strongly suggesting that exposure to benzene causes leukaemia but epidemiologically the evidence is not conclusive; moreover, the evidence in experimental animals is also limited. In 1983, Decouflé et al. reported the results of a small cohort study of 259 male chemical plant workers in the USA who had been heavily exposed to benzene.[48] Three deaths from lymphoreticular malignancies were observed against 1·1 expected. Two years later (1985) a study of almost 4000 petroleum refinery workers in Illinois reported 22 deaths from leukaemia and related diseases compared with 15·2 expected,[49] and in 1986 the results of a small but extended study of previously reported chemical employees exposed to benzene produced supportive evidence.[50] In 1987, the results of a large cohort study based on almost 30 000 Chinese workers exposed to benzene and a similar number of controls found 30 cases of leukaemia in the former and four in the latter

21

(SMR 5·74, p < 0·01).[51] While there remains little doubt that benzene exposure is a potent cause of leukaemia, the quantitative aspects of risk in relation to exposure intensity and duration remain unanswered.

Chloromethyl methyl ether (CMME)

A cohort study of 125 male chemical manufacturing workers, by Figueroa *et al.* in 1973, reported 14 cases of lung cancer, 12 confirmed histologically as oat cell in type; three of the men had never smoked.[52] The authors estimated this to be eight times higher than might be expected. The only common denominator in the exposure of these men was thought to be CMME. The cohort was followed to the end of 1979 by which time there had been 16 cases of lung cancer and two of laryngeal cancer, which entirely accounted for the overall excess mortality from all causes (SMR 1·68).[53 54] Of considerable interest is the fact that the epidemic peaked 15–19 years after onset of exposure and then subsided.

Exposure–response was investigated in two American studies, one among employees of a chemical plant in Philadelphia[55] and the other in CMME-exposed workers in the production plants of seven American companies.[56] In the first of these studies, 19 deaths from lung cancer were observed against 5·6 expected, using the experience of unexposed workers as reference. A zero to six scale based on subjective assessment of airborne intensity was used with recorded duration to derive a time-weighted estimate of exposure. Significant correlations were found between lung cancer risk and both total duration and the time-weighted index. It is unclear, however, whether the intensity component improved the correlation. In the second study, an association was found in one plant between risk and duration of exposure, not improved by allowance for estimated intensity.

Ethylene oxide

Ethylene oxide has been produced since the 1920s for various intermediate purposes in the chemical industry and as a sterilising agent for hospital use. It is a powerful mutagen in laboratory studies but less convincingly a human carcinogen. In consequence of a small number of case reports of leukaemia in persons who had been exposed in the manufacture or use of ethylene oxide in Sweden, a cohort mortality study was undertaken by Högstedt *et al.* of 241 men, 89 exposed full time, 86 exposed intermittently and 66 never exposed, to ethylene oxide.[57] In those with full time exposure during the years 1961–77 there were 23 deaths against 13·5 expected but no excess in the other two groups. The excess was attributable to tumours (observed 9, expected 3·4) and diseases of the circulatory system (observed 12, expected 6·3); the tumour excess was of the stomach (3 cases) and leukaemia (2 cases). Results of a further follow-up, through 1982, of employees in the same plant, and of two other plants

22

(one of which was the source of the original case reports) yielded evidence which at face value pointed to excess risk of leukaemia.[58] There have been a considerable number of other investigations of workers employed in the manufacture of ethylene oxide but they have generally been exposed to many other chemical compounds. Studies of people employed in sterilisation work are less seriously confounded by multiple exposures and, of these, the one in the USA by Steenland et al.,[59] with further analysis by Stayner et al.[60] is probably the most informative. This investigation was based on a cohort of 18 254 employees, 1177 of whom had died against 1454·3 expected (SMR 0·81). There were also fewer deaths than expected from cancer at all sites (SMR 0·90) but a slight excess of lymphatic and haemopoietic cancer (observed 36, SMR 1·06). Detailed regression analysis indicated a weak trend between individual estimates of exposure and mortality from these two malignancies $(p < 0·05)$.[60] The extensive but inconsistent body of epidemiological evidence has been recently considered by IARC as *limited*; however, taking into account evidence that the agent acts through a relevant mechanism of carcinogenicity, the agent has been classified (as the evaluation criteria exceptionally allow) as Group 1.[61]

Shale and mineral oils

For well over a century it has been evident that long-term occupational skin contact with mineral oils, for example in mule spinning, metal machining, and jute processing, were strongly associated with squamous cell cancers of the skin, especially of the scrotum. The oils in question were not well defined and far from pure. This type of causal association is analogous to those mentioned earlier where suspicion is on some aspect of the industrial environment rather than on specific chemical agents. There have been numerous cohort and other epidemiological surveys which have inquired into the effects of mineral oil exposure without important clarification of specific etiological relationships.[62] Several investigators have studied the question of whether exposure to mineral oil mists is associated with malignant disease at sites other than the skin. There is little evidence of any increase in respiratory cancer but possibly there is some increase in tumours of the gastrointestinal tract.[63]

An important source of mineral oil in Scotland and in the USA (Colorado) is from deposits in shale. Oils obtained in this way were not distinguished in the epidemiological evaluation of the other types of mineral oil mentioned above. Shale oils have certainly played their part in the aetiology of scrotal and other skin cancers in the cotton textile, jute, and metal machining industries. Studies of shale oil workers in the USA,[64] Scotland,[65] and Estonia[66] do not suggest that the carcinogenic effects on the skin or other organs differ from those attributed to other mineral oils.

23

Vinyl chloride

Vinyl chloride monomer is one of several chemicals used in the plastics industry, in particular in the manufacture of polyvinyl chloride (PVC) by polymerisation, a process introduced in the 1920s. Its carcinogenic potential was first recognised in 1974 by Creech and Johnson who reported three cases of angiosarcoma of the liver from an American plant.[67] Several reports of this rare tumour immediately followed from a number of industrial countries and, in due course, by systematic cohort studies. Tabershaw and Gaffey were perhaps the first to report that in a cohort of 8384 male employees from 33 plants there was probably excess mortality from cancer at other sites, including brain and lung.[68] An extended follow-up of this cohort, somewhat enlarged, strengthened the suspicion about tumours of the brain but not of other organs. However, of four other cohorts, only one from the USA provided support for a causal association with lung cancer,[69] whereas those in Canada,[70] Norway,[71] and Sweden[72] did not.

Group 2A carcinogens

Acrylonitrile

Acrylonitrile, an organic liquid compound, volatile and flammable, is used industrially in the production of plastics, resins, synthetic rubber, and acrylic fibres. The compound is carcinogenic in rats by oral administration and by inhalation. These findings have prompted a number of studies of workers in the chemical industry for evidence of cancer excess. So far there have been nine cohort studies published, mostly quite small and focused mainly on lung cancer.[73–81] The SMRs have ranged from 0·60 to 1·95, all well within 95% confidence intervals; overall a total of 86 deaths from lung cancer were observed against 81·8 expected. In addition there is some evidence, based again on small numbers of a small excess of incident cases[73] and possibly some indication of a relationship between risk and exposure intensity.[77] An increasing incidence of prostatic cancer has also been reported in four of the studies but in the absence of statistical significance or an exposure–response gradient interpretation is doubtful.[78–81] Taken together, there is thus some evidence, but obviously limited, for carcinogenicity of acrylonitrile in humans.

1–3 butadiene

1–3 butadiene, a four carbon hydrocarbon mostly derived as a byproduct of petroleum cracking in the production of ethylene, is used mainly, on a large scale, as a monomer in the manufacture of a wide range of polymers and co-polymers, particularly with styrene. Styrene-butadiene rubber, the largest single product of butadiene, is used for tyres and tyre products. The rubber industry, in which exposure to a variety of chemicals including butadiene may occur, has been evaluated by the IARC as entailing a risk of cancer (see table 2.2). On the other hand, 1–3 butadiene has been shown to be carcinogenic by inhalation in mice and rats, the likely responsible compound being its metabolite 1,2 epoxy 3-butane, which in *in vitro* experiments was generated from butadiene by human liver tissue.

With this background, evidence for carcinogenicity of 1–3 butadiene in humans has been sought mainly in one study of workers employed in the manufacture of butadiene monomer and in three studies in the rubber industry. Among 2582 monomer production workers in Texas an excess risk, in comparison with United States white men, was observed by Divine for deaths certified as due to lymphosarcoma and reticulosarcoma (ICD 8, code 200); nine deaths were observed, with an SMR of 229 (95% CI: 104 to 435); seven of the nine workers were employed before 1946, but no trend with length of employment was detected.[82] A subgroup analysis yielded an elevated SMR (1·85; 95% CI: 0·68 to 4·03) for leukaemia (ICD 8, code 204) among workers with intermittent exposure (and possibly high peaks) to 1–3 butadiene.

An almost fourfold increase in lymphatic leukaemia (RR 3·9; 99% CI: 1·6 to 8·0) was reported by McMichael *et al.* in one of three studies in the rubber industry.[83] This was carried out as a case-control analysis nested within a cohort of 6678 United States workers (this study reported a relative risk of 6·2 (99% CI: 4·1 to 12·5) for the whole class of lymphatic and haemopoietic cancers (ICD 8, code 200–209). The other two studies of styrene-butadiene rubber production also found an excess of leukaemia. The first was by Meinhardt *et al.* at two plants in the USA, with 1662 and 1994 workers.[84] They reported five deaths from leukaemia, (SMR 1·78, 95% CI: 0·65 to 4·72) in a subgroup of workers first employed between January 1943 and December 1945, before the production process was changed from batch to continuous feed operation at one of the two plants; no information on the work history of these subjects was available. The second study, at eight plants in the United States and Canada by Matanoski *et al.*, was based on a cohort of 12 113 subjects and suggested an increase in leukaemia in production workers, judged by the authors to be those with the highest exposure to 1–3 butadiene.[85] This indication was then explored in depth by comparing, within the cohort, 59 workers with lymphohaemopoietic cancers and 193 workers without cancer matched to the cases for plant, age, sex, date of hire, duration of work, and survival to date of death. Cumulative past exposure to butadiene and to styrene were estimated for each worker from job descriptions and job histories by four industrial hygienists without knowledge of the case or control status. For leukaemia (ICD 8, code 204–207) a relative risk of 7·39 (95% CI: 1·32 to 41·33) was found for exposure to butadiene (above *versus* below the mean) after adjustment for styrene, whereas after adjustment for butadiene the relative risk for styrene was 1·06 (95% CI: 0·23 to 4·95).

Thus the available studies, the last of which appeared least subject to bias or confounding, are quite consistent in pointing to an increased risk of leukaemia, as an aggregate group of conditions, associated with exposure to 1–3 butadiene. However, the lack of clear exposure–response gradient and the possible role of other chemicals in the rubber industry limits the confidence with which 1–3 butadiene can be regarded as a human carcinogen.

Creosote

Creosotes (creosote oils) are blended products of primary distillation fractions of high-temperature coal tars, which are derived from the destructive carbonisation (coking) of coal. Creosote oils are mainly used as wood preservatives. Whereas there is sufficient evidence that occupational exposure to coal tars is causally associated with skin cancer in humans (see table 2.2) the epidemiological data on creosotes are scarce. Apart from case reports of cutaneous epitheliomas in subjects exposed to creosote, one study in the UK by Henry in 1946 reported a crude mortality rate for scrotal cancer, 1911–1948, in brickmakers exposed to "creosote oil" of 29 per million, as contrasted with a rate of 4·2 per million for the general population.[86] Three cases of cancer (leukaemia, pancreas, stomach) against 0·8 expected on the basis of the rates in the general population were reported by Axelson and Kling in a group of 21 workers exposed only to creosotes in wood applications.[87] The evidence for carcinogenicity of creosote oils in humans remains obviously quite limited.

Diethyl sulphate

Diethyl sulphate is manufactured from ethylene and sulphuric acid and is used chiefly as an intermediate ethylating agent in the manufacture of dyes and pigments, and as a finishing agent in textile production. It is an obligatory intermediate in the indirect hydration (strong acid) process for the preparation of synthetic ethanol from ethylene: epidemiological observations derive mainly from cohorts of workers operating this process.

In a study by Lynch *et al.* of a cohort of 355 workers in ethanol and isopropanol manufacturing units an increased incidence of laryngeal cancer was observed (compared with the rate in the general United States population derived from the Third National Survey).[88] The relative risk was 5·04 (95% CI: 1·3 to 6·6) based on four cases. However, a subsequent case-control study within an expanded cohort at this plant indicated that the increased risk, of the size previously observed, was related to exposure to sulphuric acid and persisted even after exclusion of cases in the ethanol and isopropanol units.[89] In another study of ethanol and isopropanol process workers at two plants in the United States increased risks were found for laryngeal, buccal, and pharyngeal cancers, based on small numbers of deaths (respectively two and three) among workers more heavily exposed to sulphuric acid and diethyl sulphates, no cancer cases being observed among those less exposed.[90] In a third study fatal cases of brain tumour among workers at a petrochemical plant in the United States were compared both with dead controls (no increased risk for diethyl sulphate exposure being found[91]) and with live or dead non-cancer controls (relative risk 2·10 (90% CI: 0·57 to 7·73)[92]). Duration of exposure was not related to risk. Overall, the epidemiological data provide limited evidence of a carcinogenic effect of diethyl sulphate in humans.

Formaldehyde

Formaldehyde was discovered in 1859 and has been manufactured commercially since the beginning of this century. Its uses range from plastics and resin production, to disinfection and fumigation, to animal organ embalming, and to wood preservation. The spread of these uses and the presence of products such as urea-formaldehyde foam—which may release the compound—in buildings and mobile homes entail extensive opportunities for exposure of both workers and the general population. Beside its acute irritant and contact allergenic effects formaldehyde is carcinogenic in rats, producing (by inhalation) nasal tumours.

The possible carcinogenicity of formaldehyde in humans has been investigated in some 40 epidemiological studies but, despite this wealth of information, the question is still not conclusively settled. One group of studies has investigated mortality from cancers at several sites in anatomists, pathologists, physicians, embalmers, funeral directors, and other professionals in comparison with the general population of the same age and sex. These studies suffer from the limitation that the assessment of exposure to formaldehyde is generally based on job titles alone, often broadly defined, and that in most studies other exposures are ignored: at most the evidence they provide is only suggestive.

A second group of studies has taken the case-control approach, investigating exposure to formaldehyde in a variety of circumstances in cases of cancer, for instance of nasal cavity or lung, and comparable controls: here the assessment of exposure varies from reliance on job titles, a major limitation already noted, to reconstruction of personal work histories for each subject and inference of past exposures by expert industrial hygienists. This approach produces information more specific to formaldehyde, though less specific and quantitative than in some of the best quality studies of the third type, namely those of cohorts of industrial workers exposed to the compound. In these studies industrial hygiene investigations were carried out at the plants and, in addition, quantitative

27

Table 2.4 Relative risks of nasopharyngeal cancer by level or duration of exposure to formaldehyde (O = observed number of cases, E = expected number of cases, RR = relative risk). Based on Blair et al.[93] (Table 6)

First author	Year	Unexposed			Lower level/duration			Higher level/duration			χ² for trend
		O	E	RR	O	E	RR	O	E	RR	
Blair[94 a]	1987	1	0.5	2.0	2	0.5	4.0	2	0.3	7.5*	0.83
Roush[95 b]	1987	126	126	1.0	21	21	1.0	7	3.1	2.3*	1.29
Vaughan[96 c]	1986	16	16	1.0	7	5.8	1.2	4	2.9	1.4	0.65

(χ² for trend bracket: 2.02)

a Unexposed = <0.5 ppm-years, lower level = 0.05- <5.5 ppm-years, higher level = ≥5.5 ppm-years (all among those also exposed to particulates)
b Lower level = probably exposed, higher levels = probably exposed to some higher levels ≥20 years before death
c Relative exposure scale, low = low, high = medium and high
*P≤0.05

monitoring data were often available, both current and past. These studies thus provide the soundest evidence of a possible link between formaldehyde exposure and cancer. As it happens, tumours at some of the likely target sites of the compound, typically the nasal mucosa, are rare even in large industrial cohorts, limiting in this way the informative character of these studies in practice (see table 2.4).

In 1990 a detailed review by Blair et al. of over 30 studies was carried out.[93] It was apparent from this review that the highest risks were found where exposure to formaldehyde was classified in terms of professional categories (for example pathologists and embalmers), which is the criterion weakest in respect to specificity and confounding exposures. When, on the other hand, exposure information was more reliably derived from different classes of workers within industries, the risk appeared to be small. Guided by a priori knowledge, from animal experiments, that formaldehyde is likely to act first, or even exclusively, at the contact tissue (respiratory tract) the increases in relative risk of cancer in nasopharynx, nose, and lung deserve attention, based overall on some 22 studies. When the studies that contained enough information were used to classify three categories of increasing exposure, a gradient was found for nasopharyngeal cancer, a doubtful gradient for nasal cancer, but no gradient at all for lung cancer.

It is pertinent to note that most data on nasal cancer were obtained through case-control studies where it has proved difficult to control fully for concurrent exposure to wood dust, itself suspected to cause nasal cavity tumours in the furniture industry. For instance, Hayes et al. reported detailed occupational histories of 116 male cases of histologically confirmed epithelial cancer of the nasal cavity and paranasal sinuses and 259 population controls, which were evaluated independently by two industrial hygienists.[97] They found a large relative risk (26·3) of adenocarcinoma leaving, however, only six cases (n = 6) with sufficient exposure to wood dust for a meaningful analysis. Similar difficulties were encountered in the two other main case-control studies of nasal cancer by Olsen and Asnaes[98] and Luce et al.[99] the latter not being included in the previously quoted review. Within the limitations imposed by the small number of cases not exposed to wood dust, these studies indicate an increased risk of nasal adenocarcinomas rather than of nasal squamous carcinoma, the latter, however, being associated with exposure to formaldehyde alone.[74] The picture for nasopharyngeal cancer is clearer, the gradient with duration or level of exposure, shown in table 2·4, is replicated in all three studies (two case-control, one cohort) and was also present in a recent study by West et al.[100] Moreover, the issue of confounding by wood dust is less critical for nasopharyngeal cancer, because wood dust has been linked to cancers only of the nasal cavity and perinasal sinuses. Lung cancer risk shows no gradient with exposure and detailed analyses of the two large multicentre studies in the United

States[93] and the United Kingdom[101-104] did not detect consistent patterns of increased risk. In the American study of industrial workers at 10 plants producing and using formaldehyde, an excess of lung cancer occurred among workers with 20 or more years of latency in six plants and a deficit in four plants, the former not always with the highest level of exposure.[93]

From all these considerations it can be concluded that there is limited evidence of carcinogenicity of formaldehyde in humans. The observed excesses of nasopharyngeal cancer are likely to have been caused by exposure to formaldehyde. The association with nasal cancer on the other hand remains plausible but is less supported by the available evidence, somewhat inconsistent between studies and—more important—difficult to interpret because of incomplete control of confounding by exposure to wood dust. Still less supported, though in principle biologically plausible, is the evidence of a link with lung cancer.

Polychlorinated biphenyls

Polychlorinated biphenyls (PCBs) are a family of about 130 congeners occurring in commercial products. Since the 1930s they have been used in electric capacitors, heat exchange fluids, plasticisers, organic diluents, adhesives, and flame retardants (table 2.5). They have become widely distributed in the environment throughout the world; they are persistent and accumulate in food chains, being found in particular in fatty tissues of humans and animals. Studies in mice and rats have shown that certain PCBs, particularly those with greater than 50% chlorination (as, for instance, "Aroclor 1254") produce benign and malignant liver neoplasms when given by mouth. In humans the highest exposures to PCBs have resulted from consumption of contaminated food or from inhalation and skin absorption in the work environment. Both these have been investigated epidemiologically. The former was studied in relation to contamination of cooking oil with a mixture of PCBs ("Kanechlor 400") in Japan, where a large population was intoxicated ("Yusho" or "rice oil disease," with severe skin and mucosal symptoms).[105] Among 887 male and 874 female "Yusho" patients, significant increases in mortality were noted—in men—for all malignancies (33 Observed, 15·5 Expected), liver cancer (9 Observed; 1·6 Expected) and for lung cancer (8 Observed; 2·5 Expected). The edible rice oil was, however, also contaminated by polychlorinated quaterphenyls and polychlorinated dibenzofurans so these observations are difficult to interpret in terms of PCB exposure. Contamination, mostly from the general environment, was investigated in a study that suggested an increase in PCB concentrations in subcutaneous adipose tissue of deceased subjects with cancers of the stomach, colon, pancreas, ovaries, and prostate.[106] Two other studies did not detect an association between PCB content in breast fat and blood

Table 2.5 Mortality from selected causes in three cohorts exposed to polychlorinated biphenyls

First author	Year	Country	Cohort	All causes Observed	SMR	All cancers Observed	SMR	Gastrointestinal cancers Observed	SMR	Lymphohaemopoietic cancers Observed	SMR
Bertazzi[109]	1987	Italy	2100	M 30	101	14	183*	6	274*	3	263
				F 34	206*	12	226*			4	377*
Brown[110]	1987	US	2588	M 141	88	17	54	1	143**	1	29
				F 154	98	45	93	4	333**	4	100
Sinks[111]	1993	US	3588	M 192	70*	54	80	1	110**	7	100

*P < 0.05
**liver, gallbladder and biliary passages only

tissue and breast cancer.[107 108] Current—as opposed to past—levels in tissues may not, however, be those that are aetiologically relevant.

Three studies have investigated cancer mortality in workers employed in the manufacture of electrical capacitors (see table 2.5). In the study by Bertazzi et al. significant excesses of cancer were noted for all malignancies in men and women, lymphatic and haematopoietic cancers in women, and gastrointestinal cancers in men (one death being from liver cancer and another from cancer of the biliary passages).[109] No relation of these excesses with duration of exposure or time since first exposure was apparent. In partial agreement with this investigation Brown et al. found, against a background of low mortality in the exposed cohort (which may reflect selection of healthy workers), an excess of liver, gallbladder, and biliary tract cancers.[110] This increase was mainly attributable to deaths of women in one of the two plants where four of the five deaths occurred, this being the plant with higher past levels of exposure. Because of small numbers, trends with duration of exposure or time since first exposure could not be explored. No such increases were found in the third study by Sinks et al. in which, however, eight malignant melanomas (not shown in table 2.5) were observed against at most two expected (SMR, 4·10; 95% CI: 1·80 to 8·00): no relation with cumulative exposure to PCB was detectable.[111] Two cases of melanoma, regarded as an excess, were reported among 72 workers exposed to PCBs (and other agents) by Bahn et al.,[112] whereas two other studies on small cohorts of workers (respectively 89 and 142) did not detect increases in any cancer.[113 114]

Taken together the results on cancer of the liver (with gallbladder and bile ducts) and melanoma provide some evidence for carcinogenicity of PCBs, limited by the inconsistency of trends with duration and intensity of exposure and time since first exposure and by potential confounding by concurrent exposures to other chemicals such as dibenzofurans.

Conclusion

During the past 25 years the IARC has assessed the carcinogenicity for humans and animals of almost 800 agents and industrial exposures. It is perhaps surprising that of those specifically identified, excluding therapeutic drugs, the total number of agents in the workplace considered to be definite or probable human carcinogens is only around 50. There are others that have been seriously suspected but it is usually the epidemiological evidence that is insufficient for acceptance; even among the Group 2A carcinogens the interpretable data are often scanty. This may derive not only from sheer inadequacy or non-existence of epidemiological data but also from the fact that a good quality epidemiological study may be inherently limited by small size of the exposed population, short period of observation, or close concurrence of multiple exposures. Of greater concern is the dearth of information on quantified risk in relation to duration and intensity of exposure. If no safe substitute for a suspected carcinogen is available and the product is regarded as socially important, this may present a major problem for occupational health as well as for industry.

1 *IARC monographs on the evaluation of carcinogenic risks to humans.* Lyon, International Agency for Research on Cancer, Volumes 1 to 60, 1972–1994.
2 International Agency for Research on Cancer. *Overall evaluations of carcinogenicity: an updating of IARC monographs Volumes 1 to 42.* Lyon, International Agency for Research on Cancer, 1987.
3 Kazantzis G. Carcinogenic effects of metals. In: McDonald JC, ed, *Recent advances in occupational health 1.* Edinburgh: Churchill Livingstone, 1981, 15–25.
4 Sontag JM (ed). *Carcinogens in industry and the environment.* New York: Marcel Dekker, 1981.
5 Lee AM, Fraumeni JF. Arsenic and respiratory cancer in man: an occupational study. *J Natl Cancer Inst* 1969; **42**: 1045–52.
6 Pinto SS, Henderson V, Enterline PE. Mortality experience of arsenic-exposed workers. *Arch Environ Health* 1978; **33**: 325–31.
7 Tokudome S, Kuratsune M. A cohort study on mortality from cancer and other causes among workers at a metal refinery. *Int J Cancer* 1976; **17**: 310–17.
8 Wall S. Survival and mortality patterns among Swedish smelter workers. *Int J Epidemiol* 1980; **9**: 73–87.
9 Lubin JH, Pottern LM, Blot WJ, Tokudome S, Stone BJ, Fraumeni JF. Respiratory cancer among copper smelter workers: recent mortality statistics. *J Occup Med* 1981; **23**: 779–84.
10 Enterline PE, Marsh GM. Cancer among workers exposed to arsenic and other substances in a copper smelter. *Am J Epidemiol* 1982; **116**: 895–911.
11 Welch K, Higgins I, Oh M, Burchfield C. Arsenic exposure, smoking, and respiratory cancer in copper smelter workers. *Arch Environ Health* 1982; **37**: 325–35.
12 Lee-Feldstein A. Cumulative exposure to arsenic and its relationship to respiratory cancer among copper smelter employees. *J Occup Med* 1986; **28**: 296–302.
13 Greaves WW, Rom WN, Lyon JL, Varley G, Wright DD, Chiu G. Relationship between lung cancer and distance of residence from non-ferrous smelter stack effluent. *Am J Ind Med* 1981; **2**: 15–23.
14 Rom WN, Varley G, Lyon JL, Shopkow S. Lung cancer mortality among residents living near the El Paso smelter. *Br J Ind Med* 1982; **39**: 269–72.
15 Brown LM, Pottern LM, Blot WJ. Lung cancer in relation to environmental pollutants emitted from industrial sources. *Environ Res* 1984; **34**: 250–61.
16 Pershagen G. Lung cancer mortality among men living near an arsenic-emitting smelter. *Am J Epidemiol* 1985; **122**: 684–94.
17 Mabuchi K, Lilienfeld AM, Snell LM. Cancer and occupational exposure to arsenic: a study of pesticide workers. *Prev Med* 1980; **9**: 51–77.
18 Matanoski GM, Landau E, Tonascia J, Lazar C, Elliott EA, McEnroe W *et al.* *Environ Res* 1981; **25**: 8–28.
19 Lüchtrath H. The consequences of chronic arsenic poisoning among Moselle wine growers. *J Cancer Res Clin Oncol* 1983; **105**: 173–82.
20 Chen C-J, Chuang Y-C, Lin T-M, Wu H-Y. Malignant neoplasms among residents of a blackfoot disease-endemic area of Taiwan: high-arsenic artesian well water and cancers. *Cancer Res* 1985; **45**: 5895–9.
21 Chen C-J, Chuang Y-C, You S-L, Lin T-M, Wu H-Y. A retrospective study on malignant neoplasms of bladder, lung and liver in a blackfoot disease-endemic area in Taiwan. *Br J Cancer* 1986; **53**: 399–405.
22 *IARC monographs on the evaluation of carcinogenic risks to humans.* Lyon, International Agency for Research on Cancer, Volume 58, 1993, 41–117.

23 Ward E, Okun A, Ruder A, Fingerhut M, Steenland K. A mortality study of workers at seven beryllium processing plants. *Am J Ind Med* 1992; 22: 885–904.

24 Mancuso TF. Mortality study of beryllium industry workers' occupational lung cancer. *Environ Res* 1980; 21: 48–55.

25 Wagoner JK, Infante PF, Bayliss DL. Beryllium: an etiologic agent in the induction of lung cancer, non-neoplastic respiratory disease, and heart disease among industrially exposed workers. *Environ Res* 1980; 21: 15–34.

26 Steenland K, Ward E. Lung cancer incidence among patients with beryllium disease: a cohort mortality study. *J Natl Cancer Inst* 1991; 83: 1380–5.

27 Sorahan T. Mortality from lung cancer among a cohort of nickel cadmium battery workers: 1946–84. *Br J Ind Med* 1987; 44: 803–9.

28 Elinder C-G, Kjellström T, Hogstedt C, Andersson K, Spång G. Cancer mortality of cadmium workers. *Br J Ind Med* 1985; 42: 651–5.

29 Kazantzis G, Blanks RG, Sullivan KR. Is cadmium a human carcinogen? In: Nordberg GF, Herber RFM, Allesio L, eds, *Cadmium in the human environment: toxicity and carcinogenicity*. Lyon, IARC Scientific Publications No 118, 435–46.

30 Stayner L, Smith R, Thun M, Schnorr T, Lemen R. A dose-response analysis and quantitative assessment of lung cancer risk and occupational cadmium exposure. *Annals of Epidemiology* 1992; 2: 177–94.

31 Hayes RB, Lilienfeld AM, Snell LM. Mortality in chromium chemical production workers: a prospective study. *Int J Epidemiol* 1979; 8: 365–74.

32 Alderson J, Aaseth J, Norseth T. Uptake of chromium by rat liver mitochondria. *Toxicology* 1982; 24: 115–22.

33 Satoh K, Fukuda Y, Torii K, Katsuno N. Epidemiological study of workers engaged in the manufacture of chromium compounds. *J Occup Med* 1981; 23: 835–8.

34 Korallus U, Lange H-J, Neiss A, Wüstefeld E, Zwingers T. Relationships between environmental hygiene control measures and mortality from bronchial cancer in the chromate producing industry (Ger). *Arbeitsmed Sozialmed Präventivmed* 1982; 17: 159–67.

35 De Marco R, Bernardinelli L, Mangione MP. Death risk due to cancer of the respiratory apparatus in chromate production workers (Ital). *Med Lav* 1988; 79: 368–76.

36 Frentzel-Beyme R. Lung cancer mortality of workers employed in chromate pigment factories. A multicentric European epidemiological study. *J Cancer Res Clin Oncol* 1983; 105: 183–8.

37 Davies JM. Lung cancer mortality among workers making lead chromate and zinc chromate pigments in three English factories. *Br J Ind Med* 1984; 41: 158–69.

38 Hayes RB, Sheffet A, Spirtas R. Cancer mortality among a cohort of chromium pigment workers. *Am J Ind Med* 1989; 16: 127–33.

39 Sorahan T, Burges DCL, Waterhouse JAH. A mortality study of nickel/chromium platers. *Br J Ind Med* 1987; 44: 250–8.

40 Report of International Committee on Nickel Carcinogenesis in Man. *Scand J Work Environ Health* 1990; 16: 1–84.

41 Redmond CK. Site specific cancer mortality among workers involved in the production of high nickel alloys. In: Sunderman FW, ed, *Nickel in the human environment*. Lyon, IARC Scientific Publications No 53, 73–86.

42 *IARC monographs on the evaluation of carcinogenic risks to humans*. Lyon, International Agency for Research on Cancer, Volume 42, 1987.

43 *IARC monographs on the evaluation of carcinogenic risks to humans*. Lyon, International Agency for Research on Cancer, Volume 1, 1972.

44 *IARC monographs on the evaluation of carcinogenic risks to humans*. Lyon, International Agency for Research on Cancer, Volume 52, 1991.

45 *IARC monographs on the evaluation of carcinogenic risks to humans*. Lyon, International Agency for Research on Cancer, Volume 23, 1980.

46 *IARC monographs on the evaluation of carcinogenic risks to humans*. Lyon, International Agency for Research on Cancer, Volume 58, 1993.

47 Alderson MR, Rattan NS. Mortality of workers in an isopropyl alcohol plant and two MEK dewaxing plants. *Br J Ind Med* 1980; 37: 85–9.

48 Decoufflé P, Blattner WA, Blair A. Mortality among chemical workers exposed to benzene and other agents. *Environ Res* 1983; 30: 16–25.

49 McCraw DS, Joyner RE, Cole P. Excess leukaemia in a refinery population. *J Occup Med* 1985; 27: 220–2.

50 Bond GG, McLaren EA, Baldwin CL, Cook RR. An update of mortality among chemical workers exposed to benzene. *Br J Ind Med* 1986; 43: 685–91.

51 Yin S-N, Li G-L, Tain F-D, Fu Z-I, Jin C et al. Leukaemia in benzene workers: a retrospective cohort study. *Br J Ind Med* 1987; 44: 124–8.

52 Figueroa WG, Raszkowski R, Weiss W. Lung cancer in chloromethyl methyl ether workers. *N Engl J Med* 1973; 288: 1096–7.

53 Weiss W, Moser RL, Anerbach O. Lung cancer in chloromethyl ether workers. *Am Rev Resp Dis* 1979; 120: 1031–7.

54 Weiss W. Epidemic curve of respiratory cancer due to chloromethyl ethers. *J Nat Cancer Inst* 1982; 69: 1265–70.

55 De Fonso LR, Kelton SC. Lung cancer following exposure to chloromethyl methyl ether. *Arch Environ Health* 1976; 31: 125–30.

56 Pasternack BS, Shore RE, Albert RE. Occupational exposure to chloromethyl ethers. *J Occup Med* 1977; 19: 741–6.

57 Högstedt C, Rohlén O, Berndtsson BS, Axelson O, Ehrenberg O. A mortality study of mortality and cancer incidence in ethylene oxide production workers. *Br J Ind Med* 1979; 36: 276–80.

58 Högstedt C, Aringer L, Gustavsson A. Epidemiologic support for ethylene oxide as a cancer-causing agent. *JAMA* 1986; 255: 1575–8.

59 Steenland K, Stayner L, Greife A, Halperin W, Hayes R, Hornung R et al. Mortality among workers exposed to ethylene oxide. *N Engl J Med* 1991; 324: 1402–7.

60 Stayner L, Steenland K, Greife A, Hornung R, Hayes RB, Nowlin S et al. Exposure-response analysis of cancer mortality in a cohort of workers exposed to ethylene oxide. *Am J Epidemiol* 1993; 138: 787–98.

61 *IARC monographs on the evaluation of carcinogenic risks to humans.* Lyon, International Agency for Research on Cancer, Volume 60, 1994, 139.

62 *IARC monographs on the evaluation of carcinogenic risks to humans.* Lyon, International Agency for Research on Cancer, Volume 33, 1984.

63 Decoufflé P. Further analysis of cancer mortality patterns among workers exposed to cutting oil mists. *J Nat Cancer Inst* 1978; 61: 1025–30.

64 Costello J. Morbidity and mortality study of shale oil workers in the United States. *Environ Health Perspect* 1979; 30: 205–8.

65 Miller BG, Cowie HA, Middleton WG, Seaton A. Epidemiologic studies of Scottish oil shale workers: III, Causes of death. *Am J Ind Med* 1986; 9: 433–46.

66 Purde M, Rahu M. Cancer patterns in the oil shale area of the Estonian SSR. *Environ Health Perspect* 1979; 30: 209–10.

67 Creech JL, Johnson MN. Angiosarcoma of liver in the manufacture of polyvinyl chloride. *J Occup Med* 1974; 16: 150–1.

68 Tabershaw IR, Gaffey WR. Mortality study of workers in the manufacture of vinyl chloride and its polymers. *J Occup Med* 1974; 16: 509–18.

69 Waxweiller RJ, Smith AH, Falk H, Tyroler HA. Excess lung cancer risk in a synthetic chemicals plant. *Environ Health Perspect* 1981; 41: 159–65.

70 Theriault G, Allard P. Cancer mortality in a group of Canadian workers exposed to vinyl chloride monomer. *J Occup Med* 1981; 23: 671–6.

71 Storetvedt Heldaas S, Langård SL, Anderson A. Incidence of cancer among vinyl chloride and polyvinyl chloride workers. *Br J Ind Med* 1984; 41: 25–30.

72 Byrén D, Engholm G, Englund A, Westerholm P. Mortality and cancer morbidity in a group of Swedish VCM and PVC production. *Environ Health Perspect* 1976; 17: 167–70.

73 O'Berg M. Epidemiologic study of workers exposed to acrylonitrile. *J Occup Med* 1980; 22: 245–52.

74 Kieselbach N, Korallus UH, Lange A, Neiss T. Zwingers acrylonitrile-epidemiologic study, *Zbl Arbeitsmed* 1977; 10: 257–9.

75 Thiess AM, Frentzel-Beyme R, Link R, Wild H. Mortalitätsstudie bei Chemiefacharbeitern verschiedener Produktionsbetriebe mit Exposition auch gegenüber Acrylonitrile. *Zbl Arbeitsmed* 1980; 30: 259–67.

76 Werner JB, Carter JT. Mortality of United Kingdom acrylonitrile polymerisation workers. *Br J Ind Med* 1981; **38**: 147–53.

77 Delzell E, Monson RR. Mortality among rubber workers: VI. Men with potential exposure to acrylonitrile. *J Occup Med* 1982; **24**: 767–9.

78 O'Berg MT, Chen JL, Burke CA, Walrath J, Pell S. Epidemiologic study of workers exposed to acrylonitrile; an update. *J Occup Med* 1985; **27**: 835–40.

79 Chen JL, Walrath J, O'Berg M, Burke CA, Pell S. Cancer incidence and mortality among workers exposed to acrylonitrile. *Am J Ind Med* 1987; **11**: 157–63.

80 Collins JJ, Page LC, Caporossi JC, Utidjan HM, Lucas LJ. Mortality patterns among employees exposed to acrylonitrile. *J Occup Med* 1989; **31**: 368–71.

81 Swaen GMH, Bloemen LJN, Twisk J, Scheffers T, Slangen JJM, Sturmans F. Mortality of workers exposed to acrylonitrile. *J Occup Med* 1992; **34**: 801–9.

82 Divine BJ. An update on mortality among workers at a 1–3 butadiene facility—preliminary results. *Environ Health Perspect* 1990; **86**: 119–28.

83 McMichael AJ, Spirtas R, Gamble JF, Tonsey PM. Mortality among rubber workers: relationship to specific jobs. *J Occup Med* 1976; **18**: 178–85.

84 Meinhardt TJ, Lemen RA, Crandall MS, Young RJ. Environmental epidemiologic investigation of the styrene-butadiene rubber industry. Mortality patterns with discussion of the haematopoietic and lymphatic malignancies. *Scand J Work Environ Health* 1982; **8**: 250–9.

85 Matanoski GM, Santos-Burgoa C, Schwartz L. Mortality of a cohort of workers in the styrene butadiene polymer manufacturing industry (1943–1982). *Environ Health Perspect* 1990; **86**: 107–17.

86 Henry SA. *Cancer of the scrotum in relation to occupation.* New York, Oxford University Press, 1946.

87 Axelson O, Kling H. Mortality among wood preservers with creosote exposure (Swed) (Abstract), 1983. In: *32nd Nordic Occupational Hygiene Conference, Solna, Arbetarskyddsstyrelsen (National Board of Occupational Safety and Health)*, 125–6.

88 Lynch J, Hanis NM, Bird MG, Murray KJ, Walsh JP. An association of upper respiratory cancer with exposure to diethyl sulfate. *J Occup Med* 1979; **21**: 333–41.

89 Soskolne CL, Zeighani EA, Hanis NM, Kupper LL, Herrmann N, Amsel J, et al. Laryngeal cancer and occupational exposure to sulfuric acid. *Am J Epidemiol* 1984; **120**: 358–69.

90 Teta MJ, Perlman GD, Ott MG. Mortality study of ethanol and isopropanol production workers at two facilities. *Scand J Work Environ Health* 1992; **18**: 90–6.

91 Austin SG, Schnatter AR. A case-control study of chemical exposures and brain tumors in petrochemical workers. *J Occup Med* 1983; **25**: 313–20.

92 Leffingwell SS, Waxweiler R, Alexander V, Ludwig HR, Halperin W. Case-control study of gliomas of the brain among workers employed by a Texas City, Texas chemical plant. *Neuroepidemiology* 1983; **3**: 179–95.

93 Blair A, Saracci R, Stewart PA, Hayes RB, Shy C. Epidemiologic evidence on the relationship between formaldehyde exposure and cancer. *Scand J Work Environ Health* 1990; **16**: 381–93.

94 Blair A, Stewart PA, Hoover RN, et al. Cancers of the nasopharynx and oropharynx and formaldehyde exposure. *J Natl Cancer Inst* 1987; **78**: 191–2.

95 Roush GC, Walrath J, Stayner LT, Kaplan SA, Flannery JT, Blair A. Nasopharyngeal cancer, sinonasal cancer, and occupations related to formaldehyde: A case-control study. *J Natl Cancer Inst* 1987; **79**: 1221–5.

96 Vaughan TL, Strader C, Davis S, Daling JR. Formaldehyde and cancers of the pharynx, sinus and nasal cavities: 1. occupational exposures. *Int J Cancer* 1986; **38**: 677–88.

97 Hayes RB, Raatgever JW, De Bruyn A, Gérin M. Cancer of the nasal cavity and paranasal sinuses and formaldehyde exposure. *Int J Cancer* 1986; **37**: 487–92.

98 Olsen JH, Asnaes S. Formaldehyde and the risk of squamous cell carcinoma of the sinonasal cavities. *Br J Ind Med* 1986; **43**: 769–74.

99 Luce D, Gérin M, Leclerc A, Morcet JF, Brugère J, Goldberg M. Sinonasal cancer and occupational exposure to formaldehyde and other substances. *Int J Cancer* 1993; **53**: 224–31.

100 West S, Hildesheim A, Dosemeci M. Non-viral risk factors for nasopharyngeal

carcinoma in the Philippines: results from a case-control study. *Int J Cancer* 1993; **55**: 722–7.

101 Acheson ED, Gardner MJ, Pannett B, Barnes HR, Osmond C, Taylor CP. Formaldehyde in the British chemical industry. *Lancet* 1984; **1**: 611–16.

102 Acheson ED, Barnes HR, Gardner MJ, Osmond C, Pannett B, Taylor CP. Cohort study of formaldehyde process workers. *Lancet* 1984; **2**: 403.

103 Acheson ED, Barnes HR, Gardner MJ, Osmond C, Pannett B, Taylor CP. Formaldehyde process workers and lung cancer. *Lancet* 1984; **1**: 1066–7.

104 Gardner MJ, Pannett B, Winter PD, Cruddas AM. A cohort study of workers exposed to formaldehyde in the British chemical industry: an update. *Br J Ind Med* 1993; **50**: 827–34.

105 Kuratsune M, Yoshimara T, Matsuzaka J, Yamaguchi A. Epidemiologic study on Yusho, a poisoning caused by ingestion of rice-oil contaminated with a commercial brand of polychlorinated biphenyls. *Environ Health Perspect* 1972; **1**: 119–28.

106 Unger M, Olsen J, Clausen J. Organochlorine compounds in the adipose tissue of deceased persons with and without cancer: a statistical survey of some potential confounders. *Environ Res* 1982; **29**: 371–9.

107 Wolf MS, Toniolo PG, Lee EW, Rivera M, Dubin N. Blood levels of organochlorine residues and risk of breast cancer. *J Nat Cancer Inst* 1993; **85**: 648–52.

108 Unger M, Kiaer H, Blichert-Toft M, Olsen J, Clausen J. Organochlorine compounds in human breast fat from deceased persons with and without breast cancer and in a biopsy material from newly diagnosed patients undergoing breast surgery. *Environ Res* 1984; **34**: 24–8.

109 Bertazzi PA, Riboldi L, Pesatori A, Radice L, Zochetti C. Cancer mortality of capacitor manufacturing workers. *Am J Ind Med* 1987; **11**: 165–76.

110 Brown DP. Mortality of workers exposed to polychlorinated biphenyls: an update. *Arch Environ Health* 1987; **42**: 333–9.

111 Sinks T, Steele G, Smith AB, Watkins K, Shults RA. Mortality among workers exposed to polychlorinated biphenyls. *Am J Epidemiol* 1992; **136**: 389–97.

112 Bahn AK, Rosenwaike I, Herrmann N, Grover P, Stellman J, O'Leary K. Melanoma after exposure to PCBs. *N Engl J Med* 1976; **295**: 450.

113 Zack TA, Musch DC. *Mortality of PCB workers at the Monsanto Plant in Sanget, Illinois, St Louis, MO*, Monsanto International Report, 1979.

114 Gustavsson P, Hogstedt C, Rappe C. Short-term mortality and cancer incidence in capacitor manufacturing workers exposed to polychlorinated biphenyls (PCBs). *Am J Ind Med* 1986; **10**: 341–4.

3 Ionising radiation

YUTAKA HOSODA

Introduction

Ionising radiation is a known carcinogen. The epidemiology of radiation-induced malignancies has recently focused on cancer risks in low dose ranges. However, sufficient data have so far not been available to assess cancer risks directly. Such risks have therefore to be estimated from models by extrapolation from effects observed at high doses. This chapter will deal with studies of radiation cancers, risk estimates, prevention, and future priorities.

Man-made versus natural radiation

28 December 1995 will be celebrated as the centennial of the discovery of x rays by Wilhelm Roentgen of Wurzburg. Subsequently, uranium was discovered by Antonie Becquerel (1896) and radium by Marie Curie

(1898). Soon after these discoveries scientists themselves started to experience work-related radiation injuries such as erythema, epilation, and non-malignant conditions. The first case of skin cancer was demonstrated by Frieben at a Hamburg medical meeting in 1902 on the hand of an employee who had worked at an x ray tube manufacturing factory[1][2]. With the development of the radiation industry, osteomyelitis of the jaw bones among American dial painters (radium jaw) was reported by Theodor Blum in 1924[3] and later osteogenic sarcoma among the same group by Martland *et al.* in 1929 in New York.[4] In uranium mines of Joachimstal, Czechoslovakia, eight cases of lung cancer detected among miners were carefully examined by Sikl of Prague, who suggested that the cancer was caused not by silicosis but by radium emanation.[5] Although a series of valuable case reports appeared, these pioneers' observations remained in the realm of clinical medicine rather than epidemiology.

In August 1945, the 50th anniversary year of the discovery of x rays the human race first experienced catastrophic radiation casualties from atomic bombs on Hiroshima and Nagasaki. The energy released from these bombs was in the form of blast (50%), heat (35%), and radiation (15% only). Thus radiation was merely an accessary to the weapon. Gamma rays reached out to about 2 km and neutrons to a much shorter distance, but the blast waves extended to a distance of 4 km and heat to 3·5 km.[6] It can be said that radiation epidemiology came into being in the ruins of these two cities, largely through the cooperation of atomic bomb survivors. Studies on the cohort of survivors are a basic reference for radiation risk estimates. In recent years, however, scientific interest has shifted from the effects of high dose to those of low dose radiation.

No less than 87% of the total radiation exposure to mankind comes from natural radioactivity such as ground and buildings (14%), food and drink (12%), radon and thoron (51%), and cosmic rays (10%). Only 13% comes from man-made sources, with a little variation from one area to another.[6][7] After the creation of the earth 4·6 billion years ago, most radioactive nuclei with shorter half lives decayed, while ^{238}U with a half life of about $4·5 \times 10^9$ years and ^{40}K with one of about $1·3 \times 10^9$ years were left on the earth's surface. Radon (^{222}Rn, with a half life of 3·82 days), a decay product of ^{238}U is released into the air and contributes rather more than 50% of natural background radiation. Cosmic rays are reduced considerably when passing through the ozone layer before reaching the earth's surface.

Human exposure[7][8][9]

Radiation generally denotes the transfer of energy. If the energy is sufficient, it is transferred to atoms in human tissue, causing ejection from the atom of an electron. This process is termed ionisation. Ionising radiation includes electromagnetic radiations such as x rays and various types of particulate radiation such as α particles, β particles and neutrons. The amount of energy deposited in the tissue is measured as a function of distance along the radiation track. Linear Energy Transfer (LET), categorised as high or low, refers to the amount of energy deposited per unit of track length. Low LET radiations, such as γ and x rays cause relatively sparse ionisation along the radiation track, while high LET radiations, such as γ particles or neutrons cause dense ionisation.

Radiation may come from outside the body (external exposure) or from inside (internal exposure).[8] With exposure from external sources of γ or x rays, the body has usually no contact with the radiation source. When the source is taken away or turned off, no radiation remains in the body. On the other hand, internal exposure results from radioactive material which enters the body through inhalation, ingestion, direct absorption from the skin, or through open wounds. A person with internal exposure remains radioactive until the source is removed or has decayed. External radiation is usually monitored by film badges, automatic thermoluminescent dosimeters, alarm pocket dosimeters and so on, while internal radiation dose is measured by whole body counters and sometimes by measurement of samples of faeces and urine. Lymphocytic chromosomal aberrations are also well correlated with exposure dose and so allow biological dosimetry.[10]

The measurement of radiation dose is made using International Units (SI units). Previously popular units such as rad, rem and curie have been replaced by: the gray (Gy) for absorbed unit (1 Gy = 100 rad, 1 rad = 0·01 Gy = 10 mGy), the sievert (Sv) for radiation protection (1 Sv = 100 rem, 1 rem = 0·01 Sv = 10 mSv) and the becquerel (Bq) (1 Bq = $2\cdot7 \times 10^{-11}$ Ci, 1 Ci = $3\cdot7 \times 10^{10}$ Bq) for radiation activity. For radiological protection, the "effective dose (Sv)" as recommended by the International Commission on Radiological Protection is useful in practice.[9] The effective dose is formed by weighting the equivalent dose (according to radiation type and energy) by a tissue weighting factor.

Table 3.1 The average magnitude of the effective radiation dose encountered in various circumstances

Natural[7]	Radon	2 mSv/Yr
	Terrestrial + cosmic + intake	1 mSv/Yr
Occupational[87]	Reactor operators	2·5 mSv/Yr
	Uranium miners	4 mSv/Yr
	Non-uranium miners	1–6 mSv/Yr
	Air crew	3 mSv/Yr
Medical	Chest radiography	<0·1 mSv/exam
	Barium meal	2–5 mSv/exam
	Thorax computed tomogram	8–9 mSv/exam

In the case of intake of a radionuclide, the time integral of the effective dose rate is referred to as the "committed effective dose" and is used to reflect the integration time in years following the intake. For the general information of non-specialists, the magnitude of effective doses in circumstances close to ordinary life is shown in table 3.1, though such doses may vary widely depending on circumstances.

Biological and health effects

The absorption of radiant energy causes excitation and ionisation along the tracks of the charged particles, resulting in direct interaction between the charged particles and the DNA molecule, or indirect interaction between hydroxy radicals produced by ionising radiation and DNA.[6 7 8] With sparsely ionising radiations such as x ray and γ ray, most of the biological effects are produced by the indirect interaction modified by physical and chemical factors. As the quality of the radiation changes from low to high LET, the balance shifts the interaction from indirect to direct.

If the cell damage is not adequately repaired, the cells are prevented from surviving or reproducing, or the living cell may be modified. If the number of cells damaged or killed is large enough, the severity of harm increases when the dose exceeds some threshold (deterministic effect)[9]. Radiation cataract is an example. The threshold to low LET radiation is probably in a range 2–10 Gy.[9] On the other hand, if the irradiated cells are modified rather than killed, the clone of cells induced by reproduction of modified living somatic cells may result in a cancer, after a prolonged latent period. The probability of cancer usually increases with dose, probably without threshold, and its severity is unaffected by dose. If the damage occurs in a cell that transmits genetic information, the effects may be shown in the children of the person exposed. This type of effect on cancers or heredity where only the probability is a function of dose is termed stochastic.[9] Given the same dose, a single exposure may have larger biological effect than protracted exposures.

Lessons from the Hiroshima-Nagasaki survivors

Mortality study

The life-span study cohort of atomic bomb survivors comprised some 100 000 persons of both sexes over a wide range of ages, sampled from a total of about 280 000 survivors notified at the 1950 national census. The mortality in this cohort was examined retrospectively to 1950 and prospectively since 1959 by the Atomic Bomb Casualty Commission (ABCC), and its successor the Radiation Research Foundation (RRF) in

Hiroshima and Nagasaki. No information is available for the first five years after the bombing, 1945–1950. The recent mortality study (1950–1985) analysed 5900 deaths among the 76 000 survivors for whom the exposure doses were estimated according to the 1986 dosimetry system (DS 86).[11] To obtain this dosimetry, the US-Japan joint team estimated doses by using data from explosion experiments in the USA, other physical techniques, and interviews with survivors to inquire about shielding conditions at the time of bombing. For the dose-response curve for all cancers except leukaemia, the linear (L) model showed a good fit and for leukaemia when the high dose range was excluded, the linear quadratic (LQ) model fitted better than the L model.

Excess relative risks

The excess relative risk (relative risk minus one) for leukaemia per Gy (organ absorbed dose) was 5·21 (95% confidence interval 3·83 to 7·12) and that for non-leukaemic cancers (all cancers except for leukaemia) per Gy 0·41 1(95% CI 0·32 to 0·51). When the observation was limited to low exposures 0 to 0·5 Gy, excess relative risks per Gy were 2·40 for leukaemia and 0·38 for all cancers except leukaemia. The malignancies which showed a significant increase in mortality with increasing dose (P < 0·05) were cancers of the oesophagus, stomach, colon, lung, breast, ovary, urinary bladder, and multiple myeloma (table 3.2). No significant increase has as yet been shown for cancers of the rectum, gallbladder, pancreas, uterus, and prostate, or for malignant lymphoma. The study of non-fatal cancers such as thyroid,[12] parathyroid,[13] and skin[14] had to depend on information from clinical examination in adult health studies which began in 1958 of a 20% sample of the life span study cohort.[15] Tumour registry data were also then available. The foregoing three non-fatal cancers proved also to have a dose relationship.

Life time risks

The life time risk is estimated to be 0·4 per Sv (90% CI 0·3 to 0·6) for leukaemia and 4·0 per Sv (90% CI: 3·0 to 5·0) for non-leukaemic cancers according to the International Committee on Radiation Protection (ICRP) by applying the dose effective factor (DDEF) to data on survivors.[34]

Latency of cancer occurrence

The cancers appeared many years after the bombing, and the latent period or lag time differed between leukaemia and solid tumours. Leukaemia mortality occurred two to three years after exposure and peaked at six to eight years. The excess has continued to decline with time, but still remained significantly increased in Hiroshima even in 1981–1985 (except for chronic lymphatic leukaemia which had no dose dependency). Thus, the period of occurrence of radiation-induced leukaemia may last

Table 3.2 Organ absorbed radiation dose-response for significant excess mortality among atomic bomb survivors, 1958–85 (Shimizu et al.)[11]

Site of cancer	Relative risk at 1 Gy	Excess deaths per 10^4 person years Gy
Leukaemia	6·21 (4·83 to 8·12)	2·94 (2·43 to 3·49)
All cancers except leukaemia	1·41 (1·32 to 1·51)	10·13 (7·96 to 12·44)
Oesophagus	1·58 (1·13 to 2·24)	0·45 (0·10 to 0·88)
Stomach	1·27 (1·14 to 1·43)	2·42 (1·26 to 3·72)
Colon	1·85 (1·39 to 2·45)	0·81 (0·40 to 1·30)
Lung	1·63 (1·35 to 1·97)	1·68 (0·97 to 2·49)
Female breast	2·19 (1·56 to 3·09)	1·20 (0·61 to 1·91)
Ovary	2·33 (1·37 to 3·86)	0·71 (0·22 to 1·32)
Urinary tract	2·27 (1·53 to 3·37)	0·68 (0·31 to 1·12)
Multiple myeloma	3·29 (1·67 to 6·31)	0·26 (0·09 to 0·47)

Numbers in parentheses = 90% confidence interval

for at least 35–40 years. For cancers other than leukaemia, excess deaths continued to increase with time in proportion to the natural age adjusted cancer mortality. The mortality from radiation-induced solid cancer did not reach a level of significance until 1960 and the relative risk for all cancers except leukaemia increased significantly with time after 1960. Thus, the minimum latent period was 15 years or longer for all cancers except leukaemia: 15–19 years for stomach cancer, 20–24 years for cancer of the lung and breast, 25–29 years for cancer of the ovary and 30–34 years for cancers of colon and urinary tract and multiple myeloma.

Sex and age

Radiation cancer risks were modified by sex, age at the time of bombing and at death, and also by other carcinogenic agents such as smoking. When age-specific mortality was examined, the younger the age at time of bombing, the larger was the relative risk. For the youngest cohort, 0–9 years of age at the time of bombing, the interval from exposure to death was shortened for all cancers combined, except leukaemia in the high dose group. Women had a higher relative risk than men for all cancers except leukaemia, where no sex difference was found. The association of lung cancer with smoking appeared to be additive; therefore, the contribution of confounders such as smoking should be taken into consideration.

Contribution to cancers

Since not all cancers among atomic bomb survivors were caused by radiation effects, the attributable risks were calculated for 42 000 survivors exposed to 10 mGy or more. During the period 1950–85, about 80 of 144 deaths from leukaemia (55%) were estimated to be attributable to radiation. Likewise, the contribution of radiation was estimated at 6%

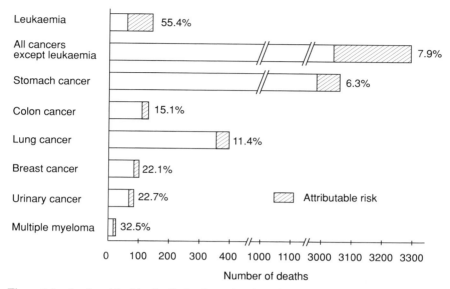

Figure 3.1 Attributable risk of radiation for major sites of cancer death among atomic bomb survivors.[11 16]

for stomach cancer, 11% for lung cancer, and 33% for multiple myeloma (figure 3.1).[16]

Incidence study

Cancer incidence data based on tumour registries in Hiroshima and Nagasaki cities have recently been available during the period 1958–87 for solid tumours. The excess relative risk/Sv in incidence is estimated to be 0·63 (90% CI: 0·52 to 0·74) against 0·45 (90% CI: 0·34 to 0·57) in mortality. The excess relative risk in incidence rates has been shown for the first time for non-fatal malignancies such as salivary gland 1·8 (0·2 to 6·0), non-melanoma skin 1·0 (0·4 to 1·9), and thyroid 1·2 (0·5 to 2·1). There was no longer any excess of multiple myeloma which previously showed a significant increase.[17–20]

Lessons from work populations with protracted exposures

Nuclear industry workers

Nuclear power and weapon industries have been developing since the second world war, drawing public attention to the risks of ionising radiation from man-made sources, though the nuclear fuel cycle is responsible for only 0·1% of total radiation exposures to mankind.

Analytic epidemiological studies have been recognised as essential for assessing late health effects of low dose radiation exposure in man. Major reports related to nuclear industry workers have been available mainly from the USA and the UK since the 1970s, with a remarkable increase since the latter half of the 1980s.

In general, the workers' average cumulative exposure doses have been relatively low, for example, about 30 mSv in the nuclear industry against more than 250 mSv among atomic bomb survivors. As the size of each population is small, a combined analysis has been attempted by Beral, Gilbert and others of eight cohort studies in the United Kingdom and the United States, comprising 120 000 workers in the nuclear industry.[21-29] In all these cohorts, the overall mortality was below their respective national rates and the pooled SMR was below unity, probably as a result of a healthy worker effect: 0·82 for all causes, 0·86 for all cancers, and 0·90 for leukaemia. The mortality from multiple myeloma was significantly higher in relation to cumulative exposure among workers at the Hanford and Sellafield plants and that from prostatic cancer was also dose-related in workers in the United Kingdom Atomic Energy Authority. The paper by Beral *et al.* concluded as follows: "Despite the large number of workers studied, the data are still too sparse to permit precise statements to be associated with repeated exposure to low levels of ionising radiation. The findings thus far are compatible with there being no increase in risk at all, or with an increase about ten times that predicted by the risk estimated on the International Commission on Radiological Protection (ICRP)."[21]

Another combined analysis was made of mortality of 36 000 white male workers in three cohorts at nuclear facilities in the United States: Hanford through 1981, Oak Ridge National Laboratory (ORNL) through 1977, and Rocky Flats Weapon Plant through 1979.[30] Although earlier analyses among Hanford workers suggested an increase in mortality from multiple myeloma correlated with cumulative radiation dose, a significant excess was seen only in the Hanford component. No evidence of increased mortality from all cancers or site-specific cancers was found either in the combined study or in the three separate components. On the other hand, an extended follow-up of the ORNL cohort through 1984 indicated that the SMRs were less than expected for most causes, except for leukaemia which showed a significantly elevated SMR of 1·63.[31] External radiation with a 20 year exposure lag was related to all causes of death (2·68% increase per 10 mSv) primarily as a result of an association with cancer mortality (4·94% increase per 10 mSv). The authors reported that the radiation cancer dose response was 10 times higher than estimates from the follow-up of atomic bomb survivors. Against this report, the most recent Hanford site study, 1945–86, showed little evidence of a positive correlation between cumulative occupational radiation dose and mortality from leukaemia and all other cancers.[32] There was no excess relative risk per 10 mSv for both leukaemia and all other cancers, but these estimates were consistent with either no risk or with estimates obtained from extrapolation from high dose data. In the updated analyses of combined mortality data for workers at the Hanford Site, ORNL, and Rocky Flats the excess relative risk estimate was negative (−1·0/Sv) for leukaemia and 0·0/Sv for all cancers except leukaemia.[33]

The British National Radiation Protection Board (NRPB) examined mortality in a cohort of about 95 000 radiation workers registered with the National Registry for Radiation Workers.[34] SMRs for most causes of death were below 1·00, except for cancer of the thyroid, which showed no trend with external recorded radiation dose. There was evidence of an association between cumulative radiation dose and mortality from leukaemia (excluding chronic lymphocytic leukaemia which is not related to radiation) and multiple myeloma. The central estimates of lifetime risk derived from the data were 10·0% per Sv for all cancers and 0·76% per Sv for leukaemia excluding chronic lymphocytic leukaemia: 2·5 times and 1·9 times the risk estimates of the 1990 International Commission on Radiological Protection (ICRP). These NRPB estimates lie above those most recently reported by the ICRP for leukaemia (excluding chronic lymphatic leukaemia) and for all malignancies, but fall well within the 90% confidence intervals. A study of employees of the UK Atomic Weapons Establishment also revealed an excess relative risk of 7·6% per 10 mSv.[35]

A Canadian cohort study, 1950–1981, of about 13 600 workers employed by Atomic Energy of Canada also found no excess risk in

Table 3.3   Excess relative risks (%) per 10 mSv among nuclear workers.

Cohort	All cancer* (90% confidence interval)	Leukaemia**
Atomic bomb survivors[11]	0·40 (0·3 to 0·5)	5·2 (3·8 to 7·1)
US Hanford site[33]	−0·1 (<0 to 0·8)	−1·1 (<0 to 1·9)
Rocky Flats[33]	<0 (<0 to 1·1)	−7·2 (<0 to 42)
Oak Ridge		
National Lab.(1)[33]	1·2 (<0 to 3·7)	<0 (<0 to 7)
(2)[31]	3·27 (1·26 to 5·28)	6·9 (−11·2 to 24·9)*
UK Atomic Energy[38]	+0·8 (−1·0 to 3·1)***	−4·2 (−5·7 to 2·6)***
	(except leukaemia)	
Atomic Weapons[32]	7·6 (0·4 to 15·3)***	
National Radiological Protection Board[34]	0·47 (−0·12 to 1·2)	4·3 (0·40 to 13·6)
Canada Atomic Energy[37]	0·36 (−4·6 to 2·45)	7·0 (−0·54 to 47·4)
Combined US[33]	−0·0 (<0 to 0·8)	−1·0 (<0 to 2·2)
UK[39]	0·03 (−5 to 0·7)***	4·18 (0·4 to 13·4)***
		(except CLL)
US–UK–Canada[40]	−0·07 (−0·4 to 0·3)	2·2 (0·1 to 5·7)
	(except leukaemia)	(except CLL)

mortality from any cause.[36] However, a more recent Canadian study on cancer mortality, 1956–1985, showed an excess relative risk of 0·36% per 10 mSv (90% confidence interval, −0·46 to 2·45) among male employees of the same company in relation to external Low Linear Energy Transfer ionising radiation.[37] There was also a positive association (p = 0·058) between radiation dose and death from leukaemia (excluding chronic lymphatic leukaemia). The paper concluded that for cancer as a whole, risk estimates based on high-dose studies were unlikely to underestimate risks substantially for low-dose and low-dose-rate exposures. Table 3.3 summarises the excess relative risks reported in the several papers to date.[38-40]

A case control study of UK atomic energy authority employees showed a significant increased risk of prostatic cancer among workers who were internally contaminated with or who worked in an environment potentially contaminated by tritium, $_{51}$chromium, $_{59}$iron, $_{60}$cobalt or $_{65}$zinc.[41]

In summary,[88] the cancer risk estimates in the reports on nuclear workers are controversial, probably because of weak statistical power in the populations observed. Most findings did not differ greatly from the extrapolation estimates from atomic bomb survivors, except for a few papers, though much depended on the models used.[31-42] Population studies with more statistical power may help to clarify the question.

Children of nuclear industry workers

Since a Yorkshire television documentary suggested in 1983 that there was an excess of leukaemia among children in the village of Seascale, near the Sellafield nuclear processing plant in West Cumbria, United Kingdom, there has been much concern about childhood leukaemia in the vicinity of nuclear installations. Governmental studies (Committee on Medical Aspects of Radiation in the Environment) confirmed a real excess of childhood leukaemia near Sellafield. A birth cohort study of children born between 1950 and 1983 to mothers resident in Seascale reported five deaths from leukaemia against 0·53 expected at national rates, a rate ratio of 9·36, (95% confidence interval; 3·04 to 21·84).[43] Furthermore, a case control study, commissioned by the Black inquiry, showed that the relative risk of the disease was higher in children born near Sellafield, particularly to parents who had high radiation dose recordings before conception of the children.[44] The relative risks were 6·42 (95% confidence interval 1·57 to 26·3) for children of fathers who received a total preconceptional exposure of 100 mSv or more, 2·44 (95% CI 1·04 to 5·71) for children of fathers who were employed at the time of their conception and 0·17 (95% CI 0·05 to 0·53) for children born further than 5 km from Sellafield.

The increased risk of the disease proved to be unrelated to environmental contamination from the Sellafield discharges, including eating seafood or home grown vegetables or playing on the beach.[45] An

Oxford study found that the relative risk of childhood leukaemia in relation to fathers' external radiation was close to unity but 2·87 in relation to fathers' internal radiation.[46] In Dounreay, UK, where a nuclear fuel reprocessing plant is located, a birth cohort study was made of children born to local mothers and a schools cohort study of those who moved to the area after birth and attended school there.[47] The birth cohort showed no significant excess of childhood leukaemia, whereas the schools cohort showed a significantly raised incidence, suggesting that the place of birth is not as important as the place of residence in the aetiology of the disease. Another paper reported that the incidence of childhood leukaemia is increased by population mixing, particularly in rural areas.[48] A further extensive study in the UK was made on the geographical distribution of preconceptional dose to fathers employed at the Sellafield nuclear installation, with a follow-up on more than 10 000 children born between 1950 and 1989.[49] The authors concluded that it is highly unlikely that the association between paternal external exposure to radiation before conception and childhood leukaemia is a direct causal relation.

In other countries, such as the USA, France, Germany, and Canada, no excess of childhood leukaemia has been reported in the vicinity of nuclear installations.[50] A Canadian case-control study of childhood leukaemia in offspring near the nuclear facility in Ontario found no evidence of an increased risk in relation to exposure before conception.[51] It was subsequently concluded by Doll *et al.* that in view of new evidence since the Gardner reports the paternal radiation hypothesis was wrong.[52] The hypothesis is not supported by most of recent epidemiological data,[53] or by leukaemia data among 7400 children of Hiroshima-Nagasaki atomic bomb survivors;[54] also the magnitude of the paternal preconceptional dose is not consistent with other genetic molecular biological results.[55–57]

Emergency personnel for nuclear accidents

Major radiation accidents worldwide totalled 290 from 1944 to 1987, with 65 acute fatalities, according to the records of the US Radiation Emergency Assistance Center/Training Site (REAC/TS) Registry in Oak Ridge.[8] Large accidents may affect not only employees at work sites but also nearby inhabitants. The Chernobyl nuclear power accident is an example of heavy contamination of workers, inhabitants, animals and food stuffs.[58 59] Workers and emergency personnel at the site were exposed to extensive β radiation, causing extensive skin burns and many deaths. Of about 1000 rescue personnel, 115 were admitted to hospital with acute radiation syndrome and 28 of these died. The combination of β burns and whole body radiation was lethal. The burns that became manifest two weeks after the injury in parallel with suppression of the haematopoietic system provided easy access for pathogenic microorganisms, and many died of sepsis. Although personnel at the site were exposed to radioactive aerosols, internal contamination was far less important than external exposure in causing the acute radiation syndrome.[8]

From a total of some 148 000 workers who worked at the Chernobyl site, mostly in 1986 and 1987, 6% were exposed to 250 mSv or more (Tsyb'A, at a Russia-Japan conference, Tokyo, 1992) and are probably at a high risk of developing cancer at a later date. In addition, 135 000 inhabitants within 30 km of the site were presumably exposed to about 120 mSv on average. In 1989, the International Atomic Energy Agency Chernobyl International Advisory Committee, chaired by I. Shigematsu, was convened to examine health effects of the inhabitants at the request of the then USSR.[60] Preliminary studies showed no difference in health status between inhabitants in contaminated areas and control areas. In the contaminated area, the estimated 70 years exposure ranged from 80 to 160 mSv for both external and internal doses. The team predicted that a slight increase in the incidence of thyroid cancer could not be excluded and a recent Belarus report suggested an increase in childhood thyroid cancer based on histological examination.[61] As the radiation dose for cases and the population at risk has not been reported, it is difficult to discuss the dose-response relationship. In other papers, the Chernobyl-related cancer risk over the next 70 years has been estimated by radiation specialists, with an extremely wide range of excess deaths, from 5100 to 100 000, against 9 500 000 deaths from all other causes.[8]

Aeroplane and space ship crew

Aeroplane crew and travellers and space ship crew are exposed to more cosmic radiation than those who stay on the ground. Flying during a large solar proton event, the so-called solar flare, would significantly increase the dose especially for the crew of a space ship. The estimated annual dose equivalents for air crew from cosmic radiation range from 0·2 to 9·1 mSv.[62] Crew on flights between Minneapolis and New York in 1987 received 5 mSv in a representative work year flying approximately 19 one-way flights every two weeks for 11 months, equivalent to 455 one-way flights.[63] After 20 years, their lifetime dose would be 100 mSv. Passengers are also exposed to a similar amount of radiation, proportional to flight hours. In pregnancy, the dose to the unborn child from occupational exposure should not be more than 0·5 mSv in any month according to the US National Council on Radiation Protection and Measurement recommendation 1987.[63] Exposures to air and space ship crew are new aspects of the radiation hazard and few surveys have yet been undertaken.

Miners

Exposures to natural radiation in mining have received much less attention than those arising in other industries and from medical uses. The number of miners in the world is estimated at about five million, of whom more than 80% are coal miners and less than 20% miners of other types. Miners' exposure to radiation is mainly internal from the inhalation of radon gas and thoron progeny and also of dusts containing radioactive materials. Miners are at higher risk from inhaling radon during underground work. The worldwide average annual dose is thought to be about one mSv in coal mines and about 10 mSv or more in other mines.[64] Not only uranium ore but mineral sands and phosphate ores are radioactive in some localities.[65] The processing and transportation of these minerals is also a source of radiation. The oldest observation on radioactive ore dates back to the 15th century in the Erz Mountains, on the German side known as the Schneeberg and on the Czechoslovakian as the Joachimsthal.[2] After the 1940s, the uranium industry everywhere grew rapidly.

Because of the complexity of measurement techniques radon exposure is often assessed in terms of working levels (WL) and cumulative exposure in working level months (WLM).[65] For uranium miners in Canada, Sweden, USA and Czechoslovakia, epidemiological studies have been conducted to examine dose-response relationship and the modifying effect of factors such as smoking, diesel exhaust, and rock dust.[64] Excess lung cancer deaths have been reported in relation to working-level months among the American, Canadian, French, and Czechoslovakian uranium miners, and also among Chinese and English tin miners and Swedish iron miners. In almost all mines, SMRs for lung cancer were considerably raised: 4·82 among Colorado uranium miners, 4·58 among Eldorado and Ontario miners, and 3·42 among Swedish iron miners.[65]

In the United States uranium mining began in the late 1940s on the Colorado Plateau and there have been several reports on health effects among the workers.[65–67] A quantitative risk assessment of lung cancer was made using a cohort of 3300 mine workers. Based on the Cox proportional hazards model, with an internal referent group, it was concluded that the exposure response relationship followed a slightly convex curve. Relative risks ranged from 1·42 at 30 WLM to 2·07 at 120 WLM. A recent report on a cohort of 4300 uranium miners in West Bohemia, followed for an average of 25 years, showed significantly raised risk ratios for lung cancer (5·07) and for gallbladder and extrahepatic bile ducts (2·36) with a trend related to cumulative radon exposure.[68]

There have also been reports of excess risk of lung cancer among non-uranium miners exposed to radiation sources. For example, Norwegian niobium miners showed a higher rate of lung cancer mortality with relative risks of 0, 6·0, 6·9, 28·6, and 37·5 in relation to cumulative WLM groups of 0, 1 to 38, 40 to 158, 160 to 238, and 240 +, respectively.[69] Niobium itself is not carcinogenic but the ore contains ^{238}U and ^{232}Th. In Swedish mines radon dissolved in water is thought to be a major source of radon for the miners.[70] Although silica is regarded by IARC as a weak carcinogen, which may cause miners' lung cancer, these studies need also to consider the effects of radioactive materials such as radon.

Radon effects have been investigated in ordinary dwellings.[71] Concentrations of radon progeny are much higher in stone than in wooden buildings. A few case-control studies showed raised odds ratio for lung cancer, but these results remain controversial. The inhabitants of Misasa hot spa in Japan where radon levels are reported to be high, showed significantly lower death rates from cancers at all sites than in the control area.[72]

Medical personnel

Pioneer radiologists received much higher doses of radiation than in recent times. British radiologists who entered the profession during the period 1897 to 1920 had a cancer mortality 75% higher than that of other medical practitioners, with significantly raised risk ratios for cancers of the pancreas (3·23), lung (2·18) and skin (7·79) and for leukaemia (6·15).[73] On the other hand, those who entered from 1921 to 1954 showed no significant excess of all or site-specific cancers. Lifetime radiation exposures in the early days are estimated to have been in the range of one to five Gy. In a US study, radiologists' lifetime exposures were estimated to be from at least two to as much as 20 Gy.[74] During the period 1920–1939, SMRs for prostate cancer were 1·24 for members of the Radiological Society of North America, while during a later period, 1940–1969, they fell to 101, though neither figure was significantly different from controls. Among pioneer radiologists who entered practice in the US during the 1920s, deaths from brain malignancies were three times higher than in other specialists.[75] In a Chinese study, about 26 000 diagnostic x ray workers who started work during the period 1950–1980, showed a 50% higher risk of developing cancer (RR 1·2, 95% CI: 1·3 to 1·7) in comparison with other specialists.[76] Interventional radiology has been developing in recent years and exposures during such procedures have to be carefully monitored and staff protected. For example, the mean projected yearly dose in interventional cardiac radiology was 50 mSv over the lead apron compared with 0·9 mSv under it and, in some procedures, exposure to the eyes exceeded the annual limit of 150 mSv.[77 78] However, excess cancer has yet to be reported among interventional radiologists. Image intensifiers, computed tomography and the moderately high speed film-intensifier systems reduce radiological exposure of staff and patients to a minimum. Medical personnel, helpers and nurses, who wear no film badges, may also be exposed to radiation in caring for patients treated with radioisotopes or assisting children during diagnostic radiography.[10]

Cancer risk estimates for radiation workers

Radiation cancer risk estimates are derived mainly from the Hiroshima-Nagasaki atomic bomb survivors,[11] Marshall islanders, uranium and other miners, and persons exposed during medical diagnosis and radiotherapy. Of these, the cohort of Hiroshima-Nagasaki atomic bomb survivors (lifespan study) is the largest and has the longest follow-up. Data based on the 1986 dosimetry system have been used as the major source of information by international bodies such as the United Nations Scientific Committee on the Effects of Atomic Radiation (UNSCEAR),[87 88] the International Commission of Radiological Protection (ICRP) and the National Research Council Committee on Biological Effects of Ionising Radiations (BEIR V).[79] For a simple guide to radiation protection, it may be useful to refer to the ICRP recommendations (see table 3.4) which are primarily concerned with workers' radiation protection.[9] The Commission relied mainly on studies of atomic bomb survivors and on their assessment by the bodies listed above. These committees have estimated lifetime cancer risks by considering the Hiroshima-Nagasaki accumulated data to 1985, the new dosimetry (DS86) and projection to lifetime from multiplicative or modified multiplicative models, at high dose rates of exposure (dose rate is taken as the quantity of absorbed dose delivered per unit time).

The Commission introduced the concept of "nominal fatality probability coefficient" which refers to the estimated probability of a fatal cancer per unit effective dose. They also adopted a multi-dimensional concept for stochastic effects using the term "detriment" which covers the

Table 3.4   Recommended radiation dose limits[1] (ICRP 1990)[9]

Application	Dose limit	
	Occupational	Public
Effective dose	20 mSv per year averaged over defined periods of 5 years[2]	1 mSv per year[3]
Annual equivalent dose in the lens of the eye	150 mSv	15 mSv
the skin[4]	500 mSv	50 mSv
the hands and feet	500 mSv	–

1. The limits apply to the sum of the relevant doses from external exposure in the specified period and the 50 year committed dose (to age 70 years for children) from intakes in the same period.
2. With the further provision that the effective dose should not exceed 50 mSv in any single year. Additional restrictions apply to the occupational exposure of pregnant women.
3. In special circumstances, a higher value of effective dose could be allowed in a single year, provided that the average over five years does not exceed 1 mSv per year.
4. The limitation on the effective dose provides sufficient protection for the skin against stochastic effects. An additional limit is needed for localised exposures to prevent deterministic effects.

53

probability of attributable fatal cancer, the weighted probability of non-fatal cancer, the weighted probability of severe hereditary effects, and the length of life lost if harm occurs. From this, they concluded that the most probable response is linear quadratic in form at low LET radiation levels. The linear coefficient at low dose or low dose rates is obtained from the high dose. The high dose rate risk is estimated by applying a dose or dose rate effectiveness factor (DDREF) of two. Thus, the nominal probability coefficient for adult workers (10^{-2} Sv^{-1}) is 5·6 for total detriment; 4·0 for fatal cancer, 0·8 for non fatal cancer, and 0·8 for severe hereditary effect. Exposure limits thus derived are recommended by agreement among international experts; however, perceptions of radiation risk may vary with persons, communities, and countries.

Primary prevention of radiation cancer and non-malignant disease

It is recognised that not only cancers but also benign tumours were dose-related among atomic bomb survivors.[15] Primary prevention thus has two aspects; one is to reduce radiation doses to as low as reasonably achievable (ALARA) and the other to consider host factors.

Radiation protection[9]

This aims to minimise such stochastic effects as cancer and hereditary defects and to avoid such deterministic effects as cataract, sterility and skin disorders by setting dose limits below the threshold. The principles of radiation protection as recommended in 1990 by ICRP are:

- Justification of practice dependent on level of benefit to exposed individuals or to society;
- Optimisation of practice in which the dose received by workers is kept as low as reasonably achievable (ALARA);
- Individual dose and risk limits to be kept for all workers within limits set to ensure that no individual is exposed to a radiation risk judged to be unacceptable.

For external exposure, the Commission recommended an effective dose limit of 20 mSv per year, averaged over five years (100 mSv in five years), with the further provision that this should not exceed 50 mSv in any single year. No restriction of dose is proposed for medical examinations made for patients' benefit. For internal exposure, annual limits on intake are based on a committed effective dose of 20 mSv to be averaged over a period of five years, taking into account the 50 year committed dose in the same period. Once pregnancy is recognised, the conceptus should be protected by applying a supplementary equivalent dose limit to the surface of the woman's abdomen of two mSv for the remainder of the pregnancy and by limiting intakes of radionuclides to about 1/20 of the annual limit. During emergency work in accidents some relaxation of the exposure limit can be permitted without lowering the long-term level of protection, but not exceeding an effective dose of 500 mSv except in life-saving activities.

Host related factors

Few epidemiological studies of radiation effects make any allowance for differences in individual susceptibility.[80] In radiotherapy of breast cancer, substantial differences in radiosensitivity of the skin have been shown.[81] Even when exposed to the same dose, people who lost their hair early after the atomic bombing had a higher risk of leukaemia than those who did not.[82]

As a result of an interaction between ionising radiation and water molecules in the human body, molecules are broken into aqueous electrons, hydroxyl radicals and proton radicals. Of these, the hydroxyl radical OH is believed to be the most potent in causing DNA damage. Agents that generate free radicals such as smoking, nitrogen oxides, and asbestos, can therefore act as tumour promoters, whereas inhibitors of free radical reactions—the so called scavengers, such as green vegetables, fish oil, and antioxidants enzymes—may suppress tumour promotion.[7] These factors deserve to be taken into account in framing general guidelines for cancer prevention, not only for workers but also for patients having radiotherapy. Further research along these lines is warranted.

The future epidemiology of low dose radiation

The epidemiology of low dose radiation is a controversial subject on which there is little consensus. Though the studies of atomic bomb survivors have provided irreplaceable information for extrapolation of risk estimates from high to low dose exposures, such estimates are inevitably uncertain and limited.[83] Developments in statistical methodology may well improve the analyses but, in the future, low dose radiation risks may be better calculated directly from low dose data. In such studies, the following points would need to be kept in mind:

Dose monitoring

The radiation dose of atomic bomb survivors was estimated according to the 1986 dosimetry system by US-Japan scientists using the best available techniques. On the other hand, doses in nuclear industries have been measured directly by personal dosimeters, which give much more accurate and precise information. These dosimeters are worn by workers whenever they enter a controlled area. To obtain an accurate cumulative dose for every worker individually, especially for those who move frequently from one facility to another, it is necessary to establish national central dose registries, as has been done in several countries.

Health monitoring

Modern medicine has made it increasingly possible to detect and diagnose cancers before death. Cancer statistics may be seriously influenced by these chronological changes in diagnostic methods. The developments can improve quality and precision but if not recognised and appropriately dealt with can result in bias.

Atomic bomb survivors' data are based mainly on life span mortality studies, but are less satisfactory for non-fatal cancers and non-malignant diseases. With improvements in treatment, patients with cancers which were fatal in the past may now have a prolonged survival time or even be cured. Mortality studies may therefore underestimate cancer risk and survival time. Cancer and histological registration systems offer a potential source of valuable information on cancer incidence, especially for employed populations under regular health surveillance. The US Department of Energy has recently introduced a health surveillance system to identify new or unexpected health hazards at any of its nuclear facilities; a first report of the results has been published.[84 85]

The continuity of study over decades also has its problems. Local interest in a specific disease may lead to the addition of special examination methods and tests for certain members of the cohort. For example, the screening of thyroid disease by measuring related hormones and by ultrasound examination, or of parathyroid disease by measuring serum concentrations of calcium and related hormones, may increase the number of the diseased people found in a specific survey year. The continuity of screening methods and diagnostic criteria must therefore be considered carefully.

Confounding factors

During a long-term follow-up of a cohort, many confounders may affect the occurrence of cancer among workers. The longer the observation period, the stronger the potential influence of such factors as smoking, food, life style, medical procedures, and other occupational and environmental exposures. It may be important to find out the extent to which such confounders influence radiation effects, and whether the effect is additive or multiplicative. For example, virus-related malignancies such as hepatitis-related liver cancer or adult T-cell leukaemia require this type of consideration. To deal adequately with confounders is difficult, only possible if the system of health surveillance is of high quality.

International collaborative research[86]

A large cohort is needed to obtain adequate statistical power, yet in any nuclear plant the number of workers is limited. To overcome this weakness an international collaborative study on radiation effects among nuclear workers has been coordinated by the International Agency for Research of Cancer (IARC), with probable participation of 14 countries; Australia, Belgium, Canada, Finland, France, Germany, Hungary, Japan, Slovakia, Spain, Sweden, Switzerland, United Kingdom, and, we hope, the United States. In preparation for this international study, a separate combined analysis of workers in Canada, United Kingdom, and United States has been conducted by the IARC. If the 11 (or 12) country joint study succeeds in collecting standardised data from all participants as planned, the resulting cohort of nearly a million workers will be the largest ever. Two important international reports on the effects of atomic radiation have recently been reported.[87][88]

Molecular epidemiology

The epidemiological potential of developments in molecular biology has yet to be realised in studies of industrial groups. The approach will entail the definition and use of appropriate molecular markers, and methods that are feasible in practice. Eventually, these studies may be expected to elucidate factors concerning individual radiation susceptibility and to augment the range of preventive measures against radiation carcinogenesis.

I gratefully acknowledge the scientific assistance of Dr S Sasagawa, Institute of Environmental Sciences and Dr K Neriishi, Radiation Effects Research Foundation, in completing this paper. I also wish to acknowledge a friend, the late Martin Gardner, who worked so hard on childhood leukaemia near Sellafield and many other problems in occupational epidemiology.

1 Tateno Y. Original papers on radiation injuries, 1896–1944. Tokyo: University of Tokyo Press, 1988 (Japanese).
2 Frieben. Aerztlich Verein Hamburg 21, X, 1902. *Fortsch Geb Roentgenstr.* 1902; **6**: 106.
3 Blum T. Osteomyelitis of the mandible and maxilla. *J Amer Dental Assoc* 1924; **11**: 802–5.
4 Martland HS, Humphries RE. Osteogenic sarcoma in dial painters using luminous paint. *Arch Pathol* 1929; **7**: 406–17.
5 Sikl H: Ueber den Lungenkrebs der Bergleute in Joachimstal (Tschecoslowakei). *Zeitschrift f Krebsforsch* 1930; **32**: 609–13.
6 Nias AHW. *An introduction of radiobiology.* Chichester: John Wiley & Sons, 1990.
7 Committee on the biological effects of ionizing radiations, Board on radiation effects research, Commission on life sciences, National research council: *Health effects of exposure to low levels of ionizing radiation, BEIR V*, Washington DC; National Academy Press, 190.
8 Mettler Jr FA, Kelsey C, Ricks RC. *Medical management of radiation effects.* Boca Raton: CRC Press Inc, 1990.
9 The International Commission on Radiological Protection: *Recommendations of the*

International Commission on Radiological Protection 1990 ICRP publication 60; Oxford: Pergamon Press, 1991.

10 Awa AA, Sofuni T, Honda T, Itoh M, Neriishi S, Otake M. Relationship between radiation dose and chromosome aberrations in atomic bomb survivors in Hiroshima and Nagasaki. *J Rad Res* 1978; **19**: 126–40.

11 Shimizu Y, Kato H, Schull WJ. *Lifespan study report 11, part 2, cancer mortality in the years 1950–85 based on the recently revised doses (DS86). Technical report RERF TR 5–88*; Hiroshima: Radiation Effects Research Foundation, 1988.

12 Akiba S, Lubin J, Ezaki H, Ron E, Ishimaru T, Asano M. *Thyroid cancer incidence among atomic bomb survivors. 1958–79. RERF TR 591*, Hiroshima: Radiation Effects Research Foundation, 1991.

13 Fujiwara S, Sposto R, Akiba S, Neriishi K, Kodama K, Hosoda Y, et al. Hyperparathyroidism among atomic bomb survivors in Hiroshima and Nagasaki. *Radiat Res* 1992; **130**: 372–8.

14 Sadamori N, Otake M, Honda T. *Study of skin cancer incidence in Nagasaki atomic bomb survivors. 1958–85, RERF TR 10–91*, Hiroshima: Radiation Effects Research Foundation, 1991.

15 Wong FL, Yamda M, Sasaki H, Kodama K, Akiba S, Hosoda Y, et al. *Adult health study report 7, noncancer disease incidence in the atomic bomb survivors, 1958–86 (Cycle 1–14) RERF TR 1–92*, Hiroshima: Radiation Effects Research Foundation, 1992.

16 Shigematsu I. Ionizing radiation and health. *Jpn J Epidemiol* 1992; **2**: 21–9.

17 Mabuchi K, Soda M, Ron E, Tokunaga M, Ochikubo S, Sugimoto S, et al. Cancer incidence in atomic survivors. Part I: Use of the tumour registries in Hiroshima and Nagasaki for incidence studies. *Radiation Research* 1994; **137**: S1–S16.

18 Thompson DE, Mabuchi K, Ron E, Soda M, Tokunaga M, Ochikubo S, Sugimoto S, et al. Cancer incidence in atomic survivors. Part II; Solid tumours, 1958–1987, *Radiation Research* 1994; **137**: S17–S67.

19 Preston DL, Kusumi S, Thompson M, Iumi S, Ron E, Kuramoto A, et al. Cancer incidence in atomic bomb survivors. Part III. Leukaemia, lymphoma and multiple myeloma, 1950–1987. *Radiation Research* 1994; **137**: S68–S97.

20 Ron E, Preston DL, Mabuchi K, Thompson DE, Soada M. Cancer incidence in atomic bomb survivors. Part IV. Comparison of cancer incidence and mortality. *Radiation Research* 1994; **137**: S98–S112.

21 Beral V, Fraser P, Booth M, Carpenter L. Epidemiological studies of workers in the nuclear industry. In: *Radiation and Health*, Jones R and Southwood R eds; London: John Wiley, 1987.

22 Beral V, Inskip H, Fraser P, Booth D, Coleman D, Rose G. Mortality of employees of the United Kingdom Atomic Energy Authority, 1946–1979. *BMJ* 1985; **291**: 440–7.

23 Smith PG, Douglas AJ. Mortality of workers at the Sellafield plant of British Nuclear Fuels. *BMJ* 1986; **293**: 845–54.

24 Wilkinson ES, Volez L, Acquavella JF, Tietjen GL, Reyes M, Brackbill R, Wiggs LD. *Mortality among plutonium and other workers at a nuclear facility Los Alamos National Laboratory document LUR-83-266*, Los Alamos, New Mexico, 1983.

25 Gilbert ES, Marks S. An analysis of the mortality of workers in a nuclear facility. *Radiat Res* 1979; **79**: 112–23.

26 Rinsky RA, Zumwalde RD, Waxweiler RJ, Murray Jr WE, Bierbaum PJ, Landrigan PJ, et al. Cancer mortality at a naval nuclear shipyard. *Lancet* 1981; **1**: 231–5.

27 Hadjimichael OC, Ostefeld AM, D'Atri DA, Brubaker RE. Mortality and cancer incidence. Experience of employees in a nuclear fuels fabrication plant. *J Occup Med* 1983; **25**: 48–61.

28 Chekoway H, Mathew CM, Shy CM, Watson Jr JE, Tankersley WG, Wolf SH, et al. Radiation work experience and cause-specific mortality among workers at an energy research laboratory. *Br J Ind Med* 1985; **42**: 525–33.

29 Acquavella JF, Wiggans LD, Waxweiler RJ, MacDonell DG, Tietjen GL, Wilkinson GS. Mortality among workers at the Pantex weapons facility. *Health Phys* 1985; **48**: 735–46.

30 Gilbert ES, Fry SA, Wiggs LD, Voelz GL, Cragle DL, Petersen GR. Analysis of combined mortality data on workers at the Hanford Site, Oak Ridge National Laboratory and Rocky Flats Nuclear Weapons Plant. *Radiat Res* 1989; **120**: 19–35.

31 Wing S, Shy CM, Wood JL, Wolf S, Cragle DL, Forme EL. Mortality among workers at Oak Ridge National Laboratory: Evidence of radiation effects in follow-up through 1984. *JAMA* 1991; **265**: 1397–402.

32 Gilbert ES, Omohundro E, Buchanan JA, Holter NA. Mortality of workers at the Hanford Site, 1945–1986. *Health Phys* 1993; **64**: 577–90.

33 Gilbert ES, Cragle DL, Wiggs LD. Updated analyses of combined mortality data at the Hanford Site, Oak Ridge National Laboratory and Rocky Flats Weapon Plant. *Radiat Res* 1993; **136**: 408–21.

34 Kendall GM, Muirhead CR, MacGibbon BH, O'Hagen JA, Conquest AJ, Goodill AA, *et al.* Mortality and occupational exposure to radiation: First analysis of the National Registry for Radiation Workers. *BMJ* 1992; **304**: 220–5.

35 Beral V, Fraser P, Carpenter L, Booth M, Brown H, Rose G. Mortality of employees of the Atomic Weapons Establishment, 1951–1982. *BMJ* 1988; **297**: 757–70.

36 Howe GR, Weeks L, Miller AB, Chiarelli AM, Etazadi-Amoli J. *A study of the health of the employees of Atomic Energy of Canada Limited. IV: Analysis of mortality during the period 1950–1981. Report 9442.* Atomic Energy of Canada Limited, 1987.

37 Gribbin Ma, Weeks JL, Howe GR. Cancer mortality (1956–1985) among male employees of Atomic Energy of Canada Limited with respect to occupational exposure to external low-Linear-Energy Transfer ionising radiation. *Radiat Res* 1993; **133**: 375–80.

38 Fraser P, Carpenter L, Maconochie N, *et al.* Cancer mortality and morbidity in employees of the United Kingdom Atomic Energy Authority, 1946–86. *Br J Cancer* 1993; **67**: 615–24.

39 Carpenter L, Higgins C, Douglas A, *et al.* Combined analysis of mortality in three United Kingdom nuclear industry workforces, 1946–1988. *Radiat Res* 1994; **138**: 224–38.

40 IARC Study Group on Cancer Risk Among Nuclear Industry Workers. Direct estimates of cancer mortality due to low doses of ionizing radiation: an international study. *Lancet* 1994; **344**: 1039–43.

41 Rooney C, Beral V, Maconochie N, Fraser P, Davis G. Case control study of prostatic cancer in employees of the United Kingdom Atomic Energy Authority. *BMJ* 1993; **307**: 1391–7.

42 Kneale GW, Stewart AM. Reanalysis of Hanford data, 1944–1986 deaths. *Am J Ind Med* 1993; **23**: 371–89.

43 Gardner MJ, Hall AJ, Downes S, Terrell JD. Follow up study of children born to mothers resident in Seascale, West Cumbria (birth cohort). *BMJ* 1987; **295**: 822–7.

44 Gardner MJ, Snee MP, Powell CA, Downes S, Terrell JD. Results of case-control study of leukaemia and lymphoma among young people near Sellafield nuclear plant in West Cumbria. *BMJ* 1990; **300**: 423–9.

45 Beral V. Leukaemia and nuclear installations: Occupational exposure of fathers to radiation may be the explanation. *BMJ* 1990; **300**: 411–2.

46 Soharan T, Roberts PJ. Childhood cancer and paternal exposure to ionising radiation: Preliminary finding from the Oxford survey of childhood cancers. *Am J Indust Med* 1993; **23**: 343–5.

47 Black RJ, Urquhart D, Kendrick SW, Bunch KJ, Waren J, Jones DA. Incidence of leukaemia and other cancers in birth and schools cohorts in the Dounreay area. *BMJ* 1992; **304**: 1401–5.

48 Kinlen LJ, O'Brien F, Clarke K, Balkwill A, Mathews F. Rural population mixing and childhood leukaemia; effects of the North Sea oil industry in Scotland, including the area near Dounreay nuclear site. *BMJ* 1993; **306**: 743–8.

49 Parker L, Craft AW, Smith J, Dickinson H, Wakeford R, Binsk K, *et al.* Geographical distribution of preconceptional radiation dose to fathers employed at the Sellafield nuclear installation, West Cumbria, *BMJ* 1993; **307**: 966–71.

50 McLaughlin JR, Anderson TW, Clarke EA, King W. *Occupational exposure of fathers to ionising radiation and the risk of leukaemia in offspring: A case control study.* Canada: Atomic Energy Control Board, 1992. (AECB Project No 7, 157, 1.)

51 McLaughlin JR, Clarke EA, Nishri ED, Anderson TW. Childhood leukaemia in the vicinity of Canadian nuclear facilities. *Cancer Causes and Control* 1993; **4**: 51–8.

52 Doll R, Evans HJ, Darby SC. Paternal exposure not to blame. *Nature* 1994; **367**: 678–80.

53 *HSE Investigation of leukaemia and other cancers in the children of male workers at Sellafield*, London: HMSO, 1993.
54 Yoshimoto Y. Cancer risk among children of atomic bomb survivors: A review of RERF epidemiological studies. *JAMA* 1990; **264**: 596–600.
55 Nomura T. Leukaemia in children whose parents have been exposed to radiation. *BMJ* 1993; **306**: 1412.
56 Abrahamson S. Risk estimates; Past, present and future. *Health Phys* 1990; **59**: 99–102.
57 Barverstock KF. DNA instability, paternal irradiation and leukaemia in children around Sellafield. *Int J Radiol Biol* 1991; **60**: 581–95.
58 WHO Regional Office for Europe, Copenhagen. Nuclear accidents and epidemiology. Reports on two meetings. Epidemiology related to the Chernobyl nuclear accident and appropriate methodologies for studying possible long-term effects of radiation in individuals exposed in a nuclear accident. Nuclear accident and epidemiology. *Environmental Health* 1987; **25**.
59 IAEA-TEC DOC-516. *Medical aspects of the Chernobyl accident*. International Atomic Energy Agency, 1989.
60 The International Chernobyl Project: Technical Report. *Assessment of radiological consequences and evaluation of protective measures. Report by an international advisory committee*: Vienna, 1991.
61 Kazakov VS, Demidchik EP, Astakhova LN, Baverstock K, Egloss B, Pinchera A, et al. Thyroid cancer after Chernobyl. *Nature* 1992; **359**: 21–2.
62 Friedberg W, Faulkner DN, Snyder L, Darden FB. Galactic cosmic radiation exposure and associated health risks for air carrier crew members. *Aviation* 1989; **60**: 1104–8.
63 Nagda NL, Forman RC, Koontz MD, Baker SR, Ginevean ME. *Airliner cabin environment: Contaminant measurements, health risk, and mitigation options. Final report prepared for US Department of Transportation Office Secretary. Report NO-DOT-P-15-89*. Washington DC, 1989.
64 Committee on the Biological Effects of Ionising Radiations. *Health risks of radon and other internally deposited alphaemitters, BEIR IV*. Washington DC, National Academy Press, 1988.
65 Chekoway J, Mathew RM, Hickey LS, Shy CM, Harris RL, Hunt EW. Mortality among workers in the Florida phosphate industry. I. Industry-wide cause-specific mortality patterns. *J Occup Med* 1985; **27**: 885–92.
66 Lundin Jr FD, Wagoner JK, Archer VE. *Radon daughter exposure and respiratory cancer. Quantitative and temporal aspects. Joint monographs No 1*, Washington DC. US Public Health Service, 1971.
67 Hornung RW, Meinhart TJ. Quantitative risk assessment of lung cancer mortality in US uranium miners; *Health Phys* 1987; **52**: 417–30.
68 Tomasek I, Serdlow A. Radon exposure and cancers other than lung cancer among uranium miners in West Bohemia. *Lancet* 1993; **341**: 919–23.
69 Soli M, Anderson A, Straden E, Langand SA. Cancer incidence among workers exposed to radon and thoron daughters at a niobium mine. *Scand J Work Environ Health* 1985; **ii**: 7–13.
70 Radford EP, St Clair-Renard KG. Lung cancer in Swedish iron miners exposed to low dose radon daughters. *N Engl J Med* 1984; **310**: 1485–94.
71 Nero AV. Airborne radionuclides and radiation in buildings. A review. *Health Phys* 1983; **45**: 303–22.
72 Mifune M, Sobue T, Arimoto H, Komoto Y, Kondo S, Tanaooka H. Cancer mortality survey in a spa area (Missa Japan) with a high radon background. *Jps J Cancer Res* 1992; **83**: 1–5.
73 Smith PG, Doll R. Mortality from cancer and all causes among British radiologists. *Br J Radiol* 1981; **54**: 187–94.
74 Matonoski GM, Startwell P, Elliot E, Tonascia J, Sternberg A. Cancer risks in radiologists and radiation workers in radiation carcinogenesis. In: Boice JD, ed. *Epidemiology and biological significance*. New York: Raven, 1984; 83–96.
75 Matanoski GM. The current mortality rates of radiologists and other physician specialists: death rate from all causes and from cancer. *Am J Epidemiol* 1975; **101**: 199–210.

76 Wang JX, Boice JD Jr, Li BX, Shang JY, Fraumeni Jr JF. Cancer among diagnostic x ray workers in China. *J Nat Cancer Inst* 1988; **80**: 344–50.

77 Marx MV, Niklason L, Mauger EA. Occupational radiation to interventional radiologists; a prospective study. *J Vascular and Interventional Radiol* 1992; **3**: 597–606.

78 Renaud L. A 5-year follow up of the radiation exposure to in room personnel during cardiac catheterisation. *Health Phys* 1992; **62**: 10–64.

79 Roesch WC. *US-Japan joint reassessment of atomic bomb radiation dosimetry in Hiroshima and Nagasaki. Final reports 1 and 2*. Hiroshima: Hiroshima Radiation Effects Research Foundation, 1986.

80 Sasagawa S, Yoshimoto Y, Neriishi S, Yamakido M, Matsuo M, Hosoda Y, *et al*. Phagocytic and bacterial activities of leucocytes in whole blood from atomic bomb survivors. *Radiat Res* 1990; **124**: 103–6.

81 Tucker SL, Turesson I, Thomas HD. Evidence for individual differences in the radioactivity of human skin. *Eur J Cancer* 1992; **28A**: 1783–91.

82 Neriishi K, Stram D, Vaeth M, Mizuno S, Akiba S. The observed relationship between the occurrence of acute radiation sickness and subsequent cancer mortality among a-bomb survivors in Hiroshima and Nagasaki. *Radiat Res* 1991; **125**: 206–13.

83 Schull WJ: Radiation epidemiology: where do we stand and where are we going? In: *Low dose radiation and biological defense mechanism*. New York: Elsevier, 1992: 39–46.

84 Strader CH, Peterson GR. Use of return-to-work medical clearance data for health surveillance. *J Occup Med* 1989; **31**: 326–30.

85 Vaughan TL, Lee JAH, Strader CH. Breast cancer incidence at a nuclear facility: demonstration of a morbidity surveillance system. *Health Phys* 1993; **64**: 349–54.

86 International Agency for Research on Cancer. IARC meeting recommends international study of nuclear industry workers. *Health Phys* 1992; **63**: 465–6.

87 United Nations Scientific Committee on the Effects of Atomic Radiation. *Sources and effects of ionizing radiation, UNSCEAR 1993 report to the General Assembly, with scientific annexes*. New York; United Nations; 1993.

88 United Nations Scientific Committee on the Effects of Atomic Radiation. *Sources and effects of ionizing radiation, UNSCEAR 1994 report to the General Assembly, with scientific annexes*. New York; United Nations; 1994.

4 Electromagnetic fields

GILLES THERIAULT

Introduction

The production of goods is often accompanied by the generation of some undesired byproducts. The production, transportation, and use of electricity is no exception to this rule. Its byproducts are extremely low frequency electromagnetic fields (EMF) (60 Hz in North America and 50 Hz in Europe). These fields have two components, the electric (E) fields and the magnetic (B) fields. E fields flow at the surface of objects and are perturbed by the presence of other objects in their environment and are therefore unstable. B fields are more stable, travel across structures with almost no disturbance and consequently can be measured with a good degree of reliability. Both E and B fields are able to generate an induced current in people exposed. At high intensity, these currents produce well documented effects but at levels encountered in daily life, no known nor perceptible effects are believed to exist. Among people exposed at work are electric utility workers, electricians, and welders. In the residential environment, the exposure depends on several variables: the proximity to transmission and distribution lines or both, the use of electric appliances, and the grounding of electric wires to water pipes. People have called the environment created by electromagnetic fields the "invisible landscape." Today's question is to understand whether this invisible landscape represents a human health risk.

The first suspicion of a health effect came from Russian scientists in the mid-sixties who reported that workers exposed to high voltages complained of non-specific illnesses such as headache, fatigue, excitability, and decrease of libido.[1][2] These effects were not substantiated by later studies and consequently they lost public attention.[3] This was to be revived in 1979 when Wertheimer and Leeper observed an association between residing near electric wires and the presence of cancer in children.[4] Since then, the hypothesis of exposure to EMF as a cause of cancer in human beings has been tested in many studies and is still being debated today.

Although they constitute only part of the overall research domain (other approaches being residential exposure from electric power lines and domestic wirings, exposure from electrical appliances and paternal occupational exposure in relation to cancer in the offspring) occupational epidemiological studies have contributed substantially to improving our knowledge on this question. In a review, it is convenient to group this research under several sub-titles: hypothesis generating studies, leukaemia case control studies, brain cancer case control studies, cohort studies of workers in electrical occupations, leukaemia among welders, and male breast cancers.

Hypothesis generating studies

The author who first reported the results of an occupational study was Samuel Milham in 1982.[5] He analysed the leukaemia mortality of Washington State white men occupationally exposed to electric and magnetic fields. His results are reported in table 4.1 (p 65).

He observed significantly greater proportional mortality ratios (PMRs) for all types of leukaemia in several trades known to be exposed to EMF: electricians (PMR = 1·38), power station operators (PMR = 2·59), aluminium workers (PMR = 1·89) and all electrical occupations (PMR = 1·37). He suggested that his findings implied that electrical and magnetic fields may cause leukaemia. Since then, no less than 13 exploratory studies have been published, most of them as short communications or letters to editors.[6-18]

Figure 4.1 shows that most of these reports indicated an excess of leukaemia in broadly defined electrical occupations and this excess was higher for acute myeloid leukaemia (figure 4.2).

Pooled analysis has established a significant excess of all leukaemia with a risk estimate of 1·18 (95% CI: 1·09 to 1·29) and a significant excess of acute myeloid leukaemia with a risk estimate of 1·46 (1·27 to 1·64).[19]

Table 4.1 Leukaemia mortality in men occupationally exposed to electrical and magnetic fields (Washington State white males, 1950–1979)

Occupation	Mortality					
	all leukaemia (204*)			acute leukaemia (204·3*)		
	observed	expected†	PMR‡	observed	expected†	PMR‡
electronic technicians	6	4·0	149	3	1·9	162
radio & telegraph operators	5	4·5	111	3	1·3	239
electricians	51	37·0	138§	23	12·9	178§
linemen (power & telephone)	15	9·4	159	6	3·3	183
television & radio repairmen	5	3·2	157	4	1·4	291§
power-station operators	8	3·1	259§	3	1·1	282
aluminum workers	20	10·6	189§	11	4·3	258§
welders & flame cutters	12	17·9	67	4	7·1	56
motion picture projectionists	4	1·7	234	1	0·9	111
electrical engineers	7	6·1	114	2	2·1	97
streetcar & subway motormen	3	1·7	175	0	0·4	0
Total	136	99·2	137§	60	36·7	163§

* Coded according to the International Classification of Diseases (7th ed)
† Based on proportional mortality for Washington State white males (PMR values are exact: "expected" values have been rounded off)
‡ Proportional mortality ratio (observed/expected × 100)
§ P < 0·01
Source: Milham 1982 (5)

Results presented in figures 4.1 and 4.2 are for all leukaemia, acute myeloid leukaemia, and for all electrical workers. More spectacular excesses were noted for specific leukaemia types and specific occupational groups but these excesses varied between studies and no findings were clearly consistent. Everyone, including the authors themselves, recognized that these exploratory studies were gross, that numbers were small, that exposure was ill-defined, that statistical analyses often were weak, that there may exist at the workplace carcinogenic agents other than EMF responsible for the observed excesses, that there has been no control for confounders. Consequently, the results could only be indicative of an association and needed to be reassessed by more powerful and better designed studies.

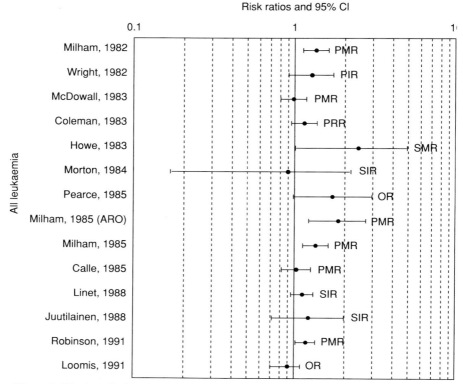

Figure 4.1 Leukaemia risks among electrical workers: exploratory studies
PMR = proportional mortality ratio; PIR = proportional incidence ratio; PRR = proportional registration ratio; SMR = standardised mortality ratio; SIR = standardised incidence ratio; OR = odds ratio

Leukaemia case-control studies

Several case-control studies have explored the risk of leukaemia and sub-types of leukaemia among workers occupationally exposed to EMF.[20–27] They are summarized in table 4.2 (p 68). In general, these studies were well designed, carefully conducted, and included large numbers of leukaemia cases. On three occasions the association of leukaemia with EMF was an incidental observation by authors whose objective was to test a different hypothesis.[20–23] Table 4.2 (p 68) shows that odds ratios were higher than those observed in the exploratory surveys. Several studies have observed significantly raised odds ratios for all leukaemia and acute myeloid leukaemia; chronic lymphocytic leukaemia is also reported to have raised odds ratios. These studies, however, are plagued by one weakness: exposure assessment. Exposure is estimated by occupational history secured through postal questionnaires or transcribed from registry forms. Gilman[20] for

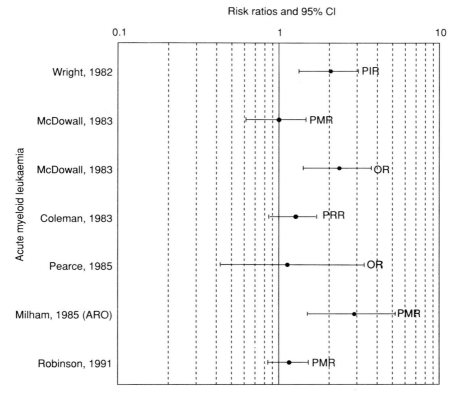

Figure 4.2 Leukaemia risks among electrical workers: exploratory studies
PIR = proportional incidence ratio; PMR = proportional mortality ratio; OR = odds ratio; PRR = proportional registration ratio

example, used time spent underground as a surrogate for EMF exposure in coal miners. These case-control studies seem to support and even strengthen the possible association between leukaemia and working in electrical occupations but because of the crude estimate of exposure, they say little about its association with EMF.

Brain cancer case-control studies

Brain is the second cancer site that has attracted the attention of occupational epidemiologists. Since 1985, at least nine case-control studies of brain cancer and occupational exposure to EMF have been published (table 4.3).[24-26 28-33] Most of these studies showed increased odds ratios for electricity-related occupations, some being remarkably high.[30] Speers[30] observed an odds ratio (OR) of 13·10 among Texas utility

67

Table 4.2 Occupational exposure to EMF and leukaemia: summary of case-control studies

Reference	Cases/controls	Exposure assessment		OR (95% CI)
Gilman, 1985[20]	underground coal miners 40 leukaemia deaths 160 non-cancer deaths	time spent underground	all L	2·53 (40)*
			AL	2·85 (22)
			CL	8·22 (14)*
			CLL	6·33 (11)*
			ML	4·74 (17)*
			AML	3·80 (14)
Stern, 1986[21]	naval shipyard workers 53 leukaemia deaths 212 members of cohort alive at dx of cases	job histories plus years of employment	all L ⎫ ML ⎬ for electricians LL ⎭	3·00 (1·29 to 6·98) 2·33 (0·77 to 7·06) 6·00 (1·47 to 24·45)
			all L ⎫ ML ⎬ for welders LL ⎭	2·25 (0·92 to 5·53) 3·83 (1·28 to 11·46) 0 (— — —)
Flodin, 1986[22]	in hospital cases 59 AML alive 334 general population controls	postal questionnaire	AML for electrical workers	3·8 (1·5 to 9·5)
Flodin, 1990[23] Coggon, 1986[24]	updating of same study male cancers in 3 UK counties 29 AML	occupational history through postal questionnaires	AML AML—a cluster of 5 electrical workers in these 29 cases	2·1 (0·7 to 5·9)
Pearce, 1989[25]	2913 other cancers male cancers from New Zealand Cancer Registry 534 leukaemia all other cancers	occupation on registry forms	for all electrical workers all L	1·62 (1·04 to 2·52)
			AL	1·25 (0·62 to 2·54)
			CL	2·12 (1·19 to 3·76)
			ML	1·22 (0·60 to 2·48)
			LL	1·73 (0·89 to 3·37)
			AML	1·16 (0·48 to 2·84)

Loomis, 1990[26]	deaths in 16 US states 3400 leukaemia deaths 10 controls from other deaths	occupation from death certificates	all L 1·0 (0·8 to 1·2) AML 1·1 (0·7 to 1·7) ALL 1·5 (0·7 to 3·4) CLL 0·6 (0·3 to 1·1) } for electrical workers; no excess seen for any specific occupational group for electrical engineers
Richardson, 1992[27]	hospitalised cases 185 alive acute leukaemia	occupational history plus exposure to EMF assessed by industrial hygienist	AL 5·2*
	513 hospitalized controls		AML 4·83 (1·48 to 15·80)*

* $P < 0.05$

AL = acute leukaemia; AML = acute myeloid leukaemia; CL = chronic leukaemia; CLL = chronic lymphocytic leukaemia; L = leukaemia; LL = lymphocytic leukaemia; ML = myeloid leukaemia

Table 4.3 Occupational exposure to EMF and brain cancer: summary of case-control studies

Reference	Cases/controls	Exposure assessment		OR (95% CI)
Lin, 1985[28]	Maryland residents −519 glioma/astrocytoma deaths −519 random non cancer deaths	occupation on death certificates—panel rating	Exposure to EMF definite probable possible no	2·15 (1·1 to 4·1) 1·95 (0·9 to 3·9) 1·44 (1·1 to 2·0) 1·00
Coggon, 1986[24]	male cancers in 3 UK counties −97 brain cancers −2845 other cancers	occupational history through postal questionnaires	for electrical engineers for electrical & electronics workers	1·9 (0·4 to 5·6) 2·0 (0·8 to 4·1)
Thomas, 1987[29]	Louisiana, New Jersey, Pennsylvania residents −435 brain cancer deaths −386 non brain cancer deaths	occupational history from next of kin—panel rating	for exposure to MW/RF for exposure to MW/RF in electrical & electronics jobs for electronics workers	1·6 (1·0 to 2·4) 2·3 (1·3 to 4·2) 3·9 (1·6 to 9·9)
Speers, 1988[30]	East Texas residents −202 glioma deaths −238 random non-brain tumour deaths	occupation on death certificates	for transportation, communication, utility workers for employment in occupations with electricity or EMF fields for utility workers	2·26 (1·18 to 4·32) 3·94 (1·52 to 10·20) 13·10 (1·3 to 128·9)
Pearce, 1989[25]	male cancers from New Zealand Cancer Registry −452 brain cancers −all other cancers	occupation on registry forms	for all electrical workers for electrical engineers for electricians	1·01 (0·6 to 1·8) 4·74 (1·7 to 13·6) 1·91 (0·8 to 4·3)

Study	Cases/controls	Source of occupation	Result (95% CI)
Loomis, 1990[26]	deaths in 16 US states −2173 brain cancer deaths −10 controls from other deaths	occupation on death certificates	for any electrical occupation: 1·4 (1·1 to 1·7)
Brownson, 1990[31]	white males cancers from Missouri Cancer Registry −312 brain cancers −1248 other cancers	occupation from hospital records (usual and longest)	for electrical engineers & technicians: 2·7 (2·1 to 3·4) for electric power workers: 1·7 (1·1 to 2·7) for electrical workers in manufacturing industry: 2·1 (1·3 to 3·4) for utilities and sanitary services workers: 0·5 (0·1 to 1·7)
Ryan, 1992[32]	adults from Adelaide hospitals −110 adult glioma cases −2 controls randomly selected	occupational history through interview questionnaires	for work in electrical/electronics industry: 0·75 (0·3 to 1·9) for female workers in EMF jobs: 4·1 (1·3 to 13·2)
Preston-Martin, 1993[33]	male cancers from New Zealand Cancer Registry −1113 male brain cancers −all other cancers	occupation on registry forms	for electrical/electronics engineers: 8·2 (2·0 to 34·7) for electrical/electronics technicians: 3·3 (0·9 to 12·1) for engineering technicians: 2·5 (0·8 to 7·4) for electricians: 4·6 (1·7 to 12·2)

MF = micro-waves; RF = radio-frequency

71

employees and Preston-Martin[33] an OR of 8·2 among electrical and electronics engineers from the New Zealand Cancer Registry.

At least three authors mentioned the presence of an exposure-response correlation between EMF exposure and brain cancer. As with the leukaemia studies, these case-control studies of brain cancer are quite impressive. They included reasonably large numbers of cases among exposed workers; they have yielded several significantly raised odds ratios and exposure-response correlations were observed more than once. However, as for leukaemia, exposure has been based on job title and assessed from sources such as cancer registry forms, death certificates, or postal questionnaires, in which information on work history is of poor reliability.

Cohort studies of workers in electrical occupations

Occupations

Cohort studies that compare the risk of cancer between groups of exposed and non-exposed workers are usually considered more powerful than case-control studies in establishing a causal relationship between an exposure and a cancer. Fortunately, several cohort studies of electrical workers have been reported. The occupational cohorts studied were: telephone operators, electronics industry workers, electrical engineers, telecommunications workers, linemen, station operators, electricians, amateur radio operators, telephone company workers, electrical utility workers, and radiomen. In most of them, the sample size was large and observation periods extended over many years. Several of these studies are summarized in table 4.4.[34-36]

These studies show a remarkable methodological development over time. In the early 1980s, they were simple straightforward mortality or incidence studies of cohorts of workers broadly defined as members of a trade or an industry which lump together several occupational groups. Since 1990, studies have become much more refined, looking at specific electrical occupations separately and regrouping them into categories believed to correspond to different levels of exposure. Two trends are noticeable in the results: until 1990, few excesses were significant, although several risk ratios for leukaemia and brain cancer were over 1·0. Only one observed a significant excess of acute myeloid leukaemia and no brain cancers were significantly in excess.[39] Since 1990, many more significant excesses of leukaemia and brain cancer have been observed. In particular, studies that have analysed risks in categories of increasing levels of exposure have observed an increase in risk of leukaemia (not so evident for brain cancers) with increasing estimated exposure to EMF.[42 45 46] As exposure in large cohort studies is usually diluted, the observation of increased risks of leukaemia and brain cancer further supports the possibility of an association between these cancers and working in electrical occupations.

Table 4.4 Cohort studies of workers in electrical occupations

Reference Type of analysis Occupational cohort	All cancers	Brain cancer	All leukaemia	AML	CLL
1. Wiklund 1981, SIR telephone operators[34]	NR†	NR	1·03 (12)	NR	NR
2. Vagero 1983, RR electronics industry[35]	1·15 (1855)*	<1·0	<1·0	NR	NR
3. Olin 1985, SMR electrical engineers[36]	0·5 (24)*	1·0 (2)	0·9 (2)	0	0
4. Vagero 1985, SMR telecommunications industry[37]	1·03 (102)	1·0 (5)	1·0 (5)	0	0
5. McLaughlin 1987, SIR electricians	NR	0·8 (42)	NR	NR	NR
powerline workers	NR	1·0 (13)	NR	NR	NR
telecommunications[38]	NR	1·1 (13)	NR	NR	NR
6. Milham 1988, SMR amateur radio operators[39]	0·89 (741)*	1·39 (29)	1·24 (36)	1·76 (15)*	1·09 (6)
7. Guberan 1989 electricians[40] SMR	1·14 (52)	1·54 (2)	1·43 (2)	NR	NR
SIR	0·92 (78)	1·18 (2)	1·25 (2)	NR	NR
8. Garland 1990, SIR young males in Navy electrician's mate	NR	NR	2·4 (7)*	NR	NR
electronics technicians	NR	NR	1·1 (5)	NR	NR
radiomen[41]	NR	NR	1·1 (4)	NR	NR

73

Table 4.4—continued

Reference Type of analysis Occupational cohort	All cancers	Brain cancer	All leukaemia	AML	CLL
9. Juutilainen 1990, SIR					
probably exposed to EMF	NR	1·31 (13)	1·85 (10)*	1·47 (3)	NR
possibly exposed to EMF	NR	1·29 (149)*	1·42 (94)*	1·37 (34)	NR
electricians installers	NR	0·75 (10)	0·95 (7)	0·74 (2)	NR
telephone installers	NR	2·37 (9)	1·43 (3)	1·23 (1)	NR
linemen and cable jointers[42]	NR	0·91 (2)	3·08 (4)	2·08 (1)	NR
10. Tornqvist 1986, 1991, SIR					
electrical/omics engineers	NR	0·9 (39)	1·3 (62)*	0·8 (6)	1·7 (26)*
linesmen	NR	1·1 (18)	1·3 (25)	0·8 (3)	2·0 (12)*
power station operators	NR	1·1 (7)	1·2 (10)	0·6 (1)	2·8 (7)*
TV radio repairs[43][44]	NR	2·9 (7)*	0·8 (2)	2·1 (1)	1·3 (1)
11. Tynes 1992, SIR					
all electrical workers	1·06 (3806)*	1·09 (119)	1·41 (74)*	1·56 (29)*	1·26 (20)
heavy EMF exposure	NR	1·37 (18)	1·79 (20)*	NR	NR
weak EMF exposure[45]	NR	2·20 (9)*	0·92 (3)	NR	NR
12. Guenel 1993, SIR					
intermittently > 0·3 μT[†]	NR	0·94 (339)	0·94 (282)	NR	NR
continually > 0·3 μT[46]	NR	0·69 (23)	1·64 (39)*	NR	NR

* p < 0·05
† NR = not reported
SIR = standardised incidence ratio; RR = relative risk; SMR = standardised mortality ratio
‡ μT = micro tesla
AML = acute myeloid leukaemia; CLL = chronic lymphocytic leukaemia

One must, however, exercise caution in maintaining that the cause of any excess was exposure to EMF. There could be other reasons, either inherent to the work in electrical occupations, such as occupational confounders, or inherent to the source population such as the socioeconomic status of electrical workers, that could possibly account for the increased cancer risks observed. Only precise and reliable measures of EMF exposure will permit EMF to be incriminated.

Table 4.5 Studies of leukaemia incidence in welders

	All leukaemia		Acute leukaemia		Lung cancer		
	O^a	RR	O^c	RR	O	RR	reference
	6	0.96	4(m)	1.71			(10)
	–	–	0(I)	0.66			(10)
	20	0.83	13(a)	1.04			(1)
	7	2.25					(36)
			$-^d$(M)	(3.8)			(35)
	19	0.89	6(A)	0.67			(45)
subtotal	52	0.93	23	0.94			
	0	–			6	0.95	(38)
	0	–			17	1.5	(39)
	4	4.2			10	2.2	(41)^e
	4	0.35			50	1.32	(37)
	1	2.5			7	1.38	(40)
			6(a)	1.81	27	0.99	(43)
	43	0.99			193	1.42	(45)
all	15	1.14			12	1.60	(44)
high exposure	(4)	0.6					(44)
low exposure	(11)	1.7					(44)
	27	0.85	7(m)	0.76	381	1.46	(42)
subtotal	95	0.90	17	0.90	305	1.27	(42)
pooled data RR^h	146	0.92^f	40	0.92^i	10.08	1.34	
pooled subtotal for studies with both all and acute leukaemia data							
	72	0.86	34	0.85			

[a] Observed
[b] Expected
[c] (m), acute myeloid; (l), acute lymphoid; (a), all acute leukaemia. All leukaemia minus all acute leukaemia = nonacute leukaemia (where listed): O = 38; E = 44.37; RR = 0.86. For studies without acute leukaemia data, O = 74; E = 75.06; RR = 0.99
[d] Number of welders not given
[e] Gas welders
[f] Standardised mortality ratio < 65 years
[g] Proportional mortality ratio 65–75 years
[h] For meta analysis, RR* showed no trend for all leukaemia and acute leukaemia; for lung cancer, RR* = 1.37; x^2 = 41.4; p* < 10^{-10}
[i] Nonsignificant
Source: Stern 1987[47]
Reprinted by permission of the *New England Journal of Medicine*

Leukaemia among welders

Welders are exposed to electric and magnetic fields of several frequencies and intensities; indeed, they are among the workers most exposed to EMF. If leukaemia is associated with EMF, it is reasonable to think that an excess of leukaemia should be observed in welders. To examine this hypothesis, Stern wrote an extensive review of 15 studies of cancers in welders.[47] Table 4.5 shows that there was a significant excess of lung cancer in a pooled analysis of all the welder studies. However, when Stern repeated his analysis for all leukaemia and acute leukaemia, he observed risk ratios of only 0·92 and 0·92, respectively. As he did not find an increased pooled risk ratio for welders and as this was contrary to his stated hypothesis, he concluded that there was no association between EMF exposure and leukaemia. As against this, in a case-control study of chronic myeloid leukaemia reported recently, Preston-Martin observed a greatly increased odds ratio of 25·4 (95% CI 2·78 to 232·54) in welders.[48] This finding was remarkably different from that of the series studied by Stern.

To what do we owe the fact that welders, who are among the most exposed workers, do not show an excess of leukaemia? Could it be that their exposure is different from that of electrical workers? Could this be the result of natural selection among welders or reflect differences in socioeconomic status between the two groups? We do not know the answer. Understanding it will certainly help explain any association that may exist between electrical occupations and increased risks of leukaemia.

Male breast cancer

When the question was first raised, the carcinogenicity of EMF was believed to be biologically impossible: scientists stated that EMF did not carry enough energy to interact with the cell and cause changes across the cell membrane. Since then, some effects of EMF on the cell have been reported such as changes in calcium transfer across the cell membrane and alteration in the replication of RNA proteins. But the most intriguing and worrisome effect noted so far has been the ability of EMF to reduce the concentration of circulating melatonin in exposed animals and humans. Experimental work in the laboratory has shown that mean night time circulating melatonin hormone in rats exposed to 39 kV/m electrical fields were lower than in sham exposed rats and returned to normal within three days after cessation of exposure. Electric fields of 10, 65, and 130 kV/m led to a similar response in rats exposed *in utero*. A similar phenomenon was observed in human volunteers. These observations led Stevens to propose a mechanism by which EMF may contribute to cancer.[49] According to him, the reduced melatonin production in exposed individuals is accompanied by an increase in oestrogen secreted by the ovary and prolactin secreted by the pituitary gland. Animal studies show that increased concentrations of oestrogen and prolactin contribute to the turnover of breast epithelial stem cells. This results in the accelerated growth of hormone sensitive cancers. By doing the reverse, that is by increasing melatonin or decreasing oestrogen and prolactin, one can delay and even reverse the development of hormone sensitive cancers. If the melatonin theory is correct, an increase in hormone sensitive cancers among people exposed to EMF would be expected.

Recently, in a study conducted among telephone workers in the United States, Matanoski observed two cases of breast cancer among men in a cohort of 9561 office technicians whereas none would have been expected.[50] As these office technicians were exposed to EMF fields at work it was suggested that this observation provided support for Stevens' hypothesised mechanism. In 1990, in an attempt to confirm Matanoski's observation, Demers looked at the occupational history of 227 cases of male breast cancer and compared them with 300 controls from the general population.[51] He found an increased odds ratio of 1·8 (95% CI 1·0 to 3·2) for all electricity-exposed jobs, an odds ratio of 6·0 (95% CI 1·7 to 21·5) for electricians, telephone linemen, and electrical power workers and an odds ratio of 2·9 (95% CI 0·8 to 10·2) for radio and communication workers. The risk was highest among subjects who were first employed in such jobs before the age of 30 years and who were initially exposed at least 30 years before diagnosis. Another recent report on male breast cancer came from Norway in a cohort of workers described as electrical workers in both the 1960 and the 1970 censuses. Twelve cases of male breast cancer were observed, whereas 5·81 were expected, the SIR being 2·07 (95% CI 1·07 to 361).[52] The observations made in these three studies of excess risk of male breast cancer among electrical workers are, to say the least, intriguing and appear to support the melatonin theory.

EMF personal exposure meters

The major limitation of past studies has been the lack of adequate methods for measuring personal exposure. In the late 1980s, there arrived on the market, almost simultaneously in three countries—Sweden, USA, and Canada—50 Hz/60 Hz personal exposure meters. These meters, some specifically designed for the conduct of epidemiological studies, are efficient, reasonably accurate, and easy to carry. Although each dosimeter features some differences, a prototype was described by Deadman et al. as follows:

> The electromagnetic dosimeter is a pocket-sized, battery operated device worn by the worker to monitor personal exposure to electric and magnetic fields at 50 or 60 Hz and to transient electric fields in the 5 to 20 MHz range.

The worker logs start and stop times of his or her activities in a diary to enable reconstruction of exposure history. Once a minute, for up to 18 days, the instrument takes a series of instantaneous readings of the E field perpendicular to the body surface; the X, Y and Z components of the B field; and the high-frequency transient electric (HFTE) field and stores them sequentially in the dosimeter's memory. The dosimeter can be configured to sample exposures at rates of up to once a second.[53]

The magnetic field is measured by a triaxial transducer in which each of the three orthogonal windings records a vectorial component of the magnetic field. Values for the three components are later integrated into a single figure by the software. The electric field is measured using a parallel-plate transducer. Only one transducer is used, as the dosimeter is worn against the body, ensuring that the E field is in the correct direction to induce a current across the plates. Both E and B-field measurements are sensitive to a frequency of 50 or 60 Hz only. The B-field measurement system is protected against induction from the earth's geomagnetic field. The electromagnetic transducer consists of a conductive foam antenna

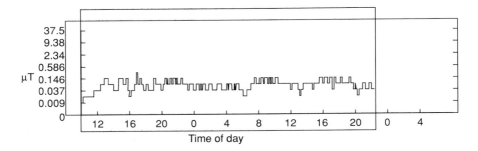

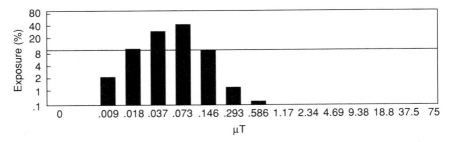

Figure 4.3 Sample of data for 60 Hz magnetic fields*
* Below the menu is basic information identifying the dosimeter, its user, start time, sampling rate (period) and enhancement factor used for the electric field measurements. In the low-resolution chronological record beneath, 8 hours of exposure are shown; each data point of the graph represents the average of 100 readings. The histogram shows the number of readings in each of the 16 exposure categories, expressed on the Y axis as a percentage of the total number of readings. Printed above the histogram are the total number of readings (n), start and stop times of the monitoring period, and average (μT) and cumulative (μT*h) field values.
Source: Adapted from Deadman 1988.[53]

with a volume and placement such that the sensitivity is independent of the dosimeter's orientation when the unit is worn. The HFTE measurement circuit is designed to detect the proportion of time over one minute (or the alternative sampling period) that an electric field threshold (approximately 200 volts/metre) is exceeded in a frequency band extending from 5 to 20 MHz.

Measurements for the three fields are classified into 16 amplitude classes (or bins) for each field: the lower limit of each bin being twice that of the preceding bin for E and B fields and 4 times for HFTE fields. Each measurement is assigned the midpoint value of the bin. The lower and upper limits of detection are 0·31 and 15 000 volts/metre; 15 nanotesla (nT) and 75 microtesla (μT); and 0·8 ppb, 335, 550 ppm for the E, B, and HTFE fields, respectively. Following retrieval of the dosimeters from the workers, the stored data are copied to a microcomputer where exposure histories for the three fields can be reconstructed by the software. The data can be displayed as a chronological record of exposure or compiled into histograms of frequencies of readings in each bin, according to user-defined time spans, periods of the day, and weekdays. With the help of the worker's activity diary, time spent at home can be separated from that spent at work, and time at work can be divided according to tasks undertaken. A sample of magnetic field exposure data is shown in figure 4.3.

Results from recent studies

Before the arrival on the market of personal meters such as the prototype just described, studies suffered from major limitations in exposure assessment. Exposure was entirely inferred from job titles; this was imprecise and the source of important exposure misclassification. Furthermore, most studies did not control for exposure to other potential carcinogens present in the workplace. Recently, three large studies were published that substantially improved over those made previously by having extensive and meticulous electromagnetic fields exposure assessment and assessment of exposure to potentially confounding chemical and physical agents encountered at the workplace.[54–56] In the first of those, by Floderus el al.[54] the base population included all men aged 20 to 64 employed in 1980 in two Swedish counties. Among these men, the author identified 250 leukaemias and 261 brain cancers diagnosed in the period 1983–87. As controls, 1121 men were selected at random from the study base. The controls were matched to cases for age and were alive at the time of investigation.

Among all subjects were identified, through work histories collated from questionnaires, the job held longest during the ten years preceding the diagnosis. Magnetic field exposure was measured for a full representative day on 50% of subjects and each was assigned the average value for his job. The author adjusted for possible confounding by place of residence and smoking and for exposure to benzene, ionizing radiation, pesticides, and solvents. The resulting analysis showed an association between exposure to EMF and chronic lymphocytic leukaemia with an exposure, response relationship. The odds ratios and 95% confidence intervals for three consecutive levels of exposure were: 1·1 (CI: 0·5 to 2·3); 2·2 (CI: 1·1 to 4·3); 3·0 (CI: 1·6 to 5·8), respectively. No association was observed with acute myeloid leukaemia. For brain tumours, the corresponding risk estimates were 1·0 (CI: 0·7 to 1·6); 1·5 (CI: 1·0 to 2·2) and 1·4 (CI: 0·9 to 2·1).

The second study was published by Sahl et al. from the Southern California Edison Company.[55] In a cohort of 36 221 people who worked for the electrical utility company for at least one year between 1960 and 1988, 44 deaths from leukaemia, 31 from brain cancer, and 63 from lymphoma were identified. For each case, 10 controls from the same source population were matched on birth date, sex, and ethnicity and were alive at time of death of the case. Summary lifetime cumulative exposures were calculated for each individual based on job history and magnetic field measurements performed on the job to which each subject had been assigned. Results were essentially negative for both leukaemia and brain cancer. Odds ratios for magnetic field exposure based on the median, mean, 99th percentile and fraction exceeding 10 μT and 50 μT were all close to or less than 1·0.

The third study, from my department was also a case-control study, within three cohorts of electric utility workers: Electricité de France, 170 000 men; Ontario Hydro, 31 543 men; and Hydro-Québec, 21 741 men.[56] It included 4151 new cases of cancer observed among these workers during the period 1970–1989. Each subject's cumulative exposure to magnetic fields was estimated from measurements of current exposure made on 2066 workers performing similar tasks to those in the cohorts, using personal dosimetry. Estimates were also made of past exposure based on knowledge of current loading, work practices, and usage. The analysis was controlled for potential occupational confounders.

Workers exposed above median cumulative exposure to magnetic field (3·1 μT years) had a higher risk of acute non-lymphocytic leukaemia (OR 2·41, CI: 1·07 to 5·44). The same observation held for acute myeloid leukaemia (OR 3·15, CI: 1·20 to 8·27). There was also an increased risk for mean exposure above 0·2 μT for acute non-lymphocytic leukaemia, (OR 2·36, CI: 1·00 to 5·58) acute myeloid leukaemia; (OR 2·25, CI: 0·79 to 6·46). However, there was no exposure-response trend with increasing exposure nor consistency in the results between the three utilities. Among men exposed above the 90th percentile of cumulative magnetic field (15·7 μT years), there was an increased risk of brain cancer (OR 1·95, CI: 0·76 to 5·0), but this was not significant. No association with magnetic

Table 4.6 Comparison of results between the Sahl and Thériault studies

	First author	Cumulative exposure OR (CI)	Cumulative exposure OR (CI)
all leukaemia			
	Sahl[55]	3·5 μT years 1·01 (0·75 to 1·36)	25·0 μT years 1·07 (0·80 to 1·45)
	Thériault[56]	3·1 μT years 1·54 (0·90 to 2·63)	15·7 μT years 1·75 (0·77 to 3·96)
brain cancer			
	Sahl[55]	3·5 μT years 0·95 (0·62 to 1·47)	25·0 μT years 0·81 (0·48 to 1·36)
	Thériault[56]	3·1 μT years 1·54 (0·85 to 2·81)	15·7 μT years 1·95 (0·76 to 5·00)

OR = Odds ratio
CI = 95% confidence interval
μT = micro tesla

fields was observed for any of the other 29 cancer types recorded, including skin melanoma, male breast cancer and prostate cancer.

Comparative analysis of the three recent studies

It is not easy to compare directly the result of these three investigations. They used different methodologies, the analyses were sophisticated but different and the results were expressed differently. At first glance, the results appear contradictory. Floderus observed an association between EMF and chronic lymphocytic leukaemia and, to a lesser degree, brain cancer, but no association with acute myeloid leukaemia. We observed an association with acute myeloid leukaemia, and a questionable one with brain cancer. Sahl's results were completely negative. Any attempt to reconcile these results may result in sterile speculation; consequently, much caution should be exercised when seeking and interpreting similarities and differences. Nevertheless, there exist points that can allow some comparison between our study and each of the other two.

In Table 4.6, I report what I think are comparable elements between Sahl's study and our own. For all leukaemia, Sahl observed an odds ratio (OR) of 1·01 for cumulative exposure above 3·5 μT years and 1·07 above 25·0 μT years; we observed an OR of 1·54 above 3·1 μT years and 1·75 above 15·7 μT years. None of these ratios are significantly different from controls although ours were higher than Sahl's. For brain cancer, Sahl observed an OR of 0·95 and 0·81 for cumulative exposure above 3·5 and 25·0 μT years, respectively; our ORs were 1·54 and 1·95 for cumulative exposure above 3·1 and 15·7 μT years, respectively. Here again, our results yielded higher odds ratios, although none was significant. Sahl analysed the mortality of his subjects, assessed their exposure up to time of death and, because of small numbers, limited his analysis to all leukaemias.

Table 4.7 Comparison of results between the Floderus and Thériault studies

	Floderus[54]	Thériault[56]
	OR* 95% CI**	OR 95% CI
All leukaemia		
mean exposure $\geqslant 0.2\ \mu$T	1·2 (0·8 to 1·9)	1·6 (0·9 to 2·8)
mean exposure $\geqslant 0.3\ \mu$T	1·6 (1·1 to 2·4)	1·1 (0·7 to 2·0)
AML		
mean exposure $\geqslant 0.2\ \mu$T	0·8 (0·4 to 1·6)	2·25 (0·8 to 6·5)
mean exposure $\geqslant 0.3\ \mu$T	1·0 (0·6 to 1·9)	1·91 (0·7 to 5·2)
CLL		
mean exposure $\geqslant 0.2\ \mu$T	2·2 (1·1 to 4·3)	1·4 (0·5 to 3·8)
mean exposure $\geqslant 0.3\ \mu$T	3·0 (1·6 to 5·8)	0·9 (0·3 to 2·3)
exposure in last 5 years before diagnosis		4·06 (0·7 to 22·4)
exposure in last 20 years before diagnosis		4·07 (0·9 to 18·0)
Brain cancer		
mean exposure $\geqslant 0.2\ \mu$T	1·5 (1·0 to 2·2)	1·6 (0·9 to 3·2)
mean exposure $\geqslant 0.3\ \mu$T	1·4 (0·9 to 2·1)	1·5 (0·8 to 2·8)
exposure in last 5 years before diagnosis		1·2 (0·6 to 2·2)
exposure in last 20 years before diagnosis		1·9 (0·9 to 3·8)
Astrocytoma✶		
mean exposure $\geqslant 0.2\ \mu$T	1·7 (1·1 to 2·7)	4·28 (0·6 to 28·5)
mean exposure $\geqslant 0.3\ \mu$T	1·5 (1·0 to 2·4)	1·31 (0·3 to 5·7)
exposure in last 5 years before diagnosis		1·2 (0·4 to 3·2)
exposure in last 20 years before diagnosis		4·0 (0·7 to 22·0)

✶ astrocytoma III-IV in Floderus' study, all astrocytoma in Thériault's study
μT = micro tesla
* OR = odds ratio
** CI = 95% confidence interval
AML = acute myeloid leukaemia; CLL = chronic lymphocytic leukaemia

We studied incident cases, assessed exposure to time of diagnosis, and scrutinised leukaemia by subtypes. This could account in part for the differences noted. Had we limited our analysis to all leukaemias, we would have observed an OR somewhat elevated but not significantly so (OR above median [3·1 μT years] 1·54, CI: 0·90 to 2·63) which is compatible with Sahl's result.

Because of major differences in study design, source population, exposure assessment and statistical analysis, any direct comparison between Floderus' study and ours is hazardous. Such comparisons, wherever possible, are summarized in table 4.7. For all leukaemias, Floderus observed a 20% increase in risk for men exposed to a daily average of 0·2 μT and a significant 60% increase for exposure of 0·3 μT or above. Our observation was the complete reverse with a 60% increase for men exposed to 0·2 μT (almost significant) and a 10% increase for exposure to 0·3 μT or above. For acute myeloid leukaemia, we found an increased OR, although not significant, for both 0·2 and 0·3 μT exposures whereas Floderus' results were quite negative. For chronic lymphocytic leukaemia Floderus observed significantly elevated odds ratios for exposure to both 0·2 and 0·3 μT with an exposure-response trend. When we calculate the average exposure over the entire workers' lifetime, we do not find such a high risk but when we consider the exposures in the previous five years, and 20 years before diagnosis (our closest analysis to that of Floderus) the ORs for above-median exposure are 4·06 and 4·07, quite close to conventional levels of significance (P = 0·11 and 0·06). For brain cancer, our ORs are similar to those of Floderus, with a risk slightly lower among workers exposed to 0·3 μT or above than among those exposed to 0·2 μT or above. As with Floderus, these increased odds ratios relate to astrocytomas. However, the ratios show wide confidence intervals, which indicates that no reliable conclusion can be drawn.

Thus after close scrutiny, apart from acute myeloid leukaemia, the results of the two studies, of Floderus and our own, are compatible. Even the differing results of chronic lymphocytic leukaemia could be explained by the dissimilar age structure of the two study groups. The proportion of chronic lymphocytic leukaemia among all leukaemias was much lower in our study than in that of Floderus; (41/140: 29%, compared with 112/250: 45%). This was inherent in the structure of our collaborative cohort— Électricité de France did not include subjects after age 60—and diminished our ability to observe an association with chronic lymphocytic leukaemia if it existed. When looking at the two other companies, Ontario Hydro and Hydro-Québec, trends seemed to confirm that the age of the cohort played an important part in our observations. The Ontario Hydro cohort, which had the oldest age group (mean age at diagnosis: 62·6) yielded a non-significant trend for chronic lymphocytic leukaemia with increasing exposure (4·9 μT years, OR 1·0; 4·9 to 9·1 μT years, OR 1·72, CI: 0·37 to 8·09; 9·1 to 27·2 μT years, OR 2·67, CI: 0·53 to 13·51; 27·2 + μT years, OR 3·34, CI: 0·35 to 31·90). On the other hand, subjects in the Hydro-Québec cohort (mean age at diagnosis: 57·1) were also followed to death but did not yield any indication of an increase in chronic lymphocytic leukaemia with increasing magnetic field exposure (6·1 μT years, OR 1·0; 6·1 to 11·8 μT years, OR 0·76, CI: 0·13 to 4·31; 11·8 to 23·6 μT years, OR 2·69, CI: 0·47 to 15·35; 23·6 + μT years, 0 cases, 3 controls).

There remains the necessity to explain the difference between Floderus's findings and ours concerning acute myeloid leukaemia, for which, at present, we see no obvious reason. In other publications, there are several studies that have shown the presence of an increased risk of acute myeloid leukaemia among electrical workers,[6 7 12 16 27 39 45] yet some have not observed it[26 44 54] and others have yielded results that are difficult to interpret.[8 11 17 23 25] The presence of this association therefore remains to be confirmed.

Conclusion

In spite of the great hopes that were raised by the arrival of newly developed EMF personal meters and their use in three large projects, recent research has not brought a clear answer to the suggestion of an association between occupational exposure to EMF and the development of cancer among workers. Some critics have proposed that concerns raised by previous findings were a mirage brought about by faulty research designs and publication bias. This hardly holds any longer. Recent studies which have been planned to achieve adequate power and minimum methodological weaknesses and to which the above mentioned comments cannot be attached are yielding results in all respects similar to those of previous studies. These results remain inconsistent and puzzling. They do not confirm nor do they reject the hypothesis of an association between EMF and cancer. Something is going on that still evades our comprehension. This may be the result of the underestimated difficulty of arriving at an accurate exposure estimate (because EMF is ubiquitous, everyone is exposed) or it can indicate that among the several variables that accompany EMF exposure (resonances, high frequency transients, and composites of radiation) those that have been measured so far are not appropriate. More research is needed.

1 Asanova TP, Rakov AN. The health status of people working in the electric field of open 400–500 kV switching structures. *Gig Tr Prof Zabol* 1966; 10: 50–2.
2 Bonnell JA, Cabanes J, Hauf R, Malboysson E. Electric and magnetic fields and man. *J Soc Occup Med* 1980; 30: 135–7.
3 Wilson BW, Steven RG, Anderson LE. *Extremely low frequency electromagnetic fields: the question of cancer*. Richland, Wa: Battelle Press, 1990; 3–8.
4 Wertheimer N, Leeper E. Electrical wiring configurations and childhood cancers. *Am J Epidemiol* 1979; 109: 273–84.
5 Milham S. Mortality from leukaemia in workers exposed to electric and magnetic fields. *N Engl J Med* 1982; 307: 249.
6 Wright WE, Peters JM, Mack TM. Leukaemia in workers exposed to electrical and magnetic fields. *Lancet* 1982; 2: 1160–4.
7 McDowall ME. Leukaemia mortality in electrical workers in England and Wales. *Lancet* 1983; 1: 246.
8 Coleman M, Bell J, Skeet R. Leukaemia incidence in electrical workers. *Lancet* 1983; 1: 982–3.
9 Howe GR, Lindsay JP. A follow-up study of a ten-percent sample of the Canadian Labour Force 1. Cancer mortality in males. 1965–73. *J Natl Cancer Inst* 1983; 70: 37–44.
10 Morton W, Marjanovic C. Leukaemia incidence by occupation in Portland-Vancouver metropolitan area. *Am J Ind Med* 1984; 6: 185–205.
11 Pearce NE, Sheppart AR, Howard JK, Fraser J, Lilley BM. Leukaemia in electrical workers in New Zealand. *Lancet* 1985; 1: 811–2.
12 Milham S. Silent keys: Leukaemia mortality in amateur radio operators. *Lancet* 1985; 1: 811.
13 Milham S. Mortality in workers exposed to electromagnetic fields. *Environ Health Perspect* 1985; 62: 297–300.
14 Calle E, Savitz DA. Leukaemia in occupational groups with presumed exposure to electrical and magnetic fields. *N Engl J Med* 1985; 313: 1476–7.
15 Linet M, Malker H, McLaughlin J, Weiner J, Stone BJ, Blot W *et al.* Leukemias and occupation in Sweden: a registry-based analysis. *Am J Ind Med* 1988; 14: 319–30.
16 Juutilainen J, Pukkala E, Laara E. Results of epidemiological cancer study among electrical workers in Finland. *J Bioelectricity* 1988; 7: 119–21.
17 Robinson CF, Lalich NR, Burnett CA, Sestito JP, Frazier TM, Fine LJ. Electromagnetic field exposure and leukaemia mortality in the United States. *J Occup Med* 1991; 33: 160–2.

18 Loomis DP, Savitz DA. Occupation and leukaemia mortality among men in 16 states: 1985–1987. *Am J Ind Med* 1991; **19**: 509–21.

19 Coleman M, Beral V. A review of epidemiological studies of the health effects of living near or working with electricity generation and transmission equipment. *Int J Epidemiol* 1988; **17**: 1–13.

20 Gilman PA, Ames RG, McCawley A. Leukaemia risk among US white male coal miners. *J Occup Med* 1985; **27**: 669–71.

21 Stern FB, Waxweiler RA, Beaumont JJ, Lee ST, Rinsky RA, Zumwalde RD, et al. A case-control study of leukaemia at a naval nuclear shipyard. *Am J Epidemiol* 1986; **123**: 980–92.

22 Flodin U, Fredriksson M, Axelson O, Persson B, Hardell L. Background radiation, electrical work, and some other exposures associated with acute myeloid leukaemia in a case-referent study. *Arch Environ Health* 1986; **41**: 77–84.

23 Flodin U, Fredriksson M, Persson B, Axelson O. Acute myeloid leukaemia and background radiation in an expanded case-referent study. *Arch Environ Health* 1990; **45**: 364–6.

24 Coggon D, Pannett B, Osmond C, Acheson ED. A survey of cancer and occupation in young and middle aged men. II Non-respiratory cancers. *Brit J Ind Med* 1986; **43**: 381–6.

25 Pearce N, Reif JS, Fraser J. Case-control studies of cancer in New Zealand electrical workers. *Int J Epidemiol* 1989; **18**: 55–9.

26 Loomis DP, Savitz DA. Mortality from brain cancer and leukaemia among electrical workers. *Br J Ind Med* 1990; **47**: 633–8.

27 Richardson S, Zittoun R, Bastuji-Garin S, Lasseve V, Guihenneuc C, Cadiou M, et al. Occupational risk factors for acute leukaemia: a case-control study. *Int J Epidemiol* 1992; **21**: 1063–73.

28 Lin RS, Dischinger PC, Conde J, Farrell KP. Occupational exposure to electromagnetic fields and the occurrence of brain tumours: an analysis of possible associations. *J Occup Med* 1985; **27**: 413–19.

29 Thomas TL, Stolley PD, Stemhagen A, Fontham ETH, Bleecker ML, Stewart PA, et al. Brain tumour mortality among men with electrical and electronics jobs: a case-control study. *J Natl Cancer Inst* 1987; **79**: 233–8.

30 Speers MA, Dobbins JG, Miller VS. Occupational exposures and brain cancer mortality: a preliminary study of East Texas residents. *Am J Ind Med* 1988; **13**: 629–38.

31 Brownson RC, Reif JS, Chang JC, Davis JR. An analysis of occupational risks for brain cancer. *Am J Public Health* 1990; **80**: 169–72.

32 Ryan P, Lee MW, North JB, McMichael AJ. Risk factors for tumours of the brain and meninges: results from the Adelaide adult brain tumour study. *Int J Cancer* 1992; **51**: 20–7.

33 Preston-Martin S, Lewis S, Winkelmann R, Borman B, Auld J, Pearce N. Descriptive epidemiology of primary cancer of the brain, cranial nerves and cranial meninges in New Zealand, 1948–88. *Cancer Causes and Control* 1993; **4**: 529–38.

34 Wilklund K, Einhorn J, Eklund G. An application of the Swedish Cancer Environment Registry. Leukaemia among telephone operators at the telecommunication administration in Sweden. *Int J Epidemiol* 1981; **10**: 373–6.

35 Vagero D, Olin R. Incidence of cancer in the electronics industry: using the new Swedish Cancer Environment Registry as a screening instrument. *Brit J Ind Med* 1983; **40**: 188–92.

36 Olin R, Vagero D, Ahlbom A. Mortality experience of electrical engineers. *Brit J Ind Med* 1985; **42**: 211–2.

37 Vagero D, Ahlbom A, Olin R, Sahlsten S. Cancer morbidity among workers in the telecommunications industry. *Brit J Ind Med* 1985; **42**: 191–5.

38 McLaughlin JK, Malker HSR, Blot WJ, Malker BK, Stone BJ, Weiner JA, et al. Occupational risks for intracranial gliomas in Sweden. *J Natl Cancer Inst* 1987; **78**: 253–7.

39 Milham S. Increased mortality in amateur radio operators due to lymphatic and haematopoietic malignancies. *Am J Epidemiol* 1988; **127**: 50–4.

40 Guberan E, Usel M, Raymond L, Tissot R, Sweetman PM. Disability, mortality and incidence of cancer among Geneva painters and electricians. *Brit J Ind Med* 1989; **46**: 16–23.

41 Garland FC, Shaw E, Gorham ED, Garland CF, White MR, Sinsheimer P. Incidence of

leukaemia in occupations with potential electromagnetic fields exposure in United States Navy personnel. *Am J Epidemiol* 1990; **132**: 293–303.

42 Juutilainen J, Laara E, Pukkala E. Incidence of leukaemia and brain tumours in Finnish workers exposed to ELF magnetic fields. *Int Arch Occup Environ Health* 1990; **62**: 289–93.

43 Tornqvist S, Norell S, Ahlbom A, Knave B. Cancer in the electric power industry. *Brit J Ind Med* 1986; **43**: 212–3.

44 Tornqvist S, Knave B, Ahlbom A, Persson T. Incidence of leukaemia and brain tumours in some "electrical occupations." *Br J Ind Med* 1991; **48**: 597–603.

45 Tynes T, Andersen A, Langmark F. Incidence of cancer in Norwegian workers potentially exposed to electromagnetic fields. *Am J Epidemiol* 1992; **136**: 81–8.

46 Guénel P, Raskmark P, Bach Anderson J, Lynge E. Incidence of cancer in persons with occupational exposure to electromagnetic fields in Denmark. *Br J Ind Med* 1993; **50**: 758–64.

47 Stern RM. Cancer incidence among welders: possible effects of exposure to extremely low frequency electromagnetic radiation (ELF) and to welding fumes. *Environ Health Perspect* 1987; **76**: 221–9.

48 Preston-Martin S, Peters JM. Prior employment as a welder associated with the development of chronic myeloid leukaemia. *Brit J Cancer* 1988; **58**: 105–8.

49 Stevens RG. Electric power use and breast cancer, a hypothesis. *Am J Epidemiol* 1987; **125**: 556.

50 Matanoski GBM, Breysse PN, Elliott EA. Electromagnetic field exposure and male breast cancer. *Lancet* 1991; **337**: 737.

51 Demers PA, Thomas DB, Rosenblatt KA, Jimenez LM, McTiernan A, Stalsberg H, *et al.* Occupational exposure to electromagnetic radiation and breast cancer in males. *Am J Epidemiol* 1991; **134**: 340–7.

52 Tynes JT, Andersen A. Electromagnetic fields and male breast cancer. *Lancet* 1990; **336**: 1596.

53 Deadman JE, Camus M, Armstrong BG, Héroux P, Cyr D, Plante M, *et al.* Occupational and residential 60 Hz electromagnetic fields and high-frequency electric transients: exposure assessment using a new dosimeter. *Am Ind Hyg Assoc J* 1988; **49**: 409–19.

54 Floderus B, Persson T, Stenlund C, Wennberg A, Ost A, Knave B. Occupational exposure to electromagnetic fields in relation to leukaemia and brain tumours. A case-control study in Sweden. *Cancer Causes and Control* 1993; **4**: 465–76.

55 Sahl JD, Kelsh MA, Greenland S. Cohort and nested case-control studies of haematopoietic cancers and brain cancer among electric utility workers. *Epidemiology* 1993; **4**: 104–14.

56 Thériault G, Goldberg M, Miller AB, Armstrong B, Guénel P, Deadman J, *et al.* Cancer risks associated with occupational exposure to magnetic fields among electric utility workers in Ontario and Quebec, Canada, and France: 1970–1989. *Am J Epidemiol* 1994; **139**: 550–72.

5 Mineral dusts and fibres

CORBETT McDONALD

Introduction

Early evidence of dust-related malignant disease was recorded by Agricola and Paracelsus in the 16th century among miners in the mountains of Bohemia, but its nature and cause were not then understood. It seems probable that these men suffered from silicosis and died of lung cancer, primarily caused by uranium and arsenic; even today the correlation between fibrogenesis and carcinogenesis in this and other circumstances has yet to be resolved. Since the 18th century exposure of chimney sweeps to soot has been recognised as a cause of skin cancer and in recent years the inhalation of chimney dust has been seen also as a cause of lung cancer. The experience of workers with bituminous shale and pitch dust has been similar. In these examples cancer was caused not by the dust alone but by simultaneous exposure to a primary chemical carcinogen or to ionizing radiation. It was not until 1935 when a case of lung cancer was reported by Lynch and Smith in a weaver with asbestosis from a textile plant in Charleston, South Carolina that dust was itself suggested as carcinogenic.[1] It may be no accident that this first association of lung cancer with asbestos was in a tobacco producing state and coincided with suspicion that the rising incidence of lung cancer might be due to the cigarette smoking epidemic of the first world war. This chapter will be limited to an assessment of the extent to which occupational exposure to the more important mineral dusts—asbestos, crystalline silica and man-made mineral fibres—causes cancer, primarily of the respiratory tract.

Asbestos

No material used in industry has been the object of more epidemiological research than asbestos, a name given to describe any fibrous mineral silicate used commercially. The main stimulus for this activity was a conference held in New York in November 1964 where it became abundantly evident that the "magic mineral," with all its innumerable and invaluable uses, was a potent cause of lung cancer, mesothelioma and perhaps other malignancies. It was recognised that asbestos comprised at least five distinct types of mineral fibre, which might well differ in their biological properties but that what constituted a hazardous exposure was quite unclear. At the close of the conference an expert working party identified priorities for epidemiological research as fibre type differences, exposure-response in various industries, comprehensive studies of mesothelioma, and effects of removal from further exposure. The extent to which these issues have been resolved provides the focus for this chapter.

Lung cancer

During the twenty years that followed the initial observations by Lynch and Smith in 1935[1] and by Gloyne[2] in the same year, case reports and case series were published with increasing frequency until in 1955 the association of asbestos and lung cancer was confirmed by Doll[3] in a small cohort study of textile workers in Rochdale and independently by Breslow in a case-control study in California.[4] Since then there have been about 50 cohort surveys of varied size and complexity in various industries, virtually all showing excess risk of lung cancer. Apart from putting the basic causal question beyond reasonable doubt, the value of these studies is limited because their findings are difficult to compare due to confounding by fibre type, industrial process, and level of exposure. The general pattern in terms of proportional mortality has, however, suggested that the risk overall may have been three or four times greater in cohorts exposed to amphiboles (crocidolite or amosite) and to chrysotile-amphibole mixtures than to chrysotile alone.[5] It is worth mentioning here that chrysotile as mined, milled, and used commercially usually contains small but variable amounts (1–2%) of the fibrous amphibole, tremolite, the potential importance of which will be discussed later in relation to mesothelioma.

A smaller number of studies, which allow conclusions to be drawn on fibre type and industrial process, are those in which intensity and duration of exposure were estimated for each cohort member. Findings from these

88

Table 5.1 Estimated increase in relative risk from lung cancer in male cohorts with individual estimates of cumulative exposure

Reference	Place		Fibre type	Lung cancer deaths	Increase in relative risk fibres/ml × years
Mining and milling					
McDonald et al., 1980[6]	Quebec		Chrysotile	230	0·0004
McDonald et al., 1986[7]	Montana		Tremolite	23	0·01
Amandus and Wheeler, 1987[8]	Montana		Tremolite	20	0·006
Armstrong et al., 1989[9]	Western Australia		Crocidolite	92	0·01
Textiles					
Dement et al., 1982[10]	South Carolina		Chrysotile	26	0·01
McDonald et al., 1983[11]	South Carolina		Chrysotile	59	0·01
McDonald et al., 1983[12]	Pennsylvania		Mixed	53	0·009
Peto et al., 1985[13]	Rochdale		Mixed	93	0·01
Cement products					
Henderson and Enterline, 1979[14]	USA		Mixed	63	0·001
Hughes et al., 1987[15]	Louisiana	Plant 1	Mixed	22	0·0003
		Plant 2		73	0·0076
Friction products					
Berry and Newhouse, 1983[16]	UK		Mixed	143	effectively
McDonald et al., 1984[17]	Connecticut		Chrysotile	73	zero

89

studies, summarised in table 5.1, are relatively more reliable than those without exposure estimates, but two problems remain. In the first place, cumulative exposure, the index used in all of them, is an unsatisfactory measure, which depends on the questionable assumption that duration and intensity are biologically equivalent; the resulting error may not be serious over the middle range of values for these variables but is increasingly unjustified at their extremes. In the second place, although assessments of exposure intensity used in these studies are expressed in fibres per cubic centimetre (f/cc), the primary measurements (or estimates) were made in millions of dust particles per cubic foot (mpcf) and only later converted to fibre concentrations, a difficult procedure because of enormous variation in the conversion factors associated with particle size and intensity. As a result the discriminating power of cumulative exposure is determined mainly by duration, which can be measured fairly accurately, rather than by concentration, which is always approximate. The assumed linearity in exposure-response correlation is thus uncertain and the question of whether or not there is a safe threshold even more so.

Problems of interpretation are further compounded by the general difficulty of estimating risk in cohort studies, depending as it does on there being a comparable basis for estimation. No external reference population is ever truly comparable and standardised mortality ratios (SMRs) at zero exposure commonly range from about 0·6 to 1·5 probably for this reason alone. Internal comparisons, whether obtained by the person-years approach or by regression methods are able to estimate risk only relative to cohort members with least exposure. Much therefore depends on the shape of the exposure-response correlation and how good is the evidence for a threshold. Resolution of this problem may depend on methods of statistical analysis that effectively separate the contributions of duration and intensity of exposure. Preliminary work on these lines has thrown further doubt on the validity of a linear model, pointing rather to a sigmoid relationship with threshold.[18] These issues are less relevant to the control of occupational risk than to the question of how seriously the health effects of low level exposure should be regarded, for example in the urban environment or in public buildings which contain asbestos in construction materials.[19]

From inspection of the enormous range in levels of risk shown in table 1 certain groupings emerge. The seven highest, which stand out from the rest, are based on four cohorts of asbestos textile workers[10-13] and two of miners and millers exposed to amphiboles, one to crocidolite[9] and the two others to fibres in the tremolite series.[7 8] At the other extreme are two cohorts of friction product workers at low or doubtful excess risk.[16 17] Somewhat higher are the chrysotile miners and millers,[6] and perhaps higher still, three cohorts of cement product workers.[14 15] Of the four textile cohorts, two were from a factory in Charleston, South Carolina, where exposure was essentially to commercial chrysotile only;[10] [11] in the other two, one in Mannheim, Pennsylvania[12] and the other in Rochdale, England,[13] important amounts of amphibole fibre were also used in the manufacturing process. At least for lung cancer, the varied nature of the exposures did not materially affect the high level of risk evident in all four cohorts. On the other hand, the four cohorts of miners and millers showed a clear difference between those working with amphiboles and those working with chrysotile. The experience of friction product and cement product workers is less easy to interpret; both the friction product cohorts were essentially exposed only to chrysotile and their experience of lung cancer was certainly low, but workers in two cement plants in the USA which used variable amounts of crocidolite were at lower risk in the one where the opportunity for amphibole exposure was less.

It would thus appear that after allowing for level of exposure and type of industrial process there may well be a higher lung cancer risk associated with amphiboles than chrysotile. The high risk observed in textile plants has yet to be explained; that it was not caused by errors in exposure estimation was shown by electron microscopic analysis of lung tissue taken at necropsy from chrysotile textile and production workers.[20] This study drew attention to the possibility that mineral oil used to control dust in textile plants deserved further investigation, but there has been no further support for this hypothesis. The proportion of very long fibres (> 20 μm), although low, was higher in the lungs of textile workers; this could conceivably explain the difference but only if shorter fibres make little contribution to risk.

It was suggested by Selikoff et al. in 1968 that the lung cancer excess in American insulation workers might be confined to smokers but at that time the number of non-smokers in their cohort was too low to be sure of this.[21] In 1979, with larger numbers, their data pointed to an interaction between asbestos and smoking that appeared to be multiplicative.[22] However, it will be seen in table 5.2, based on the work of Berry et al., that the general pattern, although more than additive, is probably less than multiplicative and not simple.[23]

Of both theoretical and practical importance is the connection between asbestosis and lung cancer, a question on which the evidence is conflicting. Martischnig and colleagues, in a case control study based on occupational histories, found a significant association between asbestos exposure and lung cancer in the absence of radiological fibrosis.[24] These findings were questioned, however, because of inadequate control for smoking and potential recall bias. Later a longitudinal study from Louisiana examined lung cancer mortality in relation to chest radiographic abnormalities in 642 male asbestos cement workers.[25] After controlling for age, smoking and asbestos exposure, an excess of lung cancer was observed only in workers with small opacities on the chest radiograph. This finding was in line with

Table 5.2 Lung cancer and smoking in studies of asbestos workers

| | Relative risk of lung cancer | | | |
	Non-smokers (NS)	Smokers (S)	Ratio of risks (NS:S)	Confidence interval (95%)
American insulation workers	5·3	5·4	1·0	0 to 5·0
Amosite factory workers	25·0	4·7	5·3	0·3 to 2·6
UK factory workers (women)	5·0	7·4	0·7	0·1 to 3·4
UK factory workers (men)	7·3	2·4	3·0	0·8 to 7·5
Quebec miners and millers	3·0	1·7	1·8	0·7 to 5·4
Five studies combined	—	—	1·8	1·1 to 2·8

Derived from Table 8 of Berry et al.[23]

results from a necropsy series of amphibole asbestos miners in South Africa in which standardised proportional mortality ratios for lung cancer showed an excess only among those with asbestosis.[26] In a longitudinal study of Quebec miners and millers,[27] 49 of an estimated 52 excess deaths from lung cancer were in men whose last chest radiograph was abnormal, 33 showing small parenchymal opacities, but the films had been taken many years before death.

More recently, however, chest radiographs in men admitted to a London hospital with lung cancer and from two control series, were classified 'blind' by three readers. Analysis of detailed work and smoking histories from these subjects disclosed a significantly raised relative risk for probable asbestos exposure in the absence of radiographic evidence of fibrosis and a somewhat higher risk in those with such evidence.[28]

Mesothelioma

In failing to take more seriously the paper published by Wagner *et al.* in 1960 the world made a costly mistake.[29] That study showed clearly that occupational and environmental exposure associated with crocidolite production in the early days of mining in the north-west Cape Province of South Africa resulted in many deaths from malignant mesothelial tumours 30–40 years later, whereas similar cases were not seen in the amosite and chrysotile mining areas. By 1960, production of crocidolite had increased many fold and continued to grow for at least 15 more years, paralleled after a 30–40 year lag by the widespread occurrence of cases of mesothelioma. Mortality from this cause continues to rise steeply in most industrialised countries in men, but not women, at 5–10% per annum and seems likely to go on doing so from its present level of at least 5000 deaths annually well into the next century.[30] The unfolding of this story is less simple than this brief account might suggest, largely as a result of confusion over the contribution of the different asbestos fibre types, conflict between epidemiological and experimental findings, and much bitter controversy among investigators. One lesson at least from this unfortunate episode must surely be that failure to act rapidly on what was clearly evident more than 30 years ago has been disastrous. Although the use of crocidolite was discontinued in the UK and Eire in 1970, and in most countries of western Europe by 1980, in many countries this has yet to be achieved.

Whereas in the 1960s peritoneal tumours comprised up to 30% of the total, in recent years the proportion has fallen to about 10%. It is not that peritoneal tumours have become less common but rather that the steady increase has been in pleural tumours. It has been suggested, on slender evidence, that the explanation may lie in the intensity of exposure. Much research has been directed at aetiological questions relating to mesothelioma and most of what was predictable from the work of Wagner *et al.* 35 years ago is now clear enough.

At first sight the epidemiological problems of mesothelioma and asbestos should have been easier to solve than those of lung cancer—the former until recently a rare tumour unrelated to smoking habit and distributed occupationally and geographically in a far from random manner, the latter extremely common, almost ubiquitous, and in some respects just one more complication of cigarette smoking. The difficulty is that the aetiology of mesothelioma has been dominated by fibre type, and mineral fibres seldom occur in nature or in industry unmixed. This problem is compounded by the fact that the disease has a long latency, seldom less than 20 years and usually 30 to 40; thus it has been well nigh impossible to determine with any confidence the exact nature and degree of exposure, occupationally or otherwise, so far back in time. More recently, however, analytical electron microscopy on lung tissue has helped to break through this barrier. This technique too has its limitations but despite difficulty in the interpretation of mineral fibres in tissue at necropsy the results of well-controlled studies have proved informative. These investigations have consistently failed to show any important difference between mesothelioma cases and controls in chrysotile concentrations at autopsy although these correlate reasonably well with lifetime exposure estimates, for example, in both mine workers and in textile plant workers.[20] The substantially higher concentrations of amphibole fibres, including tremolite, in cases than controls is equally consistent. It is hard to escape the conclusion from these studies that amphibole fibres are the major cause of mesothelioma with some or all of the cases in chrysotile workers due to fibrous tremolite.[31]

Surveys of mesothelioma in specific occupations have provided estimates of risk but few investigations have been designed to assess the relative importance of various types of work in the general population. One study with this objective was based on fatal cases and matched controls ascertained from all pathologists in Canada, 1960–72, and in the USA, 1972, with detailed employment histories from next of kin.[32] An analysis of occupations ten or more years before death was made in 344 male cases and their controls. This showed that by far the greatest relative risk was for insulation work (46·0), following in descending order by asbestos production and manufacture (6·1), heating trades (4·4), shipyard work (2·8) and construction work (2·6). Mining and asbestos cement manufacturing and demolition work made little contribution. Occupations in which evidence of increased risk was not detected included garage work, building maintenance, carpentry, and transport.

Wherever the exposure has been predominantly to crocidolite mesothelioma rates have been high; this has been well documented in South African and Australian crocidolite miners and millers, in British and Canadian gasmask filter assembly and in American cigarette filter manufacture.[33] It has also been evident in two asbestos textile plants where some crocidolite was used,[8 9] in contrast to one where it was not.[10 11] It can explain the high rates of the disease in dockyard areas, where crocidolite was a common constituent of naval insulation materials; it is reflected in the aggregation of cases in the vicinity of large crocidolite-using plants in London[34] and in Hamburg.[35] Other studies have shown the high incidence of the disease in South Africa and Western Australia, largely attributable to the crocidolite mining industries in these countries.

Although there can be no reasonable doubt that amosite asbestos is an important cause of mesothelioma, there are anomalies. There is relatively little evidence that the mining and milling of this fibre in South Africa has produced many cases of the disease,[36] but workers in a large insulation products plant in New Jersey, which reputedly used amosite only, were badly affected.[37] For many years it was maintained that the high incidence of mesothelioma in North American insulation workers was due to the chrysotile content of insulation materials rather than to a high, or higher, content of amosite. This hypothesis was less easy to sustain in the light of experience in the New Jersey plant and controlled lung burden studies in North America which have shown an amosite excess of similar order to that for crocidolite.[38] Two of the lung burden studies indicated that discrimination between cases and controls rested on fibres more than $8\mu m$ in length, with little or no contribution from shorter fibres.[38 39]

The remaining amphibole asbestos fibre types—anthophyllite and tremolite—have always been of minor commercial value and have received correspondingly little epidemiological investigation. Anthophyllite, mined and milled only in Finland, and now no longer, has produced few if any cases of mesothelioma.[40] Fibrous tremolite is widespread in the earth's crust but mined commercially only on a limited scale. With the exception of small cohorts of mine workers in Montana engaged in the exploitation of a vermiculite deposit heavily contaminated with fibres in the tremolite series there is little direct evidence that such exposure has caused mesothelioma.[8 9] On the other hand controlled studies of lung burden in Canada suggest that a large proportion of all cases are attributable to fibrous tremolite, probably as a contaminant of chrysotile, and perhaps other minerals.[37]

The tremolite question

The extensive programme of epidemiological research in Quebec chrysotile miners and millers begun in 1965 was conducted largely because it was believed that exposure in that industry was to chrysotile only. While investigating the uneven distribution of pleural changes among workers in the various mines and mills, Gibbs was probably the first to suggest that the explanation might lie with minerals other than chrysotile.[41] Some years earlier, when Pooley examined by electron microscopy lung tissue taken at necropsy from a small number of former miners, chrysotile and tremolite fibres were seen in surprisingly similar concentrations.[42] More systematic examination soon raised the question of the extent to which the fibrogenic and carcinogenic consequences of exposure were attributable to tremolite, chrysotile, or both.[43] The fact that tremolite fibre may have greater durability or ability to penetrate the lung has little epidemiological significance unless there is also evidence of greater pathogenicity.[31] That this may be so was shown in a small cohort of 406 vermiculite miners and millers in Montana where among 165 deaths there was a substantial excess of lung cancer and four probably due to mesothelioma.[7] There is, however, no certainty that the fibres to which these workers were exposed, although classified mineralogically as in the tremolite series, were biologically the same as those found in association with Quebec chrysotile. In the cohort of male Quebec miners and millers, some 10 000 of whom were alive in 1930, 33 cases of mesothelioma were identified among over 7000 deaths before 1989,[44] Of these, five were from a small asbestos products factory where commercial amphiboles had also been used and the remaining 28 were miners and millers, 20 being from the region of Thetford Mines and eight from the large mine in nearby Asbestos. There is reason to believe that the proportion of tremolite in asbestos was 2–3 times higher in the former than the latter but it remains uncertain whether tremolite contributed to this apparent difference in risk.[44]

The question of whether and to what extent malignant mesothelioma occurred before the industrial exploitation of asbestos is of considerable scientific interest. Without this knowledge it is possible only to assess the absolute and not the attributable risk of the disease under specified conditions of exposure. Evidence recently reviewed suggests that there is and has been a background incidence of the disease, low in childhood, but rising with age and perhaps more common in men than in women.[45] The cause of these background cases is not known.

Crystalline silica

Background

Crystalline silica occurs in nature in several forms (or polymorphs); the best known of which are quartz, cristobalite and tridyimite. The first is by far the most common, and is widely distributed in metamorphic rock; the other two varieties are relatively rare and comprise about 5% and 1% of the total, respectively, but may be produced when quartz or amorphous silica are heated to a high temperature. Amorphous silica is similarly distributed and in roughly equal quantities; it is not known to have any adverse health effects and will not be discussed further here. For the sake of brevity, and unless otherwise indicated, the word silica will be used in the rest of this review to connote the crystalline varieties. Silica dust is one of the oldest and most serious occupational hazards known to man, with destructive and fibrotic effects on the lung which have been recognised though not precisely defined since metal mining began, perhaps even among tool makers in the stone age. Silicosis and silico-tuberculosis, under conditions of uncontrolled dust, were rapidly progressive and often fatal which, together with many other dangers, was the reason that in early times mining was not an occupation for free men, a view discernible even to this day. Exposure to silica in metal mining is in a sense accidental but with the exploitation of sandstone as a building material, as an abrasive and in the manufacture of glass it became inherent; this is increasingly so in the many uses of silica for its specific properties throughout modern industry.

Despite occupational health legislation and the application of increasingly strict measures of dust control, silicosis still remains a fairly common disease, but during the past decade the question of lung cancer has unexpectedly been raised again. It is indeed curious that as the fibrogenic effects of silica exposure have decreased in incidence and severity, this carcinogenic possibility should come into prominence, particularly in workers with silicosis. The somewhat analogous situation, which arose with asbestos in the 1930s coincided with the developing epidemic of tobacco-related lung cancer; for silica, the comparable phase was in the 1980s when the latter epidemic was already at its peak. Before that time it was generally believed that, if anything, workers exposed to silica had less than their share of lung cancer. An extensive review of studies undertaken mainly between 1950 and 1970, published in 1984 by Heppleston, supported this point of view.[46] The evidence then available was derived mainly from large necropsy series in gold, iron and coal miners in South Africa and Western Europe and from statistical analyses of mortality in a variety of occupational groups exposed to silica. These studies showed little or no association between malignant tumours and the presence or severity of silicotic changes in the lung at necropsy. The variation observed in lung cancer mortality by occupation appeared better related to the varied distribution of such recognised carcinogens as radon, arsenic, and polycyclic hydrocarbons than to silica.

The need for reassessment of the question came in 1982 with a paper by Goldsmith et al. entitled "Does occupational exposure to silica cause lung cancer."[47] There followed a conference in 1984, proceedings of which were published in 1986, where a considerable number of studies, some negative but a larger number positive, were presented.[48] In consequence of this controversy and its important implications, an expert working group met in Lyon in 1986 under the auspices of the International Agency for Research on Cancer (IARC). After a comprehensive review of the published reports then available the group concluded that although evidence for carcinogenicity in experimental animals was *sufficient*, in man it was *limited*.[49] In IARC parlance this implied that a causal interpretation was credible, but that chance, bias, and confounding could not be excluded. This cautious conclusion stemmed largely from the fact that occupational exposure to silica has nearly always included other carcinogens, such as asbestos, radon, metals, and polycyclic hydrocarbons and that evidence from studies of people compensated for silicosis was susceptible to various sources of bias, in particular to unrepresentative case selection. Nevertheless, the IARC later assigned the overall classification of crystalline silica to 2A—probably carcinogenic to humans.[50] It may be useful to examine the epidemiological evidence before and since the IARC working group met in 1986. The studies fall into two categories, those primarily concerned with the carcinogenic effects of occupational exposure to crystalline silica dust and those that sought to establish whether silicosis predisposed to lung cancer. Both silicosis and lung cancer may be caused by many factors other than or in addition to silica exposure so an association between them would not in itself necessarily imply cause and effect.

Silica exposure and lung cancer

For a summary of the many papers considered by the working group in Lyon in 1986 the reader is referred to IARC Monographs Volume 42;[49] among these, seven cohort and two case control studies, listed in table 5.3, were the more convincing attempts to assess the impact of silica exposure alone. All but three of these studies were in gold or other metal miners, two were in pottery or ceramic workers, and one in members of a granite cutters union. Data from five substantial cohort studies are shown, two in the same gold mine in South Dakota and one each in gold or metal miners in Western Australia, Ontario and the North West Cape Province of South Africa.

The study in Western Australia by Armstrong *et al.* was based mainly on available records of a health survey of 1974 gold miners conducted in 1961–62.[52] Almost all had 10 years or more mining experience, mostly underground, and about two thirds were cigarette smokers. By 1976, 500 of the gold miners were dead, 59 from respiratory cancer (standardised mortality ratio (SMR) 140) and 15 from pneumoconiosis or tuberculosis (SMR 455). Respiratory cancer mortality was about 40% higher in those who had worked underground and 13% higher in men with radiographic evidence of silicosis, but risk was not related to duration of exposure.

Analysis of 6757 deaths, 1955–1977, among 50 201 metal miners in Ontario was reported in 1983 by Müller *et al.*[54] Excess mortality from silicosis, silico-tuberculosis and cancer of the respiratory tract was

Table 5.3 Selected studies published before 1988 on silica exposure and lung cancer

Reference	Country	Study design	Industry	Lung cancer risk	Comments
McDonald et al., 1978[51]	USA	cohort	gold mining	SMR 1·03	see below*
Armstrong et al., 1979[52]	Australia	cohort	gold mining	SMR 1·40	unrelated to duration of exposure
Thomas, 1982[53]	USA	proportional mortality	potteries	PMR 1·21	excess almost all in sanitary ware
Müller et al., 1983[54]	Canada	cohort	metal mining	SMR 1·45	excess in gold, uranium and mixed ore; not in nickel, copper or iron
Wyndham et al., 1986[55]	RSA	cohort	gold mining	SMR 1·61	in case-referent analysis smoking identified as main factor
Brown et al., 1986[56]	USA	cohort	gold mining	SMR 1·00	see below*
Hessel et al., 1986[57]	RSA	case-referent	gold mining	no increase	limited power
Steenland & Beaumont, 1986[58]	USA	proportional mortality	granite	PMR 1·19	unrelated to duration of employment
Forestiere et al., 1987[59]	Italy	case-referent	ceramics	RR 2·0	with silicosis 3·9; without silicosis 1·4

* Same mine; substantial mortality from silica-related diseases

observed in miners of gold, uranium and mixed ore but not of nickel, copper, or iron. In non-uranium miners, excess deaths from malignant and non-malignant respiratory disease were confined to gold mining. In 1991, some years after the Lyon conference, further data and analyses were reported by Kusiak et al.[60] These investigators concluded that, mainly because of dose-response relationships, exposures to arsenic and radon were to blame, rather than crystalline silica.

A similar study by Wyndham et al.[55] of 3971 white South African gold miners also showed a substantial lung cancer excess (SMR 1·61) but after further analysis the authors concluded that smoking rather than mining exposure was probably responsible. The results from three further studies of the same working population, the first published in 1986[57] (see table 5.3), and the other two in 1990[61] and 1991[62] are difficult to interpret. The first two were analyses of intensity and duration of silica exposure in cases of primary lung cancer, almost all confirmed by necropsy, compared with deaths from other causes closely matched for age and smoking habit. These studies showed no association of exposure with lung cancer but, with pulmonary fibrosis, defined radiographically and pathologically, the relationship was clear. As against this, a study of a second cohort selected from the same work-force by some of the same investigators in 1991 showed a significant correlation between death from lung cancer and particle-years of silica exposure standardised for age and smoking.[62] However, further analyses have since revealed that only cases of small cell type were related to respirable silica exposure; as cases of this type were not associated with silicosis alone, the authors suggest that radiation may have been the responsible factor.[63]

Arising out of a national silicosis survey in the USA, 1958–61, and some suggestive findings from a small cohort study by Gillam et al. of underground workers in a South Dakota gold mine, two larger and partially overlapping investigations were undertaken in the same population.[64] The first of these was a cohort mortality study by McDonald et al. of 1321 men with 21 years or more employment reported in 1978.[51] The results showed a considerable excess in all cause mortality (SMR 1·15), wholly due to benign silica-related cardiorespiratory diseases, systematically related to estimated silica exposure but with no overall excess from lung cancer (Observed 17, Expected 16·5). Later, a larger study of 3328 full-time underground workers reported by Brown et al. in 1986, with more extensive data on dust exposure, showed closely similar findings.[56] The all cause mortality was again raised (SMR 1·12), largely explained by non-malignant respiratory disease, but again there was no excess of lung cancer (Observed 43, Expected 42·9). There was thus close independent confirmation of the earlier study, despite suspected exposure in the mine to low levels of arsenic and radon.

Among several studies in granite workers was an analysis by Steenland

and Beaumont of mortality, 1949–1982, in members of the US Granite Cutters Union.[58] Of 2274 deaths, the certified cause was obtained for 1911 (84%) and their proportional mortality was compared with that for the USA with due allowance for age. There was a large excess mortality from silicosis and silico-tuberculosis but only a small non-significant increase in lung cancer (Observed 97, Expected 81·1, PMR 1·19). Although the lung cancer mortality was unrelated to duration of employment, there was evidence from a case-control analysis of an association with silicosis as recorded on death certificates.

A similar analysis of proportional mortality among members of the US Potters and Allied Workers Union was reported by Thomas in 1982.[53] Tuberculosis as a cause of death was grossly in excess (Observed 62, Expected 18·3), and to lesser degree other non-malignant respiratory diseases (Observed 268, Expected 173·7). There was also some excess of lung cancer (Observed 178, Expected 146·6; PMR 1·21), almost entirely explained by work in the sanitary ware divisions (Observed 62, Expected 34·4) where non fibrous talc was also used.

A case-referent study was conducted by Forestiere et al. among the male residents of a small town in central Italy where pottery was the predominant industry and sanitary ware and crockery the main product.[59] Silica exposure was known to be heavy, but talc and chromates were also used. The case series comprised 84 subjects certified to have died of carcinoma of the lung in the period 1968–1984. A total of 334 referents, four for each case, were selected from the same source of people who died from other causes, matched for age and year of death. Work histories and smoking habits were sought blind for each subject by three nurses and all names were checked against the official register of people compensated for silicosis. The ratio of cases to referents for ceramic work, standardised for age, smoking and period of death was 2·0 (95% CI: 1·1 to 3·5)–1·4 (95% CI: 0·7 to 2·8) without silicosis and 3·9 (95% CI: 1·8 to 8·3) with silicosis; the corrected ratio for quarry work was 1·0. Thirty five deaths from pneumoconiosis or chronic bronchitis had been excluded from the referent series, on the grounds that silica might have been a contributory factor. Had these cases not been removed, the standardised rate ratio for ceramic work would have been reduced to 1·5 (95% CI: 0·9 to 2·6), that for silicosis would also have been reduced but have remained significant (2·1, 95% CI: 1·0 to 4·4).[65]

Among more recent studies, results of which were not available to the IARC working group in 1986 (see table 5.4), was one of a series by Koskela et al. on mortality in 1026 employees of granite quarries in Finland where, by the end of 1985, 296 had died.[66] Deaths from silicosis and non-malignant respiratory disease were in excess (observed 40, expected 15·7) as were those from lung cancer (observed 31, expected 19·9; SMR 15·6). Gastrointestinal cancers were also in excess (observed 18,

101

Table 5.4 *Selected studies published since 1987 on silica exposure and lung cancer*

Reference	Country	Study design	Industry	Lung cancer risk	Comments
Kusiak et al., 1991[60]	Canada	cohort	gold mining	SMR 1·29	attributed to arsenic and radon exposure
Hessel et al., 1990[61]	RSA	case-referent	gold mining	RR 1·1	no association with either silicosis at necropsy or cumulative silica exposure
Hnizdo and Sluis-Cremer, 1991[62]	RSA	cohort	gold mining	RR 1·02	per 1000 particle years; excess confined to small cell cancers, possibly attributable to radiation (63)
Koskela et al., 1990[66]	Finland	cohort	granite quarries	SMR 1·56	substantial deficiency of cancer at other sites
Thomas, 1990[67]	USA	cohort	potteries	SMR 1·43	deficiency of cancer at other sites
Winter et al., 1990[68]	UK	cohort	potteries	SMR 1·32	SMR=1·32 against local rates; some deficiency of cancer at other sites
Amandus and Costello, 1991[69]	USA	cohort	metal mining	SMR 1·23	silicotics 1·73; non-silicotics 1·18; other causes of death not reported
Merlo et al., 1991[70]	Italy	cohort	refractory brick manufacture	SMR 1·51	risk increased with years since first employment
Carta et al., 1992[71]	Italy	cohort	metal mining	SMR 1·12	ns; risk higher in those with lower silica but higher radon exposures
McLaughlin et al., 1992[72]	China	case-referent	metal mining and potteries	not stated	complex pattern of results providing "only limited support for an aetiological association"
Checkoway et al., 1993[73]	USA	cohort	diatomaceous earth	SMR 1·43	RR increased steadily with exposure to silica (mainly cristobalite)
Cherry et al., 1993[74]	UK	cohort	potteries	SMR 1·91	SMR 1·28 against local rates

expected 11·5) and there was an unexplained deficiency of cancers at other sites (observed 10, expected 22·9. A similar type of deficiency was observed in two other studies, both in pottery workers. In the first of these from the USA (64), the SMR for lung cancer was 1·43 (observed 52, expected 36·4) but at other anatomic sites there were 72 cancer deaths against 85·7 expected. In the second study, from the UK, the SMR for lung cancer was 1·32 and for gastro-intestinal cancer 1·14 and again there was some deficiency at other sites (observed 28, expected 35·8).[65]

Some recent studies reported by Merlo et al.[70] and Checkoway et al.[73] provide rather stronger evidence. The study by Merlo et al. was of a cohort of 1022 men employed for six months or more in an Italian factory engaged in the manufacture of refractory bricks from crystalline silica. There was no evidence of exposure to asbestos or polycyclic hydrocarbons in the plant. By the end of 1986, 243 (24%) had died; 732 (72%) were alive and 47 (5%) were lost to follow-up. Analysis of mortality by cause showed a significant excess of respiratory tract cancer (observed 33; expected 21·9; SMR 1·51) and of non-malignant respiratory disease (observed 40; expected 16·6; SMR 2·41). The data were insufficient, however, for adequate examination of the contribution of cigarette smoking or for analysis of risk in relation to level of exposure.

The cohort of Checkoway et al. comprised 2570 white men employed for one year or more in the mining and heat processing of diatomaceous earth in California, where the predominant exposure was to the product, cristobalite.[73] By the end of 1987, 628 deaths were observed from all causes (SMR 1·12), 59 from lung cancer (SMR 1·43) and 77 from non-malignant respiratory disease (SMR 2·27); cancer deaths at other sites were close to expectation (73, SMR 0·92). An approximate index of cumulative exposure was calculated from measures of duration, estimates of intensity and opinions as to the effectiveness of respirator use. Parallel trends in relative risk against this index were found for lung cancer and non-malignant respiratory disease. These findings support the conclusion that cristobalite exposure was causally related to the lung cancer excess but rather less convincing evidence for the gradients in exposure-responses. It seems unlikely that cigarette smoking was an important confounder in this study, but there remains some question as to whether sufficient account was taken of possible exposure to asbestos in the plant. It is clear that even after allowance for excess deaths attributed to lung cancer (17·6) and non-malignant respiratory disease there was no deficiency in deaths from other causes (567, SMR 1·01).[73] Of the remaining studies in table 5.4 that by Amandus and Costello showed a small excess of lung cancer (SMR 1·23) in US metal miners largely among men with silicosis, but no data were reported on deaths from other causes.[69]

Among the negative studies, that by Carta et al. of two rather small cohorts of Sardinian metal miners was quite convincing.[71] In one mine where exposure to quartz was high but low to radon there was no lung cancer excess whereas in the other mine where the exposure pattern was reversed the SMR was raised, although not significantly so. Findings from a case-control analysis based on a cohort of 68 285 pottery and metal mine workers in China were complex and seriously confounded by exposures to arsenic, polycyclic hydrocarbons, and radon.[72] In pottery workers risk of lung cancer was related to silica but not to silicosis and the dose-response gradient showed no significant trend. Preliminary findings from a recent cohort mortality study of some 5000 British pottery workers gave an SMR for lung cancer of 1·91 against national rates falling, but still significantly raised, against local rates (SMR 1·28; 90% CI: 1·04 to 1·57).[74]

An emerging source of speculation concerns possible differences in the toxicity and carcinogenicity of quartz, cristobalite, and tridyimite. It has always been suspected that quartz was less fibrogenic than the other two varieties, both of which result from exposure of silica to high temperatures. It is thus of interest that the strongest evidence of carcinogenicity has been associated with refractory brick and cristobalite production, rather than mining and quarrying. Resolution of this question will depend on detailed analyses of dust and exposure response.

Silicosis and lung cancer

Studies of the association between silicosis and lung cancer, whether cohort or case-referent, provide evidence at two levels. Most reliable are the studies in which the cases of silicosis are ascertained by some objective screening procedure; much less reliable are studies in which the identification of cases is subject to self-selection or to potentially biased judgement. In the latter category are all studies based on compensated cases of silicosis. There are many reasons why a person may or may not be compensated for an occupational disease and case series derived from compensation registers can seldom, if ever, be considered representative of all cases which have occurred as a result of a given exposure. Of 13 epidemiological surveys of people with silicosis reviewed by the IARC Working Group in 1986, and seven reported more recently, only one, that of Amandus et al. was possibly free from this type of potential bias.[75] In this study of silicosis ascertained radiographically among silica exposed workers routinely examined by the Industrial Commission for North Carolina an SMR of 2·6 for lung cancer was observed. Even so, the Commission had also available a questionnaire which included work history, medical symptoms, and smoking habits and could well have used this additional information in making a diagnosis. The effects of selection bias inherent in studies of people compensated for silicosis were discussed in the paper by Infante-Rivard et al., in particular the increased cancer risk if compensation was associated with cigarette smoking.[76] However, the problem is not simply a matter of smoking level, but that men whose smoking has led to respiratory symptoms may be more likely to seek compensation. Other mechanisms that might possibly link lung cancer, silicosis and smoking have been reviewed by Swaen and Meijers who presented evidence that heavy smoking considerably increased the risk of silicosis in Dutch ceramic workers.[77] In a large study of nearly 7000 Ontario dust exposed workers Finkelstein[78] found that smokers were about 50% more likely to develop silicosis than non-smokers (relative risk 1·45; 90% CI: one tailed 1·04 to 2·04).[78]

Man-made mineral fibres

Production and exposure

Asbestos fibres and crystalline silica exist in forms that are naturally limited both mineralogically and in physicochemical characteristics. Whatever the health effects to date of exposure to man-made mineral fibres (MMMF), industrial ingenuity and demand put virtually no limit on the variety of fibres that could be produced and for which there would be a market. Herein lies the potential danger of these fibres, particularly with regard to diseases of long latency, such as cancer. As it is hardly acceptable to wait to see whether a problem develops 30 years later, ongoing cooperation between epidemiological and toxicological research is therefore mandatory.

Before considering the epidemiological evidence the nature, production, and uses of man-made mineral fibres need to be understood. As these are highly technical subjects, reference should be made to the appropriate sections of IARC Monograph Volume 43[79] and to Dodgson et al.[80] A brief description may nevertheless be helpful. From early beginnings in south Wales in the 1840s, production of fibrous wool from rock and slag reached a commercial scale in Britain, Germany and the USA by the end of the last century and accelerated after the first world war. The manufacture of wool and filaments from glass began in the 1930s and of ceramic fibres in the 1940s. In Europe, the term "mineral wool" is applied whatever the material, whereas in the USA a distinction is made between mineral (rock or slag) wool and glass wool. The range of minerals used is wide; for example, in one Swedish plant, some 60 varieties of rock and slag were used over a 10 year period, some containing potentially hazardous substances such as arsenic and asbestiform fibres.[81] Almost equally varied are the sources of energy used to bring these raw materials to a molten state, and the fibre dimensions which result from the various production processes.

From the epidemiological point of view it is important to recognize that in the early days of this industry rock and slag wool were generally produced in small, dirty, and dusty plants and entailed exposure of the employees to many potentially carcinogenic agents. On the other hand the more recent manufacture of glass and ceramic fibres and filaments has more usually been in large, clean, modern factories. The health effects of exposure to rock and slag wool may therefore tend to reflect the chemical composition of raw materials and of contaminants during production whereas with glass and ceramic fibres, size and physical qualities might well be factors of relatively greater importance. Ceramic fibres are mostly 2–4 μm in diameter and are usually produced by blowing or spinning high temperature melts of alumina and silica, with further additives for use at very high temperatures. High performance ceramic fibres are manufactured for specified purposes from pure silica and from a variety of oxides, carbides and nitrides of boron, silicon, aluminium and zirconium.

Occupational exposure to man-made mineral fibres can occur in their production or in any one of the innumerable places where they are used. These exposures are generally at much lower concentrations than occur, even today, in the production and use of asbestos. These levels vary enormously and lack any clear pattern related to type of work or type of fibre, but usually they are several fold higher with rock or slag wool than with glass fibre.[82]

Early epidemiological evidence

With the exception of a few small studies almost all that is known about the carcinogenic risks of man-made mineral fibres has been obtained from two major multicentre cohort mortality surveys, one in the USA and one in Europe. The results from these investigations were presented for discussion at two international conferences in Copenhagen, the first in 1982 on mortality mainly to the end of 1977[83] and the second in 1986 after follow-up to the end of 1982.[84] Previously, five well-designed but small cohort studies of American production workers had been published between 1975 and 1982. None of these showed any important lung cancer excess; however, there were only 69 deaths from this cause in all, against 73·6 expected, among 1169 deaths (all causes).[85] Given the limited size of these cohorts, and the low exposure levels prevailing in man-made mineral fibre production plants, only high risks would have been detectable.

Copenhagen 1982

Of the four cohort mortality analyses presented at this conference, that conducted by Enterline and Marsh carried the greatest weight.[86] Their cohort comprised 16 730 men employed for six to 12 months during the years 1945–63 in 17 of America's oldest and largest mineral fibre production plants, eleven of which manufactured fibrous glass and six mineral wool. Using various methods, vital status was established for 98% of the cohort to the end of 1977 and cause of death ascertained for 3653 (97%) of the 3761 known to have died. Environmental surveys were conducted to help estimate the fibre concentrations to which cohort members had been exposed over their years of employment and cumulative exposures were calculated for each man. Compared with fibre concentrations experienced by asbestos workers, these exposures were low—0·059 fibres per cubic metre in the fibrous glass plants and 0·352 in mineral wool production. Duration of employment averaged 11·2 years in the former and 11·1 years in the latter. For fibrous glass workers, SMRs calculated against mortality rates for the US white population were: all causes, 96·2; respiratory cancer, 99·3; and non-malignant respiratory disease, 105·4. For mineral wool workers the corresponding figures were 106·6, 160·1 and 117·1. Although the SMRs for respiratory cancer 20–29 and 30 or more years from first employment respectively were 98·4 and 130·4 for fibrous glass and 145·8 and 172·7 for mineral wool, there was little evidence that risk was related to accumulated exposure or to duration of employment in either group. No death from mesothelioma was confirmed in the entire cohort.

The second major study was that reported by Saracci *et al.* on the mortality of a cohort of 20 766 men and 4380 women employed in seven rock wool, six glass wool and two continuous filament factories in seven European countries.[87] These subjects were followed from first employment until at least the end of 1977, but to the end of 1978 in two plants, and to the end of 1979 in two others. The mean duration of employment in the 13 factories ranged from 2·3 to 11·3 years—overall 5·1 years—and, as in the American study, environmental surveys had been conducted to estimate exposure intensities. The average respirable fibre concentrations/m^3 were stated to have been approximately 0·04 in the rock wool plants, 0·02 in the glass wool plants and 0·006 in the continuous filament plants. Despite the large size of this cohort, of which only 3% were lost to follow-up, the total number of deaths available for analysis was only 1609—1505 in men and 154 in women. In men overall, SMRs were: all causes 90·3, lung cancer (ICD 162, 163) 102·6, and non-malignant respiratory disease 85·4; deaths in women were too few to be meaningful. In men, further analyses by type of fibre were inconclusive but, for lung cancer, the risk appeared slightly higher in the production of rock wool (SMR 111) than of glass wool or filament (SMR 103); overall, the SMR 30 or more years after first employment was raised (SMR 193), though not to a significant extent.

The findings from two smaller cohorts of glass fibre production workers were also reported at the 1982 Conference. One in the USA, by Morgan *et al.*,[88] was based on 294 deaths to the end of 1977 in 4399 men; there were 37 deaths from lung cancer (SMR 135), 11 in men with 20 years' employment and 30 years' latency (SMR 177). Neither of these SMRs was statistically significant. The second cohort study by Shannon *et al.* was from Ontario where 2576 men were identified and 97·2% were traced to the end of 1977.[89] Only seven lung cancer deaths were observed in

Table 5.5 *Observed deaths and SMRs for respiratory cancer (ICD 160–163) by process, average exposure and time since first exposure. American plants*[92]

Process	Average exposure (fibres/cm³)	<20 yr				20+yr	
		Observed	SMR 1	SMR 2	Observed	SMR 1	SMR 2
Fibrous glass filament	0·011	15	64·9	66·2	49	110·7	105·2
Fibrous glass wool	0·033	27	97·4	104·2	52	109·8	110·8
Fibrous glass, both	0·059	33	92·9	105·6	155	129·5†	110·6
Mineral wool	0·352	15	155·9	142·6	45	146·1*	130·8

SMR 1 based on US expected deaths. SMR 2 based on local expected deaths
† P < 0·01
* P < 0·05

production workers against 4·22 expected. Finally, a study by Engholm *et al.* of Swedish construction workers, although of considerable size, was preliminary in nature and seriously confounded by uncertainty over the nature of their exposure.[90] Thus, in 1982, the need was clear for more conclusive evidence than was then available, and there was general agreement that the major cohorts should be followed for a longer period.

Copenhagen 1986

At this second conference, data were presented on mortality in the US and European MMMF cohorts to the end of 1982, in the Canadian cohort to the end of 1984 and from an intensive analysis of the large Swedish cohort of construction workers. Results from the Canadian study gave a significantly high SMR for lung cancer (observed 21; SMR 176), concentrated in production workers 15 or more years from first employment.[91] The Swedish study, despite its size—135 000 subjects observed for 10 to 12 years—was again inconclusive, due mainly to the high correlation between man-made mineral fibre and asbestos exposure. Again, therefore, data from the two major multicentre surveys provided the main source of evidence.

In the American survey the same high levels of tracing (98%) and ascertainment of cause of death (97%) were maintained and by the end of 1982, 4986 men or 30% of the original cohort had died.[92] Observed deaths and SMRs for causes of main interest are presented in table 5.5 by era and type of plant. Two measures of risk are shown: SMR 1 is based on expected deaths from US national statistics and SMR 2 on deaths expected from rates in counties selected to reflect the distribution of cohort members by home address. In general, the SMRs were lower when based on local mortality rates. The pattern was greatly confused by considerable variation between individual plants; the authors, commenting on the importance of one particular plant, stated that "the overall study is being driven to some extent by the experience of Plant 9." The importance of another plant (Plant 17) was later demonstrated in a study of lung dust analyses at autopsy from cohort members. In this plant, which had a high lung cancer SMR (200) and a probable mesothelioma, amosite at > 1·0 fibres per microgram was found in four of six workers examined but in none of their matched controls.[93]

In the European study, where the follow-up was also extended to the end of 1982, the results were similar to those from the US.[94] Lung cancer mortality was increased above expectation in both rock or slag wool and glass wool production, particularly among subjects 20 or more years from first employment. These findings are summarised in table 5.6, again analysed against both national and local mortality rates. SMRs for glass wool workers, based on local rates, were appreciably higher than those based on national rates but for rock or slag wool workers there was little

Table 5.6 Observed deaths and SMRs for lung cancer (ICD 162) by process, average exposure and time since first exposure. European plants[94]

Process	Average exposure[a] (fibres/cm³)	<20 year			20 + year		
		Observed	SMR 1	SMR 2	Observed	SMR 1	SMR 2
Continuous filament	not stated	15	145·6	115·4	0	–	–
Glass wool	0·03	47	116·6	95·3	46	139·0[b]	111·3
Rock/slag wool	0·06[c]	47	114·4	114·4	34	140·0[b]	140·0[b]

SMR 1 based on national expected deaths. SMR 2 based on local expected deaths.
[a] approximate values based on Dodgson et al. 1987[80]
[b] p < 0·05
[c] much higher in the early technological phase

difference between the two. The substantial excess observed in the latter group was largely concentrated in men employed during the early years of production from slag when fibre levels were probably higher but exposure may also have included arsenic or furnace fumes. As in the American study there was no evidence of a mesothelioma risk, only one case being observed in a man employed for less than one year who died 13 years after first exposure.

The interpretation of these various studies based on cohorts exposed for the most part to low airborne fibre concentrations is difficult. It is unlikely that men with similar levels of exposure to asbestos, even in textile manufacture, would show more convincing evidence of a lung cancer risk than was observed in either the American or European man-made mineral fibre cohorts. The problem is increased by the use of SMRs calculated against both local and national mortality rates without clear indication of which is the more appropriate. The general tendency for the observed risks to be related to time since first exposure cannot be ignored, nor confidently attributed to other exposures in the more distant past, as these were also times when fibre concentrations were higher. After review of the available evidence, the IARC concluded in 1988 that with the exception of glass filaments, which were not classifiable, glass wool, rock wool, slag wool and ceramic fibres were all possibly carcinogenic to humans.[95] This conclusion was reached without data on exposure in man to ceramic fibres, but whatever uncertainty remains regarding lung cancer there has so far been no sign whatever of a link between man-made mineral fibre exposure and mesothelioma, although this would certainly have been noted had cohorts of this size been exposed to similar concentrations of amphibole fibres. Even for lung cancer serious questions have been raised as to the validity of the evidence for cause and effect.[96]

Conclusions

The three groups of mineral dust considered in this review, each of major economic and industrial importance, have collectively and perhaps individually been the object of more intense epidemiological research over the past 40 years than any other agents in the workplace. Within each group the constituent elements vary considerably in their chemical and physical characteristics but exposure to respirable concentrations of all three carries at least the possible risk of lung cancer. With all types of asbestos fibre the risk is definite, for crystalline silica increasingly probable, but with man-made mineral fibres it remains less certain. The clear interaction between asbestos and cigarette smoking, the variation with industrial process and the concentration of risk in persons with pulmonary fibrosis, whether related to asbestos fibre or silica particles, all suggest that in the absence of these additional circumstances their carcinogenicity is low, even doubtful. In contrast, the clear ability of fine amphibole fibres—crocidolite and tremolite in particular—to cause malignant mesothelial tumours in the absence of pulmonary fibrosis or any obvious co-carcinogen, implies that these fibres possess qualities which are inherently hazardous. Both epidemiological and experimental findings point to fibre dimensions and long term durability in biological tissues as the main determinants. Since the carcinogenicity of asbestiform fibres and crystalline silica particles is almost certainly related to intensity and duration of exposure, quite probably with an effective threshold, these risks should be controllable. It is almost anomalous, therefore, that man-made mineral fibres, so far without proven risk of lung cancer and none whatever of mesothelioma, deserve nevertheless to be regarded with continuing caution. It is unfortunately not beyond the power of humans to create elongated inorganic particles which approximate even more closely to the requirements for maximal risk than crocidolite, or even fibrous erionite.[49] It is to be hoped that it will never be the task of epidemiology to show that this warning too should have been taken more seriously.

1 Lynch KM, Smith WA. Pulmonary asbestosis III: Carcinoma of the lung in asbestos-silicosis. *Am J Cancer* 1935; 24: 56–64.
2 Gloyne SR. Two cases of squamous carcinoma of the lung occurring in asbestosis. *Tubercle* 1935; 17: 5–10.
3 Doll R. Mortality from lung cancer in asbestos workers. *Br J Ind Med* 1955; 12: 81–6.
4 Breslow L. Industrial aspects of bronchogenic neoplasms. *Dis Chest* 1955; 28: 421–30.
5 McDonald JC. Cancer risks due to asbestos and man-made fibres. In: Band P, ed. *Recent results in cancer research*. Vol 120, Berlin-Heidelberg, Springer-Verlag. 1990: 122–31.
6 McDonald JC, Liddell FDK, Gibbs GW, Eyssen G, McDonald AD. Dust exposure and mortality in chrysotile mining, 1910–75. *Br J Ind Med* 1980; 37: 11–24.
7 McDonald JC, McDonald AD, Armstrong B, Sébastien P. Cohort study of mortality of vermiculite miners exposed to tremolite. *Br J Ind Med* 1986; 43: 436–44.
8 Amandus HE, Wheeler R. The morbidity and mortality of vermiculite miners exposed to tremolite-actinolite: Part II Mortality. *Am J Ind Med* 1987; 11: 15–26.
9 Armstrong BK, DeKlerk NH, Musk AW, Hobbs MST. Cancer mortality in relation to measures of occupational exposure to crocidolite at Wittenoom Gorge in Western Australia. *Br J Ind Med* 1988; 46: 529–36.
10 Dement JM, Harris RL, Symons MJ, Shy C. Estimate of dose-response for respiratory cancer among chrysotile asbestos workers. *Ann Occup Hyg* 1982; 26: 869–87.
11 McDonald AD, Fry JS, Woolley AJ, McDonald JC. Dust exposure and mortality in an American chrysotile textile plant. *Br J Ind Med* 1983; 40: 361–7.
12 McDonald AD, Fry JS, Woolley AJ, McDonald JC. Dust exposure and mortality in an American factory using chrysotile, amosite and crocidolite in mainly textile manufacture. *Br J Ind Med* 1983; 40: 368–74.
13 Peto J, Doll R, Hermon C, Binns W, Clayton R, Goffe T. Relationship of mortality to measures of environmental asbestos pollution in an asbestos textile factory. *Ann Occup Hyg* 1985; 29: 305–55.
14 Henderson V, Enterline PE. Asbestos exposure: factors associated with excess cancer and respiratory disease mortality. *Ann NY Acad Sci* 1979; 330: 117–26.
15 Hughes JM, Weill H, Hammad YY. Mortality of workers employed in two asbestos cement manufacturing plants. *Br J Ind Med* 1987; 44: 161–74.

16 Berry G, Newhouse ML. Mortality of workers manufacturing friction materials using asbestos. *Br J Ind Med* 1983; **40**: 1–7.

17 McDonald AD, Fry JS, Woolley AJ, McDonald JC. Dust exposure and mortality in an American chrysotile friction products plant. *Br J Ind Med* 1984; **41**: 151–7.

18 Vacek PM, McDonald JC. Risk assessment using exposure intensity: an application to vermiculite mining. *Br J Ind Med* 1991; **48**: 543–7.

19 McDonald JC. An epidemiological view of asbestos in buildings. *Toxicol Ind Health* 1991; **7**: 187–93.

20 Sébastien P, McDonald JC, McDonald AD, Case BW, Harley R. Respiratory cancer in chrysotile textile and mining industries: exposure inferences from lung analysis. *Br J Ind Med* 1989; **46**: 180–7.

21 Selikoff IJ, Hammond EC, Churg J. Asbestos exposure, smoking, and neoplasia. *JAMA* 1968; **204**: 104–10.

22 Hammond EC, Selikoff IJ, Seidman H. Asbestos exposure, cigarette smoking and death rates. *Ann NY Acad Sci* 1979; **330**: 473–90.

23 Berry G, Newhouse ML, Antonis P. Combined effects of asbestos exposure and smoking on mortality from lung cancer and mesothelioma in factory workers. *Br J Ind Med* 1985; **42**: 12–8.

24 Martischnig M, Newell DJ, Barnsley WR, Cowan WK, Feinmann EL, Oliver E. Unsuspected exposure to asbestos and bronchogenic cancer. *BMJ* 1977; **1**: 746–9.

25 Hughes JM, Weill H. Asbestosis as a precursor of asbestos related lung cancer: results of a prospective mortality study. *Br J Ind Med* 1991; **48**: 229–33.

26 Sluis-Cremer GK, Beziudenhout BN. Relation between asbestosis and bronchial cancer in amphibole asbestos miners. *Br J Ind Med* 1989; **46**: 537–40.

27 Liddell FDK, Thomas DC, Gibbs GW, McDonald JC. Fibre exposure and mortality from pneumoconiosis, respiratory and abdominal malignancies in chrysotile production in Quebec, 1926–75. *Ann Acad Med Singapore* 1984; **13**(Supplement): 345–52.

28 Wilkinson P, Hansell DM, Janssens J, Rubens M, Rudd RM, Taylor AN, McDonald JC. Is lung cancer associated with asbestos exposure without small opacities on the chest radiograph? *Lancet* 1995; **345**: 1074–8.

29 Wagner JC, Sleggs CA, Marchand P. Diffuse pleural mesothelioma and asbestos exposure in the North Western Cape Province. *Br J Ind Med* 1960; **17**: 260–71.

30 McDonald JC. Health implications of environmental exposure to asbestos. *Environ Health Perspect* 1985; **62**: 319–28.

31 McDonald JC. Epidemiological significance of mineral fibre persistence in human lung tissue. *Environ Health Perspect* 1994; **102S5**: 221–4.

32 McDonald AD, McDonald JC. Malignant mesothelioma in North America. *Cancer* 1980; **46**: 1650–6.

33 McDonald JC, McDonald AD. Epidemiology of mesothelioma. In: Liddell D, Miller K, eds. *Mineral fibers and health.* Boca Raton: CRC Press, 147–68.

34 Newhouse ML, Thompson H. Mesothelioma of pleura and peritoneum following exposure to asbestos in the London area. *Br J Ind Med* 1965; **22**: 261–9.

35 Bohlig H, Dabbert AF, Dalquen P, Hain E, Hinz I. Epidemiology of malignant mesothelioma in Hamburg. A preliminary report. *Environ Res* 1970; **3**: 365–72.

36 Sluis-Cremer GK, Liddell FDK, Logan WPO, Bezuidenhout BV. The mortality of amphibole miners in South Africa, 1946–80. *BMJ* 1992; **49**: 566–75.

37 Seidman H, Selikoff IJ, Hammond EC. Short-term asbestos work exposure and long-term observation. *Ann NY Acad Sci* 1979; **330**: 61–89.

38 McDonald JC, Armstrong B, Case BW, Doell D, McCaughey WTE, McDonald AD, *et al.* Mesothelioma and asbestos fibre type: evidence from lung tissue analyses. *Cancer* 1989; **63**: 1544–7.

39 Rogers AJ, Leigh J, Berry G, Ferguson DA, Mulder HB, Ackad M. Relationship between lung asbestos fibre type and concentration and relative risk of mesothelioma. *Cancer* 1991; **67**: 1912–20.

40 Meurman LO, Kiviluoto R, Hakama M. Mortality and morbidity among the working population of anthophyllite asbestos miners in Finland. *Br J Ind Med* 1974; **31**: 105–12.

41 Gibbs GW. Etiology of pleural calcification: a study of chrysotile asbestos miners and millers. *Arch Environ Health* 1979; **34**: 76–83.

42 Pooley FD. An examination of the fibrous mineral content of asbestos lung tissue from the Canadian chrysotile mining industry. *Environ Res* 1976; **12**: 281–98.

43 Rowlands N, Gibbs GW, McDonald AD. Chrysotile fibres in the lungs of ex-asbestos miners and millers. *Ann Occup Hyg* 1981; **26**: 411–5.

44 McDonald JC, Liddell FDK, Dufresne A, McDonald AD. The 1891–1920 birth cohort of Quebec chrysotile miners and millers: mortality 1976–88. *Br J Ind Med* 1993; **50**: 1073–81.

45 McDonald JC, McDonald AD. Mesothelioma: is there a background? *Eur Respir Rev* 1993; **11**: 71–3.

46 Heppleston AG. Silica, pneumoconiosis, and carcinoma of the lung. *Am J Ind Med* 1985; **7**: 285–94.

47 Goldsmith DF, Guidotti TL, Johnston DR. Does occupational exposure to silica cause lung cancer? *Am J Ind Med* 1982; **3**: 423–40.

48 Goldsmith DF, Winn DM, Shy CM, eds. Silica, silicosis and cancer. *Controversy in occupational medicines*. New York: Praeger, 1986.

49 International Agency for Research on Cancer. Monographs on the evaluation of the carcinogenic risk of chemicals to humans. *Silica and some silicates*, Lyon: IARC 1987; Vol 42.

50 IARC Working Group on the Evaluation of Carcinogenic Risks to Humans. *Overall evaluations of carcinogenicity: an updating of IARC monographs*. Supplement 7, Lyon: WHO 1987; Vols 1–42.

51 McDonald JC, Gibbs GW, Liddell FDK, McDonald AD. Mortality after long exposure to cummingtonite-grunerite. *Am Rev Respir Dis* 1978; **118**: 271–7.

52 Armstrong BK, McNulty JC, Levitt LJ, Williams KA, Hobbs MST. Mortality in gold and coal miners in Western Australia with special reference to lung cancer. *Br J Ind Med* 1979; **36**: 199–205.

53 Thomas TL. A preliminary investigation of mortality among workers in the pottery industry. *Int J Epidemiol* 1982; **11**: 175–80.

54 Müller J, Wheeler WC, Gentleman JF, Suranyi G, Kusiak RA. *Study of mortality of Ontario miners, 1955–1977. Part 1*, Toronto: Ministry of Labour/Ontario Workers' Compensation Board/Atomic Energy Control Board of Canada, 1983.

55 Wyndham CH, Benzuidenhout BN, Greenacre MJ, Sluis-Cremer GK. Mortality of middle-aged white South African gold miners. *Br J Ind Med* 1986; **43**: 677–84.

56 Brown DP, Kalplan SD, Zumwalde RD, Kaplowitz M, Archer VE. Retrospective cohort mortality study of underground gold mine workers. In: Goldsmith DF, Winn DM, Shy CM, eds, *Silica, silicosis and cancer. Controversy in occupational medicine*. New York: Praeger, 1986: 335–50.

57 Hessel PA, Sluis-Cremer GK, Hnizdo E. Case-control study of silicosis, silica exposure and lung cancer in white South African gold miners. *Am J Ind Med* 1986; **10**: 57–62.

58 Steenland K, Beaumont J. A proportionate mortality study of granite cutters. *Am J Ind Med* 1986; **9**: 189–201.

59 Forastiere F, Lagorio S, Michelozzi P, Cavariani F, Arca M, Borgia P, *et al.* Silica, silicosis and lung cancer among ceramic workers: a case-referent study. *Am J Ind Med* 1986; **10**: 363–70.

60 Kusiak RA, Springer J, Ritchie AC, Muller J. Carcinoma of the lung in Ontario gold miners. *Br J Ind Med* 1991; **48**: 808–17.

61 Hessel PA, Sluis-Cremer GK, Hnizdo E. Silica exposure, silicosis, and lung cancer: a necropsy study. *Br J Ind Med* 1990; **47**: 4–9.

62 Hnizdo E, Sluis-Cremer GK. Silica exposure, silicosis and lung cancer. *Br J Ind Med* 1991; **48**: 53–60.

63 Hnizdo E, Murray J, Klempman S. Histological type of lung cancer in relation to silica dust and silicosis in South African gold miners. *Proceedings of Second International Symposium on Silica, Silicosis, and Cancer*, San Francisco, 1993. *Scand J Work Environ Health in press.*

64 Gillam JD, Dement JM, Lemen RA, Wagoner JK, Archer VE, Blejer HP. Mortality patterns among hard rock gold miners exposed to an asbestiform mineral. *Ann NY Acad Sci* 1976; **271**: 336–44.

65 Forastiere F, Lagorio S, Michelozzi P, Perucci CA, Axelson O. Letter to Editor. *Am J Ind Med* 1987; **12**: 221–2.

66 Koskela RS, Klockars M, Järvinen E, Rossi A, Kolari PJ. Cancer mortality of granite workers, 1940–1985. In: Simonato L, Fletcher AC, Saracci R, Thomas TL, eds. *Occupational exposure to silica and cancer risk*. Lyon: IARC Scientific Publications No 97, 1990: 43–53.

67 Thomas TL. Lung cancer mortality among pottery workers in the United States. In: Simonato L, Fletcher AC, Saracci R, Thomas TL, eds. *Occupational exposure to silica and cancer risk*. Lyon, IARC Scientific Publications No 97, 1990: 75–81.

68 Winter PD, Gardner MJ, Fletcher AC, Jones RD. A mortality follow-up study of pottery workers: preliminary findings on lung cancer. In: Simonato L, Fletcher AC, Saracci R, Thomas TL, eds. *Occupational exposure to silica and cancer risk*. Lyon, IARC Scientific Publications No 97, 1990, 83–94.

69 Amandus HE, Costello J. Silicosis and lung cancer in United States metal miners. *Arch Environ Health* 1991; **46**: 82–9.

70 Merlo F, Costantini M, Reggiardo G, Ceppi M, Pantoni R. Lung cancer risk among refractory brick workers exposed to crystalline silica: a retrospective cohort study. *Epidemiology* 1991; **2**: 299–305.

71 Carta P, Cocco PL, Picchiri G. Lung cancer and airway obstruction among metal miners exposed to silica and low levels of radon daughters. Proceedings of 9th International Symposium on Epidemiology in Occupational Health, DHHS (NIOSH) Publication No 94–112, 1994, Cincinnati, 151–7.

72 McLaughlin JK, Chen J-Q, Dosemeci M, Chen R-A. Rexing SK, Wu Z, et al. A nested case-control study of lung cancer among silica exposed workers in China. *Br J Ind Med* 1992; **49**: 167–71.

73 Checkoway H, Meyer NJ, Demers PA, Breslow NE. Mortality among workers in the diatomaceous earth industry. *Br J Ind Med* 1993; **50**: 586–97.

74 Cherry NM, McNamee R, Burgess G, Turner S, McDonald JC. Initial findings from a cohort mortality study of British pottery workers. *Appl Occup Environ Hyg* 1995 (in press).

75 Amandus HE, Shy C, Wing S, Blair A, Heineman EF. Silicosis and lung cancer in North Carolina dusty trades workers. *Am J Ind Med* 1991; **20**: 57–70.

76 Infante-Rivard C, Armstrong B, Petitclerc M, Cloutier LG, Thériault G. Lung cancer mortality and silicosis in Quebec, 1938–85. *Lancet* 1989; **2**: 1504–7.

77 Swaen MH, Meijers JMM. Lung cancer risk among workers with silicosis: potential confounding by smoking habits. *Am J Ind Med* 1987; **12**: 223–5.

78 Finkelstein MM. *Silicosis surveillance in Ontario: detection rates, modifying factors, and screening intervals*. Health and Safety Studies Unit, Ontario Ministry of Labour, 1993.

79 International Agency for Research on Cancer (IARC). *Man-Made Mineral Fibres and Radon*, IARC Monographs on the Evaluation of the Carcinogenic Risk of Chemicals to Humans, Vol 43, Lyon: IARC, 1988.

80 Dodgson J, Cherrie J, Groat S. Estimates of past exposure to respirable man-made mineral fibres in the European insulation wool industry. *Ann Occup Hyg* 1987; **31**: 567–82.

81 Öhberg I. Technological development of the mineral wool industry in Europe. *Ann Occup Hyg* 1987; **31**: 529–45.

82 Meek ME. Lung cancer and mesothelioma related to man-made mineral fibres: the epidemiological evidence. In: Liddell FDK, Miller K, eds, *Mineral fibers and health*. Boca Raton: CRC Press, 1991, 175–85.

83 *Biological effects of man-made mineral fibres. Proceedings of a WHO/IARC Conference*, Copenhagen: World Health Organization, Regional Office for Europe, 1984.

84 Man-made mineral fibres in the working environment. Walton WH, ed. *Ann Occup Hyg* 1987; **31(No 4B)**: 517–34.

85 McDonald JC. Mortality of workers exposed to man-made mineral fibres—current evidence and future research. In: *Biological Effects of Man-Made Mineral Fibres*. Copenhagen: World Health Organization, Regional Office for Europe, 1984, Vol 1: 369–80.

86 Enterline PE, Marsh GM. The health effects of workers in the MMMF industry. In: *Biological Effects of Man-Made Mineral Fibres. Proceedings of a WHO/IARC Conference*, Vol 1, Copenhagen: World Health Organization, Regional Office for Europe, 1984, 311–39.

87 Saracci R, Simonato L, Acheson ED, Andersen A, Bertazzi PA, Claude J, *et al.* The IARC mortality and cancer incidence study of MMMF production workers. In: *Biological Effects of Man-Made Mineral Fibres. Proceedings of a WHO/IARC Conference*, Vol 1, Copenhagen: World Health Organization, Regional Office for Europe, 1984, 279–310.

88 Morgan RW, Kaplan SD, Bratsberg JA. Mortality in fibrous glass production workers. In: *Biological Effects of Man-Made Mineral Fibres. Proceedings of a WHO/IARC Conference*, Vol 1, Copenhagen: World Health Organization, Regional Office for Europe, 1984, 340–6.

89 Shannon HS, Hayes M, Julian JA, Muir DCF. Mortality experience of glass fibre workers. In: *Biological Effects of Man-Made Mineral Fibres. Proceedings of a WHO/IARC Conference*, Vol 1, Copenhagen: World Health Organization, Regional Office for Europe, 1984, 347–9.

90 Engholm G, Englund A, Hallin N, Schmalensee Gv. Incidence of respiratory cancer in Swedish construction workers. In: *Biological Effects of Man-Made Mineral Fibres. Proceedings of a WHO/IARC Conference*, Vol 1, Copenhagen, World Health Organization Regional Office for Europe, 1984, 350–65.

91 Shannon HS, Jamieson E, Julian JA, Muir DCF, Walsh C. Mortality experience of Ontario glass fibre workers—extended follow-up. *Ann Occup Hyg* 1987; 31: 657–62.

92 Enterline PE, Marsh GM, Henderson V, Callahan C. Mortality update of a cohort of US man-made mineral fibres workers. *Ann Occup Hyg* 1987; 31: 625–56.

93 McDonald JC, Case BW, Enterline PE, Henderson V, McDonald AD, Plourde M, Sébastien P. Lung dust analysis in the assessment of past exposure of man-made mineral fibre workers. *Ann Occup Hyg* 1990; 34: 427–41.

94 Simonato L, Fletcher AC, Cherrie JW, Andersen A, Bertazzi P, Charnay N, *et al.* The International Agency for Research on Cancer historical cohort study of MMMF production workers in seven European countries: extension of the follow-up. *Ann Occup Hyg* 1987; 31: 603–23.

95 International Agency for Research on Cancer. Monographs on the evaluation of carcinogenic risks to humans. *Man-made mineral fibres and radon.* Lyon: IARC 1988, Vol 43.

96 Wong O, Musselman RP. Carcinogenicity of insulation wools: further comments and some new data. *Regul Tox Pharmacol* 1993; 18: 202–5.

NON-MALIGNANT DISEASES

6 Asthma

ANTHONY NEWMAN TAYLOR

Research objectives

Asthma is commonly defined as airway narrowing which is reversible over short periods of time, either spontaneously or as a result of treatment. This definition emphasises the variability of airflow limitation which distinguishes asthma from less reversible causes of airway narrowing, particularly associated with chronic bronchitis and emphysema. A further characteristic of asthma is airway hyper-responsiveness—an exaggerated narrowing of the airways provoked by a variety of non-specific stimuli such as exercise, inhaled cold dry air, sulphur dioxide, histamine, and methacholine. These characteristics of asthma—reversible airway narrowing and airway hyperresponsiveness—are probably manifestations of a characteristic and defining pattern of airway inflammation—desquamative eosinophilic bronchitis.

Agents that cause this pattern of airway inflammation and increase airway responsiveness have been described as "inducers," to distinguish them from "inciters," which provoke acute airway narrowing in people with hyperresponsive airways, without inducing airway inflammation.

Table 6.1 Occupational asthma: inducers and inciters

Inducers		
Irritant:	Hypersensitivity	
chlorine	Proteins:	enzymes
ammonia		animal urine proteins
toluene di-isocyanate		flour
		latex
	Low molecular weight chemicals: isocyanates	
		platinum salts
		acid anhydrides
Inciters		
exercise		
cold dry air		
sulphur dioxide		

Both inducers and inciters of asthma may be encountered in the workplace. Conceptually, exposure to inducers may increase the incidence of asthma, whereas inciters increase the frequency of episodes of asthma in those with pre-existing disease. Examples of occupational inducers and inciters are given in table 6.1. Inducers may initiate asthma as the consequence of direct toxic damage to the airway epithelium or of a specific hypersensitivity reaction. Inciters provoke acute airway narrowing in asthmatics by many different mechanisms, including pharmacological, immunological, and neurogenic.

Unlike many diseases caused by agents that are inhaled at work, cause and effect correlations in asthma can be investigated, at least for hypersensitivity induced asthma, by experimental studies in patients by inhalation challenge testing with the putative cause. The aim in these studies is to compare, usually with the subject "blind," the effect of exposure to a specific agent compared with an appropriate control exposure, in provoking acute airway narrowing. Ideally the results of the tests should be both reproducible in the subject tested and consistent with others whose asthma is considered to have the same cause. Showing that the particular agent provokes acute airway narrowing and increases non-specific airway responsiveness but does not, in the exposure concentrations tested, provoke airway narrowing in others with a similar level of airway responsiveness, provides evidence that the agent is a hypersensitivity inducer rather than an inciter of asthma. The results of such inhalation tests have been considered to be the gold standard both for identifying a specific agent and for diagnosing an occupational cause of asthma in individual cases. Much of the scientific literature comprises case reports of asthma caused by agents encountered in the workplace, the number of which now exceeds 200.[1] A classification of some of the more important causes is given in table 6.2.

Case series, although attesting to the considerable number of different causes of asthma, provide no information about the number of cases of

118

Table 6.2 Some agents responsible for "hypersensitivity induced" occupational asthma

	Proteins	Low molecular weight chemicals
animal	excreta of rats, mice and other laboratory animals	
	locusts	
	grain mites	
vegetable	grain/flour	plicatic acid (western red cedar)
	castor bean	colophony (pinewood resin)
	green coffee bean	
	ispaghula	
	latex	
microbial	harvest moulds	antibiotics such as penicillins, cephalosporins
"mineral"		acid anhydrides
		isocyanates
		complex platinum salts
		polyamines
		reactive dyes

asthma attributable to exposures at work, to the relative importance of correlations between the development of disease and the nature of exposure to its cause or of the factors, such as atopy and tobacco smoking, that may modify these relationships. These questions, which are of considerable importance to occupational and public health, can be addressed only by studying cases in relation to the populations from which they are drawn. Such studies are of necessity observational in design; the most common have been cross-sectional surveys of the frequency of work-related asthma in groups of workers exposed to recognised causes, such as laboratory animals, enzymes, flour dust, and isocyanates. These studies, although potentially susceptible to survivor bias, provide some estimate of the size of the problem in the occupations studied. They are not comprehensive and have used different methods of case ascertainment. They have therefore not been able to assess the relative importance of different causes or to provide an estimate of the number of cases of asthma attributable to occupational agents. The first of these requirements has been provided for several years in Finland through a national survey of occupational diseases and within the last six years in the United Kingdom through a national surveillance scheme, SWORD (Survey of Work-related and Occupational Respiratory Disease) and a local scheme in the Birmingham region.

Exposure-response correlations and potentially modifying factors have been less systematically investigated. Ideally these questions need to measure the connection between disease incidence and exposure. Few such studies have been reported although exposure-response correlations and modifying influences have been assessed in some cross-sectional studies. Most formal studies of occupational asthma have defined their study populations by exposure; the case-referent approach has been used to analyse correlations within a cross-sectional or longitudinal design.

Methodological issues

Case ascertainment

There is no consensus on the best means of identification of occupational asthma in epidemiological studies. The gold standard in clinical diagnosis has been the inhalation test with a specific agent, but with few exceptions this method has not been considered feasible for survey work. The most commonly used survey method has been the questionnaire, frequently supplemented by measures of lung function, forced expiratory volume in one second (FEV_1), airway response to inhaled histamine or methacholine and, when feasible, specific immunological response to the relevant agent, by skin test or measurement of specific IgE in serum.

The most widely used questionnaires—those of the United Kingdom Medical Research Council and American Thoracic Society—although standardised, were designed to identify not cases of asthma, but of chronic mucus hypersecretion and associated airflow limitation. Various investigators have either modified these questionnaires or introduced their own. The same questionnaire has seldom been used in more than a few surveys and validity against any reasonable standard has seldom been reported. Burney et al. examined the correlation in 256 subjects between the bronchial symptoms questionnaire of the International Union against Tuberculosis and Lung Disease (IUATLD) and non-specific airway responsiveness to inhaled histamine.[2] They derived a discriminant predictor function from symptoms which included shortness of breath at night and tightness of the chest in dusty parts of the house or with animals or feathers, which had a sensitivity of 53% and specificity of 90%. In a similar study, Venables et al. examined in 211 subjects the relationship between nine questions on symptoms such as wheeze and difficulty with breathing in defined circumstances, such as exercise, sleep, and exposure to tobacco smoke, dust, and other irritants.[3] They found that with one reported symptom sensitivity for airway hyperresponsiveness was 90% but specificity was 65%. Specificity increased with two or three symptoms (87% and 94%), but sensitivity was reduced (79% and 69%). The reproducibility of the questionnaire was tested by repeating it on three separate days. Reproducibility, measured as agreement of two or more symptoms, was 94% and 98% and, of three or more symptoms, 96% and 96%.

The identification of occupational asthma from a questionnaire has generally been based on symptoms such as wheeze, breathlessness, and chest tightness, which follow exposure to the causal agent and which improve during absences and deteriorate during periods at work. Malo and colleagues assessed the validity of cases identified by response to questionnaire in cross-sectional studies of snow crab process workers,[4] of manufacturers of the laxative psyllium,[5] and of the staff of four chronic care hospitals where psyllium was widely used.[6] They compared case identification based on symptoms obtained by questionnaire, and lung function tests, which included spontaneous variability ($> 10\%$ in FEV_1) against increased airway responsiveness to inhaled histamine. In addition they used indicators of occupational asthma which included serial self-recorded peak flow measurements, increase in airway responsiveness after return to work and evidence of a specific immunological response by skin prick test and specific IgE, for comparison with the results of inhalation testing against snow crab extract and psyllium. On the assumption that the tests were more likely to provide false positives than false negatives, they were undertaken in a stepwise fashion; thus inhalation tests were used only in those with an appropriate response to the questionnaire or evidence of airway or immunological response. The distribution of cases identified by questionnaire, immunological test and specific inhalation test is summarised in table 6.3. The proportion of cases diagnosed by questionnaire and confirmed by inhalation tests varied between 52% in snow crab process workers and 10% in hospital employees. In part this could have reflected the use of different questionnaires in the snow crab and psyllium workers. In the two psyllium studies where the same questionnaire was used the proportions of cases confirmed by inhalation test were similar—10% and 13%.

Almost all epidemiological studies of occupational asthma have been cross-sectional in design, repeatability within and between observers of the measures used for case identification seldom being studied. Venables *et al.*,[7] in another study of repeatability within and between four observers in the identification of asthma from 61 serial peak flow records, found that agreement within individual observers varied between 90% and 100%. Agreement occurred between all four observers in 69% and between at least three of the four in 97%.

Exposure assessment

The finding of an exposure-response gradient provides important evidence of causation, as does a reduction in attack rate following an effective intervention to reduce exposure. The focus of many epidemiological studies of occupational asthma has been on the host factors that influence immunological and airway responses. In part, this has reflected the emphasis of much asthma research—on mechanisms rather than on

Table 6.3 Validation of questionnaire diagnosed occupational asthma

Reference	Occupational group	Number studied	Questionnaire diagnosed occupational asthma	Specific immunological response		Specific inhalation test (% of questionnaire diagnosed)
				skin test	specific E	
Cartier[4]	snow crab process workers	303	64	65		33/64 tested (51·5%)
Bardy[5]	psyllium manufacture	130	39	23	31	5/18 tested (13%)
Malo[6]	hospital staff	197	29	10	24	8/10 tested (10%)

causes—but also the absence until recently of reliable methods for measuring aero-allergen concentrations. Most studies that have examined exposure-response relationships have used surrogates of severity of exposure such as job title, proximity to the source or, in one case, frequency of exposure (table 6.3). Few studies have measured concentrations of the relevant agent in air, but this has been done for isocyanates, colophony, wood dust, flour dust, and rat urine proteins.

Although the development of immunoassays to measure specific proteins in air is an important advance, the fundamental need is to use a sampling strategy that provides a valid and reliable estimate of exposure for all members of the study population to the specific agent. The technique of exposure zoning is a valuable tool, which fulfils the needs of a sampling strategy suitable for epidemiological purposes.[8] An exposure zone has been described as "a characteristic grouping of workers based on the similarity of their job and the environments in which they work." Each zone fulfils four basic attributes:

(1) Work similarity (similar tasks).
(2) Similarity with regard to hazardous agents.
(3) Environmental similarity (potential for exposure to same agents for all people in the zone, including similar ventilation).
(4) Identifiability (to ensure that workers are allocated to only one zone).

Zoning does not require the characterisation of each worker but work with regard to exposure. The exposure experienced by any worker in the zone can therefore be estimated from the values obtained from air samples taken from a representative sample of workers in the zone.

Exposure has two major components—intensity and duration. Information about duration is usually available but estimates or measurements of intensity are often lacking. This is particularly important in occupational asthma where those who develop disease may leave and those who accumulate exposure are those who survive to do so. The use of cumulative exposure (intensity × duration) which assumes their equivalence is almost certainly not justified as a biologically relevant measure. It is also unclear whether intermittent peak concentrations or exposure accumulated during the early period of employment are of equal importance. These issues need to be considered in the analysis of studies, particularly of asthma incidence.

Estimated incidence

In the United Kingdom information about the number of cases of asthma caused by agents inhaled at work, and their relative importance has, until recently, been confined to official statistics of industrial injuries benefit. Surveys of disease prevalence in specific occupational groups and even the few longitudinal studies that have been reported give no indication of incidence rates in terms of age, sex, agent, or industry. In Finland a register of occupational diseases (including occupational asthma) was set up about 30 years ago. Case registration was based on a legal requirement for doctors to report all cases of occupational disease or disease related to work. In the United Kingdom, two formal surveillance schemes, one national (Surveillance of Work-related and Occupational Respiratory Diseases—SWORD[9]) and one local (a notification scheme for occupational asthma in the West Midlands Region—SHIELD[10]) were inaugurated in 1989. SWORD is a voluntary reporting scheme that provides estimates of case frequency by cause and disease incidence by occupational group, which has achieved almost complete coverage of chest physicians and a similar number, but unknown proportion, of occupational physicians. Participants regularly report new cases of work-related respiratory disease that they have identified each month with information about age, sex, residence, occupation, and suspected cause. In 1989, 2101 cases of occupational lung disease were notified[8] but as a result of a sampling scheme introduced in 1992 the annual number of new cases is estimated around 3500.[11] Asthma which accounted for 28% of cases, was the single most common diagnostic category. Isocyanates have been consistently the most commonly reported agent, accounting for about 22% of cases; flour/grain dust, wood dust, solder flux, and laboratory animals have together accounted for a similar proportion (22%). Disease incidence has varied considerably by occupational group. Meredith et al. also reported a more detailed survey which included cases in workers employed in the chemical and plastics industry.[12] Eighty five of the 95 patients studied had respiratory symptoms that improved on days away from work, 45 had serial measurements of lung function; inhalation test or specific IgE or both were undertaken in 11. In only two cases was there no corroboration for the diagnosis. It is unusual, however, for chest physicians to investigate the place of work and they are likely to attribute asthma to its well recognised causes. Rates by occupational group may therefore be more reliable than attribution to specific causes.

In another study Meredith presented a detailed analysis of occupational asthma reported to the SWORD scheme during 1989 and 1990, which showed considerable consistency in the total number of cases and distribution by cause and occupational group in these two years.[13] The overall annual incidence was 22/million working population. Table 6.4 gives annual incidence rates by occupational set and sex. These varied from three/million for those in orders one to 10 (except cleaners, hairdressers, farmers and laboratory technicians) to 658/million for coach and other spray painters, with little difference between men and women in the same occupational set. Analysis by region also showed wide variation

Table 6.4 *Incidence of occupational asthma in relation to occupational set and sex**

Order	Occupational set	Women		Men		Sexes combined	
		Cases	Rate million/year	Cases	Rate million/year	Rate million/year	(95% CI)
1–10	Professional, clerical and service work						
	laboratory technicians and assistants	25	203	25	174	188	139 247
	cleaners	10	9	5	13	10	5,16
	nurses	22	17	0	0	16	10 24
	farmers and farm workers	7	43	16	24	28	18,41
	hairdressers	16	87	0	0	81	46,131
	remainder	45	3	52	3	3	2,4
11	Material processors (excluding metal and electrical)						
	wood workers	1	35	50	54	54	40,70
	food processors (excluding bakers)	15	146	20	90	108	75,150
	bakers	22	364	28	314	334	248,440
	plastic workers	5	163	42	386	337	248,448
	chemical processors	5	271	49	377	364	274,475
	remainder	31	41	63	53	49	39,60
12	Metal and electrical processing and making						
	welding, soldering and electronic assembly	44	268	34	120	175	138 218
	metal treatment	2	174	41	275	267	194 360
	remainder	10	48	122	28	29	24,35
13	Painting, assembly and packing						
	painters (excluding spray painters)	4	510	24	58	66	44,95
	coach and other spray painters	1	450	64	663	658	508,839
	remainder	18	31	23	41	36	26,49
14	Construction and mining	1	64	21	11	11	7,17
15	Transport and storage	0	0	23	8	8	5,11

*based on data from the SWORD scheme[13]

which was not explained by the geographical distribution of high risk industries, suggesting differences in ascertainment and reporting. The authors estimated that if the incidence of occupational asthma was as high as that in regions with the highest rates the true annual incidence would be about three times that reported nationally. The scheme includes only cases reported by consultant chest and occupational physicians; cases not seen or seen only by general practitioners would not have been reported.

The West Midlands reporting scheme provided results which were in general compatible with those from the SWORD scheme. The most common causes of new cases in that region were isocyanates, colophony, flour, and oil mists.[10]

Comparison of the results of the SWORD scheme with those from Finland suggest that the reported incidence of occupational asthma in Finland is appreciably higher than the rate reported to SWORD in United Kingdom. This is the result, at least in part, of more complete case ascertainment by all physicians and not only specialists. The most common cause of occupational asthma in Finland was allergy to cow epithelium, a reflection of the greater proportion of the population employed in agriculture and with animal contact; the incidence of allergic alveolitis was also many times higher in Finland than in the UK.[14]

The strength of the SWORD scheme (see also Chapter 14) has been the high level of participation of respiratory and occupational physicians. Validation of reported cases is difficult to establish, but the participants are specialist occupational and respiratory physicians and the validation exercise undertaken found corroboration of case status in most cases.[12] Under-ascertainment will inevitably occur to the extent that cases do not come to the attention of respiratory or occupational physicians or, if they do, an occupational cause is not recognised. The best estimate at present suggests that perhaps one half of all new cases of occupational asthma are now being reported to this scheme.

Irritant-induced asthma (RADS)

Irritant induced occupational asthma (or RADS—reactive airways dysfunction syndrome) is chronic asthma which persists after a single, usually short, inhalation of a respiratory irritant in toxic concentrations. The development of respiratory symptoms and the presence of airway hyperresponsiveness within a few hours of an identifiable exposure distinguishes irritant induced from hypersensitivity induced occupational asthma. In most reported cases caused in this way, respiratory symptoms and airway hyperresponsiveness have persisted for more than a year from the time of onset.

Most descriptions of RADS have been in case series. The original report described 10 patients, none of whom had evidence of pre-existing respiratory disease.[15] All developed persistent asthma after a single exposure—usually of a few minutes duration, but in one for twelve hours—to a variety of irritants which included a spray paint containing ammonia, heated acid, floor sealant, uranium hexafluoride, and smoke. The onset of respiratory symptoms was immediate in three and after an average interval of nine hours in the others. Duration of symptoms to the time of follow up ranged from one to 12 years, at which time static lung function tests were normal in three but there was evidence of airflow limitation in the remaining seven; all 10 had increased airway responsiveness to inhaled methacholine. Subsequent reports of RADS have documented asthma induced by a single inhalation in toxic concentration of a variety of agents which have included sulphur dioxide,[16] toluene di-isocyanate,[17] anhydrous ammonia fumes,[18] and smoke.[19]

The case reports in the medical literature suggest that acute inhalation of an irritant chemical in concentrations toxic to the airway epithelium can induce asthma and airway hyper-responsiveness. However, in general the cases reported have been highly selected and have not provided information on lung function prior to the inhalation accident. One study of hospital employees exposed to 100% acetic acid after a spill in a hospital laboratory was able to overcome these problems by:

(1) Studying a random sample of the exposed population
(2) Demonstrating an exposure-response relationship between the estimated intensity of exposure and the prevalence of acute irritant symptoms and measured airway hyper-responsiveness: the risk of developing RADS was some tenfold higher in those most highly exposed to acetic acid, as compared with those least exposed, following the spill
(3) Partial validation of respiratory health before the accident by examination of pre-employment health questionnaires.[20]

During its first five years, 1989–93 the SWORD scheme received reports of 904 cases of inhalation accidents among 8586 newly diagnosed occupational respiratory diseases. By taking into account the sampling system in place during 1992–1993, the authors estimated that a total of about 250 inhalation accidents occurred annually during these two years. Numerous agents were implicated, 85% of which were chemicals, the most common being chlorine (13%), smoke/combustion gases (9%), and oxides of nitrogen (5%).[20] The highest rates occurred among metal and electrical processors (162/million/year) and chemical processes (75/million/year). Preliminary results from a more detailed investigation of a selected series of over 700 inhalation accidents (1990–1993) indicate that symptoms lasted for more than one month in 142 cases, including 42 new cases with asthmatic symptoms.[21] Spills, leaks and faulty processes accounted for over one third of these accidents and failure to observe safety guidelines—including both failure to use respiratory protection and inappropriate procedures when mixing chemicals—for a further third.

The connection between RADS and recognised risk factors for hypersensitivity-induced occupational asthma, such as atopy and smoking has not been reported.

Hypersensitivity induced asthma

Cross-sectional studies

Cross-sectional studies estimate the prevalence of disease in a defined population at a particular point in time. Estimates of exposure tend also to be limited to the present time, and these may differ considerably from the exposures of the past that were responsible for the disease. Unlike cohort studies they are confined to the investigation of people currently available, a potentially serious drawback for a disease that causes acute symptoms that may be clearly associated with a particular exposure. This provides a reason to avoid further ill health by changing job, whereas employees who accumulate exposure are those who remain healthy. Cross-sectional studies can be strengthened considerably, however, by the introduction of the time dimension to both the development of disease and the estimation of past exposure.[22]

Most cross-sectional studies of occupational asthma have been undertaken primarily to describe disease prevalence or its various manifestations, in populations exposed to recognised causes. The findings have only occasionally been compared with a similar but unexposed population. The most commonly used measure of outcome has been an index of work-related respiratory symptoms based on response to questionnaires which to date have not been standardised, making difficult any comparison between findings in different populations exposed to the same or other agents.

Notwithstanding these limitations, cross-sectional studies can be instructive and to date represent most epidemiological observations on occupational asthma. In addition to providing an estimate of the size of the problem in different occupational settings, their results have been used to analyse the connection between respiratory symptoms and indices of specific immunological response, measures of lung function (including airway responsiveness), host factors such as atopy, personal habits (particularly tobacco smoking), and on occasion assessments of exposure. The results of some of the more informative cross-sectional studies are set out in table 6.5. Surveys of those working with enzymes, low molecular weight chemicals such as isocyanates and acid anhydrides and with laboratory animals are described below as examples of cross-sectional studies from which useful inferences can be drawn.

Table 6.5 Some informative prevalence studies of occupational asthma

Reference	Exposure	Occupation	Population	Asthma (usually defined as work-related respiratory symptoms)	
				Prevalence	Determinants identified
Venables[38]	laboratory animals	pharmaceutical company	138	11%	atopy
Slovak[50]		pharmaceutical company	141	10%	atopy
Cullinan[43]	rats	research laboratories	238	7% (new work related respiratory symptoms)	measured exposure to rat urine protein, atopy and smoking
Musk[51]	flour	bakery	279	13%	current dust exposure
Prichard[52]		bakery	176	11%	exposure
Mitchell[28]	enzymes	detergent manufacture	98	50%	measured exposure
Cartier[4]	snow crab	process workers	303	21%	smoking not atopy
Tee[53]	locust	research laboratory	35	33% (5 of 15 currently exposed)	not atopy
Coutts[40]	cimetidine	pharmaceutical company	55	14.5%	frequency of exposure
Venables[30]	isocyanates	steel coating (TDI)	241	9.5%	exposure defined by work area (proximity to TDI)
Weill[54]	isocyanates	TDI manufacture	112	8.3%	exposure defined by job
Johnson[31]	isocyanates	MDI foundry	78	18.2%	excess of asthma in foundry v. railway yard workers
Venables[32 33]	acid anhydrides	TCPA (electronics factory)	329	3.2%	exposure (proximity to TCPA) and smoking
Wernfors[55]	acid anhydrides	PA	118	18%	exposure and atopy, not smoking
Burge[56]	colophony	solder manufacture	45	11%	exposure: category by measured airborne colophony
Bardy[5]	psyllium	production workers	130	38%	probably exposure, atopy
Malo[41]	spiramycin	production workers	51	8%	
Chan Yeung[39]	W. red cedar	cedar mill workers	652	4.1%	exposure intensity and duration

MDI = diphenylmethane di-isocyanate
TDI = toluene di-isocyanate
TCPA = tetrachlorophthalic anhydride

Table 6.6   Correlation of allergic symptoms (eyes, nose and chest) with immediate skin test responses to enzyme alcalase in enzyme detergent manufacturers (after Newhouse[25])

	Allergic symptoms present	Allergic symptoms absent	Total
Skin test Positive	52	5	57
Skin test Negative	75	139	214
Total	127	144	271

Enzymes

Workers exposed to proteolytic enzymes in the detergent industry in the early 1970s were an early example of an occupation studied cross-sectionally. Asthma from this cause was first identified in 1969 when commercial production had already become widespread.[23 24] Assessment of the size of the problem was important and cross-sectional surveys were undertaken in United Kingdom,[25 26] USA,[27] and Australia.[28] All reported high rates of respiratory symptoms and skin test responses to the relevant enzymes. Newhouse *et al.* for example, found allergic symptoms in 47% of the workforce surveyed and an association between skin test response to enzymes and both allergic symptoms (table 6.6) and skin test atopy (table 6.7). These findings led to important technological advances—in particular to granulation of the enzymes used in manufacture—with marked reduction in exposure.[29]

Isocyanates and acid anhydrides

Isocyanates have been repeatedly reported as potent causes of occupational asthma but relatively few population studies have been made. A cross-sectional survey in a steel-coating plant where toluene di-isocyanate (TDI) had been introduced into the process some years earlier identified 21 cases (9·5%) of work-related asthma among 221 employees.[30] Johnson *et al.* reported 12 cases (15%) in 78 iron and steel foundry workers exposed to diphenyl methane di-isocyanate (MDI) which they considered the most probable cause.[31]

Although acid anhydrides are less often responsible for occupational

Table 6.7   Correlation of immediate skin test response to enzyme alcalase with atopy (as defined by skin test response to common inhalant allergens) (after Newhouse[25])

	Skin test Positive	Skin test Negative	Total
Atopy present	40	9	49
Atopy absent	21	33	54
Total	61	42	103

asthma than isocyanates, studies of populations exposed to them have been more widely reported, primarily because of specific identifiable immunological responses. Of the several acid anhydrides used commercially, workers exposed to trimellitic (TMA) and tetrachlorophthalic (TCPA) anhydrides have been the most extensively reported. Howe *et al.* reported an outbreak of seven cases of asthma which had developed in an electronic components factory within one year of the introduction of TCPA as a constituent of an epoxy resin plastic coat.[32] In all seven cases there was an immediate skin test response to conjugates of TCPA with human serum albumin and specific IgE was identified in their serum in concentrations significantly in excess of seven comparably exposed workers without symptoms. Specific inhalation tests with TCPA in the four cases in whom this was undertaken provoked an asthmatic response, the magnitude of which was related to the concentration of airborne TCPA used.[33] The outbreak led to a survey among workers in the factory to identify other cases and to investigate potential determinants of sensitisation to the chemical.[34] No further cases of TCPA-related asthma were identified, but several employees had an immediate skin test response to TCPA-human serum albumin (TCPA-HSA) conjugate. Specific IgE to TCPA-HSA was twice as common among workers in areas of the factory adjacent to the coating machines where TCPA was used. Cigarette smokers were some five times more likely than non or ex-smokers to have specific IgE. Although atopy-defined by skin prick test as one or more immediate response to common inhalant allergens—was not independently associated with specific IgE to TCPA-HSA, there was an interaction between atopy and cigarette smoking, the highest prevalence of specific IgE to the TCPA-HSA conjugate being among atopic smokers. A similar correlation between proximity of exposure, atopy and cigarette smoking to both sensitisation and asthma, was later observed in an epidemic associated with allergy to soya beans released during unloading in the harbour of Barcelona.[35]

Laboratory animals

Laboratory animal workers have been subject to several cross-sectional surveys. In the United Kingdom some 35 000 people encounter laboratory animals in their work, most often in universities and the pharmaceutical industry. The most commonly used animals are rats and mice; the major allergens are low molecular proteins excreted in the urine[36] but also present in saliva and sebaceous gland secretions.[37] Several such cross-sectional studies have estimated the prevalence of laboratory animal allergy at between 15 and 30%. One survey of 138 employees of a pharmaceutical company with animal contact reported a prevalence of 44% for allergic symptoms and 11% for chest symptoms.[38] This study also provided suggestive evidence of survivor bias in that no relationship of chest symptoms was found with job type and an inverse relationship with increasing duration of exposure.

Other causes

The prevalence of occupational asthma has been estimated in occupational groups exposed to well documented causes. These have included wood dust in cedar mill workers,[39] pharmaceuticals such as cimetidine,[40] psyllium,[5] and spiramycin[41] in manufacturers, psyllium in hospital staff,[6] and snow crab in process workers[4] (table 6.5). Most of these studies identified an effect either of exposure or of modifying factors or both. For many reported causes of occupational asthma, particularly those that are uncommon, such as polyamines, evidence of causation is based on case reports only, making attribution difficult and uncertain.

Cohort studies

In design, the cohort study most closely approximates the experiment. Unlike the experiment, however, allocation into work and within different categories of exposure at work are not random but subject to considerable selection and, even when the investigators can study the population without information on levels of exposure, the workers themselves are well aware of it. Nevertheless, the cohort has strengths when compared to the cross-sectional approach. In particular, definition of the population before exposure and later observations on both exposure and attack rate reduce the potential for distortion of exposure-response by survivor bias. The cohort design also provides opportunities to investigate the effect of controlling exposure to a specific agent on the subsequent attack rate. Cohort studies consume more time and resources than cross-sectional surveys and there are few in occupational asthma.

Enzyme workers

One of the earliest cohort studies reported was a seven year follow up of employees in a factory manufacturing enzyme detergents[29] where the original case of enzyme-induced asthma reported by Flindt had worked.[23] Following the case report a number of measures were taken to reduce the airborne concentration of enzyme in the factory. The study was thus able to examine the relationship of attack rate to changes in enzyme exposure.

- *Study population*: The study population was defined as those employed at the time of introduction of enzymes into the manufacturing process in 1968 and those who entered employment during the next seven years.
- *Exposure*: Dust and enzyme levels were measured in the enzyme packing area throughout the period of the study. The results showed that concentrations of both enzyme and dust were highest in 1969 and 1970, peak levels of total dust being in excess of 1200 μ/m^3. From 1972

onward concentrations fell and the total dust concentration was consistently less than 400 $\mu g/m^3$. For the purposes of analysis jobs were grouped into four exposure categories: high, (constant); high, (intermittent); intermediate; and low.

- *Outcome*: Two measures of outcome were used to analyse attack rates (i) skin prick test response to enzymes and (ii) transfer from the enzyme areas after development of respiratory symptoms.
- *Observations*: The development of skin prick test reactions to enzymes occurred primarily in the first two years of exposure. These responses occurred more commonly in those employed in the higher exposure categories and were more common in each exposure category among atopic individuals.

The proportion of non-atopic workers who developed a skin test reaction to enzymes fell with decreasing enzyme exposure in the factory. Whereas 41% of those employed in 1968/69 developed a skin test response to enzymes, among those entering employment between 1969 and 1971 it occurred in 29% compared with 11% in those joining between 1971 and 1973. Similarly the number of cases who were transferred out because of development of respiratory symptoms fell from 50 between 1968 and 1971 to one each year in 1972–74. This study, although incomplete in some aspects, remains one of the few studies of occupational allergy and asthma to have related attack rate to measured estimates of exposure and to provide evidence of the effectiveness of reducing exposure to aero-allergen at work on the attack rate of both sensitisation and respiratory symptoms.

Platinum refinery workers

Cohort studies can be undertaken on data collected in the past provided the information has been collected in a systematic and unbiased fashion. Venables *et al.* investigated the association of tobacco consumption with sensitisation and respiratory symptoms caused by complex platinum salts in a platinum refinery workforce.[42] Several cross-sectional studies, including the study of acid anhydride workers described earlier in this chapter, had suggested an association between cigarette smoking and sensitisation to occupational allergens, but no previous study had examined the association longitudinally.

- *Study population*: 91 workers who had entered employment at the platinum refinery between January 1973 and December 1974. The results of pre-employment examination, which included skin test reactions to common inhalant allergens and smoking history had been recorded on all employees at the time of joining. Individuals with a history of allergic disease, severe respiratory disease or reduced FEV_1 were excluded from employment.
- *Outcome*: Two measures of outcome were used in the analysis of attack

rates: (1) skin prick test responses to platinum salts, recorded at entry and at three to six monthly intervals; and (2) respiratory symptoms identified from contemporary records: a diagnosis by a doctor of platinum salt allergy, a request from a nurse to a doctor for a medical examination because of respiratory symptoms related to work; a record of attendance at the factory clinic with new respiratory symptoms; and sickness certificates stating respiratory symptoms.

- *Follow up*: Was from date of first employment to the end of April 1980 or date of leaving employment.
- *Observations*: The attack rate of both skin test reactions to platinum salts and of respiratory symptoms was greatest during the first year of employment falling from 9% in the first six months to 6% in the second six months, 6% in the second year, 2·5% in the third and fourth years to zero after four years.

The most important predictor of the development of a skin test response to platinum salt was smoking; the risk among smokers was four to five times greater than among non-smokers. Although the risk was increased among subjects with atopy this was not significant and there was no evidence of an interaction between atopy and smoking. Cigarette consumption was the most important predictor of respiratory symptoms, which were twice as common in smokers as in non-smokers.

This study showed the strengths of the cohort over the cross-sectional design in the study of an acute respiratory disease. The study population was defined and relevant information about smoking and atopy were recorded before the onset of exposure. Follow up was complete and measures of outcome were based on contemporary records. The medical selection process led to the exclusion of people with allergic respiratory disease, which may have attenuated any correlation of sensitivity to platinum salts with atopy.

This study did not include information on exposure to platinum salts or to chlorine gas that was known to have occurred. With the exception of the enzyme study and current studies of laboratory animal, flour, and acid anhydride workers, no other investigation has estimated the incidence of sensitisation and asthma in relation to measured exposure.

Laboratory animal workers

Attenuation or loss of exposure-response correlations in prevalence surveys because the sick, particularly those with asthma, may leave employment, can at least in part be corrected by adding a time dimension to the study. This approach was taken in a recently reported survey of allergy and asthma among laboratory animal workers.[43] A cross-sectional survey was the initial phase of a longitudinal study with observations only on those who fulfilled the cohort definition, were in current employment, or had entered employment during the previous four years. The aim was to investigate exposure-response relationships and possible modifying factors such as atopy and smoking.

- *Study population*: 238 workers employed in three animal laboratories who had entered employment during the previous four years and were still in employment at the time of the study.
- *Exposure*: Exposure was estimated by the exposure zoning technique, in groups with similar exposure (for example technicians, scientists, cage cleaners) during an eight hour working day. Air samples were analysed for both total dust and rat urine protein, estimated by an inhibition immunoassay. For analysis, the workforce was grouped into one of three categories of exposure: low, medium, and high.
- *Outcome*: Two primary measures of outcome were used: respiratory symptoms elicited by questionnaire; and immediate skin test responses to an extract of rat urine.
- *Observations*: The prevalence of reported symptoms increased with exposure to both total dust and rat urine protein. This was true of skin symptoms in relation to both current exposure and exposure at time of onset, and of chest, nose and eye symptoms only in relation to exposure category at the time of onset, suggesting that those who had developed respiratory symptoms may have moved away from higher exposures.

The prevalence of positive skin prick tests to rat urine protein increased with increasing exposure especially in atopics and current cigarette smokers.

The longitudinal analysis will provide information about the attack rate of both sensitisation and symptoms in relation to measured exposure to rat urine protein during the period of observation. Provided the attack rate is sufficiently high, it should be possible not only to show an exposure-response gradient and any modifying effect of atopy and smoking, but also to discern its shape.

Outcome of occupational asthma

Studies of the outcome of patients with occupational asthma have been reported for several of its causes. The major findings from these studies are tabulated in table 6.8. While most studies have concentrated on the long term effects on respiratory function, some more recent studies have reported financial and social consequences of the disease.

These studies need to be interpreted with caution. The study populations in several comprise hospital patients who are likely to have been referred because of the severity of their illnesses. Furthermore, those with continuing symptoms are probably over represented among those who remain in view. In four studies the cases of asthma were identified,

Table 6.8 Some studies of outcome of occupational asthma after avoidance of exposure

| | | Population | | | | Persistence of | |
Reference	Agent	Source	Number	Diagnosis	Follow-up (years)	Symptoms	Airway hyper-responsiveness
Paggiaro[57]	isocyanates	hospital patients	12	BPT	$\geqslant 2$	8/12	7/11
Lozewicz[47]		hospital patients	50	BPT	$\geqslant 4$	41/50	14/21
Chan Yeung[58]	W. red cedar	hospital patients	75	BPT	1–9	37/75	25/33
Burge[59]	colophony		20	BPT	1–4	18/20	10/20
Venables[45]	tetrachloro-phthalic anhydride	factory workforce	7	BPT 4/7 history + skin tests 3/7	$4\frac{1}{2}$	6/6	5/5
Malo[44]	snow crab	factory workforce	31	BPT	$4\frac{1}{2}$–6	31/31	26/31
Slovak[46]	azodicarbonamide	factory workforce	151	history	> 3	5/8	

BPT = bronchial provocation test

not through hospital referral, but from surveys of factory populations. These were of snow crab process workers,[44] TCPA workers,[45] azodicarbonamide workers,[46] and (within a hospital based study of isocyanate workers), twelve who were all the known cases from one factory.[47] Follow up was complete in all four. Each study reported evidence of continuing asthma—respiratory symptoms, reduced FEV_1 or increased airway responsiveness—in more than half the patients. Furthermore, in the snow crab process workers and the TCPA workers, a progressive decline in specific IgE provided confirmatory evidence that exposure to these agents had been avoided during the period of follow up. No study has provided objective evidence of normal airway function, FEV_1 or airway responsiveness, before the onset of exposure as a basis for comparison with the subsequent findings.

These studies suggest that occupational asthma persists for several years, and probably indefinitely, after avoidance of exposure to the initiating agent. However, the outcome in patients whose condition was caused by several of the other more common causes of asthma, such as laboratory animals, flour, and enzymes has not been reported. The wider social and financial consequences of occupational asthma have been investigated in two studies, both of hospital patients. In one study 59% had lost or changed their job and 74% reported loss of income.[48] In the other, one third were unemployed at the time of interview, 57% reported difficulty in finding alternative employment and 49% had lost income.[49] However, in neither study were comparable observations made in patients without asthma.

Screening

The observation that occupational asthma occurs more commonly in individuals who are atopic (usually defined as one or more immediate skin test reactions provoked by extracts of common inhalant allergens such as *Dermatophagoides pteronyssinus*, grass pollen, and cat fur) has led to the use of these tests for pre-employment screening of those whose work would bring them into contact with potential causes of occupational asthma, particularly laboratory animals, enzymes, and platinum salts. To be

Table 6.9   Correlation of atopy (skin test response to common inhalant allergens) with work related chest symptoms in cross-sectional survey of laboratory animal workers (after Venables[38])

	Chest symptoms present	Chest symptoms absent	Total
Atopy present	11	47	58
Atopy absent	4	76	80
Total	15	123	138

Table 6.10   Correlation between atopy and work related chest symptoms which developed after start of employment in survey of laboratory animal workers (after Cullinan[43])

	New chest symptoms present	New chest symptoms absent	Total
Atopy present	12	76	88
Atopy absent	4	127	131
Total	16	203	219

effective a screening test needs to fulfil certain criteria of which a high positive predictive value (a low proportion of false positives) is the most important. Most of the evidence for an association between atopy and occupational allergy and asthma comes from cross-sectional studies of workers exposed to laboratory animals and enzymes. The relationship between atopy, laboratory animal allergy, and skin test responses to complex platinum salts has been investigated in longitudinal studies. The correlations observed in some of these studies are tabulated in tables 6.7, 6.9, 6.10 and 6.11.

The study of enzyme workers (table 6.7) showed that whereas 40 of the 49 subjects with atopy (82%) in the workforce developed a skin test reaction to alcalase, so did 21 of the 54 (39%) who were not atopic.[25] On this evidence, exclusion of people with atopy from the workforce would reduce the prevalence of sensitisation to enzymes only from 59% to 39%. However, 91% of those with a positive skin test developed symptoms associated with allergy to enzymes.

The two studies of laboratory animal workers (tables 6.9 and 6.10) showed similar findings, an association between chest symptoms and atopy, but a high false positive rate and hence low positive predictive values 12/88 (13·6%) and 11/58 (19%).[43 50] In addition, both studies identified false negatives—4/131 (3%) and 4/80 (5%).

A study of the association of atopy with skin test response to platinum salts (table 6.11) showed both high false positive (19/29 (65·5%)) and high false negative (12/62 (19·5%)) rates and therefore low positive (10/29 = 35%) or negative (50/62 = 81%) predictive values.[42]

Table 6.11   Correlation between atopy and development of skin prick test response to complex platinum salts in a historical cohort study of platinum refinery workers (after Venables[42])

	Skin prick tests positive	Skin prick tests negative	Total
Atopy present	10	19	29
Atopy absent	12	50	62
Total	22	69	91

These observations, although limited, suggest that atopy as a pre-employment screening test, which would exclude more than one third of all employees is not sufficiently discriminatory for practical use. Moreover, this approach would deflect attention from environmental control to the question of individual susceptibility which, although related to some causes of occupational asthma, has generally been found to be weak.

Conclusions

Studies reported in the past 10 years have concentrated on several important epidemiological questions about occupational asthma. Surveillance schemes in the United Kingdom and Finland have provided both information about the relative importance of different causes of occupational asthma and estimates of the risks in different occupational groups. The contribution of occupational causes to the prevalence of asthma in the general population, however, remains unclear. Surveys undertaken in different occupations have been informative about the prevalence of both allergy and asthma caused by various agents, but methodological differences have limited the opportunity for comparisons of disease prevalence in different circumstances in the same industry. Cohort studies of enzyme workers and laboratory animal workers have shown exposure-response correlations and evidence of modifying influences, particularly atopy and tobacco smoking. Although which of the different components of exposure—intensity, duration, or cumulative exposure—is important in establishing the risk of developing the disease has not been clarified, there is sufficient evidence to justify studies of the effect of interventions to reduce exposure to the important causes of occupational asthma, such as isocyanates and laboratory animal excreta, on subsequent attack rates. One cohort study of enzyme workers, which showed an exposure-response gradient, reported a fall in disease incidence after enzyme concentrations in air were reduced.[29] Few other studies of occupational asthma have reported the effects on disease incidence of reductions in airborne allergen concentrations, although the introduction of methods to prevent the dissemination of soya bean dust during its unloading in the harbour of Barcelona was followed by a considerable fall in the number of emergency admissions and cases of asthma needing intensive care.[53]

There is now considerable evidence that the prevalence of asthma has increased in Western communities during the past 20 to 30 years. This does not appear to be wholly attributable to diagnostic transfer or methodological differences between surveys made at different times. Several studies have found that the increase in asthma prevalence has been accompanied by an increase in the prevalence of skin test responses to common environmental allergens and of eczema and hay fever, suggesting an increase in sensitisation. The reasons for this are obscure, but findings from studies of occupational asthma could make an important contribution to its understanding.

The incidence of occupational asthma and sensitisation is greatest during the first one to two years of exposure. The risk during this period increases with increasing exposure, and the modifying effect of tobacco smoking is greatest during this period. This suggests that the risks of respiratory allergy and asthma are greatest during the early period of exposure to a novel allergen and may be increased by exposure to both specific and non-specific factors during this vulnerable period. There is circumstantial evidence that exposure to indoor pollutants, both allergenic—house dust mite and cat—and others such as the oxides of nitrogen, has increased in recent years since the replacement of open fires by central heating and the sealing of buildings, both domestic and commercial. The increase in the prevalence of asthma has also been accompanied by an increase in tobacco consumption by women of child bearing age.

Occupational asthma is a good example of a health problem, which potentially is amenable to prevention. It is also a valuable model of asthma induced by specific environmental exposure; lessons from its study could illuminate the important public health problem of the current, as yet unexplained, increase in the prevalence of asthma.

1 Newman Taylor AJ. Occupational asthma. *Thorax* 1980; **45**: 241–5.
2 Burney PJG, Chinn S, Britton JR, Tattersfield AE, Papacosta AO. What symptoms predict the bronchial response to histamine? Evaluation in a community survey of the bronchial symptoms questionnaire (1984) of the International Union against Tuberculosis and Lung Disease. *Int J Epidemiol* 1989; **18**: 165–73.
3 Venables KM, Farrer N, Sharp L, Graneek BJ, Newman Taylor AJ. Respiratory symptoms questionnaire for asthma epidemiology: validity and reproducibility. *Thorax* 1993; **48**: 214–9.
4 Cartier A, Malo J-L, Forest F, Lafrance M, Pineau L, St-Aubin JJ, Dubois JY. Occupational asthma in snow crab process workers. *J Allergy Clin Immunol* 1984; **74**: 261–9.
5 Bardy JD, Malo J-L, Séguin P, Ghezzo H, Desjardins D, Dolovich J, Cartier A. Occupational asthma and IgG sensitisation in a pharmaceutical company processor psyllium. *Am Rev Respir Dis* 1987; **125**: 1033–8.
6 Malo J-L, Cartier A, L'Archevêque J, Ghezzo H, Lagier F, Trudeau C, Dolovich J. Prevalence of occupational asthma and immunological sensitisation to psyllium amongst health personnel in chronic care hospitals. *Am Rev Respir Dis* 1991; **142**: 1359–66.
7 Venables KM, Burge PS, Davison AG, Newman Taylor AJ. Peak expiratory flow rates in surveys: the reproducibility of observers reports. *Thorax* 1984; **39**: 828–32.
8 Corn M. Strategies of air sampling. In: McDonald JC, ed. *Recent Advances in Occupational Health 1*. Edinburgh. Churchill Livingstone, 1981: 199–209.
9 Meredith SK, Taylor VM, McDonald JC. Occupational respiratory disease in the United Kingdom 1989: a report to the British Thoracic Society and the Society of Occupational Medicine by the SWORD project group. *Br J Ind Med* 1991; **48**: 292–8.
10 Gannon PGF, Burge PS. A preliminary report of a surveillance scheme of occupational asthma in the West Midlands. *Br J Ind Med* 1991; **48**: 579–82.
11 Sallie BA, Ross DJ, Meredith SK, McDonald JC. SWORD'93. Surveillance of work-related and occupational respiratory disease in the UK. *Occup Med* 1994; **44**: 177–82.

12 Meredith S, McDonald JC. Occupational asthma in chemical, pharmaceutical and plastics processors and manufacturers in the United Kingdom, 1989–90. *Ann Occup Hyg* 1994; **38**: 833–7.

13 Meredith S. Reported incidence of occupational asthma in the United Kingdom. *J Epidemiol Community Health* 1993; **47**: 459–463.

14 Keskinen H. Registers for occupational disease. *BMJ* 1991; **303**: 597–8.

15 Brooks S, Weiss MA, Bernstein IL. Reactive airways dysfunction syndrome: persistent asthma syndrome after high level irritant exposure. *Chest* 1985; **88**: 376–84.

16 Harkonen H, Nordman H, Korhonen O *et al.* Long term effects from exposure to sulphur dioxide: lung function 4 years after a pyrite dust explosion. *Am Rev Respir Dis* 1983; **128**: 840–7.

17 Luo JCJ, Nelson K, Fischbein A. Persistent reactive airways dysfunction after exposure to toluene di-isocyanate. *Br J Ind Med* 1988; **47**: 239–41.

18 Bernstein IL, Bernstein DI, Weiss M, Campbell GP. Reactive airways disease syndrome (RADS) after exposure to toxic ammonia fumes. *J Allergy Clin Immunol* 1989; **83**: 173.

19 Moisan T. Prolonged asthma after smoke inhalation: a report of 3 cases and a review of previous reports. *J Occup Med* 1991; **33**: 458–61.

20 Kern DG. Outbreak of the reactive airways dysfunction syndrome after a spill of glacial acetic acid. *Am Rev Respir Dis* 1991; **144**: 1056–64.

21 Sallie BA, McDonald JC. Circumstances, severity and outcome of inhalation accidents in the UK. *Proceedings of Tenth International Symposium on Epidemiology in Occupational Health.* Como, 20–23 September 1994 (in press).

22 McDonald JC. Epidemiology In: Weill H, Turner-Warwick M, eds. *Occupational Lung Disease: Research Approaches and Methods.* New York: Marcel Dekker, 1981.

23 Flindt MLH. Pulmonary disease due to inhalation of derivatives of *Bacillus subtilis* containing enzymes. *Lancet* 1969; **i**: 1177–81.

24 Pepys J, Hargreaves FE, Longbottom JL, Fowkes J. Allergic reactions of the lungs to enzymes of *Bacillus subtilis.* Lancet 1969; **i**: 1181–4.

25 Newhouse ML, Tag B, Pocott SJ, McEwan AC. An epidemiological study of workers producing enzyme washing powders. *Lancet* 1970; **i**: 689–93.

26 Greenberg M, Milne JF, Watt J. Survey of workers exposed to dust containing derivatives of *Bacillus subtilis. BMJ* 1970; **ii**: 629–33.

27 Weill H, Waddell LC, Ziskind M. A study of workers exposed to detergent enzymes. *JAMA* 1979; **217**: 425–33.

28 Mitchell CA, Gandevia B. Respiratory symptoms and skin reactivity in workers exposed to proteolytic enzymes in the detergent industry. *Am Rev Respir Dis* 1971; **104**: 1–12.

29 Juniper CP, Howe W, Goodwin BFJ, Kinshott AK. *Bacillus subtilis* enzymes: a 7 year clinical epidemiological and immunological study of an industrial allergen. *J Soc Occup Med* 1977; **27**: 3–12.

30 Venables KM, Dally MB, Burge PS, Pickering CAC, Newman Taylor AJ. Occupational asthma in a steel coating plant. *Br J Ind Med* 1985; **42**: 517–24.

31 Johnson A, Chan-Yeung M, McLean L, Atkins E, Dybuncio A, Cheng F, Enison D. Respiratory abnormalities among workers in an iron steel foundry. *Br J Ind Med* 1985; **42**: 94–100.

32 Howe W, Venables KM, Dally MB, Hawkins ER, Law SJ, Newman Taylor AJ. Tetrachlorophthalic anhydride asthma: evidence for specific IgE antibodies. *J Allergy Clin Immunol* 1983; **71**: 5–11.

33 Venables KM, Newman Taylor AJ. Exposure-response relationships in asthma caused by tetrachlorophthalic anhydride. *J Allergy Clin Immunol* 1990; **85**: 55–8.

34 Venables KM, Topping MD, Howe W, Luczynska CM, Hawkins ER, Newman Taylor AJ. Interaction of smoking and atopy in producing specific IgE antibody against a hapten protein conjugate. *BMJ* 1985; **290**: 201–4.

35 Anto JM, Sunyer J, Grimal T, Acenes M, Reed C. Community outbreak of asthma associated with inhalation of soya bean dust. *N Engl J Med* 1989; **321**: 1097–103.

36 Newman Taylor AJ, Longbottom JC, Pepys J. Respiratory allergy to urine proteins of rats and mice. *Lancet* 1977; **ii**: 847–9.

37 Newman Taylor AJ, Gordon S. Laboratory Animal and Insect Allergy. In: Bernstein IL,

Chan-Yeung M, Malo J-L, Bernstein DI, eds. *Asthma in the Workplace*. New York: Marcel Dekker, 1993. 399–414.

38 Venables KM, Tee RD, Hawkins ER, Gordon DJ, Wale CJ, Farrer NM, *et al.* Laboratory animal allergy in a pharmaceutical company. *Br J Ind Med* 1988; 45: 667–71.

39 Chan-Yeung M, Vidal S, Kus J, McLean L, Enison D, Tse KS. Symptoms, pulmonary function and bronchial hyper-reactivity in Western red cedar workers compared with those in office workers. *Am Rev Respir Dis* 1984; 130: 1038–41.

40 Coutts II, Lozewicz S, Dally MD, Newman Taylor AJ, Burge PS, Flyn DAC, *et al.* Respiratory symptoms related to work in a factory manufacturing cimetidine tablets. *BMJ* 1984; 288: 14.

41 Malo J-L, Cartier A. Occupational asthma in workers of a pharmaceutical company processing spiramycin. *Thorax* 1988; 43: 371–7.

42 Venables KM, Dally MB, Nunn AJ, Stevens JF, Stephens R, Farrer N, *et al.* Smoking and occupational allergy in a platinum refinery. *BMJ* 1989; 299: 939–42.

43 Cullinan P, Lowson D, Nieuwenhuijsen MJ, Gordon S, Tee RD, Venables KM *et al.* Work-related symptoms, sensitisation and estimated exposure in workers not previously exposed to laboratory rats. *Occup Environ Med* 1994 (in press).

44 Malo J-L, Cartier A, Ghezzo H, Lafrance M, McCantz M, Lehrer S. Patterns of improvement on spirometry. Bronchial hyper-responsiveness and specific IgE antibody levels after cessation of exposure in occupational asthma caused by snow crab processing. *Am Rev Respir Dis* 1988; 138: 807–12.

45 Venables KM, Topping MD, Nunn AJ, Howe W, Newman Taylor AJ. Immunologic and functional consequences of chemical (tetrachlorophthalic anhydride) induced asthma after four years of avoidance of exposure. *J Allergy Clin Immunol* 1987; 80: 212–8.

46 Slovak AJM. Occupational asthma caused by a plastics blowing agent, azodicarbonamide. *Thorax* 1981; 36: 906–9.

47 Lozewicz S, Assoufi BK, Hawkins R and Newman Taylor AJ. Outcome of asthma induced by isocyanates. *Br J Dis Chest* 1987; 81: 14–22.

48 Weir DC, Robertson JF, Jones S, Burge PS. The economic consequences of developing occupational asthma. *Thorax* 1987; 42: 209.

49 Venables KM, Davison AG, Newman Taylor AJ. Consequences of occupational asthma. *Respir Med* 1989; 83: 437–40.

50 Slovak AJM, Hill RN. Laboratory animal allergy: a clinical survey of an exposed population. *Br J Ind Med* 1981; 38: 38–41.

51 Musk AW, Venables KM, Crook B, Nunn AJ, Hawkins R, Crook GDW, *et al.* Respiratory symptoms, lung function and sensitisation to flour in a British bakery. *Br J Ind Med* 1989; 46: 636–42.

52 Prichard MG, Ryan G, Musk AW. Wheat flour sensitisation and airway disease in urban bakers. *Br J Ind Med* 1984; 8: 450–4.

53 Tee RD, Gordon DJ, Hawkins ER, Nunn AJ, Lacey J, Venables KM, *et al.* Occupational allergy to locusts: An investigation of the sources of the allergen. *J Allergy Clin Immunol* 1988; 81: 517–25.

54 Weill H, Salvaggio JE, Neilson A, Butcher B, Ziskind M. Respiratory effects of toluene di-isocyanate manufacture: a multidisciplinary approach. *Environ Health Perspect* 1975; 11: 101–8.

55 Wernfoss S, Neilson J, Schutz A, Skerfung S. Phthalic anhydride induced occupational asthma. *Ind Arch Allergy Appl Immunol* 1986; 79: 77–82.

56 Burge PS, Edge G, Hawkins R, White V, Newman Taylor AJ. Occupational asthma in a factory making flux cured solder containing colophony. *Thorax* 1981; 36: 828–34.

57 Paggiaro PL, Loy LM, Rossi O, Ferrante B, Pardy IF, Rosselli MG, *et al.* Follow up study of patients with respiratory disease due to toluene di-isocyanate (TDI). *Clin Allergy* 1984; 14: 463–9.

58 Chan-Yeung M, Lam S, Korerner S. Clinical features and natural history of occupational asthma due to Western red cedar (Thuja plicata). *Am J Med* 1982; 72: 411–5.

59 Burge P. Occupational asthma in electronics workers caused by colophony fumes: Follow-up of affected workers. *Thorax* 1982; 37: 348–53.

7 Dermatoses

HENRIËTTE SMIT, PIETER-JAN COENRAADS,
EDWARD EMMETT

Introduction

On a visit to any manufacturing plant, one is likely to encounter workers
with hand dermatitis. Work-related dermatoses, in particular hand
dermatitis, are still among the most prevalent occupational diseases.
There is a vast literature on work-related dermatoses, particularly case
reports and investigative clinical studies; their epidemiology however, has
received little attention. The most important reason is probably that the
condition is never fatal, and only a small proportion leads to disability.
Nevertheless, contact dermatitis is a nuisance to its sufferers and often
takes a long time to heal.

The vast majority of work-related dermatoses comprises contact
dermatitis (90–95%); the rest are of other dermatoses such as contact
urticaria, oil acne, chloracne, chemically-induced leucoderma, and
infections.[1] Therefore, this chapter will focus on studies related to
contact dermatitis.

Contact dermatitis is an inflammatory reaction of the skin that may occur as a result of contact with external factors. Two aetiologically different types can be distinguished: irritant and allergic contact dermatitis. Irritant contact dermatitis results from contact with irritant substances, while allergic contact dermatitis is a delayed-type immunological reaction in response to contact with an allergen in sensitised individuals. Irritant contact dermatitis is more prevalent in "wet work" occupations like cleaning, hairdressing, nursing, and food handling while allergic contact dermatitis is predominant in, for example, the rubber, building, and plastics industries.[2] In general, irritant contact dermatitis is more prevalent than allergic contact dermatitis, although the latter more often requires medical care.[2]

Contact dermatitis results in redness, papules, pustules, vesicles, exudation, and itching. In chronic cases, the redness fades, and is replaced by fissures, thickening of the skin and exaggeration of the normal skin relief. Primary lesions are usually found at the site of contact with the irritant or allergen. The symptoms of irritant contact dermatitis remain restricted to the site of contact. In cases of allergic contact dermatitis, secondary lesions may occur in other sites of the body, even at those sites that have never been in contact with the allergen. In most cases of contact dermatitis the hands are affected, alone or in combination with other sites. This predominance of contact dermatitis in the spectrum of occupational dermatoses, and the predominance of the hands as the most common localisation, is the reason why in many statistics occupational skin disease is almost the same as hand dermatitis. In Continental Europe the term eczema is more or less equivalent to the Anglo-Saxon term dermatitis, and will therefore be used as a synonym in this text.

Frequency

Data on the incidence and prevalence of occupational dermatoses are scarce. The most important sources of data are occupational disease registries, case series of patients visiting dermatology clinics, and a limited number of cross-sectional studies in one or more occupational groups. However, none of these sources provide enough occupation-specific figures to allow identification of high risk occupations. Occupational disease registries provide national data or nationally representative data but suffer from underdiagnosis and underreporting. Observational studies are often restricted to a limited number of occupations. The case definition and study design differs from study to study, hampering comparison of prevalence figures across studies. Case series (patient populations visiting dermatology clinics) provide information only on the numerator and are therefore inadequate for determining incidence or prevalence. Nevertheless, most of the current knowledge on high risk occupations stems from case-series. Also, assuming that the source population of dermatology clinics remains fairly constant over time, reports of case studies over a prolonged period of time, may reflect changes in exposure that have occurred in the source population.

Occupational disease registries

Occupational disease registries provide national data based on the notification of occupational skin diseases and are available in many countries. National registries are usually incomplete as a result of underdiagnosis and underreporting of the disease.[3][4] It has been estimated that the incidence of occupational skin diseases in the USA is being underestimated by 10 to 50 times,[5] the milder cases of skin disease not being registered at all. The extent of underreporting is likely to differ between countries, because each country has its own system of notification. The registration of occupational diseases in Sweden, the former Federal Republic of Germany, and Finland is based upon the notification of occupational diseases for which compensation is payable.[5-7] Criteria for compensation, and thus criteria for notification of occupational diseases, depend on the legislation on occupational diseases in each country. In the United States, the occupational disease statistics originate from an annual survey by the Bureau of Labor Statistics among a representative random sample of about 280 000 employees in private industry.[5] Data on work related injuries and illnesses are obtained from logs which must be kept in the workplace for each calendar year. For these purposes occupational illnesses have been defined as any abnormality that resulted from any work exposure in the work environment, other than an injury. Only new illnesses during the reporting year are included, so that the survey records incidence rather than prevalence data. In the United Kingdom a new initiative (EPIDERM) for recording occupational dermatoses has recently started: dermatologists in a number of centres report confirmed or suspected cases of occupational skin disease, including the occupation of the patient concerned.[8] It is a voluntary system, and operates on the principle of simplicity (ensuring compliance), more or less analogous to the SWORD project on occupational respiratory disease (see Chapter 14). The system can detect previously unreported hazards. The epidemiological limitations are well recognised, but the system corrects the virtual absence of meaningful statistics in the UK since 1983.

Skin diseases constitute up to 30% of all occupational diseases for which compensation is payable. In some countries, this proportion has declined in recent years because other diseases (in particular musculo-skeletal diseases) have been recognised as occupational diseases. This caused an increase in the total number of notified occupational diseases and a decrease of the proportion of skin diseases, while the incidence rates remained about the same. Most papers reporting results of occupational disease registries or national surveys were published in the 1980s.[5-7 9 10] To follow trends in incidence of work related dermatoses recent data are needed.

Although a formal comparison of national data is hampered by differences across countries in underreporting of occupational diseases, the incidence of registered occupational skin diseases in most countries is about 0·5–1·0/1000 full-time workers/year.[4] The incidence in agriculture and the construction and manufacturing industries is above average in most countries. Within the manufacturing industry, relatively high rates are observed in the leather, metal, food, chemical, and rubber industries. A population-based study of cases of occupational skin diseases in North Bavaria (Germany) is one of the few studies that can claim completeness in terms of new cases (numerator) and of size of the occupational groups as denominator.[11] This study showed substantially higher incidence in occupations such as hairdressers (25/1000 employees/year), bakers (10/1000) and florists (4/1000).

Case series

Much of the current knowledge about high-risk occupations and major irritating and sensitising agents comes from the accumulation of case material from specialised referral centres or practitioners with a particular interest in contact dermatitis. The most important investigative tool for contact dermatitis is patch testing and these centres have well developed patch testing (and usually phototesting) facilities, protocols, and procedures. The physicians have a particular interest in contact dermatitis so that visits to industrial plants and other investigative studies are conducted as needed. A number of such centres have published fairly large series, which give interesting data on changes over time and on the relative frequency of important causes of contact dermatitis. The data are particularly strong because the aetiology of the condition has been carefully and exhaustively evaluated leading to diagnostic precision. Such centres generally draw patients from a large urban area or region, but the coverage cannot be guaranteed to be exclusive and will depend on referral patterns and biases. There is likely to be a referral bias towards allergic contact dermatitis, and to forms of dermatitis as a group rather than conditions such as occupational skin cancer or occupational acne which will not benefit from diagnostic patch testing and other procedures available at such clinics.

Evidently, a high proportion of certain occupations within a patient population does not necessarily indicate that the occupation is at high risk of work-related dermatoses because it may also reflect the fact that a particular industry is well represented in a certain area. However, many high-risk occupations mentioned in the classic study by Fregert are also prevalent in other case series and are generally accepted as high-risk occupations.[2] The study reported on 1752 patients studied between 1960–69 in Lund, Sweden.[2] Among women, the highest ranking occupations were hospital work, cleaning, hairdressing, and occupations within the food industry, and hotels or restaurants. Most of the men were working in the metal, building, plastics, rubber, and food industries. The observation that high-risk occupations in men and women are different reflects differences in the predominant occupations that they follow.

A recent study reported 1954 cases of occupational skin disease accumulated during 1980–87 in a private practice with a particular interest in occupational skin disease in Perth, Western Australia.[12] Of 993 patients who had had a diagnosis of occupational skin disease made during this period, 954 had each been recontacted, interviewed, and examined during 1988; in addition, 147 work sites were visited. There was a substantial difference by gender in the occupational distribution. Overall, there was a predominance of men among the cases, even after allowing for the higher proportion of men in the workforce of that region. The most common occupations in men were maintenance workers, construction workers and food handlers and, in women, hairdressers, food handlers, and nurses. In some occupations, the proportion of subjects who first developed dermatitis during apprenticeship was high (notably hairdresser 97%, and food handlers, chefs, and butchers 26%). Of these patients, 4% had developed skin disease within days of starting work in that occupation, 12·5% within weeks, 21% within less than 12 months, 16% between one and two years, 15% between two and five years and 31·5% after more than 5 years.

The duration of occupational skin disease before diagnosis was 6% < 1 month, 32% 1–6 months, 19% 7–12 months, and 43% more than one year, indicating the protracted nature of the dermatitis and delays in diagnosis in a substantial proportion of cases.

Other relatively large case series of occupational contact dermatitis have been published from Italy,[13] London, England,[14] Finland,[15 16] and Singapore.[17]

Table 7.1 Major occupational activities incriminated by case series

men	women
engineering/metal work	hairdressing
food handling	nursing
construction	food handling
rubber industry	cleaning
painting	dental work
agriculture	

Table 7.2 Major occupational irritants and allergens identified in case series

irritants	allergens
metal working fluids	nickel
solvents	chromate
detergents	epoxy resin
cement	rubber chemicals
food juices	preservatives

Tables 7.1 and 7.2 show the major occupational activities and the major causative agents mentioned in published case series.

Observational studies

To identify high-risk occupations within a country or a geographically defined area, prevalence figures from a population-based cross-sectional survey are most useful, as the prevalence in all occupational groups is estimated over the same period using the same methods. A breakdown by occupation or industry was given in two major population-based studies. Coenraads *et al.*,[18] investigated a sample of 3140 men and women aged 28–71 years in an urban and a rural area in the Netherlands. All subjects were examined by a team of trained medical students who were instructed to call the authors (dermatologists) who were on standby when any skin disorder on the hands or distal arms was observed or suspected. Eczema was defined as the presence of eczematous symptoms for more than three weeks, or as recurrent eczema over the previous three years. The age-adjusted three-year prevalence of hand eczema, thus obtained, was 14·2% in the chemical industry, 11·6% in the metal industry, 7·8% in the construction industry, and 6·5% in agriculture. Another survey using the same methods in the construction industry showed age-adjusted three-year prevalence of 12·1% among bricklayers compared with 6·9% among supervisors and administrative personnel.

Meding and Swanbeck performed a large scale survey among a sample of 16 587 men and women aged 28–63 years in Gothenburg, Sweden.[19] The presence of hand dermatitis was initially assessed by a self-administered questionnaire. Those who reported that they had had hand eczema during the previous 12 months, were invited to a dermatological examination with a standardised interview and registration of objective skin signs. The overall one-year prevalence was 10·6%. The prevalence of hand dermatitis among the 12 750 subjects who were gainfully employed is shown in table 7.3. The highest prevalence was observed in medical and nursing work (15·9%), and in service occupations (15·4%). Among the latter, the prevalence in cleaners was highest (21·9%). Recently another study was performed among car mechanics by the same group. The

Table 7.3   Reported one year prevalence of hand eczema in occupations from a population-based study in Gothenburg (Sweden)

Occupational group	One-year prevalence (%)		
	men	women	total
production	8·1	13·0	8·8
administrative work	8·4	11·8	10·6
service work	9·4	17·9	15·4
medical and nursing	8·7	12·3	11·9
sales	8·1	12·3	10·2
engineering	6·6	12·3	7·4

Modified from Meding *et al.* 1990[19]

prevalence of hand eczema using the same questionnaire and study methods as in the population-based study, was 15%.[20]

In another study, surveys were performed among five occupational groups and a sample of the general population as a control group.[21] In all surveys the prevalence was assessed by a standard self-administered questionnaire,[22] allowing a valid comparison of the prevalence figures across occupational groups. The prevalence of hand dermatitis ranged from 2·9% in office workers to about 30% in nurses. The prevalence ratio of hand dermatitis in male manual workers in a chemical company, electricity company, and public works seemed to be independent of the type of exposure that occurs in these occupational groups. It was suggested that mechanical stress, which occurs frequently in manual work, in combination with low or moderate exposure to irritants, contributes to the development of hand dermatitis.

Several other cross-sectional studies have been made among specific occupational groups, for example in the metal industry,[23] construction,[24 25] rubber industry,[26] hospital work,[27-29] agriculture,[30 31] painters,[32] and fish processing.[33] The prevalence in these occupations is usually between five and 20%. However, the differences in study methods (in particular, case definition and case ascertainment) between these studies make ranking of the prevalence in these occupations meaningless. This illustrates the need for some form of standardisation in the definition of contact dermatitis in epidemiological studies, as well as methods of case ascertainment (see p 158).

Publications on properly designed follow-up studies which generate incidence-type data are virtually absent. One of the exceptions is the North-Bavaria study, which has been discussed in the paragraph on occupational disease registries.[11] In a study based on medical and employment records in a chemical works it was possible to reconstruct cumulative incidences of dermatitis.[34] There are various studies with something approaching a follow-up design, but as a result of various practical circumstances, these studies have their limitations. Some are cross-sectional at two different points in time,[24] suffer from loss of follow-up,[35] base their follow-up on questionnaires only,[36] or have selection bias.[37] For a further discussion on these limitations, see the paragraph below on methodological considerations.

Risk factors and determinants

The development of contact dermatitis is influenced by a combination of individual susceptibility and exposure characteristics. Skin contact with external factors (irritant or allergic) is a necessary condition for the development of contact dermatitis. No lesions will occur without exposure, but when contact with the irritant or allergen has occurred, the probability and severity of a reaction depend on the type and intensity of exposure. Individual susceptibility may be related to personal characteristics such as age, gender, atopic constitution, contact sensitisation, and the condition of the skin. Environmental factors may play a part in this process by influencing the individual susceptibility (condition of the skin) and the characteristics of exposure or both, but little is known about the interplay of exposure, individual susceptibility, and environmental factors.

Exposure

Case series have identified the irritants and allergens that are most common among patients suffering occupational skin disease (see table 7.2). A high ranking agent in a case series is not, however, automatically also a strong sensitiser or irritant. A wide application in industry of a weak allergen or irritant is more likely to result in a large number of cases than the use of a particular strong agent in one or more plants within an area. There is no information from epidemiological studies about the relative risk of exposure to single agents. The lack of epidemiological studies on that question may be ascribed to the difficulties in performing such studies properly.

Individual susceptibility

There are few epidemiological studies that take the effect of several risk factors (personal characteristics, exposure, and environmental conditions) into account simultaneously.

Kristensen reported a prospective study among 1564 new employees in an automobile manufacturing industry, who were followed up for one year after preemployment screening.[35] Written questionnaires were used at three and 12 months to obtain information on type of work, exposure, protection, and hand dermatitis. All patients who developed hand eczema were examined, patch tested, and followed to establish the course and consequence of their eczema. On average 4·4% of the newly employed people acquired symptoms of hand eczema during the first year of employment. The risk was higher in women than in men (6% versus 3·5%), which was suggested as the result of women being more commonly employed in "wet work" (cleaning and kitchen work). The risk was significantly higher in those with previous hand eczema (21%), atopic dermatitis (14%), wool intolerance (11%), and hay fever (9%). Most of the patients developed their eczema within the first six months of follow-up.

Meding and Swanbeck reported predictive factors for hand eczema from their large population-based study.[38] The most important risk factor was childhood eczema. Of those who reported having childhood eczema 27·3% reported hand eczema compared with 9% of the others (odds ratio adjusted for other risk factors 3·3). The second risk factor was female gender, followed by occupational exposure, atopic mucous membrane symptoms, and an occupation in the service industry. A small reduction in risk with advancing age was found.

Smit, van Rijssen, and Coenraads followed 74 apprentice hairdressers and 111 apprentice nurses from the start of first occupational exposure until the end of their apprenticeship to study the role of individual susceptibility to hand dermatitis.[39] The average incidence of hand dermatitis was 32·8/100 person-years in hairdressers and 14·5/100 person-years in nurses. The relative risk of those with a dry compared with normal skin type was 7·3 in hairdressers and 1·7 in nurses. Apprentice nurses with a history of atopic mucosal symptoms had a 3·4-fold increased risk of hand dermatitis. The increased risk of mucosal atopy in apprentice hairdressers was 2·2. The results suggested an increased risk of hand dermatitis in apprentice hairdressers with transepidermal water loss on the hand greater than 15 $g/m^2.h$; but this association was not statistically significant. No significant association was observed between age, gender, childhood eczema, or presence of a positive skin test (prick or patch test) and the risk of hand dermatitis. The lack of an association with childhood eczema in that study is inconsistent with results from other studies in which childhood eczema was the most important risk factor for hand dermatitis (see further in this paragraph: atopy). It was suggested that the study lacked power to detect a potential association, because the study population contained only a small number of persons with childhood eczema. Another explanation may be that those who had hand dermatitis at the start of the study were excluded from the analysis because they were not free of disease. These people were all atopic and their hand dermatitis (in fact atopic dermatitis) continued throughout the study.

Indications with respect to the effect of age, gender, atopy, contact sensitisation, condition of the skin, and environmental factors, obtained from other studies are summarised below.

151

Gender

The prevalence of irritant contact dermatitis is higher among women. Some physiological and anatomical differences between the skin of men and women exist, which may cause gender-related differences in susceptibility to irritants or sensitisers (dryness of the skin, subcutaneous fat, and other variables) but gender-related differences in irritability of the skin have not been observed in experimental studies.[41] [42] It is more likely that gender-related differences in exposure are responsible for a difference in the prevalence of irritant contact dermatitis. The fact that women's hands tend to be more exposed to household wet work is the most likely explanation, although this exposure has rarely been quantified in epidemiological studies.[36]

Age

In general it is believed that the sensitivity of the skin decreases with age.[42] A population-based study showed that the association between age and eczema prevalence disappeared when account was taken of occupation in the analysis, and concluded that occupation and not age was a major factor associated with eczema prevalence.[18] It is likely that during the years of employment, age related exposure variables are for the most part responsible for the alleged effect of age.

Atopy

In general terms, atopy can be defined as the presence of one or a combination of the symptoms: asthma, hay fever, and atopic dermatitis. For the ascertainment of atopic dermatitis, scoring systems are available.[43] [44] Based on Diepgen's criteria, about 10% of the general population have signs of atopic dermatitis. In recent years, evidence has accumulated that past or present atopic dermatitis is a risk factor for contact dermatitis. Earlier studies indicated that the proportion of atopic individuals among patients with hand eczema was almost three times as high as among the general population or a healthy control group. Later it appeared that a history of atopic dermatitis was particularly associated with irritant contact dermatitis. This was ascribed to reduced resistance of the atopic skin. The proportion of people with sporadic or continuous hand eczema was significantly greater in those with moderate and severe atopic dermatitis in childhood (60% and 48% respectively) compared with those with respiratory allergy only, and a group who had no atopy (14% and 11% respectively).[45] Rystedt provided evidence that exogenous factors such as exposure to irritant factors were less important in the development of hand eczema than constitutional factors like atopic dermatitis in childhood, persistent eczema on other parts of the body and dry and itchy skin.[46] A family history of atopic dermatitis, female gender, and concurrent asthma and rhinitis were of limited importance. In the follow-up study by Nilsson a history of atopic dermatitis increased the odds of developing hand eczema three fold.[36] A population-based incidence study in the food industry calculated a more than eight times increased risk of occupational skin disease in employees with an atopic skin diathesis.[47] The increased risk of more than 13 times in people with atopy reported in a study from South Carolina, USA, is derived from odds ratios generated by a type of case-control design that may have been affected by serious selection bias.[48]

Even if in epidemiological terms atopic dermatitis is an effect modifier, it can be argued that the observed irritant contact dermatitis associated with atopy is an exacerbation of underlying atopic dermatitis, rather than irritant contact dermatitis. Since atopic dermatitis is associated with respiratory atopic symptoms, one would expect that respiratory atopy is also a risk factor. The same problem arises with the risk factor "dry skin" (see below), which may be an expression of atopic dermatitis.

After childhood, atopic dermatitis has a tendency to become manifest during puberty and young adulthood. This phenomenon may have influenced the perceived association between age and contact dermatitis. Contact allergy is thought to be less common among persons with atopic dermatitis; it is as yet unresolved whether this is a feature of atopy, or whether this is a variant of the healthy worker effect: people with atopic dermatitis tend to avoid certain occupations, and hence certain exposures.

Contact sensitisation

For people with a present allergy to a substance in the workplace the importance of allergy as a risk factor is evident: a chromate sensitive person, for example, cannot be employed as a bricklayer. Most speculations on the role of contact allergy stem from cross-sectional studies such as, for example, the role of nickel dermatitis in hairdresser's hand dermatitis. Contrary to common belief, there is no evidence that the presence of a contact allergy which is not occupational, is a risk factor for the development of hand dermatitis. This may be illustrated by the problems surrounding contact allergy to nickel. The presence of nickel allergy has always been regarded as a risk factor for the development of contact dermatitis of the hands; in a prospective study there was, however, no evidence that nickel allergy was relevant.[39]

Nickel allergy is common, mostly resulting from ear-piercing, and occurs in 20% of young women. The perceived association between nickel allergy and risk of occupational contact dermatitis stems mainly from clinical observations of the numerator, where the source population has been left out of the denominator. Women with occupational hand dermatitis often have nickel allergy; the epidemiological evidence points towards an association between gender-related exposure and nickel allergy, and not towards nickel being a risk factor itself.

Nickel allergy may be associated with atopy.[11] [49] This observation supports the notion that nickel allergy has "contaminated" many observational statistics on hand dermatitis, rather than being relevant in most cases.

Chromate has been a common sensitiser in men, and clinical observations suggest that this allergy contributes to a poor prognosis. Epidemiological evidence for any role of chromate allergy as a risk factor for the development of contact dermatitis is lacking, except in specific occupations with high exposure to chromate.

False positive and false negative test results are not uncommon in skin testing for contact allergy (patch testing). Sensitivity, specificity, and the predictive value of a positive test have not been taken into account in analyses of the role of pre-existing contact allergy as a risk factor.

Condition of the skin

Dry skin is a vaguely defined condition which is mainly based on the subject's own opinion about his or her skin. Even when used in this ambiguous way, this factor shows significant impact in several studies.[41] [46] It is also a feature of atopic dermatitis, explaining, at least in part, its role as a risk factor. The quality of the barrier function of the skin is suggested as a factor with a significant role in the risk of contact dermatitis. Instruments have been developed to measure this barrier function by approximation (that is indirectly, by measuring transepidermal water loss). There are individual differences in transepidermal water loss of the unexposed skin.[50] However, there is no evidence to postulate an association between increased transepidermal water loss (as a parameter of skin barrier) and increased contact dermatitis risk.[39]

There is no epidemiological evidence of racial factors determining susceptibility, although clinical and laboratory experiments suggest racial differences in susceptibility to allergens[51] and irritants.[52]

Environmental conditions

Low humidity, high temperatures, occlusion, and sweating may damage the surface of the skin and facilitate penetration of irritants and allergens, thus provoking contact dermatitis. These factors may contribute to the development of contact dermatitis, especially in occupational settings. Seasonal variations in relation to these factors are known to occur, but no epidemiological data are available to quantify this variation. Low skin temperature of the hands in the fish processing industry is a risk factor for hand eczema.[33]

In conclusion, there is, besides atopy, little hard quantitative information on the contribution of personal ch and environmental conditions, not to mention the interaction these factors and characteristics. There is little aetiological resea quantify the contribution of exposure, individual susceptibility, a environmental conditions. This requires carefully designed prospective studies for which some considerations are given below.

Key points

- Atopic dermatitis is a risk factor, or is activated by exposure.
- Except in certain circumstances, contact allergy is not a risk factor.
- Within the time span of employment life, age is not a risk factor.
- Dry skin is probably a risk factor, a proxy for atopic dermatitis.
- Gender is not a risk factor, but is associated with exposure.
- There is no other known personal skin characteristic associated with risk.
- There is ample evidence for exposure being the most important determinant of risk.
- Quantifications of exposures and their association with disease risk are virtually absent.
- Extremes in the micro-environment (dryness, humidity, occlusion) are important effect modifiers.

Prognosis

The prognosis of contact dermatitis is notoriously poor.[4] A great number of papers, dating back to 1930, have reported on the follow-up of patients with dermatitis. A review of most of these studies by Hogan et al., showed that half or less than half of the patients had healed after several years of follow-up.[53] The percentage of eczema patients with recurring symptoms of contact dermatitis in working populations varied between 35% and 80% depending on the severity of the symptoms, the period of follow-up, and the intensity of exposure.[34] The prognosis for allergic contact dermatitis is thought to be worse than for irritant contact dermatitis.[2 40 54] Not all studies show this effect, but the greater tendency for medical consultation, sick leave, and permanent disability in persons with allergic contact dermatitis is consistent with the observation that symptoms in these patients are generally more persistent than in patients with irritant dermatitis.[2 40 54 55] It should be kept in mind, however, that information bias and selection bias may have caused the discrepancies; contact allergy to chromate in men, and to nickel in women have probably "contaminated" the statistics. A persistent and troublesome type of dermatitis is more likely to be subject to additional skin testing, creating a

: result. The relevance of these common
stence is uncertain; it can be questioned
allergy have allergic contact dermatitis,
hatitis that is complicated by allergy to the
i (see also the paragraph on risk factors).
ct allergies, it may be relatively easy to avoid

s with hand dermatitis who were identified in a
in Gothenburg, 22% reported five or more
their condition.[54] Sick leave in relation to hand
derm... by 21%. The mean duration of sick leave was four
weeks. Wall a... ier followed 954 patients with occupational skin
diseases diagnosed between 1980–1987.[37] The period from original
diagnosis until review varied from 0·5 to eight years. Sixty one percent
of the subjects reported that they had lost time from work as a result of
their skin disease. About 6% had been off work for longer than 12 months
continuously.

Opinions are divided with respect to the effect of a change of
occupation. Fregert concluded that a change of occupation did not result
in better healing than continuing in the same job, although the rate of
healing seemed to be slightly better in the group which had changed.[2] In
his discussion, Fregert noted that most of those who changed their work
had the most severe eczema, which could explain the persistence of the
condition. He therefore did not discourage advice to change jobs. Among
metal workers with soluble oil dermatitis, no significant beneficial effect
was observed from a change of occupation. Pryce *et al.* on the other hand
noted that 11 of the 15 individuals who had changed their occupation
healed within three months.[56] Rystedt found that 65–70% of the patients
with hand eczema and severe or moderate atopic dermatitis had improved
substantially after a change of job.[45] Wall and Gebauer observed a clear
beneficial effect of a change to an entirely different kind of work.[37] Over a
quarter of the patients who changed jobs because of skin problems, chose
occupations in which the work environment aggravated their occupational
skin disease. This should be taken into account in studying the effect of
change. A study of 896 Finnish farmers with hand dermatoses showed that
after 12 years of follow-up the proportion who healed was greater in those
who had given up farm work during the period of follow-up than in those
who continued farming (48% versus 71%).[57]

Wall and Gebauer found that 11·5% of the patients had persistent skin
disease for which there was no obvious present cause.[37] The major
allergens involved in these cases were chromate among men and nickel
among women. Although this is consistent with earlier reports of the
alleged bad prognosis of dermatitis from both metals,[2 58] observer bias and
selection bias, as explained above, may be a more likely explanation.

Prevention

Approaches to the prevention of work-related dermatoses are analogous to the prevention of other work-related diseases. Priority should be given to measures at the source, such as elimination of harmful exposures, with thorough encapsulation of the process as an alternative. Good occupational hygiene, including cleanliness and ventilation is the next step. Personal protection, for example by gloves, has to be the last option, but is often selected in the first place. Good epidemiological intervention studies that evaluate the relative impact of various measures, have not been published.

Clinical observations indicate that many personal protective measures do not have the desired effect, but epidemiological evidence for or against is lacking. Protective gloves, for example, are widely prescribed, but may well contribute to increased risk of contact dermatitis: inside gloves the micro-environment is drastically changed and faulty gloves are worse than no gloves at all. Barrier creams are also widely prescribed, although the effect in terms of reduction of incidence or prevalence of dermatitis has never been documented. Hairdressers, for example, are exposed to a variety of allergens and irritants, and a programme for elimination or reduction of exposure seems timely. A properly designed intervention study might help in finding the most effective strategy.

Emollient creams and ointments used during and after work are also supposed to be effective in preventing contact dermatitis of the irritant type, but the epidemiological evidence is scant.[59] An interesting debate surrounds the prevention of chromate allergy in bricklayers by the addition of ferrous sulphate to cement.[60] Scandinavian countries introduced the addition as mandatory to reduce the prevalence of chromate allergy. However, chromate allergy seems to have decreased in countries which did not introduce this measure[61] and in Sweden before the change.[62] A historical cohort, studied during the transition to chromate-free cement in Denmark, was reconstructed by Avnstorp from two cross-sectional studies in the same cement factory.[24] As the data were derived mostly from two different populations and did not give incidence-based relative risks, the evidence was indirect, but pointed towards a beneficial effect.

A thorough preemployment screening to detect a history of atopic dermatitis or contact allergy may be useful in detecting susceptible workers. These workers could receive guidance and be made aware of the importance of hygienic and protective practices. According to several publications on prevention, people with atopy should be discouraged from occupations with high risks of irritant contact dermatitis, especially wet work.[4 63] This pertains in particular to those with atopy of the skin. For a further discussion see the paragraph on risk factors and determinants.

There is no quantitative evidence supporting preemployment screening programmes; with the uncertainties surrounding the personal risk factors this is not surprising. Obviously, workers with a history of contact allergy to a specific allergen, confirmed by a positive patch test, should not be working with that allergen. Preemployment patch testing with allergens to which workers are going to be exposed does not have any predictive value; risk of sensitisation is determined by the nature of the potential allergen (sensitisation capacity), by the level of exposure, and so far as we know, not by any personal risk factor.

Methodological considerations

Case definition and case finding in observational studies

To avoid bias resulting from the method of case ascertainment, it is usually not enough to restrict case ascertainment within a defined study population to reviewing the files of dermatologists or general practitioners. In general it requires some effort to bring all cases in the study population to the attention of the investigator. Screening of the complete study population according to standardised criteria by one or more trained dermatologists is the most reliable and therefore preferred method. But it is generally not feasible, especially in large study populations. A questionnaire that can be self-administered by the whole study population as was used in several population-based studies is more cost-effective. A diagnosis of contact dermatitis based on a self-administered questionnaire is, however, significantly less valid than the diagnosis based on examination by a dermatologist. This is illustrated by experience in a study of occupational skin disease among California grape (n = 183) and tomato harvesters (n = 43).[64] The survey was prompted by reports of increased dermatitis amongst table grape growers; the tomato harvesters were chosen as a comparison as they were of similar ethnic and socioeconomic status but were engaged in mechanical harvesting without direct skin exposure to the crop. As the workforce comprised mainly migrant and seasonal workers such people are unlikely to be well represented in the usual standard sources of occupational and health data.

An interview questionnaire was prepared in English or Spanish, concerning work history, demographic variables, and general health. To evaluate skin diseases, subjects were asked "Have you had any type of skin rash or skin irritation within the last three months that has lasted two days or more?" This and similar questions were asked for the previous year. Further questions concerned appearance, duration, and symptoms. A waist-up examination was made by trained physicians, who recorded a grading of skin type and most current skin conditions, excluding certain local lesions such as moles, granulomas, cysts, warts, and others.

Fifty two percent of grape workers and 19% of tomato workers reported rashes lasting two days or more during the previous three months; a slightly greater difference was noted when the period in question was one year. No significant differences were seen between the two occupational groups, however, for prevalence of skin conditions on examination. One of the explanations raised by the authors was that rashes earlier in the growing season were reported in the questionnaire, while the symptoms had disappeared by the time of examination. Assuming that the investigators were blinded to the occupation of the workers, the authors also suggested the presence of information bias, in the sense that grape workers may have been more aware than tomato workers of dermatitis from harvest work. The sensitivity of the questionnaire for evaluating current skin conditions was 31%, indicating that only about one third of the cases was detected by the questionnaire. The low sensitivity was attributed to differences in the understanding of abnormality between examiner and respondent. The authors stated that it might also relate to the observed skin conditions being of less than two days' duration; however, given the nature of those most common (acne and variants, folliculitis and eczematous dermatitis), this seems an unlikely explanation. The authors concluded that questionnaires may be insensitive for some dermatological conditions and active surveillance would improve case finding and the validity of incidence data.

Given the practical limitations of a medical examination of large populations, a method was evaluated to combine the validity of a clinical diagnosis and the easy applicability of a self-administered questionnaire.[22] A set of three questions was developed, asking about symptoms of hand dermatitis, their duration, and whether these were recurrent. The validity was evaluated among 109 nurses and compared with a medical diagnosis made by a dermatologist. A diagnosis of hand eczema, defined as "one or more symptoms, with a recurrent character, or lasting for more than three weeks"; had a sensitivity of 100% and a specificity of 64%, resulting in a positive predictive value of 31%. This indicates that use of the questionnaire alone would result in a significant overestimation of the prevalence. Medical examination of only those who responded positively, to exclude false-positive cases, would, however, increase the specificity while maintaining the high sensitivity. It would reduce the screening effort by trained physicians. If the definition of hand eczema was based upon two or more symptoms with a recurrent character, or lasting for more than three weeks, the sensitivity remained high (80%) while the specificity increased to 89%, resulting in a positive predictive value of 63%. The definition may therefore be useful for comparing prevalence figures in different study populations, although the absolute prevalence may be overestimated.

Another issue with regard to questionnaires concerns the validity of objective signs compared with a self-diagnosis of hand eczema.[22] For current objective and past skin disorders on the face, a questionnaire was validated among employees who worked with visual display units.[65] The comparison of these studies gives some idea of the extent of information bias resulting from the use of questionnaires.

Design of observational studies

Much work needs to be done on the development of methodological aspects of prospective studies to address specifically the topic of occupational dermatitis. In particular, the following points should be given further thought.

Definition and ascertainment of incident cases Contact dermatitis is a recurrent disease; if an incident case is defined as "first time symptoms" this implies that one is studying the cause of the first occurrence of symptoms. The determinants of recurrent symptoms may be different. These can be studied by starting with people who have previously shown symptoms of hand dermatitis. Case ascertainment requires examination of the study population at short time intervals (weeks rather than months).

The subjects in a prospective study should be free of the disease The recurrent character of contact dermatitis complicates this requirement. First, the definition of "free of disease" poses the question of time frame (how long should the subject be free of disease). Secondly, the presence of previous hand eczema and atopic dermatitis is of interest, given the hypothesis that it predisposes to work related hand eczema. Exclusion of all those who ever had symptoms, would exclude all subjects with atopic eczema, which is thought to be a risk factor in itself. Moreover, a reliable assessment of "ever symptoms" is not feasible.

To evaluate the contribution of individual susceptibility, the occupational exposure is likely to be a strong confounder Given that the assessment of occupational exposure to irritants and allergens is extremely complex and not well developed, it is likely that adjustment for occupational exposure will leave ample room for residual confounding. It may therefore be efficient to study occupational groups with little or no interindividual variation in occupational exposure. In such circumstances, however, the interaction between level of exposure and individual susceptibility could not be studied.

Some of the individual risk factors, in particular condition of the skin, are also intermediates on the pathway between exposure and disease Examples are contact sensitisation, dry skin, and increased transepidermal water loss. This implies that the effect of these risk factors can be studied only prospectively and that the study subjects should be unexposed at the start of the study.

For practical reasons, follow-up studies have resorted to repeated cross-sectional assessments Odds ratios are then calculated as an approximation to the rate ratio. Logistic regression analysis to assess the correlation between risk factors and hand dermatitis in cross-sectional studies is being used more often in recent years.[36] This gives an estimate of the prevalence odds ratio (POR) for the risk factor of interest. Symptoms of hand eczema are not rare among people without no obvious exposure; in that case the POR may overestimate the size of the association. Under such conditions the Cox proportional hazards model may give a more accurate answer.[66]

Need for further epidemiological studies

Although there is a wealth of information based on clinical data and case series, the paucity of sound epidemiological data on work related dermatoses is clearly illustrated in this chapter. First of all, data on prevalence of work related dermatoses are difficult to compare across studies because of the lack of standardisation of definitions and methods. To be able to compare cross-sectional studies, it is important that some form of standardisation is reached about definitions of contact dermatitis, as well as about methods of case ascertainment. Some efforts to validate and standardise questionnaires are reported in this chapter;[22 65] recently an initiative was taken in Finland to reach consensus about case definition for epidemiological studies. Secondly, little is known about the interaction of occupational exposure, individual susceptibility, and environmental conditions. Prevention should be focused upon elimination, reduction, and avoidance of exposure to casual agents; in many instances, however, this is not feasible. Exposure of the skin of the hands in the household, for example, will always exist to a certain degree. Studies developing and using advanced exposure assessments, or job-exposure matrices, are needed to give regulatory authorities the means of enforcing a cost-effective reduction of exposure to acceptable levels. A challenging question for epidemiologists and dermatologists to solve together is: given that occupational exposure occurs, why is it that some workers develop dermatitis and others do not? This type of question requires carefully designed prospective studies for which some considerations are given above. The results will provide further clues on effective methods of protection and care for susceptible individuals, including job advice and preemployment screening, when exposure cannot be avoided or further reduced.

1 Hogan DJ, Tanglertsampan C. The less common occupational dermatoses. *Occup Med* 1992; 7: 385–401.
2 Fregert S. Occupational dermatitis in a 10-year material. *Contact Dermatitis* 1975; 1: 96–107.
3 Taylor JS. Occupational disease statistics in perspective (editorial). *Arch Dermatol* 1988; 124: 1557–8.
4 Rycroft RJG, Menné T, Frosch PJ, Benezra C (eds). *Textbook of contact dermatitis*, Berlin: Springer, 1992.
5 Mathias CGT, Morrison JH. Occupational skin disease, United States: results from the

Bureau of Labor Statistics Annual Survey of Occupational Injuries and Illnesses, 1973 through 1984. *Arch Dermatol* 1988; **124**: 1519–24.

6 Vaaranen V, Vasama M, Alho J. *Occupational diseases in Finland in 1982.* Publication office Institute of occupational health, Vantaa 1983.

7 Fabry H. Statistik der Berufskrankheiten der Hautgefährdungskataster. *Dermatosen* 1981; **29**: 42–4.

8 Cherry NM, Beck MH, Owen-Smith V. Surveillance of occupational skin disease in the United Kingdom: the OCC-DERM project. In: *Proceedings of the Ninth International Symposium on Epidemiology in Occupational Health*, DHHS (NIOSH) Publication No 94–112, Cincinnati, 1994, 608–10.

9 Eggeling F. Zur Epidemiologie der Berufskrankheiten. Eine Analyse der von den Staatlichen Gewerbeärzten dokumentierten Berufskrankheiten Meldungen 1971–1976 in der Bundesrepublik Deutschland. BAU, Dortmund 1980; **254**:

10 Laubstein H, Mönnich HT. Zur Epidemiologie der Berufsdermatosen (III). *Dermatol Mon schr* 1980; **166**: 369–81.

11 Diepgen TL, Fartasch M. General aspects of risk factors in hand eczema. In: Menné T, Maibach HI, eds. *Hand Eczema*, London: CRC Press, 1994, 141–56.

12 Wall LM, Gebauer KA. Occupational skin disease in Western Australia. *Contact Dermatitis* 1991; **24**: 101–9.

13 Meneghini CL, Angelini G. Primary and secondary sites of occupational contact dermatitis. *Dermatosen* 1984; **32**: 205–7.

14 Cronin E. *Contact Dermatitis.* Edinburgh: Churchill Livingstone, 1980.

15 Förström L. en V. Pirilä, 27 Years of occupational dermatology in Finland. *Berufsdermatosen* 1975; **23**: 207–13.

16 Kanerva L, Estlander & R. Jolanki, Occupational skin disease in Finland. An analysis of 10 years of statistics from an occupational dermatology clinic. *Int Arch Occup Environ Health* 1988; **60**: 89–94.

17 Goh CL, Soh SD. Occupational dermatoses in Singapore. *Contact Dermatitis* 1984; **11**: 288–93.

18 Coenraads PJ, Nater JP, Lende van der R. Prevalence of eczema and other dermatoses of the hands and arms in the Netherlands. Association with age and occupation. *Clin Exp Dermatol* 1983; **8**: 495–503.

19 Meding B, Swanbeck G. Occupational hand eczema in an industrial city. *Contact Dermatitis* 1990; **22**: 13–23.

20 Meding B, Barregard L, Marcus K. Hand eczema in car mechanics. *Contact Dermatitis* 1994; **30**: 129–34.

21 Smit HA, Burdorf A, Coenraads PJ. The prevalence of hand dermatitis in different occupations. *Int J Epidemiol* 1993; **22**: 288–93.

22 Smit HA, Coenraads PJ, Lavrijsen APM, Nater JP. Evaluation of a self-administered questionnaire on hand dermatitis. *Contact Dermatitis* 1992; **26**: 11–6.

23 Boer de EM, Ketel van WG, Bruynzeel DP. Dermatoses in metal workers I. Irritant contact dermatitis. *Contact Dermatitis* 1989; **20**: 212–8.

24 Avnstorp C. Prevalence of cement eczema in Denmark before and since addition of ferrous sulfate to Danish cement. *Acta Derm Venereol (Stockholm)* 1989; **69**: 151–5.

25 Kiec-Swierczynska M. Occupational dermatoses and allergy to metals in Polish construction workers manufacturing prefabricated building units. *Contact Dermatitis* 1990; **23**: 27–32.

26 Varigos GA, Dunt DR. Occupational dermatitis. An epidemiological study in the rubber and cement industries. *Contact Dermatitis* 1981; **7**: 105–10.

27 Hansen KS. Occupational dermatoses in hospital cleaning women. *Contact Dermatitis* 1983; **9**: 343–51.

28 Kavli G, Angell E, Moseng D. Hospital employees and skin problems. *Contact Dermatitis* 1987; **17**: 156–8.

29 Lammintausta K. Hand dermatitis in different hospital workers, who perform wet work. *Dermatosen* 1983; **31**: 14–9.

30 Gamsky TE, McCurdy SA, Wiggins P, Samuels SJ, Berman B, Schenker MB. Epidemiology of dermatitis among California farm workers. *J Occup Med* 1992; **34**: 304–10.

31 Susitaival P, Husman L, Horsmanheim M, Notkola V, Husman K. Prevalence of hand dermatoses among Finnish farmers. *Scand J Work Environ Health* 1994; **20**: 214–20.

32 Högberg M, Wahlberg JE. Health screening for occupational dermatoses in house painters. *Contact Dermatitis* 1980; **9**: 100–6.

33 Halkier-Sorensen L, Thestrup-Pedersen K. Skin temperature and skin symptoms among workers in the fish processing industry. *Contact Dermatitis* 1988; **19**: 206–9.

34 Williamson KS. A prognostic study of occupational dermatitis cases in a chemical works. *Br J Ind Med* 1967; **24**: 103–13.

35 Kristensen O. A prospective study of the development of hand eczema in an automobile manufacturing industry. *Contact Dermatitis* 1992; **26**: 341–5.

36 Nilsson GE, Mikaelsson B, Andersson S. Atopy, occupation and domestic work as risk factors for hand eczema in hospital workers. *Contact Dermatitis* 1985; **13**: 216–23.

37 Wall LM, Gebauer KA. A follow-up study of occupational skin disease in Western Australian. *Contact Dermatitis* 1991; **24**: 241–3.

38 Meding B, Swanbeck G. Predictive factors for hand eczema. *Contact Dermatitis* 1990; **23**: 154–61.

39 Smit HA, Rijssen van A, Vandenbroucke J, Coenraads PJ. Susceptibility to and incidence of hand dermatitis in a cohort of apprentice hairdressers and nurses. *Scand J Work Environ Health* 1994; **20**: 113–21.

40 Agrup G. Hand eczema and other dermatoses in South Sweden. *Acta Derm Venereol (Stockholm)* 1969; **61**: 1–91.

41 Tupker RA, Pinnagoda J, Coenraads PJ, Nater JP. Susceptibility to irritants: role of barrier function, skin dryness and history of atopic dermatitis. *Br J Dermatol* 1990; **123**: 199–205.

42 Patil S, Maibach HI. Effect of age and sex on the elicitation of irritant contact dermatitis. *Contact Dermatitis* 1994; **30**: 257–64.

43 Hanifin JM, Rajka G. Diagnostic features of atopic dermatitis. *Acta Derm Venereol (Stockh)* 1980; **92**: 44–7.

44 Diepgen TL, Fartasch M, Hornstein OP. Evaluation and relevance of atopic basic and minor features in patients with atopic dermatitis and in the general population. *Acta Derm Venereol (Stockh)* 1989; **Suppl. 144**: 50–4.

45 Rystedt I. Work-related hand eczema in atopics. *Contact Dermatitis* 1985; **12**: 167–71.

46 Rystedt I. Factors influencing the occurrence of hand eczema *Contact Dermatitis* 1985; **12**: 185–91.

47 Tacke J, Schmidt A, Fartasch M, Diepgen TL. Occupational contact dermatitis in bakers, confectioners and cooks. A population based study. *Contact Dermatitis* (in press).

48 Shmunes E, Keil JE. Occupational dermatosis in South Carolina: a descriptive analysis of cost variables. *J Am Acad Dermatol* 1983; **9**: 861–8.

49 Möller H, Svensson A. Metal sensitivity: positive history but negative test indicates atopy. *Contact Dermatitis* 1986; **14**: 57–60.

50 Tupker RA, Coenraads PJ, Pinnagoda J, Nater JP. Baseline transepidermal water loss (TEWL) as a prediction of susceptibility to sodium lauryl sulphate. *Contact Dermatitis* 1989; **20**: 265–9.

51 Kligman AM. The identification of contact allergens by human assay. *J Invest Dermatol* 1966; **47**: 375–92.

52 Wilson DR, Berardesca E, Maibach HI. In vitro transepidermal water loss: differences between black and white human skin. *Br J Dermatol* 1988; **119**: 647–52.

53 Hogan DJ, Dannaker CJ, Maibach HI. The prognosis of contact dermatitis. *J Am Acad Dermatol* 1990; **23**: 300–7.

54 Meding B, Swanbeck G. Consequences of having hand eczema. *Contact Dermatitis* 1990; **23**: 6–14.

55 Menné T, Bachmann E. Permanent disability from skin diseases. A study of 564 patients registered over a six year period. *Dermatosen* 1979; **27**: 37–42.

56 Pryce DW, Irvine D, English JSC, Rycroft RJG. Soluble oil dermatitis: a follow-up study. *Contact Dermatitis* 1989; **21**: 28–35.

57 Susitaival P, Hannuksela M. The 12-year prognosis of hand dermatosis in 896 Finnish farmers. *Contact Dermatitis* (in press).

58 Christensen OB. Prognosis in nickel allergy and hand eczema. *Contact Dermatitis* 1982; **8**: 7–15.
59 Halkier-Sorensen L, Thestrup-Pedersen K. The efficacy of a moisturizer (Locobase) among cleaners and kitchen assistants during everyday exposure to water and detergents. *Contact Dermatitis* 1993; **29**: 1–6.
60 Fregert S, Gruvberger G, Sandahl E. Reduction of chromate in cement by iron sulfate. *Contact Dermatitis* 1979; **5**: 39–42.
61 Burrows D, Corbett JR. Industrial dermatitis in Northern Ireland. *Contact Dermatitis* 1977; **3**: 145–50.
62 Färm G. Changing patterns in chromate allergy. *Contact Dermatitis* 1986; **15**: 298–310.
63 Griffiths WAD, Wilkinson DS (eds). *Essentials of industrial dermatology*, Oxford: Blackwell, 1985.
64 McCurdy SA, Wiggins P, Schenker MB, Munn S, Shelab A, Weinbaum Z, et al. Assessing dermatitis in epidemiologic studies: occupational skin disease among California grape and tomato harvesters. *Am J Industr Med* 1989; **16**: 147–57.
65 Berg M, Axelson O. Evaluation of a questionnaire for facial skin complaints related to work at visual display units. *Contact Dermatitis* 1990; **22**: 71–7.
66 Lee J, Chia KS. Estimation of prevalence rate ratios for cross sectional data: an example in occupational epidemiology. *Br J Ind Med* 1993; **50**: 861–2.

8 Neurobehavioural effects

OLAV AXELSON

Introduction

Neurotoxic effects of occupational exposures have long been recognised, for example, from lead, mercury, and other metals or carbon disulphide, trichloroethylene, and other solvents. Early knowledge about these hazards was usually based on clinical observations of relatively few cases. However, the symptoms had to be sufficiently dramatic or characteristic to suggest an occupational aetiology. With the development of more sophisticated examination methods and modern epidemiology, the clinically less obvious correlations between exposures in the workplace and the symptoms and signs of neurobehavioural disorder became evident. But, as with other questions in occupational health, the interpretation of the various study results has sometimes been controversial, especially perhaps with regard to solvent exposure.[1]

This review summarises achievements in occupational neuroepidemiology along with some currently uncertain and therefore scientifically interesting issues. Since the early 1970s, many case series and cross-sectional studies have been published regarding the symptoms and signs of neurobehavioural disturbances in working populations exposed to solvents and other agents. Rather few subjects may be involved, and as these studies are typically of a less clear epidemiological design, I will give them less attention in this review. Instead, I will place emphasis on results from the better designed epidemiological studies of occupational exposures and neuropsychiatric disorders.

Most neurobehavioural studies have been concerned with solvent exposure, probably reflecting the widespread use of solvents plus the fact that the results have not always been consistent. Other neurotoxic agents such as lead, mercury and other metals may be better controlled, or the exposures may be less widespread, at least in countries capable of the appropriate research.

Towards the recognition of neurobehavioural effects

Symptoms and syndromes

Cases of illness probably resulting from exposure to neurotoxic agents in the work environment have been reported for several decades. Numerous cases and case series associated with solvent exposure were reviewed by Browning in 1965.[2] Case reports are hardly more than suggestive in terms of cause and effect but certainly provide important clues for more systematic study. The symptoms noted were memory disturbances, difficulties in concentration and reading, tiredness, sleepiness, lack of initiative, emotional lability, irritability, but also dizziness, headache, alcohol intolerance, and reduced libido. The continuing appearance of clinical and epidemiological reports indicate that adverse effects from exposure to solvents are still common.

Symptoms similar to those in workers exposed to solvents have also been reported among people exposed to lead, even in the absence of lead encephalopathy.[3] Such symptoms have also been noted among welders exposed to aluminium, lead, and manganese.[4] Although less clearly documented, various neurotoxic symptoms may also be related to exposure to pesticides. With these agents, paralysis and weakness of peripheral muscles of the hands and feet, suggesting polyneurophathies, are the effects that predominate.[5] Symptoms characteristic of the neurotoxic effects of many industrial agents usually agree more or less with the so called psychoorganic syndrome or neurasthenic syndrome.[6 7] An alternative term proposed by a WHO working group which considered solvent exposure is chronic toxic encephalopathy.[8]

Methodology

The more definite referral of vague symptoms to work conditions, requires a sound epidemiological study design. This usually depends on finding an adequate reference group and on obtaining a reliable assessment of exposure. In the commonly applied cross-sectional design, current complaints are compared between exposed and unexposed workers in relation to prevailing exposure levels and, at best, with due consideration of earlier exposures, age, and other relevant factors. Long-term severe effects can easily be overlooked in such cross-sectional studies however, because those more seriously affected tend to have left the job because of their symptoms, increasing disability, or even death. Exposed groups may therefore be different from reference groups. Furthermore, the cross-sectional studies often fail to distinguish between acute and chronic effects, as functional disturbances from recent exposure may overshadow those that have developed over time.

Several outcome variables have usually been considered in these cross-sectional studies. These may have been derived from questionnaire information and the performance in psychological tests, sometimes with the addition of results from clinical and neurophysiological examinations. To obtain more valid and comparable data, at least on solvent exposure, an international working group recommended methods for the study of exposed populations.[9] These guidelines, although criticised, may also be useful in studies of agents other than solvents.[1]

Since the 1970s, various questionnaires on neuropsychiatric symptoms have been constructed more or less *ad hoc*. There have been attempts to introduce standardised questionnaires such as the so called Q16, an instrument that comprises 16 questions, which was originally intended for screening neuropsychiatric symptoms in large solvent-exposed groups.[10] It has also been used successfully in studies of workers with lead and of welders exposed to other metals.[4][11] The specificity of this questionnaire was set low so as to obtain sufficient sensitivity to defect incipient effects. This should be kept in mind as a warning against the uncritical use of Q16, or other such sensitive questionnaires, especially for diagnosis in clinical work, but also for epidemiological research. Even when information from a questionnaire is of value for both diagnosis and epidemiology, the symptoms recorded may be exaggerated or underreported and clinical judgement is often necessary.

Various neuropsychological functions, including visual perception, speed of perception, attention and concentration, eye-hand coordination, learning and memory, abstraction and reasoning, may suffer as a result of neurotoxic exposures. Test batteries, differing somewhat and recently computerised, have been used in various studies and countries with results that are often difficult to compare. Attempts have been made by WHO working groups to recommend standard test batteries suitable for this kind of study;[8][9] details and comments can be found elsewhere.[1][12] A quite extensive review on neurobehavioural test results after exposure to metals, solvents, and insecticides is also available.[13]

Findings

There are now many studies that indicate disturbed neuropsychological function after occupational exposure, for example, to carbon disulfide, tri-

and tetrachloroethylene, toluene, xylene, and various mixtures, including white spirit.[14–17] House painters,[18-20] and workers engaged in the manufacture of products from styrene-modified glass fibre-reinforced polyester plastics have been similarly affected.[21] Neuropsychological tests have indicated adverse effects in car painters,[22 23] jet fuel workers,[24] seamen on tankers,[25] rotogravure printers,[26] and others. A possible predisposition or augmentation of the neuropsychological effects of solvents by age is worth noting.[23]

The interpretation of these results is both crucial and controversial. Various circumstances other than exposure have been suggested to explain inconsistencies, especially regarding solvent exposure. A study of 21 monozygotic twins with exposure to solvents is therefore of interest. This showed that the exposed twins had lower performance in several tests, but psychomotor speed was relatively less affected compared with the unexposed co-twins as well as another unexposed twin group.[27]

Nonspecific symptoms such as irritability, tiredness, and sleep disturbance may also occur among people exposed to lead, and psychometric tests indicate effects on the central nervous system. For example, the psychological test scores were found to correlate with lead absorption, and particularly well with zinc protoporphyrin concentrations.[28] Several studies which have looked at psychomotor and cognitive functions indicate effects from relatively low lead exposure levels.[28–31] In some workers, memory and learning functions were apparently affected at blood lead levels as low as 1·45 and 1·3 micromol per litre.[11 32]

Welders with exposure to aluminium, and others to manganese and lead, were asked to answer a questionnaire (Q16) on neuropsychiatric symptoms; significantly more symptoms were reported by these people than by a control group of other welders without the specific exposures.[4] Other studies that have looked at long-term exposure to mercury at low levels have shown neurobehavioural symptoms and disturbances, for example affecting memory. Sometimes, but not always, these symptoms have been associated with poor performance in psychological testing.[33 34]

In a study that compared 84 workers exposed to mercury in a thermometer manufacturing plant with 79 unexposed controls, various neurobehavioural symptoms were slightly more common among the exposed than the referents.[35] Neurological signs such as static tremor, abnormal Romberg test, dysdiadochokinesis, and difficulty with heel-to-toe gait were also more prevalent in the exposed group. Relative risks calculated for some of the symptoms and signs were, for example, 2·8 for difficulty in sleeping and 5·8 for abnormal heel-to-toe gait.

Neurological findings such as weakening or loss of reflexes, tremors, and disturbances of equilibrium have been reported to correlate with years of exposure to organochlorine and organophosphorus insecticides in 441 apple-growers as compared with a control group.[36] Deficits in performance on psychological tests have been reported from Hawaii among apparently symptom-free people who had been exposed to organophosphates.[37] The frontal areas of the brain were reported to have been particularly affected. The presence of several behavioural sequelae from organophosphate poisoning, for example, regarding vigilance and concentration, psychomotor speed, memory deficit, and other disturbances have also been described in many case series.[38] Workers exposed to methyl bromide and sulphuryl fluoride and other fumigants have shown an increased incidence of muscle aches, incoordination, and slurred speech.[39] Performance in behavioural tests was also impaired in comparison with controls.

Comment

Neurophysiological methods have played a major part in the cross-sectional studies already mentioned but also in other studies on solvent-induced disorders that have been reviewed elsewhere.[40]

Electroencephalography has sometimes shown abnormalities, most commonly diffuse and generalised, and both among patients in hospital and in active workers. The clinical importance of these abnormal electroencephalographic findings is unclear, but they have some correlation with results of psychological tests.

Some five to ten percent of people exposed to solvents have paroxysmal electroencephalographic abnormalities in the form of spikes or spike-and-wave discharges, which might indicate a lowered threshold for seizures.[41] These findings corroborate the results from an epidemiological study showing a three-fold increase in risk of epileptic seizures among people exposed to solvents.[42] This study included 104 cases of idiopathic focal epilepsy and 312 matched controls. An increasing risk up to about four-fold was seen in relation to degree of exposure. The latter was based on job titles drawn from census data and consequently somewhat crude, and likely to reduce the risk rather than the opposite. Evoked potentials and cerebral blood flow have been studied in solvent exposed workers.[43] There are several such studies but with inconsistent results, possibly because of less stringent study designs and perhaps also relatively small effects.

Occupational exposures to neurotoxic agents are hazardous not only to the central nervous system but also to peripheral nerves. With solvents, the polyneuropathies are attributable particularly to carbon disulfide, n-hexane, and methyl-n-butyl ketone. Some workers have shown fairly pronounced signs of polyneuropathy, for example, Italian shoe and leather workers exposed to mixtures of n-hexane, n-heptane, other aliphatic hydrocarbons, ethyl acetate, and trichloroethylene.[44] Also affected were groups of Swedish aircraft workers who were exposed to jet fuel,[24] US painters,[45] and Swedish industrial painters and car painters.[22] Other observations suggest that styrene may affect peripheral nerve function, especially the large sensory myelinated fibres, but also the autonomic nervous system.[46] Subjects with a psychoorganic syndrome may also have symptoms that indicate an effect on the autonomic nervous system, but few studies have focused on this aspect. It has been reported, however, that the autonomic nerve regulation of the electrocardiographic P-R interval might be affected by solvent exposure, for example, in a small group of exposed Japanese workers.[47]

Epidemiology of chronic neuropsychiatric disorders

An increasing number of studies have concerned the development over time of more severe neuropsychiatric disorders related to occupational exposures, especially solvents. As outcomes, these studies have examined either a less well-defined psychoorganic syndrome, or disease entities such as Alzheimer's dementia, multiple sclerosis, amyotrophic lateral sclerosis and related conditions, and Parkinson's disease.

The psychoorganic syndrome

Epidemiologic studies of the psychoorganic syndrome or toxic chronic encephalopathy and solvent exposure appeared first from the Nordic countries, but have been followed by similar investigations from other parts of Europe and North America. These studies, which are both of case-control and cohort design, will be reviewed briefly here; in addition, some overall results are shown in tables 8.1 and 8.2.

Table 8.1 Findings in some case-control studies on exposure to white spirit or unspecified solvents

Reference	Type of effect or disorder	Typical odds ratios
Axelson et al., 1976 (Sweden)[48]	disability pension for neuropsychiatric disorders	1·8
Olsen and Sabroe 1980 (Denmark)[52]	disability pension for neuropsychiatric disorders	up to 2·8
Lindström et al., 1984 (Finland)[53]	disability pension for neuropsychiatric disorders	up to 5·5
O'Flynn et al., 1987 (UK)[64]	deaths from presenile dementia	1·1 or less
Riise and Moen, 1988 (Norway)[61]	disability pension for neuropsychiatric disorders	4·3
Brackbill et al., 1990 (USA)[58]	disability pension for neuropsychiatric disorder	up to 1·4
v. Vliet et al., 1990 (Netherlands)[59]	"neuroses"	up to 2·3
	all neuropsychiatric disorders	1·2
Cherry et al., 1992 (Canada)[49]	organic dementia, brain atrophy, psychoorganic syndrome	up to 2·3
Labrèche et al., 1992 (Canada)[60]	any psychiatric diagnosis	up to 1·1

Table 8.2   Findings in some cohort studies on exposure to white spirit or unspecified solvents

Reference	Type of effect or disorder	Typical risk or rate ratios
Mikkelsen, 1980 (Denmark)[51]	disability pension for neuropsychiatric disorder	up to 3·5
Mikkelsen et al., 1988 (Denmark)[65]	clinical dementia	up to 4·9
Guberan et al., 1989 (Switzerland)[56]	disability pension for neuropsychiatric disorders, mainly alcoholism	1·8
Hein et al., 1990 (Denmark)[62]	memory and concentration difficulties	up to 3·7 as odds ratio
Rasmussen et al., 1993 (Denmark)[63]	psychoorganic syndrome	up to 11·2

The term toxic chronic encephalopathy requires comment as such a diagnosis would obviously imply recognition that a toxic agent was responsible, making any epidemiological study of causation superfluous. Instead, the term psychoorganic syndrome appears epidemiologically more appropriate. When the diagnoses under study are thought to be less stringent, this entity may sometimes be permitted to include rather broad and diffuse neuropsychiatric conditions, including any of those conceivably resulting from chronic toxicity.

For reasons just indicated, diagnoses such as dementia, encephalopathy, and cerebral atrophy, but also neurosis, neurasthenia, and similar terms have sometimes been considered *en bloc* for epidemiological purposes. These diagnoses might well overlap in medical practice and include diseases of toxic origin.[48] With growing insight into the conditions most probably associated with exposure, more specific disease entities have been selected for study, such as organic dementia and cerebral atrophy.[49] It may be recalled that by selecting less characteristic disease entities for study, risk ratios tend to decrease rather than to increase.[50] The inclusion of less distinct diagnoses may therefore easily obscure an effect, but hardly results in a falsely positive association between exposure and disease.

In the mid 1970s, a case-control study from Sweden on chronic effects of solvents was based on a register of candidates for disability pension.[48] The study included 151 cases of neuropsychiatric disorders and 248 controls with other diseases. There were 35 subjects in each group with solvent exposure, all in occupations connected with construction work. The results showed that painters, varnishers, and carpet layers had an almost doubled risk (odds ratio 1·8) in comparison with other skilled workers.

These results were independent of whether or not alcoholism was included. Extended to all Sweden, this study implied that about three to four percent of all neuropsychiatric disorders in men 36 to 65 years of age,

171

and severe enough to entitle them to a sick pension, might be related to solvent exposure.

Similar results were obtained in two epidemiological studies from Denmark in the early 1980s, one of them a cohort and the other a case-control study.[51][52] In the cohort study, 2601 male painters were compared with 1790 bricklayers and also with Copenhagen men in general with regard to disability pensioning.[51] The painters had a relative risk of about 3·5 of a disability pension for presenile dementia of unknown cause, which was interpreted as dependent on exposure to solvents. The contemporary Danish case-control study, involving 206 cases and the same number of controls, showed an increased risk of disability or early pension in relation to solvent exposure.[52] Several analyses were made according to the exposure conditions; for example, an odds ratio (or risk ratio) of 2·8 was obtained for indoor exposure in painters.

Among the earlier studies was also a Finnish survey of 374 case-control pairs which reported an odds ratio as high as 5·5 for neurosis and psychopathic personality in relation to solvent exposure.[53] No association was seen with various other psychiatric diagnoses, however. Another Danish case-control study of 229 cases of dementia or other kinds of encephalopathy requiring social supportive facilities also showed some, but less clear, association with solvent exposure.[54]

Studies on disability from neuropsychiatric disorders followed from elsewhere, the earliest of which showed little or unclear effects. For example, in a British study there was no excess of solvent-exposure among patients who consulted general practitioners for neuropsychiatric ailments in comparison with other disorders.[55] A Swiss study of 1916 painters and 1948 electricians found an almost doubled risk of early pensioning among the painters, but mainly from alcoholism.[56]

It seemed possible from this latter study that the excess of alcoholism might have reflected less reliable diagnostic criteria. Alcoholism is not easily distinguished from solvent-induced disability and might well be the physician's first diagnostic choice for any neuropsychiatric malfunction. Notably, though, a potentiating effect of alcohol on nervous dysfunctions in solvent exposed workers has been shown.[57] It may well be, therefore, that the combined effect of solvent exposure and alcohol intake are particularly important in causing the disability seen among the exposed workers, but with the contribution of alcohol alone being covered by the diagnostic label.

This suggestion of a combined effect of solvents and alcohol is supported by a Canadian study, which had careful and detailed exposure assessment, not only for alcohol but also for other potentially neurotoxic occupational exposures and solvents.[49] This study included 309 men with organic dementia, cerebral atrophy or psychoorganic syndrome and two equally large hospital control groups with other psychiatric diagnoses and selected non-psychiatric diagnoses, respectively. Odds ratios of 1·4 were obtained for solvent exposure both by individual exposure ratings and by using a job-exposure matrix, rising to 4·0 in men with an alcohol-related diagnosis. The combined effect of solvent exposure and alcohol intake was considered as probably an important cause of organic brain damage. The observation that heavy drinkers exposed to toluene perform better than more moderate drinkers in psychological tests is not necessarily contradictory; the manifestations of short and long-term toxicity may well differ in nature and severity.[26]

Further evidence of the chronic neurotoxic effect of solvents has been obtained from a US case-control study. Among white male recipients of disability compensation, painters, except spray painters, were found to have about a 45 per cent excess of disabling neuropsychiatric disorders compared with bricklayers.[58] The numbers in this study were quite considerable, that is, 3565 cases and 83 245 controls. The exposure to solvents was assessed by means of a job-exposure matrix approach, as it was costly, if not impossible, to obtain individual exposure information for such large numbers. People who were compensated for infectious, neoplastic, musculoskeletal, circulatory, and respiratory diseases constituted the controls. More specifically the odds ratio for all painters was 1·42, and for construction painters 1·47. Unlike other studies, presenile dementia did not show an increased odds ratio.

A Dutch study also considered disability among painters and construction workers with questionnaires on exposure completed for 252 cases and 822 controls.[59] An adjusted odds ratio of 2·3 was found for "neuroses" and solvent exposure; however when several neuropsychiatric diagnoses were included, some of which could hardly be expected to have a relation to solvent exposure, the odds ratio fell to 1·2.

In a Canadian study conducted in parallel with that mentioned above[49] on psychiatric disorders requiring five nights or more in psychiatric hospitals, there was essentially no association with solvent exposure.[60] A total of 381 men, relatively few with dementia or psychoorganic syndrome, and an equal number of hospital controls were included in this study. Regarding the negative result, it seems reasonable to believe that psychiatric disorders requiring admission to hospital will include various conditions without any connection with occupational exposures. Some conditions would even be likely to appear more commonly in people without permanent jobs.

In addition to surveys of painters and similar workers, somewhat different types of job entailing exposure to petroleum products were considered in a Norwegian cohort of seamen on tankers.[61] A nested case-control analysis based on 199 cases and four matched controls for each case from within the defined cohort gave an overall odds ratio of 5·8. Mates on tankers had a higher risk than captains, suggesting an exposure-effect relationship, but alcohol intake was not recorded.

Two further studies from Denmark deserve mention; one of these included 3387 men originally enrolled in 1971 for cardiovascular research.[62] The cohort was followed through 1985/86 when those still alive were invited to participate in a clinical examination for cardiovascular disease. At this time, they also answered a questionnaire. According to information given by 3303 of the cohort, 295 had been exposed to mixed solvents for five years or more. Memory difficulties, decreased concentration ability, and headache were considered as outcome variables in an essentially cross-sectional analysis. For active workers, identical and significantly increased odds ratios of 3·7 were obtained for solvent exposure with both memory difficulties and decreased concentration ability. For retired workers the odds ratios were around 2·0, but still significant.

The second study was based on a follow-up of 96 metal degreasers with exposure especially to trichloroethylene but also to chlorofluorocarbons.[63] The outcome variable was psychoorganic syndrome, further characterised as mild dementia as assessed by psychometric tests. The risk of developing the syndrome was proportional to duration of exposure, with an adjusted odds ratio of 11·2 for the most heavily exposed subjects, who had a mean duration of full-time exposure of 11 years with a range of 3·9 to 35·6 years. Arteriosclerotic and neuropsychiatric disease, alcohol abuse, and current solvent exposure were taken into account as potential confounders.

These Danish studies were both cross-sectional in character, although longitudinal with regard to exposure. Furthermore, especially in the first study, the outcome represented a relatively weaker effect than in most of the other studies mentioned.

Although these investigations provide increasing and convincing epidemiological evidence of neurotoxicity from long term exposure to solvents, some inconsistencies remain, especially relating to severity of effect. A major difficulty is definition of the disease entities to be considered in a study. There can be the same problem even in cancer research despite the fact that cancer diagnoses are much better defined than neuropsychiatric illnesses. Some disorders are more clear than others, however, and disability is a fairly reliable indicator of disease.

Several studies of solvent exposure have considered serious conditions such as organic brain damage, dementia, and cerebral atrophy, diagnoses which are well-defined disorders and are suitable for clear-cut epidemiological study. Nevertheless, in addition to those mentioned from Denmark,[54] and Canada,[49] two other studies, one from UK,[64] and one from Denmark[65] did not show consistent results.

The UK study[64] of 557 deaths from presenile dementia found no association with solvent exposure in contrast to the Danish cohort study of painters and bricklayers.[65] In the latter, mental impairment was related to degree of exposure and, in a sub-sample of the cohort, computer tomography indicated some degree of cerebral atrophy, which seemed to increase with exposure. Under certain conditions applied in the analysis, the increase in risk of dementia was up to 4·95 for the most heavily exposed subjects.

Whether the inconsistent findings in various studies on neuropsychiatric disorders depend on differences in diagnostic criteria, chance, or some other explanation is unclear. For example, Alzheimer's dementia, as discussed below, has not been shown to have any clear association with occupation. Such cases may get included in the cohort and the effect of exposure is diluted, if seen at all; this aspect might account for the inconsistencies seen regarding studies of dementia. Somewhat similarly, it seems likely that psychiatric disorders requiring admission to hospital, as in the Canadian study,[60] represent quite different conditions from the slowly developing, relatively mild but disabling dementias associated with solvent exposure in other studies.

Finally, some peculiar and interesting observations on sleep apnoea deserve a mention. Similarity of the symptoms of psychoorganic syndrome and those reported by patients with sleep apnoea suggested study of a possible relationship.[66] In a group of 66 men exposed to solvents, the prevalence of sleep apnoea was found to be 19·7%, compared with 1·4% in the general population, suggesting a strong relationship with solvent exposure (RR 14·1). Similar observations were made in two Norwegian studies on 78 workers exposed to trichloroethylene and other solvents.[67 68]

Alzheimer's dementia

Alzheimer's dementia has been studied in relation to occupational exposure. No association was found with solvent or lead exposure in a case-control study comprising 98 cases and 162 controls,[69] nor has a recent meta-analysis of 11 case-control studies of this disorder given any suggestion of associations of this kind.[70] These negative results are in agreement with those from a follow-up of patients with neuropsychiatric symptoms and solvent exposure by departments of occupational medicine in Sweden. In this group of patients no severe dementia of the Alzheimer type was observed.[74]

In a recent study, however, by inclusion of such broad exposure categories as blue collar work compared with all other types of work, an increased risk was found.[72] Based on 98 cases and 216 controls, the odds ratio was as high as 5·3 for men after adjustment for alcohol consumption, a more evident risk factor. Further research with more specific evaluation is therefore warranted on various occupational exposures and Alzheimer's dementia. At present there is not enough evidence for any definite suspicion of a work-related association with this disorder, although there are some environmental studies suggesting the possibility of a hazard from aluminium in drinking water.

Multiple sclerosis

An association between solvent exposure and multiple sclerosis was first reported in an Italian case-control study.[73] This study suggested an association with glue solvents in the Italian shoe industry. The number of cases among those exposed was almost five times the expected, but in a series of only 41, this was not particularly convincing. However, the suspicion was strengthened by a Swedish study of 83 cases and 467 randomly selected controls which gave an odds ratio of 2·3 for solvent exposure.[74] Some other exposures were also associated with increased risks, including work with phenoxy herbicides, welding, and radiological work.

A suggestive case report of a worker who had been exposed to organic solvents and showed areas of demyelination in the temporal lobe has been published.[75] Taken together, these observations indicate the need for further epidemiological studies of occupation and multiple sclerosis, particularly perhaps the less typical forms of the disease. In a study of cerebrospinal fluid in subjects exposed to solvents an increase in the concentrations of protein, albumin, and IgG and some reduction in taurine were observed,[76] but this was not confirmed in another investigation.[77]

Parkinson's disease

Some epidemiological reports suggest that there is a higher risk of Parkinson's disease in younger people associated with rural residence.[78] Case-control studies from Canada, China, Spain, and Sweden have indicated that exposure to industrial chemicals, pesticides, and metals might play some part in the aetiology of this disorder, but no specific agents have been identified. There is no evidence of a connection between Parkinson's disease and work with solvents.

In a study from Quebec, Canada, of 42 cases of Parkinson's disease and 84 controls, an odds ratio of 2·3 was reported for exposure to manganese, iron, and aluminium.[79] There was also some association with pesticide use and with industrial work. The epidemiological association of this disease with manganese exposure is certainly in agreement with the classic observations on manganese poisoning, which even seem to have led to the rediscovery of Parkinson's "Shaking palsy".[80] In another study, some geographical clustering of Parkinson's disease in Israel was thought to depend on exposure to agricultural chemicals, but without further specification.[81]

In a study from Calgary, Canada, of 130 cases and 260 randomly selected controls, exposure being assessed by personal interview, a risk ratio of 3·1 was found for herbicide exposure. The increased risk remained after adjustment for other agricultural exposures, including insecticides.[82]

Among those who recalled the use of specific agents, these were phenoxy herbicides or thiocarbamates. One person recalled exposure to paraquat. This is of particular interest because of the molecular similarity with the chemical MPTP (N-methyl-4-phenyl-1,2,3,6-tetrahydro-pyridine), which induces a syndrome resembling Parkinson's disease. A study of paraquat workers has not revealed any occurrence of such a syndrome, however,[83] and there remain doubts as to the effect of any agricultural chemicals in this disease.[84]

Motor neurone disease

Some epidemiological attention has been given to occupation and motor neurone disease, including amyotrophic lateral sclerosis, progressive bulbar palsy, and progressive muscular atrophy. Table 8.3 shows some results from studies that have recently become available.

Female medical service workers, office workers, and farm workers appeared to be at increased risk of amyotrophic lateral sclerosis in a large Swedish case-control study. The investigation was of 1961 cases and 2245 controls but had only crude census information on occupation.[85]

Whether the use of various pesticides carries any risk for farmers is unclear. Methyl–mercury preparations have been used as a seed dressing and a few reported cases of mercury intoxication resembling amyotrophic lateral sclerosis are therefore of interest and point to the need for research.[86]

Table 8.3   Occupational factors associated with motor neurone disease in some studies, along with selected risk estimates

Reference	Type of study	Agent or exposure	Typical risk or odds ratio
Gunnarson et al., 1991 (Sweden)[84]	case-control	males:	
		office workers	1·8
		farm workers	1·7
		females:	
		medical service work	1·7
Sienko et al., 1990 (USA)[91]	cohort	physical trauma	elevated[a]
		(lead and mercury in blood)	(similar)[a]
Armon et al., 1991 (USA)[86]	case-control	lead	elevated[a]
		welding and soldering	elevated[a]
Gunnarsson et al., 1992 (Sweden)[87]	case-control	heavy metals	1·9[b]
		welding	3·7
		electricity work	6·7
		solvents	1·3[c]

[a] Risk estimate not calculated. [b] For sub-entity progressive muscular atrophy (PMA) and heavy metals 3·2. [c] For PMA and neurodegenerative thyroid disease and solvents in men 14·2.

Exposures to welding, soldering, and blue collar work in general were reported more often among cases than controls in a study from the US, but no risk estimates were given.[87] The study included 74 cases of amyotrophic lateral sclerosis and 201 matched controls. In a Swedish study, welding also appeared as a risk factor together with electricity work, potential exposure to electric shock, and work with solvents alone or in mixtures.[88] The risks were in the range of 3·5 to 6·7, and the 95% confidence interval excluded unity. The highest risk ratio was in workers with electricity. The study was based on 92 cases and 372 controls, questionnaires being used for exposure assessment.

There has been some indication that exposure to lead and solvents could be of importance in the causation of amyotrophic lateral sclerosis.[89–91] In the Swedish study mentioned above, a particularly high risk ratio of 15·6 was found for the combination of a family history of neurodegenerative and thyroid disease, male sex, and exposure to solvents.[88]

The association of lead exposure and amyotrophic lateral sclerosis has been investigated. In one early study, lead exposure was reported among 15% of cases compared with 5·4% of controls,[89] and in the US study already mentioned, the crude risk ratio was 5·5, although it was based on small numbers.[87] In a small study of a localised cluster of six cases and 12 controls, blood lead levels were similar (10·8 and 10·6 μg/100 ml, respectively).[92] Other investigators have found higher concentrations of lead in plasma from cases than controls and also higher concentrations in cerebrospinal fluid.[93 94] The few reported studies are not consistent, however.[95]

Conclusions

Although the acute and severe neurotoxic effects of many agents have been known for a long time, epidemiological research during the past two decades has shown that there are also serious effects of long term exposure at lower levels. Only for solvent exposure is there a reasonable number of epidemiological studies. Many investigations have focused on more or less isolated symptoms and signs, especially in cross-sectional studies. The extent to which continuous, long-term exposures or relatively short repeated episodes of high intensity exposure are required for the development of chronic conditions, attributable to solvents for example, remains unclear.

The pathological mechanisms which underlie associations between various exposures and neurobehavioural disorders are not within the realm of epidemiology. It is helpful nevertheless for overall judgements of risk, that publications on the mainly experimental aspects are quite extensive and that good reviews have been written.[1 5 96] Animal exposures have usually been high compared with environmental concentrations at work, which certainly hampers interpretation, as do the many inconsistencies in the experimental findings. The effects seen with various exposures appear quite complex, and there are regional differences within the central nervous system. Nevertheless, the experimental data are generally supportive of the evidence obtained from epidemiological studies of neurobehavioural effects of various industrial agents.

To mention a few examples briefly: lead and manganese both seem to influence dopaminergic functions, although in different ways; manganese toxicity may, to some extent at least, result from its ability to oxidise dopamine. The ability of organophosphates to inhibit acetylcholine esterase is well known, and both catecholaminergic and serotoninergic systems are affected by toluene, styrene, and other solvents. Degenerative morphologic changes have been identified in exposed animals, especially in the frontal cortex, and also in the hippocampal and cerebellar regions. Indications of astroglial cell proliferation have been obtained in some studies, for example after exposure to xylene and white spirit. Foci of demyelination have been found in animals exposed to white spirit with low nonane and high aromatic content. Trichloroethylene causes changes in the composition of brain lipids and infiltrates of lymphocyte-like cells in the pons and cerebellum. Further information may be obtained from the reviews listed above, and details from the original reports.

In spite of the many consistent findings from epidemiological investigations of solvent exposure, there are disturbing discrepancies concerning the specific types of defect that constitute the chronic psychoorganic syndromes. Some studies have found the strongest correlation with diffuse diseases such as neurosis, whereas others emphasise more severe effects such as dementia and cerebral atrophy. In view of the complex patterns found with different agents in experimental studies, it is likely that some of the epidemiological inconsistencies have to do with different exposure patterns and possible interactions. The concept of "solvents" is particularly unsatisfactory as a measure of exposure, although difficult to avoid, because of the many agents of this type handled as mixtures in the work place.

The few studies of occupational exposure and disorders such as Parkinson's disease, motor neurone disease, and multiple sclerosis indicate an interesting and important deficiency. It seems possible that solvents, together with metals and pesticides, may have a role in the development of these disorders; alternatively, some types of chronic neurotoxic effects may be clinically confused with these diagnostic labels. A greater use in epidemiology of metabolic data may help to unravel some of these problems. Motor neurone disease, for example, seems to be associated with a particular metabolic pattern of poor sulphoxidation and sulphation.[97 98] Parkinson's disease on the other hand has been associated with poor metabolic capacity for debrisoquine.[99] The use of this knowledge in occupational and other epidemiological research appears to be quite feasible.[50] It remains to be seen, however, whether the principle of subdividing the case series in case-control studies on the lines suggested will prove profitable in practice.

1 Arlien-Soborg P. *Solvent neurotoxicity.* Boca Raton: CRC Press, 1992.
2 Browning E. *Toxicity and Metabolism of Industrial Solvents.* New York: Elsevier North-Holland, 1965.
3 Hänninen H, Mantere P, Hernberg S, Seppäläinen AM, Kock B. Subjective symptoms in low-level exposure to lead. *Neurotoxicity* 1979; 1: 333–47.
4 Sjögren B, Gustavsson P, Hogstedt C. Neuropsychiatric symptoms among welders exposed to neurotoxic metals. *Br J Ind Med* 1990; 47: 704–7.
5 Ecobichon DJ, Davies JE, Doull J, Ehrich M, Joy R, McMillan D, *et al.* Neurotoxic effects of pesticides. In: Baker SR, Wilkinson CF, eds. *The effect of pesticides on human health.* Princeton: Princeton Scientific Publishing, 1990.
6 Bleuler M. *Lehrbuch der psychiatrie.* New York: Springer, 1969.
7 Mayer-Gross W, Slater E, Roth M. *Clinical Psychiatry*, ed 3. London: Tindall & Cassel, 1969.
8 World Health Organisation. *Organic solvents and the central nervous system and diagnostic criteria.* Environmental Health Series No 5. Copenhagen: WHO Regional Office for Europe, 1985.
9 World Health Organisation. *Solvent and the central nervous system—Core protocol.* Environmental Health Series No 36. Copenhagen: FADL Publishers, 1989.
10 Hogstedt C, Hane M, Axelson O. Diagnostic and health care aspects of workers exposed to solvents. In: Zenz C, ed: *Developments in occupational medicine.* Chicago: Year Book Medical Publishers, 1980.
11 Hogstedt C, Hane M, Agrell A, Bodin L. Neuropsychological test results and symptoms among workers with well-defined long-term exposure to lead. *Br J Ind Med* 1983; 40: 99–105.
12 Ekberg K, Hane M, Berggren T. Psychologic effects of exposure to solvents and other neurotoxic agents in the work environment. In: Zenz, C, ed. *Occupational Medicine. Principles and practical applications.* Chicago: Year Book Medical Publishers, 1988.
13 Firnhaber White R, Feldman RG, Hyland Travers P. Neurobehavioural effects of toxicity due to metals, solvents, and insecticides. *Clin Neuropharmacol* 1990; 13: 392–412.
14 Grandjean E, Münchinger R, Turrian V, Haas PA, Knoepfel HK, Rosenmund H. Investigation into the effects of exposure to trichloroethylene in mechanical engineering. *Br J Ind Med* 1955; 12: 131–45.
15 Hänninen H. Psychological picture of manifest and latent carbon disulphide poisoning. *Br J Ind Med* 1971; 28: 374–81.
16 Ng TP, Ong SG, Lam WK, Jones GM. Neurobehavioural effects of industrial mixed solvent exposure in Chinese printing and paint workers. *Neurotoxicol Teratol* 1990; 12: 661–4.
17 Bazylewicz-Walczak B, Marszal-Wisniewska M, Siuda A. The psychological effects of chronic exposure to white spirit in rubber industry workers. *Pol J Occup Med* 1990; 3: 117–27.
18 Hane M, Axelson O, Blume J, Hogstedt C, Sundell L, Ydreborg B. Psychological function changes among house painters. *Scand J Work Environ Health* 1977; 3: 91–9.
19 Fidler AT, Baker EL, Letz RE. Neurobehavioural effects of occupational exposure to organic solvents among construction painters. *Br J Ind Med* 1987; 44: 292–308.
20 Parkinson DK, Bromet EJ, Cohen S, Dunn LO, Dew MA, Ryan C, *et al.* Health effects of long-term solvent exposure among women in blue-collar occupations. *Am J Ind Med* 1990; 17: 661–75.
21 Lindström K, Härkönen H, Hernberg S. Disturbances in psychological functions of workers occupationally exposed to styrene. *Scand J Work Environ Health* 1976; 2: 129–39.

22 Elofsson S, Gamberale F, Hindmarsh T, Iregren A, Isaksson A, *et al*. A cross-sectional epidemiologic investigation on occupationally exposed car and industrial spray painters with special reference to the nervous system. *Scand J Work Environ Health* 1980; 6: 239–73.

23 Daniell W, Stebbins A, O'Donnell J, Horstman SW, Rosenstock L. Neuropsychological performance and solvent exposure among car body repair shop workers. *Br J Ind Med* 1993; 50: 368–77.

24 Knave B, Anshelm-Olson B, Elofsson S, Gamberale F, Isaksson A, Mindus P, *et al*. Long term exposure to jet fuel. II. A cross-sectional epidemiological investigation on occupationally-exposed industry workers with special reference to the nervous system. *Scand J Work Environ Health* 1978; 4: 19–45.

25 Moen BE, Riise T, Haga EM, Fossan GO. Reduced performance in tests of memory and visual abstraction in seamen exposed to industrial solvents. *Acta Psychiatr Scand* 1990; 81: 114–9.

26 Hänninen H, Antti-Poika M, Savolainen P. Psychological performance, toluene exposure and alcohol consumption in rotogravure printers. *Int Arch Occup Environ Health* 1987; 59: 475–83.

27 Hänninen H, Antti-Poika M, Juntunen J, Koskenvuo M. Exposure to organic solvents and neuropsychological dysfunction: a study on monozygotic twins. *Br J Ind Med* 1991; 48: 18–25.

28 Valciukas JA, Lilis R, Singer R, Fischbein A, Anderson HA, Glickman L. Lead exposure and behavioral changes: Comparisons of four occupational groups with different levels of lead absorption. *Am J Ind Med* 1980; 1: 421–6.

29 Grandjean P, Arnvig E, Beckman J. Psychological dysfunction in lead-exposed workers. *Scand J Work Environ Health* 1978; 4: 295–303.

30 Ryan CM, Morrow L, Parkinson D, Bromet E. Low level lead exposure and neuropsychological functioning in blue collar males. *Int J Neurosci* 1987; 36: 29–39.

31 Williamson AM, Tea RKC. Neurobehavioural effects of occupational exposure to lead. *Br J Ind Med* 1986; 43: 374–80.

32 Mantere P, Hänninen H, Hernberg S, Luukonen RA. Prospective follow-up study on psychological effects in workers exposed to low levels of lead. *Scand J Work Environ Health* 1984; 10: 43–50.

33 Piikivi L, Hänninen H, Martelin T, Mantere P. Psychological performance and long-term exposure to mercury vapors. *Scand J Work Environ Health* 1984; 10: 43–50.

34 Piikivi L, Hänninen H. Subjective symptoms and psychological performance of chlorine-alkali workers. *Scand J Work Environ Health* 1989; 15: 69–74.

35 Ehrenberg RL, Vogt RL, Blair Smith A, Brondum J, Brightwell WS, Hudson PJ, *et al*. Effects of elemental mercury exposure at a thermometer plant. *Am J Ind Med* 1991; 19: 495–507.

36 Davignon LF, St Pierre J, Charest G, Tourangeau FJ. A study of the chronic effects of insecticides in man. *Can Med Assoc J* 1965; 92: 597–602.

37 Korsak RJ, Sato MM. Effects of chronic organophosphate pesticide exposure on the central nervous system. *Clin Toxicol* 1977; 11: 83–95.

38 Levin HS, Rodnitzky RL. Behavioural effects of organophosphate pesticides in man. *Clin Toxicol* 1976; 9: 391–405.

39 Anger WK, Moody L, Burg J, Brightwell WS, Taylor BJ, Russo JM, *et al*. Neurobehavioural evaluation of soil and structural fumigators using methyl bromide and sulphuryl fluoride. *Neurotoxicology* 1986; 7: 137–56.

40 Seppäläinen AM. Neurophysiological findings among workers exposed to organic solvents. *Scand J Work Environ Health* 1981; 4(suppl): 29–33.

41 Seppäläinen AM. Neurotoxic effects of industrial solvents. *Electroencephalogr Clin Neurophysiol* 1973; 34: 702–3.

42 Littorin M, Fehling C, Attewell RG, Skerfving S. Focal epilepsy and exposure to organic solvents: A case-referent study. *J Occup Med* 1988; 30: 805–8.

43 Descamps D, Garnier R, Lille F, Tran Dinh Y, Bertaux L, Reygagne A, *et al*. Evoked potentials and cerebral blood flow in solvent induced psycho-organic syndrome. *Br J Ind Med* 1993; 50: 325–30.

44 Buiatti E, Cecchini S, Ronchi O, Dolara P, Bulgarelli G. Relationship between clinical

and electromyographic findings and exposure to solvents in shoe and leather workers. *Br J Ind Med* 1978; 35: 168–73.

45 Demers RY, Markell BL, Wabeke R. Peripheral vibratory sense deficits in solvent-exposed painters. *J Occup Med* 1991; 33: 1051–4.

46 Murata K, Araki S, Yokoyama K. Assessment of the peripheral, central, and autonomic nervous system function in styrene workers. *Am J Ind Med* 1991; 20: 775–84.

47 Murata K, Araki S, Yokoyama K, Maeda K. Autonomic and peripheral nervous system dysfunction in workers exposed to mixed organic solvents. *Int Arch Occup Environ Health* 1991; 63: 335–40.

48 Axelson O, Hane M, Hogstedt C. A case-referent study on neuropsychiatric disorders among workers exposed to solvents. *Scand J Work Environ Health* 1976; 2: 14–20.

49 Cherry NM, Labrèche FP, McDonald JC. Organic brain damage and occupational solvent exposure. *Br J Ind Med* 1992; 49: 776–81.

50 Axelson O, Söderkvist P. Characteristics of disease and some exposure considerations. *Appl Occup Environ Hyg* 1991; 6: 428–35.

51 Mikkelsen S. A cohort study of disability pension and death among painters with special regard to disabling presenile dementia as an occupational disease. *Scand J Soc Med* 1980; 16(Suppl): 34–43.

52 Olsen J, Sabroe S. A case-reference study of neuropsychiatric disorders among workers exposed to solvents in the Danish wood and furniture industry. *Scand J Soc Med* 1980; 16(Suppl): 44–9.

53 Lindström K, Riihimäkki H, Hänninen K. Occupational solvent exposure and neuropsychiatric disorders. *Scand J Work Environ Health* 1984; 10: 321–3.

54 Rasmussen H, Olsen J, Lauritsen J. Risk of Encephalopathia among retired solvent-exposed workers. *J Occup Med* 1985; 8: 561–6.

55 Cherry N, Waldron HA. The prevalence of psychiatric morbidity in solvent workers in Britain. *Int J Epidemiol* 1984; 13: 197–200.

56 Guberan E, Usel M, Raymond L, Tissot R, Sweetnam PM. Disability, mortality, and incidence of cancer among Geneva painters and electricians: a historical prospective study. *Br J Ind Med* 1989; 16: 127–32.

57 Massioui FE, Lille F, Lefèvre N, Hazemann P, Garnier R, Dally S. Sensory and cognitive event related potentials in workers chronically exposed to solvents. *J Clin Toxicol* 1990; 28: 203–19.

58 Brackbill RM, Maizlish N, Fischbach T. Risk of neuropsychiatric disability among painters in the United States. *Scand J Work Environ Health* 1990; 16: 182–8.

59 van Vliet C, Swaen GM, Volovics A, Tweehuysen M, Meijers JM, de Boorder T, *et al.* Neuropsychiatric disorders among solvent-exposed workers. First results from a Dutch case-control study. *Int Arch Occup Environ Health* 1990; 62: 127–32.

60 Labrèche FP, Cherry NM, McDonald JC. Psychiatric disorders and occupational exposure to solvents. *Br J Ind Med* 1992; 49: 820–5.

61 Riise T, Moen BE. A nested case-control study of disability pension among seamen, with special reference to neuropsychiatric disorders and exposure to solvents. *Neuroepidemiology* 1990; 9: 88–94.

62 Hein HO, Suadicani P, Gyntelberg F. Mixed solvent exposure and cerebral symptoms among active and retired workers. An epidemiological investigation of 3387 men aged 53–75 years. *Acta Neurol Scand* 1990; 81: 97–102.

63 Rasmussen K, Jeppesen HJ, Sabroe S. Solvent-induced chronic toxic encephalopathy. *Am J Ind Med* 1992; 23: 779–92.

64 O'Flynn RR, Monkman SM, Waldron HA. Organic solvents and presenile dementia: a case referent study using death certificates. *Br J Ind Med* 1987; 44: 259–62.

65 Mikkelsen S, Jörgensen M, Browne M, Gyldensted C. Mixed solvent exposure and organic brain damage. *Acta Neurol Scand* 1988; 78(Suppl): 118.

66 Edling C, Lindberg A, Ulfberg J. Occupational exposure to organic solvents as a cause of sleep apnoea. *Br J Ind Med* 1993; 50: 276–9.

67 Monstad P, Nissen T, Sulg IA, Mellgren SI. Sleep apnoea and organic solvent exposure. *J Neurol* 1987; 234: 152–4.

68 Monstad P, Mellgren SI, Sulg JA. The clinical significance of sleep apnoea in workers

exposed to organic solvents: implications for the diagnosis of organic solvent encephalopathy. *J Neurol* 1992; **239**: 195–8.

69 Shalat SL, Seltzer B, Baker EL Jr. Occupational risk factors and Alzheimer's disease: a case-control study. *J Occup Med* 1988; **12**: 934–6.

70 Graves AB, van Duijin CM, Chandra V, Fratiglioni L, Heyman A, Jorm AF, *et al*. In EURODEM Risk Factors Research Group: Occupational exposures to solvents and lead as risk factors for Alzheimer's disease: a collaborative re-analysis of case-control studies. *Int J Epidemiol* 1991; **20**(Suppl 2): 58–61.

71 Edling C, Ekberg K, Ahlborg Jr G, Alexandersson R, Barregård L, Ekenvall L, *et al*. Long-term follow up of workers exposed to solvents. *Br J Ind Med* 1990; **47**: 75–82.

72 Fratiglioni L, Ahlbom A, Viitanen M, Winblad B. Risk factors for late-onset Alzheimer's disease: A population-based, case-control study. *Ann Neurol* 1993; **33**: 258–66.

73 Amaducci L, Arfaioli C, Inzitari D, Marchi M. Multiple sclerosis among shoe and leather workers: An epidemiological survey in Florence. *Acta Neurol Scand* 1982; **65**: 94–103.

74 Flodin U, Söderfeldt B, Noorlind-Brage H, Fredriksson M, Axelson O. Multiple sclerosis, solvents and pets. A case-referent study. *Arch Neurol* 1988; **45**: 620–3.

75 Gatley MS, Kelly GA, Turnbull IW. A case of organic solvent exposure and temporal lobe demyelination. *J Soc Occup Med* 1991; **41**: 83–5.

76 Moen BE, Kyvik KR, Engelsen BA, Riise T. Cerebrospinal fluid proteins and free amino acids in patients with solvent induced chronic toxic encephalopathy and healthy controls. *Br J Ind Med* 1990; **47**: 277–80.

77 Barregård L, Wikkelslö C, Rosengren LE, Aurell A, Thiringer G, Nilson L, *et al*. Cerebrospinal fluid proteins in men with chronic encephalopathy after exposure to organic solvents. *Scand J Work Environ Health* 1990; **16**: 423–7.

78 Tanner CM. The role of environmental toxins in the etiology of Parkinson's disease. *Trends Neurosci* 1989; **12**: 49–54.

79 Zayed J, Ducic G, Campanella G, Panisset JC, André P, Masson H, *et al*. Facteurs environnementaux dans l'étiologie de la maladie de Parkinson. *Can J Neurol Sci* 1990; **17**: 286–91.

80 Raffle PAB, Lee WR, McCallum RI, Murray R. *Hunter's diseases of occupations*. London: Hodder and Stoughton, 1987.

81 Goldsmith JR, Herishanu Y, Abarbanel JM, Weinbaum Z. Clustering of Parkinson's disease points to environmental etiology. *Arch Environm Health* 1990; **45**: 88–94.

82 Semchuk KM, Love EJ, Lee RG. Parkinson's disease and exposure to agricultural work and pesticide chemicals. *Neurology* 1992; **42**: 1328–35.

83 Howard JK. A clinical survey of paraquat formulation workers. *Br J Ind Med* 1979; **36**: 220–3.

84 Bennett V, Rajput AH, Uitti RJ. An epidemiological survey of agricultural chemicals and incidence of Parkinson's disease. *Neurology* 1988; **38** (Suppl 1): 349.

85 Gunnarsson L-G, Lindberg G, Söderfeldt B, Axelson O. Amyotrophic lateral sclerosis in Sweden in relation to occupation. *Acta Neurol Scand* 1991; **83**: 394–8.

86 Adams CR, Ziegler DK, Lin JT. Mercury intoxication simulating amyotrophic lateral sclerosis. *JAMA* 1983; **250**: 642–3.

87 Armon C, Kurland LT, Daube JR, O'Brian PC. Epidemiologic correlates of sporadic amyotrophic lateral sclerosis. *Neurology* 1991; **41**: 1077–84.

88 Gunnarsson L-G, Bodin L, Söderfeldt B, Axelson O. A case-referent control study of motor neuron disease: its relation to heritability, and occupational exposures, particularly to solvents. *Br J Ind Med* 1992; **49**: 791–8.

89 Campbell AMG, Williams ER, Barltrop D. Motor neuron disease and exposure to lead. *Neurol Neurosurg Psychiatry* 1970; **33**: 877–85.

90 Hawkes CH, Cavanagh JB, Fox AJ. Motoneuron disease: a disorder secondary to solvent exposure? *Lancet* 1989; **1**: 73–6.

91 Chio A, Tribolo A, Schiffer D. Motoneuron disease and glue exposure. *Lancet* 1989; **2**: 921.

92 Sienko DG, Davis JD, Taylor JA, Brooks BR. Amyotrophic lateral sclerosis. A case-control study following detection of a cluster in a small Wisconsin community. *Arch Neurol* 1990; **47**: 38–41.

93 Conradi S, Ronnevi L-O, Vesterberg O. Increased plasma levels of lead in patients with

amyotrophic lateral sclerosis compared with control subjects as determined by flameless atomic absorption spectrophotometry. *J Neurol Neurosurg Psychiatry* 1978; 41: 389–93.

94 Conradi S, Ronnevi L-O, Nise G, Vesterberg O. Abnormal distribution of lead in amyotrophic lateral sclerosis: reestimation of lead in the cerebrospinal fluid. *J Neurol Sci* 1980; 48: 413–8.

95 Stober T, Stelte W, Kunze K. Lead concentrations in blood, plasma, erythrocytes, and cerebrospinal fluid in amyotrophic lateral sclerosis. *J Neurol Sci* 1983; 61: 21–6.

96 DeHaven DL, Mailman RB. The interactions of behaviour and neurochemistry. In: Annau Z, ed. *Neurobehavioural toxicology*. London: Edward Arnold, 1987.

97 Steventon G, Williams AC, Waring RH, Pall HS. Xenobiotic metabolism in motoneuron disease. *Lancet* 1988; 2: 644–7.

98 Loft S. Metronidazole and antipyrine as probes for the study of foreign compound metabolism. *Pharmacol Toxicol* 1990; 66: Supp VI.

99 Smith CAD, Gough AC, Leigh PN, Summers BA, et al. Debrisoquine hydroxylase gene polymorphism and susceptibility to Parkinson's disease. *Lancet* 1992; 339: 1375–7.

9 Noise and vibration

PETER PELMEAR

Introduction

Exposure to intense noise damages the human hearing process. While noise-induced hearing loss is the most important adverse health effect and is well documented, other less well reported reactions include annoyance, interference with communication and work, extra-auditory effects on the special senses, stress, and mental illness. Another physical agent, hand-arm (segmental) vibration, causes vibration white finger, now known as the hand-arm vibration syndrome. Whole-body vibration causes discomfort, gastrointestinal upsets, generalised health effects, back pain, and vertebral degeneration, the latter being the most common and disabling.

Noise

Sources

Industrial noise may arise from machines or tools within the internal working environment which directly affect workers, or the occupational activity may create a noise hazard for the community, for example road transport and aircraft. The problem of industrial noise is as old as industry itself. In the century following Ramazzini, Thackrah (1831) reported deafness among ship's carpenters, "frizzers" (who worked up the nap on

185

cloth), and shear grinders. In the same period Fosbroke (1830–1831) observed that deafness was caused by the explosion of cannons and by continued impact noise, such as that to which blacksmiths are exposed. Quantitative observations were made by Barr (1886), who reported that only 9% of the boilermakers—riveters, caulkers, platers, and "holders-on"—whom he studied in the Glasgow shipyards had normal hearing. By comparison, 79% of postmen and 46% of iron moulders (foundry men) could hear normally. Noise became a widespread hazard in the industrial revolution and has continued to be so. The rates of incidence and prevalence of hearing loss in workers have varied depending on the level of noise and the length of exposure.

Hearing loss

That workers, in particular coppersmiths, exposed to noise lose some hearing was recognised and reported by Ramazzini in 1713:[1]

> In every city, e.g. at Venice, these workers are all congregated in one quarter and are engaged all day in hammering copper to make it ductile so that with it they may manufacture vessels of various kinds. From this quarter there rises such a terrible din that only these workers have shops and homes there; all others flee from that highly disagreeable locality. One may observe these men as they sit on the ground, usually on small mats, bent double while all day long they beat the newly-mined copper, first with wooden then with the iron hammers till it is as ductile as required. To begin with, the ears are injured by that perpetual din, and in fact the whole head, inevitably, so that workers of this class become hard of hearing and, if they grow old at this work completely deaf. For that incessant noise beating on the eardrum makes it lose its natural tonus; the air within the ear reverberates its sides, and this weakens and impairs all the apparatus of hearing. In fact the same thing happens to them as to those who dwell near the Nile in Egypt, for they are all deaf from the excessive uproar of the falling water.

Thus Ramazzini almost two centuries ago was able to identify correctly one of the causes of deafness. To justify a diagnosis of occupational hearing loss today it is important to consider both occupational exposure to noise from machines, tools, vehicles, and so on, and non-occupational factors. Phaneuf and Hétu in a recent review have indicated that non-occupational factors include age; noise from recreational and modern living activities; trauma; diseases; antibiotics (for example streptomycin, neomycin, and chloramphenicol), and such drugs as aminoglycosides, salicylates and quinine (table 9.1).[2] In this century activities outside the work environment including motor racing, shooting, and disco music may contribute substantially. Lastly there is a hypothetical connection between smoking and hearing loss,[3] which may be related to raised concentrations of carbon monoxide in the blood.[4]

Table 9.1   Hearing loss from non-occupational noise and disease[2]

	Prevalence /1000 persons	Incidence /100 000 persons/ year
acoustic neuroma	0·05	8·7
brain tumour	–	12·6
congenital	<0·5 per 1000 live births	–
familial	0·25 characteristically bilateral	–
idiopathic	0·2	–
Menière's disease	10	–
otosclerosis	11	14
toxic origin	1·2	–
trauma	2·2	–

At the end of the 1960s two studies were published providing for the first time satisfactory data from which the correlation between noise exposure and hearing loss could be quantified. The Passchier-Vermeer study was an analysis of data from 4600 workers within 20 groups, derived in turn from the publications of eight authors.[5] Exposure times varied from 10 to 40 years and the noise levels were defined in terms of a noise rating, ranging from 500 to 2000 Hz. The noise rating numbers considered (75 to 98), corresponded to 79 to 102 dBA (decibels weighted according to the A scale). Damage to hearing was found to increase with increasing noise level, given a constant exposure time. The most important aspect of Passchier-Vermeer's work was that its base was derived from the data from many other researchers, making it unlikely that the entire range of results could be seriously affected by minor inaccuracies in the published work.[6] The second study, by Burns and Robinson, commissioned in 1961 by the British government, was a survey of the hearing and noise exposure of workers in British industry.[7] The final analyses were based on 759 noise-exposed workers and 97 non-exposed controls. The analyses defined the effect on hearing loss of noise levels of 75 to 120 dBA, and exposure duration of one month to 50 years, and the effect of age on hearing (presbycusis). The results of the analyses were expressed in the form of an equation, which expresses the expected decibel hearing level at frequencies from 500 to 6000 Hz for any given noise level, exposure period, and age. The concepts of the noise emission level and the total A-weighted noise energy received by the ear, were developed. The main conclusion to be drawn from both sets of data was that long-term exposure to levels below 80 dBA was not likely to injure hearing; at exposures to levels of 85 to 90 dBA the risk was minor; and at 90 dBA and higher there was a major risk. From these reports Robinson derived the equal energy principle, which states that an intensity increase of 3 dB doubles the exposure risk.

For every increase of 3 dB in noise level above 90 dBA the exposure time must be halved to equalise the risk.

Since then there has been a debate over the years as to whether the exchange rate should be 3 or 5 dB (the CHABA 5 rule) but it is now generally agreed, that the rate should be 3 dB.[8][9] Another important principle established from these reports is that the average auditory damage in a large group exposed to exactly the same noise conditions is a function of the integral over time of the instantaneous A-weighted sound intensity at the entrance to the ear canal.[10] For a review of the epidemiological strategies most suitable for evaluating noise-induced hearing loss the reader is referred to a paper by Erdreich and Erdreich published in 1982.[11]

All studies have shown that noise-induced hearing loss usually begins as a reduction in the frequency spectra at 4000 Hz, and at a later stage this widens and deepens to 3000 and 6000 Hz. Taylor et al. in their study of 401 Dundee weavers and 57 controls clearly showed this 4 kHz notch.[12] Before the development of a permanent threshold shift a short-term loss, known as temporary threshold shift, was always found. The extent to which the hearing threshold is reduced depends on the intensity and duration of the noise and is at a maximum just after the exposure is ended. Recovery occurs over some hours, is logarithmic, and is usually measured at a two minute recovery point (the TTS_2).[13] The extent to which the noise-induced loss becomes permanent and the degree of recovery are dependent on the previous permanent threshold shift. To measure the degree of hearing hazard produced by sounds of varying intensity the L_{eq} unit is used. This is the average noise level over the period of measurement. The sound pressure level is the L_{eq} value referred to one second. The "noise dose" is an L_{eq} measurement over a period of eight hours and is used in the assessment of hazard to hearing.

Susceptibility

In a group of workers with similar noise exposure, some will have negligible loss of hearing, while others will be severely impaired. Some correlation exists between susceptibility to noise-induced hearing loss and temporary threshold shift. The correlation is, however, too weak to predict permanent hearing loss from the temporary threshold shift measured after a two weeks interval free from noise. A recent study compared 56 naval aviators who had either suffered a hearing loss (hearing threshold level > 40 dB at 4 to 8 kHz), or retained normal hearing (< 25 dB at 125 Hz to 8 kHz) after many thousand hours of flying. No typical profile of the noise-susceptible or noise-resistant individuals emerged.[14] The suscep- tible group had higher systolic blood pressures, and blood concentrations of cholesterol, and triglyceride; more were current smokers and fewer had never smoked; and more had blue eyes. The resistant group had higher blood concentrations of calcium, albumin, and lactate dehydrogenase. In surveys of noise-induced hearing loss in occupationally exposed workers it is thus important to have sufficiently large numbers in the test sample to allow for considerable variation in individual susceptibility.

Smoking

Some recent studies have found a significant correlation between smoking and hearing loss, whereas in earlier studies the correlation was less clear-cut. The United States national health survey in 1964 found that the percentage of smokers with reported hearing impairments increased as the number of cigarettes smoked increased.[15] Friedman et al. working with data from self-administered questionnaires by 70 289 male and female workers found that loud noise exposure for long periods was reported more often by smokers.[16] However, neither the noise levels nor hearing thresholds were measured in these studies so the results cannot be used as a quantitative indication of the role of smoking in the association between smoking and hearing loss. In British Columbia, for example, audiometric surveillance is mandatory in industries in which workers are exposed to a noise level of 90 dBA L_{eq} (equivalent continuous sound pressure level) or higher for eight hours a day. The workers are tested by technicians trained by the Workers' Compensation Board, to which copies of the audiograms have to be submitted. Chung et al. reviewed 61 074 records and made a detailed analysis of 5440 distributed by age as follows—20 years, 584; 21 to 30, 3204; 31 to 40, 880; 41 to 50, 494; >50, 278.[17] A linear model and analysis of covariance were used to estimate the effects of age and noise exposure. A worker's lifetime exposure was calculated from the number of years in the current job and the estimated noise rating. Lifetime smoking histories were calculated from the number of cigarettes smoked each day and the number of years of smoking. The analysis showed that hearing loss was significantly related to smoking, but not to a history of cardiovascular disease or diabetes. If there is a smoking effect it is probably the result of destruction of hair cells from anoxia resulting from carbon monoxide intoxication.

Vibration

Recent studies indicate that the hearing of subjects with hand-arm vibration syndrome is excessively vulnerable to noise. Pyykkö et al. studied 72 lumberjacks in 1972 and 203 in 1978, and grouped them according to their history of vibration syndrome, age, duration of chain saw use, and use of hearing protectors.[18] They were exposed to noise at 95 to 107 dBA L_{eq}. The hearing level at 4000 Hz was used as a measure of noise induced hearing loss. A significant difference ($p < 0.001$) in hearing level was found between lumberjacks with and without hand-arm vibration syndrome. These findings were confirmed by Pelmear et al. in a study of 227 hard-rock miners exposed in 1985 and 1987 to noise levels of 107 to 117 dBA L_{eq}.[19] Multiple regression analysis showed significant associations (p < 0.003) between hearing level (at 4000 Hz) and stage of hand-arm vibration syndrome, hearing loss and age, and hearing loss and years of vibration exposure. To evaluate the association further, 18 pairs (subjects with hand-arm vibration syndrome and those without) in the 1985 survey and 16 pairs in the 1987 survey, matched for age and total years exposed, were selected and analysed. The hearing loss was significantly greater (p < 0.05) in subjects with hand-arm vibration syndrome who had less than 11 years vibration exposure. Analysis of the risk factors for the development of hearing loss in vibration-exposed workers indicates that age is the major risk factor, followed by exposure to noise and the presence of hand-arm vibration syndrome. It is unlikely that vibration from hand-held tools is transmitted to the inner ear in amounts sufficient to cause a direct mechanical effect on the cochlear structures. The explanation is presumably reflex sympathetic vasoconstriction associated with the vasospasm in the hands, with consequent ischaemia and hair cell destruction.[20]

Impact noise

Hearing loss from impulsive and impact noise, as opposed to continuous noise, has required separate evaluation. An impulsive, percussive noise is normally defined as sound of a short duration, particularly characterised by a shock waveform with short rise time. The duration of the impact is the time taken for the sound to fall by 20 dB from its initial peak; typically this is 0.1 to 2 seconds. Such noise is normally generated by explosions or gun fire, and in industry by drop forges and presses. Initially it was presumed that the risk to hearing was different from that posed by continuous noise. Risk criteria were based primarily on the assumption that the degree of temporary threshold shift produced was related to the risk of noise-induced hearing loss. This was the view of the Committee on Hearing, Bioacoustics and Biomechanics (CHABA), which defined risk in terms of maximum allowable instantaneous peak pressure, duration of the impulse and number of impulses per day.[21] Later epidemiological studies[22 23] showed that the equivalent continuous noise concept (L_{eq}) was also applicable to impact noise, and this is now generally accepted.[8 9 24] The view that industrial impact noise and steady state noise may affect hearing in systematically different ways is, however, supported by studies by Sulkowski et al. in Poland,[25 26] and Taylor et al. in the United Kingdom.[27] Sulkowski et al. found appreciably more hearing loss among men who used hammers than among weavers who were exposed to steady noise at 101 dBA L_{eq}. The difference was particularly evident at 6 kHz. Taylor et al. studied a population of 3780 drop forge men. For the final analysis 505 hammer men exposed to an L_{eq}

of 108 dBA, and 211 press men to 99 dBA were accepted. They were compared with 293 controls who were not exposed to noise. Despite the differences in equivalent level the hearing loss was nearly identical among the younger workers exposed for less than 10 years. Moreover, for the hammer operators in this age group the loss was significantly less than expected from steady noise at the same value of L_{eq}. The findings were different in older workers exposed for much longer periods of time. In this group, the hammer workers had much greater hearing loss than the press operators, and greater loss than would be expected from the difference in equivalent noise level. Moreover, in both cases, the loss was as great or greater than would be expected following exposure to steady noise at the same levels. A possible explanation is that, for exposures of less than 10 years, impact noise in the two groups had a similar effect on the hearing mechanisms, but for longer-term exposures at higher ages a latent effect, associated with the greater energy exposure level, manifests itself. Simultaneous exposure to hand-arm vibration and impact noise does not increase the risk of sensorineural hearing loss.[28] The scientific evidence and a discussion of the issues, including the exchange rate, were reviewed by Shaw in 1985.[29]

Other factors

With respect to aging the available data suggest that presbycusis and noise-induced hearing loss occur independently and are additive.[2] In animal experiments, a number of chemicals found in the workplace have been associated with sensorineural hearing loss.[30] These include carbon monoxide, heavy metals (lead, arsenic, and mercury), and organic solvents (toluene, styrene, and xylene). Apart from a direct ototoxic action, an interaction with the effect of noise exposure is likely for at least some of these agents.

The common belief that non-occupational exposure to loud music will cause severe hearing loss is not supported by the evidence,[31] although musicians who perform regularly for many years may be at some risk.[32 33] McBride et al.[34] examined 63 (70%) of 89 musicians in an orchestra and measured sound levels during rehearsals and performances. In some sections these exceeded the 90 dBA occupational exposure level but over eight hours this produced only 65% of a daily dose, suggesting a margin of safety. The musicians were divided into two groups on the basis of the sound level survey and their audiometric results were compared. No significant difference was found at high frequencies while for some unknown reason, at low frequencies the high risk group appeared to have the better hearing.

Non-auditory effects

There have been many studies on the non-auditory effects of noise on

191

health,[35] efficiency,[36] and annoyance,[37] but epidemiological research on such effects is still limited, particularly in the psychosomatic field.[38] Many studies have been directed at the relation between noise and arterial blood pressure. Dijk in a recent review reported that in about half of these a positive correlation could be shown but that firm conclusions were still not possible.[38] Recent publications continue to provide conflicting evidence. Parrot *et al.* found that heart rate responses to noise in men were significantly greater than in women.[39] Tarter and Robins studied the prevalence of hypertension and mean blood pressure in 150 white men and 119 black men and found a significant association of noise with mean blood pressure and hypertension among the black workers but no correlation among the white.[40] Yiming *et al.* in a prevalence study of blood pressure in 1101 female workers in a textile mill found by logistic regression analysis that exposure to noise was a significant determinant of hypertension, but third in order of importance after family history of hypertension and use of salt.[41] Why some studies of relatively good quality are positive and other studies of the same quality are negative is unclear. Perhaps future studies should pay more attention to noise perception, and concentrate on stress factors as a consequence of interactions between noise, task, and personality.

Pregnancy

Hartikainen-Sorri *et al.* in Finland, using a case-control design, found no correlation between low birth weight and noise exposure.[42] McDonald *et al.* who interviewed 56 000 mothers in Canada, 23 000 in full-time employment at the time of conception, found that subjective complaints of noise were significantly related to low birth weight in the health and manufacturing sectors of industry, but not in other types of work.[43] However, noise was much less strongly related than other adverse ergonomic conditions. In a later more detailed analysis these investigators concluded that any associations with occupational noise were unlikely to be causal.[44]

Special senses

Effects of noise on the senses apart from hearing are well documented.[35] There is a direct correlation between the content of melanin in the iris and resistance to acoustic trauma; subjects with blue irises are more susceptible. Vestibular function can be disturbed by high noise levels, typically 130 dB or more, leading to nystagmus and vertigo. Audio-analgesia is a well recognised phenomenon and can be used to suppress pain in dental patients.

Noise produces a number of reflex reactions, including orienting, startle, and defensive responses, which are self-evident. Reflex epilepsy is not a large problem in the sense of numbers of patients. While epilepsy affects about 1% of the population, it is estimated that only 6·5% of epileptic patients have their seizures evoked by sensory stimulation, the usual stimulus being visual.[45] Auditory stimuli included unexpected noises, specific simple noises such as the clicking of billiard balls, and complex voice or musical compositions.

Prolonged environmental noise exposure, such as from factories and airports, is thought to be associated with an increase in stress related and mental disorders. Knipschild in a series of epidemiological studies into the medical effects of aircraft noise on communities in the vicinity of Schiphol airport (Amsterdam) found that in areas with more aircraft noise, more people were under medical treatment for heart trouble and hypertension.[46] Furthermore, the use of sedatives and hypnotics, and for female patients anti-hypertensive drugs, was greater. Drug consumption decreased when the number of flights was reduced. He concluded that aircraft noise constitutes a serious threat to public health in all its aspects: affection of well being, mental disorders, somatic symptoms, and disease (especially cardiovascular disease). Noise-related annoyance in itself is probably not a cause of mental illness, although psychiatric patients are vulnerable to the adverse effects of noise. Further study is needed to discover whether noise is an important external factor in precipitating mental illness and whether noise aggravates mental states.

Noise can affect task performance, usually causing deterioration but occasionally, in specific environments, improvement. In laboratory studies of task performance the interpretation of the data is frequently limited by study design and methodological considerations. Recent research has shown that certain features of tasks make them susceptible to the effect of noise. Among these are the difficulty of the task, the requirement for long-continued concentration, and the opportunity to perform the task in several different ways.[36]

Annoyance is a response of attitude and is subjective and difficult to quantify. Hence numerous questions and scales have to be used to grade annoyance as it relates to the noise itself, including loudness, intermittency, sound character, or as it relates to the subject's psychology—for example, perception, sensory, and emotional effects. In predicting annoyance for communities, social surveys seem to suggest that the noise intensity level has more effect overall than the type of noise.[37]

Prevention and control

The results of well conducted cohort and case-control studies, clearly showing the adverse effect of noise on hearing, have led to the introduction of voluntary hearing conservation programmes in industry, which fulfil statutory regulations at the same time. The results of environmental studies have been less definite scientifically. Therefore environmental noise suppression and attenuation have been accomplished largely through emotional and political pressures. Concerning the European Union directives (regulations) on noise in the environment, which are binding on member states, further studies are needed if the directives are to have scientific validity.[5]

Sophisticated forms of hearing protection[47] have been available for over 30 years and if used as part of a hearing conservation programme, hearing loss can be prevented.[48] Therefore it is disturbing to read that miners are still losing their hearing,[49] and that risks to farmers[50 51] and high school farm students[52] remain to be addressed. While it is common to see airport workers using hearing protection, as it is well recognised that they and airport fire fighters are at risk,[53 54] the same is not true of policemen on traffic duty,[55] or road and gas mains repair men using pneumatic drills.

Vibration

Vibration is a physical agent to which many people are exposed at work, in the home and in their social activities. This review is restricted to the epidemiology of whole body and hand-arm vibration. For an understanding of the physics of vibration, the units of measurement, and the pathophysiological changes that result, the reader must refer to comprehensive textbooks.[56–58]

The human body, like other physical structures, responds characteristically to certain critical vibration frequencies at which there is maximum energy transfer from source to receiver. At specific resonant frequencies, which vary for the different organs, adverse effects from vibration exposure are exacerbated by resonance. Resonance is the tendency of the human body (or other mechanical system) to act in concert with externally generated vibration and so to amplify the impinging vibration. In general the larger the mass of the system the lower the resonant frequency. In man, the principal whole-body resonance when sitting occurs at 4 to 7 Hz, while in the chest it is in the 4 to 6 Hz range, and in the eyes in the 20 to 25 Hz range. The existence of resonance always leads to increased strain and greater tissue damage.

It is common to distinguish two varieties of vibration exposure, (1) whole-body vibration, when the body is supported on a vibrating surface (usually a seat or floor) and (2) hand-arm vibration syndrome, when contact with the source is through the fingers and hands. They will be discussed separately.

Whole-body vibration

To suffer adverse effects from whole-body vibration exposure the frequency range 1–100 Hz is critical. In the occupational setting several vibration frequencies are usually present simultaneously, with one or more predominant. Depending on the magnitude, direction (axis), frequency, and duration of exposure to vibration, the effects will range from sensations of pleasure, discomfort or pain to interference with performance in reading or hand control, to acute or chronic illness with physiological and pathological changes to body structures.

The occupational groups most exposed to whole body vibration fall into four main categories: (1) drivers, for example of tractors, trucks, buses, and heavy construction vehicles (2) workers on vibrating stationary or quasi-stationary equipment such as cranes, excavators, and drilling platforms (3) helicopter pilots and (4) sea and air travellers, including those in space crafts.[59-65]

Knowledge of the health effects of whole body vibration is incomplete because of the difficulty in mounting well designed epidemiological studies.[66] The principal acute adverse health effect is motion sickness. Ship motion studies have shown that whole-body vibration exposure in the region of 0·1–0·5 Hz is generally associated with motion sickness (kinetosis) in susceptible subjects. The incidence is at a maximum after two to three hours at sea, and increases as the frequency decreases at constant acceleration.[67] Despite comprehensive reports on motion sickness, many of high quality, knowledge of the illness and the effect of various stress factors on the receptor systems is incomplete. Acclimatisation occurs as days at sea increase.[68] Prophylactic measures include a reduction in vibration, stabilisation, modification of the conduct of the person affected, and pharmacological treatment. Heavy-equipment operators do not suffer motion sickness because their exposure to vibration is for short periods only. Transient disequilibrium, postural sway and tremor may occur following exposure to excessive levels of vibration such as long drives over bumpy roads, turbulent flights, sea journeys, space exploration, and by tractor drivers covering rough terrain.

Dupuis and Zerlett have reviewed many epidemiological studies, the results of which indicate that the most common long-term effects of exposure to whole body vibration are low back pain and degenerative changes in the spine.[65] The symptoms and signs may be aggravated or caused by adverse ergonomic factors related to machine design and seating, or bad driving posture. These factors and the movements of the worker enhance the likelihood that the spine will buckle and degenerate.[69] Human experiments have shown that the spinal system has a characteristic response to compressive vibrational inputs in a seated posture, and that the response is most apparent at 4·5 to 6 Hz.[70] The degenerative changes are usually localised in one part of the spine, such as the middle and lower thoracic spine, the upper lumbar, and to a lesser extent in the lower lumbar spine. Intense vibration at or near 20 Hz seems to be the critical frequency for spinal degeneration, while vibration at 40 to 50 Hz has caused osteoporosis and arthrosis of the feet.[71]

A higher incidence of inguinal hernia, muscular insufficiency, scoliosis (mainly lumbar), and disorders of the digestive system including peptic ulcers, pain, discomfort, and gastritis have also been reported. Exposures to frequencies above 20 Hz appear to cause fewer disorders of the digestive system.[71]

In women exposed to whole body vibration a higher risk has been reported of menstrual disorders, proneness to abortion, and other complications of pregnancy, including hyperemesis gravidarum and varicose veins.[71] It is also associated with an increase in blood volume during the phases of ovulation and menstruation. Other effects on the circulatory system have been reported, including varicose veins, haemorrhoids, varicoceles, ischaemic heart disease, hypertension, and a variety of other diseases and symptoms.[71] These studies are often without adequate control groups.

Following long-term exposure in both sexes there is decreased vestibular excitability and a higher incidence of other vestibular disturbances, including subjective complaints of dizziness. As mentioned earlier, interaction with noise may be an important factor. The question of the effects of long-term exposure to vibration below 20 Hz on the central nervous system remains open, mainly because of poor study design and lack of appropriate controls.[71] Clinically, it is recognised that after an intense period of exposure to vibration, general malaise, lassitude, and disablement occur but full recovery takes place after a short period of freedom from exposure. The evaluation of these vague psychosomatic effects requires sound epidemiological techniques and statistical analyses, which are generally lacking.

The National Institute for Occupational Safety and Health (NIOSH) in the United States, conducted morbidity studies in four occupational groups. A significant excess of venous, bowel, respiratory, muscular, and back disorders was found in a population of 1488 bus drivers compared with two control groups, including office workers and the general population.[72] A study of long distance truck drivers looked at 3205 drivers and a control group of air traffic controllers.[61] It was concluded that the combined effect of forced body posture, cargo handling, improper eating habits, and whole-body vibration were the factors contributing to the significant excess of vertebral pain, spinal deformities, sprains, strains, and haemorrhoids in truck drivers. A study of heavy equipment operators showed an excess of male genital, musculoskeletal, and ischaemic heart diseases, and also of obesity.[73] In a study of 371 farm tractor operators it was concluded that low back pain and gastrointestinal disorders were exacerbated by other factors such as poor seating, poor posture and long irregular hours.[74] Kelsey et al., from epidemiological studies of car and truck drivers, concluded that drivers were three times more likely to develop acute herniated lumbar discs than controls who never drove.[75 76]

Whole-body vibration research is still in its infancy. One reason for this is that many of the researchers have lacked expertise in epidemiological and statistical fields. Another problem is that many of the adverse effects are subjective, are difficult to quantify, and may be influenced by confounding variables such as stress factors. Furthermore some of the chronic changes, for example spinal, are not specific, so their causal relationship with vibration stress is difficult to prove.

Hand-arm vibration

Adverse health effects from exposure to hand-arm vibration have been recognised since 1911 when Loriga reported "dead fingers" in Italian miners using pneumatic tools.[77] Such tools had been introduced into the French mines in 1839 and were being extensively used by 1890. In the United States pneumatic tools were first introduced into the limestone quarries of Bedford, Indiana about 1886. The health risks from their use was subsequently investigated in 1918 by Alice Hamilton and her colleagues who examined 150 men.[78] Behrens and Pelmear reviewed the epidemiology of hand-arm vibration syndrome, and found that the syndrome was reported in users of compressed air tools (1911, 1918), grinding wheels (1931), cutlery grinding (1940), pneumatic drills, fettlers, riveters, caulkers, and polishers (1945), jack-leg and stoper drills (1962), chain saws (1964), brush cutters (1979), and speedway motorcycles (1982).[79]

As Raynaud's phenomenon is the predominant symptom the occupational disease was originally called vibration white finger. When the sensory component became fully recognised as a distinct entity in the 1980s, it was necessary to redefine vibration white finger as hand-arm vibration syndrome. This is a disease entity with the following separate peripheral components:[80] circulatory disturbances (vasospasm with local finger blanching—white finger); sensory and motor disturbances (numbness, loss of finger co-ordination and dexterity, clumsiness and inability to perform intricate tasks); and musculo-skeletal disturbances (muscle, bone, and joint disorders).

The vasospasm, also known as secondary Raynaud's phenomenon, is precipitated by exposure to cold and/or damp conditions, or to vibration. The time between first exposure to hand-arm vibration and the first appearance of white finger tips is termed the latent interval. The shorter this period the greater the vibration intensity and the greater the risk to vibration exposed workers, but there is considerable variation because of individual susceptibility. The blanching of the digits is accompanied by numbness, and as the circulation to the digits recovers there is usually tingling and pain. Tingling and paraesthesia may precede the onset of blanching in many subjects.[81]

The blanching is initially restricted to the tips of one or more fingers but

197

Table 9.2   The Stockholm Workshop Scale for the classification of cold-induced Raynaud's phenomenon in the hand-arm vibration syndrome*

Stage	Grade	Description
0		no attacks
1	mild	occasional attacks affecting only the tips of one or more fingers.
2	moderate	occasional attacks affecting the distal and middle fingers (rarely also proximal) phalanges of one or more fingers.
3	severe	frequent attacks affecting all phalanges of most fingers.
4	very severe	as in stage 3, with trophic skin changes in the finger tips.

* The staging is made separately for each hand. In the evaluation of the subject, the grade of the disorder is indicated by the stages of both hands and the number of affected fingers on each hand; example: "2L(2)/1R(1)," "- - -/3R(4)," etc.

progresses as vibration exposure time increases. The thumbs are usually the last to be affected. The existence of both sensory and vascular components in hand-arm vibration syndrome led to the adoption of the Stockholm classification for staging severity (tables 9.2 and 9.3), based on a subjective history and supported by the results of clinical tests.[82][83] The vascular and sensorineural symptoms and signs are evaluated for each hand separately.

In advanced cases the circulation becomes sluggish, giving a cyanotic tinge to the skin of the fingers. In severe cases ulceration and severe skin changes, even gangrene, may appear at the finger tips as a result of impaired blood flow to the fingers. In addition to tactile, vibrotactile, and thermal threshold impairment, which may be less evident in some subjects but marked in others, reduction of grip strength is a common finding in longer exposed workers. Discomfort and pain in the upper limbs is also a common complaint.

The toes may be affected if directly subjected to vibration from a local source such as vibrating platforms, or they may show reflex spasm in subjects with severe hand symptoms.[84][86] Reflex sympathetic vasoconstriction may also account for the increased severity of noise induced hearing loss in hand-arm vibrating syndrome subjects.[18][19] Bone cysts and vacuoles, although often reported, are more likely to be caused by

Table 9.3   The Stockholm Workshop Scale for the classification of sensorineural effects of the hand-arm vibration syndrome*

Stage	Symptoms
0 SN	exposed to vibration but no symptoms.
1 SN	intermittent numbness, with or without tingling.
2 SN	intermittent or persisent numbness, reduced sensory perception.
3 SN	intermittent or persistent numbness, reduced tactile discrimination and/or manipulative dexterity.

* The sensorineural stage is to be established for each hand.

biodynamic and ergonomic factors. Working while leaning on vibratory tools, for example a jack hammer, may result in abdominal injuries.[87] [88]

Whether smoking accelerates the onset of hand-arm vibration syndrome has not yet been proved conclusively, but this aggravating factor has been shown to increase the risk in several studies, presumably as a result of the action of toxic elements on the digital arteries.[89]

Field studies

The first reported study in the United Kingdom was in 1931. Seyring investigated cleaners of castings and found that the prevalence of hand-arm vibration syndrome increased with years exposed: 4% within two years, 48% within three years, 55% within 10 years, and 61% after 10 years.[90] It was most prevalent among workers who used air drills on hard material. In 1946, Agate et al. reported that 32 of 37 foundry grinders had Raynaud's phenomenon.[91] In a subsequent investigation of workers employed polishing and grinding metal castings Agate found that 70% of 233 men and 47% of 45 women were affected.[92] From a follow-up questionnaire two years later, it was estimated that 80–90% of the original 278 employees were now affected. Hunter et al. examined 286 pneumatic tool workers in various trades; the incidence in fettlers was 71%, in riveters 74%, and in caulkers 82%.[93] By the mid 60s reports of epidemiological studies from Tasmania,[94] Japan,[95] Sweden,[96] and Australia[97] had shown the hazard in chain saws. In consequence, the Forestry Commission and the University of Dundee supported an investigation by Taylor et al.[98] A questionnaire was sent to 800 randomly selected employees and 732 responded (97%). Of the 142 chain saw operators, 44% had Raynaud's phenomenon compared with 18% in non-users. The prevalence increased with greater use, reaching 75% after eight years. Taylor et al. followed-up with an extensive study of 1283 forestry, forge, and foundry workers and their findings confirmed previous reports.[99] This was a landmark in the evaluation of hand-arm vibration syndrome as it advanced knowledge in the clinical assessment of workers, proposed a classification system for severity grading that has been widely adopted, and promoted the use of vibration measurement techniques for evaluating hazard. The Taylor-Pelmear classification was modified in 1986 from the Stockholm classification.

Subsequent studies have continued to measure risk by cross-sectional prevalence and incidence studies with a view to developing safety standards. Other studies have advanced clinical assessment by introducing objective tests. Many of the prevalence studies have been conducted on large population groups in different work places.[100–102] As a result the power of these studies has been good, and the validity of the findings has been confirmed by researchers in other countries. It is apparent from these reports that almost any hand-held vibratory tool will cause hand-arm vibration syndrome to a lesser or greater extent if the vibration is sufficiently intense over the frequency range 4 to 5000 Hz for long enough. The critical factor is vibration dose, which is a product of vibration level and exposure time.

For the diagnosis and grading of hand-arm vibration syndrome, methods have to be evaluated both in the field and in the hospital. Many reports of the statistical evaluation of diagnostic instruments used in patients with hand-arm vibration syndrome are now available.[103 106] This is important to researchers because the validity of follow-up epidemiological studies depends on accurate diagnosis, using instrumentation with reference data for the respective objective tests.

Follow-up studies are now reporting a reduction in the incidence and prevalence rates when preventive measures have been taken by attenuation of vibration of the tool, reduction in work exposure time,[107 108] and the introduction of "work breaks" to avoid continuous vibration exposure throughout the shift.

Conclusion

The severity and the extent of the adverse health effects associated with the physical agents, noise and vibration, were only fully realised when researchers published the results of their epidemiological studies. The early studies on noise drew attention to the hazard in many industrial processes, but it was not possible to quantify the risk and specify the protection required until the 1960s, when the reports from Passchier-Vermeer[5] and Burns and Robinson[7] were released. These were crucial documents for promoting an advance in knowledge and conservation of hearing. An equivalent circumstance occurred in the early 1970s in respect of hand-arm vibration with the report by Taylor et al.[99] This research initiative also advanced knowledge and promoted prevention. Less dramatic but important were the studies on impact noise by Sulkowski et al.[25] and Taylor et al.[27] to clarify the risk from impact as opposed to continuous noise. Thus in respect of these occupational hazards epidemiological studies have been pivotal in promoting preventive medicine.

The non-auditory effects of noise and the health effects of whole body vibration need to be better evaluated, but as can be seen from the studies reported here there are inherent difficulties. The epidemiological method is appropriate, but the markers of disease need to be better defined if there is to be any advance in knowledge. For future studies there is a need to derive methods both to evaluate and quantify subjective symptoms more scientifically. Quantifying subjective symptomatology has in the past been the major obstacle.

The studies on noise have led to the development of safety standards and protective equipment such that noise induced hearing loss is now a preventable disease. Unfortunately, this is not true for vibration as yet.

Most of the recent epidemiological studies on the prevalence and severity of hand-arm vibration syndrome have required a multi-disciplinary team of engineers, physicians, neurologists, epidemiologists, scientists and statisticians. This will continue to be necessary, because of the complexity of the issues. If progress is to be made with safety standards and the development of anti-vibration devices, reliable dose-response data are required.

Diagnostic tests used in the examination of hand-arm vibration syndrome patients need to be standardised and the results statistically analysed. Normative data are also required. This will permit physicians to establish the severity of hand-arm vibration syndrome correctly, and the impairment in those subjects seeking compensation. There is a need also to evaluate the administrative and treatment regimens used for patients with vibration induced disease. There is at present wide variation in treatment because of the lack of fundamental epidemiological data and insufficient pathophysiological knowledge on which it should be based.

1 Ramazzini B. *Diseases of workers* (De morbis artificum diatriba. 1713). Translation of Latin text. New York; Hafner, 1964.
2 Phaneuf R, Hétu R. An epidemiological perspective of the causes of hearing loss among industrial workers. *J Otolaryngol* 1990; **19**: 31–40.
3 Zelman S. Correlation of smoking history with hearing loss. *JAMA* 1984; **223**: 920.
4 Bobin RP, Gondra MI. Effect of nicotine on cochlear function and noise-induced hair cell loss. *Ann Otol Rhinol Laryngol* 1976; **85**: 247–54.
5 Tempest W. Noise in Industry. In: Tempest W, ed. *The noise handbook*. London: Academic Press, 1985.
6 Passchier-Vermeer W. *Hearing loss due to exposure to steady state broad-band noise*. Report 35, Institute for Public Health Engineering, TNO, Netherlands, 1968.
7 Burns W, Robinson DW. *Hearing and noise in industry*. London: HMSO, 1970.
8 ISO Acoustics—*Determination of occupational noise exposure and estimation of noise-induced hearing impairment*. Draft International Standard ISO/DIS 1999, 1984.
9 Burkett KM, Lockington N, Valentine K. *Report of the Special Advisory Committee on the Noise Regulation*. Ministry of Labour, Ontario, Dec 1985.
10 Ward WD, Turner CW. The total energy concept as a unifying approach to the prediction of noise trauma and its application to exposure criteria. In: Hamernik R, Henderson D, Salvi R, eds. *New perspectives on noise-induced hearing loss*. New York: Raven Press 1982; 423–35.
11 Erdreich J, Erdreich LS. Epidemiologic strategies to understanding noise-induced hearing loss. In: Hamernik R, Henderson D, Salvi R, eds. *New perspectives on noise-induced hearing loss*. New York: Raven Press, 1982: 439–60.
12 Taylor W, Pearson JCG, Mair A, Burns W. Study of noise and hearing in jute weaving. *J Acoust Soc Am* 1965; **38**: 113–20.
13 Ward WD, Glorig A, Sklar DL. Dependence of TTS at four kHz on intensity and time. *J Acoust Soc Am* 1958; **30**: 944–54.
14 Thomas GB, Williams CE. Noise susceptibility: a comparison of two naval aviator populations. *Environment International* 1990; **16**: 363–71.
15 US Department of Health, Education, and Welfare: *Cigarette smoking and health*

characteristics: United States July 1964–June 1965, PHS Publication No 1000 Series 10, No 34, Washington DC, 1967.

16 Friedman GD, Siegelaub AB, Seltzer CC. Cigarette smoking and exposure to occupational hazards. *Am J Epidemiol* 1973; **98**: 175–83.

17 Chung DY, Willson GN, Gannon RP, Mason K. Individual susceptibility to noise. In: Hamernik R, Henderson D, Salvi R, eds. *New perspectives on noise-induced hearing loss.* New York: Raven Press, 1982; 511–9.

18 Pyykkö I, Starck J, Färkkilä M, Hoikkala M, Korhonen O, Nuriminen M. Hand-arm vibration in the aetiology of hearing loss in lumberjacks. *Br J Ind Med* 1981; **38**: 281–9.

19 Pelmear PL, Leong D, Wong L, Roos J, Pike M. Hand-arm vibration syndrome and hearing loss in hard rock miners. *Journal of Low Frequency Noise and Vibration* 1987; **6**: 49–66.

20 Iki M, Kurumatani N, Moriyama T, Ogata A. Vibration-induced white finger and auditory susceptibility to noise exposure. *Kurume Med J* 1990; **37**: 33–4.

21 Ward WD, ed. *Proposed damage-risk criterion for impulse noise (gunfire).* NAS-NRC Committee on Hearing, Bioacoustics and Biomechanics, Working Group 57, Report, Washington D.C., 1968.

22 Atherley GRC, Martin AM. Equivalent continuous noise level as a measure of injury from impact and impulse noise. *Ann Occup Hyg* 1971; **14**: 11–28.

23 Martin AM, Atherley GRC. A method for the assessment of impact noise with respect to injury to hearing. *Ann Occup Hyg* 1973; **16**: 19–26.

24 von Gierke HE, Robinson DW, Karmy SJ. Results of a workshop on impulse noise and auditory hazard. *Journal of Sound and Vibration* 1982; **83**: 579–94.

25 Sulkowski WJ, Lipowczan A. Impulse noise-induced hearing loss in drop forge operators and the energy concept. *Noise Control Engineering Journal* 1982; **18**: 24–9.

26 Sulkowski WJ, Kowalska S, Lipowczan A. Hearing loss in weavers and drop-forge hammermen: Comparative study on the effects of steady-state and impulse noise. In: Rossi G, ed. *Proceedings of the 4th International Congress on Noise as a Public Health Problem.* Turin, 1983; 171–84.

27 Taylor W, Lempert B, Pelmear PL, Hempstock J. Noise levels and hearing thresholds in the drop-forging industry. *J Acoust Soc Am* 1984; **76**: 807–19.

28 Stark J, Pekkarinen J, Pyykkö I. Impulse noise and hand-arm vibration in relation to sensory neural hearing loss. *Scand J Work Environ Health* 1988; **14**: 265–71.

29 Shaw EAG. *Occupational noise exposure and noise-induced hearing loss: Scientific issues. Technical arguments and practical recommendations.* APS 707, NRCC No 25051. National Research Council of Canada, Physics Division, 1985; 1–64.

30 Hétu R, Phaneuf R, Marien C. Non-acoustic environmental factor influences on occupational hearing impairment: a preliminary discussion paper. *Canada Acoustics* 1987; **15**: 17–31.

31 Medical Research Council Institute of Hearing Research: Damage to hearing arising from leisure noise. *Br J Audiol* 1986; **20**: 157–64.

32 Whittle LS, Robinson DW. *Discotheques and pop music as a source of noise-induced hearing loss: A review bibliography.* NPL Acoustics Report Ac66. Department of Trade and Industry, England, 1974; 1–45.

33 Axelsson A, Lindgen F. Does pop music cause hearing damage? *Audiology* 1977; **16**: 432–7.

34 McBride D, Gill F, Proops D, Harrington M, Gardiner K, Attwell C. Noise and the classical musician. *BMJ* 1992; **305**: 1561–3.

35 Pelmear PL. Noise and health. In: Tempest W, ed. *The Noise Handbook.* London: Academic Press, 1985; 31–46.

36 Davies DR, Jones DM. Noise and efficiency. In: Tempest W, ed. *The Noise Handbook.* London: Academic Press, 1985; 87–141.

37 Langdon FJ. Noise annoyance. In: Tempest W, ed. *The Noise Handbook.* London: Academic Press, 1985; 143–76.

38 van Dijk FJH. Epidemiological research on non-auditory effects of occupational noise exposure. *Environment International* 1990; **16**: 405–9.

39 Parrot J, Petiot JC, Lobreau JP, Smolik HJ. Cardiovascular effects of impulse noise, road traffic noise, and intermittent pink noise at LAeq = 75 dB, as a function of sex, age,

and level of anxiety: a comparative study. *Int Arch Occup Environ Health* 1992; **63**: 477–84.

40 Tarter SK, Robins TG. Chronic noise exposure, high-frequency hearing loss, and hypertension among automotive assembly workers. *J Occup Med* 1990; **32**: 685–9.

41 Yiming Z, Shuzheng Z, Selvin S, Spear RC. A dose response relation for noise induced hypertension. *Br J Ind Med* 1991; **48**: 179–84.

42 Hartikainen-Sorri A, Sorri M, Anttonen HP, Tuimala R, Läärä E. Occupational noise exposure during pregnancy: a case control study. *Int Arch Occup Environ Health* 1988; **60**: 279–83.

43 McDonald AD, McDonald JC, Armstrong B, Cherry NM, Nolin AD, Roberts D. Prematurity and work in pregnancy. *Br J Ind Med* 1988; **45**: 56–62.

44 McDonald A, Sloan M, Armstrong B. Noise at work and the outcome of pregnancy. In: Sakurai H, Okazaki I, Omae K, eds. *Proceedings of the 7th International Symposium on Epidemiology in Occupational Health.* Tokyo 1990; 297–300.

45 Symonds C. Excitation and inhibition in epilepsy. *Brain* 1959; **82**: 133–46.

46 Knipschild P. Medical effects of aircraft noise: Community cardiovascular surgery. *Int Arch Environ Health* 1977; **40**: 185–90.

47 Alberti PW, ed. *Personal hearing protection in industry.* New York: Raven Press, 1982.

48 National Institute for Occupational Safety and Health: *A practical guide to effective hearing conservation programs in the workplace.* U.S. Department of Health and Human Services, Centers for Disease Control, NIOSH, Cincinnati, Ohio, 1990; Publication No. 90–120.

49 Leigh J, Morgan G. Hearing loss in the NSW coal mining industry. *Journal of Occupational Health and Safety Australia and New Zealand* 1990; **6**: 387–91.

50 Crutchfield CD, Sparks ST. Effects of noise and vibration on farm workers. *Occupational Medicine: State of the Art Reviews* 1991; **6**: 355–69.

51 Marvel ME, Pratt DS, Marvel LH, Regan M, May JJ. Occupational hearing loss in New York dairy farmers. *Am J Ind Med* 1991; **20**: 517–31.

52 Broste SK, Donald DA, Strand RL, Stueland DT. Hearing loss among high school farm students. *Am J Public Health* 1989; **79**: 619–22.

53 Tubbs RL. Occupational noise exposure and hearing loss in fire fighters assigned to airport fire stations. *Am Ind Hyg Assoc J* 1991; **52**: 372–8.

54 Chen TJ, Chiang HC, Chen SS. Effect of aircraft noise on hearing and auditory pathway function of airport employees. *J Occup Med* 1992; **34**: 613–9.

55 Kamal AM, Eldamati SE, Faris R. Hearing threshold of Cairo traffic policemen. *Int Arch Occup Environ Health* 1989; **61**: 543–5.

56 Wassermann DE. *Human aspects of occupational vibration.* Amsterdam: Elsevier, 1987.

57 Griffin MJ. *Handbook of human vibration.* London: Academic Press, 1990.

58 Pelmear PL, Taylor W, Wasserman DE, eds. *Hand-arm Vibration: A comprehensive guide.* New York: Van Nostrand Reinhold, 1992.

59 Boshuizen HC, Bongers PM, Hulshof CTJ. Self-reported back pain in tractor drivers exposed to whole-body vibration. *Int Arch Occup Environ Health* 1990; **62**: 109–15.

60 Wassermann DE, Doyle TE, Asburry WC. *Whole-body vibration exposure of workers during heavy equipment operation.* 1978; DHEW (NIOSH) Publication No. 78–153.

61 Gruber GJ, Ziperman HH. *Relationship between whole-body vibration and morbidity patterns among motor coach operators.* 1974; DHEW (NIOSH) Publication No. 75–104.

62 Helmkamp JC, Talbott EO, Marsh GM. Whole-body vibration—A critical review. *Am Ind Hyg Assoc J* 1984; **45**: 162–7.

63 Bongers PM, Boshuizen HC, Hulshof CTJ, Koemeester AP. Long-term sickness absence due to back disorders in crane operators exposed to whole-body vibration. *Int Arch Occup Environ Health* 1988; **61**: 59–64.

64 Harding RM, Mills FJ. Special forms of flight. II: Helicopters. *BMJ* 1983; **287**: 346–9.

65 Dupuis H, Zerlett G. Epidemiological research on professional groups exposed to vibration. In: Dupuis H, Zerlett G, eds. *The effects of whole-body vibration.* Berlin: Springer-Verlag, 1986; 91–6.

66 Griffin MJ. Whole-body vibration and health. In: Griffin MJ, ed. *Handbook of human vibration.* London: Academic Press, 1990; 171–220.

67 Dupuis H, Zerlett G. Acute effects of mechanical vibration: Kinetosis. In: Dupuis H, Zerlett G, eds. *The effects of whole-body vibration.* Berlin: Springer-Verlag, 1986; 66–9.

68 Kanda H, Goto D, Tanabe Y. Ultra-low frequency vibrations and motion sickness incidence. *Ind Health* 1977; **15**: 1–12.

69 Wilder DG, Pope MH, Frymoyer JW. The biomechanics of lumbar disc herniation and the effect of overload and instability. *J Spinal Disord* 1988; **1**: 16–32.

70 Wilder DG, Woodworth BS, Frymoyer MD, Pope MH. Vibration and the human spine. *Spine* 1982; **7**: 243–54.

71 Seidel H, Heide R. Long-term effects of whole-body vibration: a critical survey of the literature. *Int Arch Occup Environ Health* 1986; **58**: 1–26.

72 Gruber GJ. *Relationship between whole-body vibration and morbidity patterns among interstate truck drivers.* DHEW (NIOSH) Publication No. 77–167, 1976.

73 Milby TH, Spear RC. *Relationship between whole-body vibration and morbidity patterns among heavy equipment operators.* DHEW (NIOSH) Publication No. 74–131, 1974.

74 Rosegger R, Rosegger S. Health effects of tractor drivers. *Journal of Agricultural Engineering Research* 1960; **5**: 241–75.

75 Kelsey JL. An epidemiological study of the relationship between occupations and acute herniated lumbar intervertebral discs. *Int J Epidemiol* 1975; **4**: 197–205.

76 Kelsey JL, Hardy RJ. Driving of motor vehicles as a risk factor for acute herniated intervertebral discs. *Am J Epidemiol* 1975; **102**: 63–73.

77 Loriga G. Il lavoro con i martelli pneumatici. *Bolletino Inspettione Lavoro* 1911; **2**: 35–60.

78 Hamilton A. *A study of spastic anaemia in the hands of stonecutters.* Industrial Accident Hygiene Services Bulletin 236, No. 19. U.S. Dept. of Labor, Bureau of Labor Statistics 1918; 53–66.

79 Behrens VJ, Pelmear PL. Epidemiology of hand-arm vibration syndrome. In: Pelmear PL, Taylor W, Wasserman DE, eds. *Hand-arm vibration: A comprehensive guide for occupational health professionals.* New York: Van Nostrand Reinhold, 1992; 105–21.

80 Gemne G, Taylor W. Editors foreword. In: Gemne. G. Taylor W, eds. *Hand-arm Vibration and the central autonomic nervous system.* Special Volume. J Low Freq Noise Vib 1983; XI.

81 Pelmear PL, Taylor W. Clinical picture (vascular, neurological, and musculoskeletal). In: Pelmear PL, Taylor W, Wasserman DE, eds. *Hand-arm vibration: A comprehensive guide for occupational health professionals.* New York: Van Nostrand Reinhold, 1992: 26–40.

82 Gemne G, Pyykkö I, Taylor W, Pelmear PL. The Stockholm workshop scale for the classification of cold-induced Raynaud's phenomenon in the hand-arm vibration syndrome. *Scand J Work Environ Health* 1987; **13**: 275–8.

83 Brammer AJ, Taylor W, Lundborg G. Sensorineural stages of the hand-arm vibration syndrome. *Scand J Work Environ Health* 1987; **13**: 279–83.

84 Hedlund U. Raynaud's phenomenon of fingers and toes of miners exposed to local and whole-body vibration and cold. *Int Arch Occup Environ Health* 1989; **61**: 457–61.

85 Sakakibara H, Hashiguchi T, Furuta M, Kondo T, Miyao M, Yamada S. Circulatory disturbances of the foot in vibration syndrome. *Int Arch Occup Environ Health* 1991; **63**: 145–8.

86 Toibana N, Ishikawa N. Ten patients with Raynaud's phenomenon in fingers and toes caused by vibration. In: Okada A, Taylor W, Dupuis H, eds. *Hand-arm vibration.* Kanazawa, Japan: Kyoei Press, 1990; 245–8.

87 Kron MA, Ellner JJ. Buffer's Belly. *N Engl J Med* 1988; **318**: 584.

88 Shields PG, Chase KH. Primary torsion of the omentum in a jackhammer operator: Another vibration injury. *J Occup Med* 1988; **30**: 892–4.

89 Gemne G. Pathophysiology and pathogenesis of disorders in workers using hand-held vibratory tools. In: Pelmear PL, Taylor W, Wasserman DE, eds. *Hand-arm vibration: A comprehensive guide for occupational health professionals.* New York: Van Nostrand Reinhold, 1992; 41–76.

90 Seyring M. Maladies from work with compressed air drills. *Bull Hyg* 1931; **6**: 25.

91 Agate JN, Druett HA, Tombleson JBL. Raynaud's phenomenon in grinders of small castings. *Br J Ind Med* 1946; **3**: 167–74.

92 Agate JN. An outbreak of cases of Raynaud's phenomenon of occupational origin. *Br J Ind Med* 1949; **6**: 144–63.

93 Hunter D, McLaughlin AIG, Perry KMA. Clinical effects of the use of pneumatic tools. *Br J Ind Med* 1945; **2**: 10–6.

94 Grounds MD. Raynaud's phenomenon in users of chain saws. *Med J Aust* 1964; **1**: 270–2.

95 Miura T, Kimura K, Tominaga Y, Kimotsuki K. *On the Raynaud's phenomenon of occupational origin due to vibrating tools—its incidence in Japan.* Report of the Institute for Science and Labour. No. 65, 1966; 1–11.

96 Axelsson S. *Analysis of vibration in power saws.* No. 59, Skogshogskolan, Royal College of Forestry Monograph, Stockholm, 1968.

97 Barnes R, Longley EO, Smith ARB, Allen JG. Vibration disease. *Med J Aust* 1969; **1**: 901–5.

98 Taylor W, Pearson J, Kell RL, Keighley GD. Vibration syndrome in Forestry Commission chain saw operators. *Br J Ind Med* 1971; **28**: 83–9.

99 Taylor W, Pelmear PL, eds. *Vibration white finger in industry.* London: Academic Press, 1975.

100 Hellstrom B, Andersen KL. Vibration injuries in Norwegian forest workers. *Br J Ind Med* 1972; **29**: 255–63.

101 Thériault G, DeGuire L, Gingras S, Larouche G. Raynaud's phenomenon in forest workers in Quebec. *Can Med Assoc J* 1982; **126**: 1404–8.

102 Pyykkö I. The prevalence and symptoms of traumatic vasospastic disease among lumberjacks in Finland. A field study. *Scand J Work Environ Health* 1974; **11**: 118–31.

103 Pelmear PL, Roos J, Leong D, Wong L. Cold provocation test results from a 1985 survey of hard-rock miners in Ontario. *Scand J Work Environ Health* 1987; **13**: 343–7.

104 Bovenzi M. Finger systolic pressure during local cooling in normal subjects aged 20–60 years: reference values for the assessment of digital vasospasm in Raynaud's phenomenon of occupational origin. *Int Arch Occup Environ Health* 1988; **61**: 179–81.

105 Lundborg G, Sollerman C, Stromberg T, Pyykkö I, Rosen B. A new principle for assessing vibrotactile sense in vibration-induced neuropathy. *Scand J Work Environ Health* 1987; **13**: 375–9.

106 Katims JJ, Rouvelas P, Sadler BT, Weseley SA. Current perception threshold reproducibility and comparison with nerve conduction in evaluation of carpal tunnel syndrome. *Transactions of the American Society of Artificial Internal Organs* 1989; **XXXV**: 280–4.

107 Futatsuka M, Uneo T. A follow-up study of vibration-induced white finger due to chain saw operation. *Scand J Work Environ Health* 1986; **12**: 304–6.

108 Pyykkö I, Korhonen OS, Färkkilä MA, Starck JP, Aatola SA, Jäntti V. Vibration syndrome among Finnish forest workers, a follow-up from 1972 to 1983. *Scand J Work Environ Health* 1986; **12**: 307–12.

10 Back and limb disorders

HILKKA RIIHIMÄKI

Introduction

Back and limb disorders are one of the most important occupational health problems in the industrialised countries. These disorders are seldom life threatening but they impair the quality of life of a large proportion of the adult population. Back and limb disorders cause considerable losses in productivity and high expenses as a result of short term and long term disability and use of health care services. During the past two decades statistics from many countries have shown that there has been a steeply increasing trend in the pecuniary costs of musculoskeletal disorders.

During the same time working methods have gone through a drastic change as a result of mechanisation, automation, and the introduction of personal computers. For many heavy tasks machines have been designed to take over the burden from workers, but often dynamic manual work has been replaced by monotonous static or repetitive work—a jump out of the frying pan into the fire. The impact of these changes on musculoskeletal morbidity is largely unknown but it probably explains only part of the increase in cost. Other suggested factors are improved social security benefits and health services and a change in attitude towards musculoskeletal pain.

A need for effective preventive action against musculoskeletal disorders is widely acknowledged. For the planning of preventive programmes it is necessary to know the work-related and other factors that affect these disorders.

Interest in epidemiological research on musculoskeletal diseases has increased during the past decade, and this has improved the understanding of the occurrence and risk factors of these disorders. In this chapter the occurrence, impact, and risk factors are described for low back disorders, osteoarthritis of the two load-bearing joints—the hip and knee—and for upper limb complaints. The first two groups are responsible for a high proportion of long-term disability. In 1992, almost 3% of the Finnish population aged 18–64 years were receiving premature pensions on account of musculoskeletal diseases, the leading cause being back disease (14/1000) followed by osteoarthritis (6/1000).[1] Upper limb disorders appear to be a new epidemic and they have caused considerable controversy.

Low back disorders

In many cases of acute low back pain the cause cannot be found by routine physical examination or imaging techniques. The underlying cause may range from muscular fatigue and soft tissue sprains to injuries and herniations of the intervertebral discs or osteoarthritis of the facet joints. Essentially, a distinction can be made between local low back pain and radicular pain or sciatica indicating entrapment of a spinal nerve.[2] In chronic low back pain the underlying cause often remains uncertain but it is clear that not only structural derangements but also psychological factors play their part.

The vague concept of low back pain conceals many kinds of complaint, which differ from each other in aetiology and in prognosis. The most common disorder for epidemiological research has been degeneration of the lumbar spine. Only a few case-referent or cohort studies on clinically verified sciatica or herniated intervertebral disc have been reported. Most information is based on prevalence; definition of a new incident case is problematic for common symptoms as well as for degenerative changes.

Occurrence and impact

The prevalence estimates of low back pain vary depending on the methods of assessment and the characteristics of the population. The lifetime prevalence of low back pain in different populations is 50 to 70%, one year prevalence 25%, and point prevalence 12 to 30%.[3] In a national sample of the US population the lifetime prevalence of low back pain on most days for at least two weeks was 14%, the lifetime prevalence of back pain along with the features of sciatica was 2%, and the same percentage of patients had been told that they had a ruptured disc in the low back.[4] The prevalence rates of radiographically detectable degenerative changes of the lumbar spine in the UK were described by Lawrence in 1969.[5] The prevalence of spondylophytes with or without disc space narrowing and end-plate sclerosis (disc degeneration grades 1–4) was 51% in men aged 35–44, increasing to 91% at 65 or older. In women the prevalence rates were 40% and 78%, respectively. The corresponding rates for more severe disc degeneration (grades 3 and 4) were 5% and 38% in men and 3% and 24% in women. Magnetic resonance imaging, a more sensitive method of detection, confirmed the high prevalence of disc degeneration even in symptom-free subjects: 6% in women aged 20 years or younger and 79% in those 60 years or older.[6]

Time trends in prevalence of low back pain have been reported from 1978 to 1992 in Finland, based on health questionnaires sent annually to random samples of 5000 Finns 15–64 years of age.[7] The questionnaire asked about degenerative or other back disease verified or treated by a doctor during the previous year, and back pain during the previous 30 days. Although the coding was changed in 1985, on average the one year prevalence of back disease was about 15%, and there was no significant trend before or after that date. Likewise, the one month prevalence was about 36% in women and 34% in men, again without any significant time trend. These results support the view that no major changes have occurred in morbidity from back pain during the past 25 years.

In tables 10.1 and 10.2 the occurrence and impact of back disorders in the general population are presented. The data are from the Mini-Finland Health Survey, a comprehensive health survey of a representative sample of 3322 men and 3895 women aged 30 years or more.[8] The point prevalence of low back pain syndrome diagnosed by a doctor was 17·5% in men and 16·3% in women and of sciatica or prolapsed intervertebral disc 5·1% and 3·7%. Back disorders increased with age up to 65 years after which there was a decline. Also in accordance with several other population statistics, peak rates for sciatica and herniated intervertebral disc were at age 45–54 years in men and 55–64 years in women.

Table 10.1   Age-adjusted prevalence rates (%) of back disorders in the Finnish population over 30 years of age. (Adapted from Heliövaara et al. 1993.)[8]

	Men	Women
Lifetime prevalence of back pain	76·3	73·3
Lifetime prevalence of sciatic pain	34·6	38·8
Five-year prevalence of sciatic pain requiring bedrest		
for at least two weeks	17·3	19·4
One-month prevalence of low back or sciatic pain	19·4	23·3
Point prevalence of clinically verified		
low back pain syndrome	17·5	16·3
sciatica or herniated disc	5·1	3·7*

*p = 0·005

On physical examination by a physician, about half the people with a back syndrome had some, and 5% had severe, functional impairment (table 10.2). Back problems accounted for a greater proportion of inability to work than any other syndrome; 19% for complete disability and 24% for any grade. About 10% of those with back syndromes were heavy consumers of health care services as compared with 4% of those without. People with sciatica had been in hospital more often than those with unspecified back complaints and one in five had had surgical treatment. The consequences of low back pain are thus substantial, and this is confirmed in table 10.3, which shows statistics from the United Kingdom.[9]

Table 10.2   Impact of clinically verified back disorders in the Finnish population (Adapted from Heliövaara et al. 1993.)[8]

	Sciatica	Other back syndrome	No back syndrome	Population attributable fraction* (%)
Impairment (%)				
at least slight	55·6	53·4	29·3	14·4
severe	5·2	4·6	2·9	9·9
Inability to work (%)				
at least slight	58·2	46·1	18·1	23·8
complete	14·5	11·1	6·4	19·0
Consultations with a doctor				
in past 12 months				
mean number	3·8	3·4	2·3	8·6
at least 10 times	10·8	8·0	3·8	16·4
In hospital for any reason,				
past 12 months (%)	20·3	19·4	15·0	5·4
Ever in hospital as a result of				
a back disorder (%)	31·9	8·4	1·8	56·3
a back operation (%)	21·4	1·4	0·5	70·9

* The proportion of the impact in the population attributable to the observed back morbidity

Table 10.3   Consequences of back pain in the United Kingdom. (Adapted from Frank 1993.)[9]

Sickness absence	52·6 million certified working days (1988–9)
	12·5% of total sick days
Lost output	Estimated loss £2000 million (1987–8)
General practitioner consultations	Estimated 2 million annually
Hospital outpatient consultations	Estimated 300 000 annually
Hospital inpatient episodes	Estimated 100 000 annually (1989–90)
Severe disability	50–1000 people severely affected in an average health district of 250 000 population

Work-related risk factors

Since the 1950s many original articles and reviews have addressed the question of work-related risks for low back disorders. Here I give a summary of four recent reviews, supplemented with evidence from publications that have since appeared.[10–13]

Heavy physical/manual work

There is strong evidence that heavy physical work is associated with an increased risk of low back pain. The four reviews cited a total of 28 studies; in only two was no association detected and even in these the reviewers' interpretations were contradictory. Most of the studies were cross-sectional with job title as the indicator of exposure.

Eight cross-sectional studies, cited in all four reviews showed an association between heavy physical work and radiographically detectable lumbar disc degeneration.[10–13] A case-referent study on herniated lumbar disc[14] reported an uncertain result and a prospective study on hospital admission for this disease showed an association with heavy physical work.[15] In the Mini-Finland Health Survey a summary index of occupational physical stress was introduced, to include lifting and carrying heavy objects in awkward work postures, whole body vibration or use of vibrating equipment, and paced work determined by a machine.[16] A graded correlation was found between the index and low back syndromes, unconfounded by covariates. For sciatica the odds ratio increased from 1·6 to 2·0 and for unspecified low back syndrome from 1·3 to 3·2.

Heavy physical work is an nonspecific concept often measured in energy expenditure which may not adequately reflect physical load on the back. Heavy manual work includes the handling of materials in combination with postural load and it is not easy to differentiate the effects of these two factors. Loading on an afflicted back provokes symptoms, and pain in the back is more troublesome in jobs with high physical demands. Thus those employed in physically demanding jobs are more likely to report symptoms than those in lighter jobs. In studies on low back pain it is

211

therefore impossible to decide whether the results depict pain provocation or aggravation or an effect of heavy work on back morbidity. Moreover in cross-sectional studies there is obviously a negative bias resulting from worker selection. Yet the evidence for an association between heavy manual work and disc degeneration is convincing and indicates its adverse effect on the lumbar spine.

Manual handling

The four reviews cited 26 references relating to the handling of materials, including heavy or frequent lifting, pulling, pushing, or carrying, nearly all showing a positive association with low back pain.[10-13] Ten studies were mentioned in two or more reviews; eight were positive, one negative, and one study cited by all four reviews gave contradictory interpretations. In most of the studies exposure was a subjective assessment based on a questionnaire or an interview. In few was there any quantitative data on lifting. In only one study was workers' strength assessed in relation to job requirements; a mismatch was found to increase the risk of back injuries.[17] In a case-referent study, cases of low back pain were twice as likely as the referents to have lifted 4·5 kg or more at least once a minute throughout the work day;[18] the assessment was based on interview. Likewise among men aged 18–55 years those who declared that they lifted at least 20 kg more than twice a day were at increased risk of low back pain.[19]

Herniated intervertebral disc was not related to lifting in a case-referent study[14] cited in two reviews whereas all four reviews cited a later case-referent study suggesting a correlation.[20] Further analysis of the latter study indicated that lifting while twisting the body was associated with a three fold increased risk of herniated disc, and a six fold increase if the knees were straight. A case-referent study on non-occupational lifting supported these findings.[21] Assessment of exposure was based on interview and restricted to two years before the health problem began. Exposure was regarded as positive if objects weighing at least 10 kg were lifted, on average, at least once a week during the two years. Frequent lifting with knees straight and back bent was associated with increased risk, particularly among cases confirmed by operation or imaging techniques (risk ratio 4·0). Among the latter, positive associations were also found for frequent lifting with arms extended (risk ratio 1·9) and for twisting while lifting (risk ratio 1·9). Occupational lifting did not confound these findings.

Material handling carries a risk of back injury resulting from overloading of tissues. In the past, the load on the back entailed by lifting was calculated from simple static two-dimensional models even though the task is mostly dynamic in nature.[22] The influence of dynamic movement on joint loading was previously ignored because of difficulties in assessment but recently it has become possible.[23] In a study of three-dimensional dynamic trunk movements covering over 400 industrial lifting jobs in 48 industries, trunk movement and workplace factors that predicted risk of low back disorders were found to include lifting frequency, load moment, trunk lateral velocity, trunk twisting velocity, and trunk sagittal angle.[23] When three of these five dynamic predictors were increased in magnitude the probability of being associated with a high-risk job was multiplied by over 11 times. In comparison with prediction based on the assumption of static, sagitally symmetrical postures according to the National Institute of Occupational Safety and Health (NIOSH) Guide,[22] the power of the dynamically based assessment was over three times greater.

Twisting and bending

In one of the four reviews[10] postures were considered only in conjunction with lifting, whereas the other three[11–13] cited seven studies on non-neutral postural load associated with an increased risk of low back pain. The most convincing evidence was obtained from a case-referent study in an automobile assembly plant where exposure was assessed by video recording of each employee, although for some a proxy assessment was used.[18] The results showed that back disorders were related to mild trunk flexion (odds ratio 4·9), severe trunk flexion (odds ratio 5·7), and trunk twist or lateral bend (odds ratio 5·9). The risk increased with multiple exposures and increasing duration; the effect of postural load was almost four times greater than the effect of lifting. In a study among workers in the manufacture of prefabricated concrete elements, low back pain was related to the time spent in a bent or twisted posture but no correlation was detected with lifting.[24] Objective assessment of postural load on the back is difficult and the quality of exposure data in epidemiological studies is poor.[25] Variation of exposure to postural load in five different occupational groups was studied by Burdorf who estimated the time spent in trunk flexion and rotation.[26] He noted that occupational group was the main source of variation but within worker variation (29% of the total for flexion and 16% of that for rotation) and between worker variation (24% and 12%, respectively) were also considerable. Moreover, he estimated that the bias resulting from misclassification of exposure can easily be up to 50%.[27]

Whole body vibration

Evidence that motor vehicle driving is a risk factor for low back pain was consistent in 14 studies reviewed.[10–13] There is also evidence that motor vehicle driving is associated with increased risk of sciatic pain and in two studies with lumbar disc degeneration. In a retrospective 10-year follow-up it was found that disability from back trouble was more common

213

among crane operators with more than five years of exposure to vibration than in a control group and pensionable disability as a result of disc disease almost three-fold more common.[28] In study of tractor drivers, the prevalence of low back pain increased with duration of exposure to vibration but not with its mean estimated magnitude.[29] Two other studies showing an exposure-effect correlation have been published. The first was of helicopter pilots, in whom transient low back pain was strongly related to the average hours of flying per day and chronic back pain to 2000 hours or more of flying or an accumulated vibration dose of 400 m^2h/s^4.[30] The second was a one-year follow-up study of commercial travellers, among whom the first occurrence of low back pain was related to driving ten or more hours a week.[31]

The four reviews cited five studies indicating that herniated lumbar intervertebral disc is also related to motor vehicle driving.[10-13] Two were case-referent studies, one of which indicated that the risk increases with weekly hours spent driving.[32 33] In a prospective 11-year follow-up study of hospital admissions for herniated disc, exposure assessment being based on job title, professional drivers had the highest risk among all occupational groups.[15]

Experimentally, vibration of spinal tissues can impair nutrition of the disc[34] and cause muscle fatigue.[35] Vibration in motor vehicles often coincides with the natural frequency of the human lumbar spine thus rendering the tissues vulnerable to injury from resonance.[35] In motor vehicle driving whole-body vibration is combined with prolonged sitting which in itself seems hazardous to the back. Many drivers must also handle materials, the hazardous effect of which may be enhanced by muscular fatigue after exposure to vibration.

Sedentary work

Evidence for a connection between low back disorders and sedentary work is contradictory. With regard to low back pain, 13 studies were cited in the four reviews, seven with a positive result, five with a negative result, and one for which the interpretations in two reviews were contradictory.[10-13] Altogether four studies were cited regarding herniated intervertebral disc, two showing and two not showing an association between sedentary work and disc herniation. In a recent study of construction workers exposure to different work-related loading factors were classified in four categories (never; less than 1 hour/day; 1–4 hours/ day; and more than 4 hours/day) based on subjective statements in an interview. No association was detected between sitting and the prevalence of severe or any low back pain.[36]

There are many problems in the interpretation of the results from these studies. Health-dependent selection of workers is likely to cause bias and confounding by factors that are difficult to control. Furthermore, sedentary occupations may differ from each other in characteristics that may be pertinent to the risk of back disorders. In some sedentary occupations people can move relatively freely when they feel uncomfortable or fatigued whereas in others sitting posture is constrained. An example of the former is ordinary office work, and of the latter kind motor vehicle driving or operating a sewing machine. Evidence from experimental research supports the view that movement is necessary for the well-being of the back but there have been few quantitative investigations.

Trauma

Injuries are an obvious cause of acute back pain, but the long-term effects have received little study even though repeated minor and major trauma are thought to contribute to disc degeneration.[13] Some cross-sectional studies point to back accidents as a causal factor for sciatica and other back syndromes.[16 37 38] A general population survey suggests that back injuries contribute substantially to chronic low-back pain and sciatica; the estimated attributable fraction was 16·5% for sciatica and 13·7% for unspecified low back pain.[16] In all these studies information on back accidents was based on self-reports. Differentiation of truly accidental injuries from other acute episodes of low back pain may not be easy, particularly in retrospect. Thus the evidence of a relationship between back accidents and back morbidity may partly reflect the well-established fact that previous low back pain is the best predictor of low back pain in the future. Accidental back injuries occur too seldom for easy objective assessment.

Psychosocial factors

Bongers *et al.* have recently published an exhaustive review of the connection between psychosocial factors and musculoskeletal disease, classifying such factors at work into two categories: demands and control, and social support.[39] In the former category, musculoskeletal symptoms were associated with monotonous work, time pressure, high concentration, high responsibilities, high workload, little opportunity to take breaks, lack of clarity, and low control or little autonomy.

Factors in the second category were poor social support from colleagues and from superiors. Seven cross-sectional studies were thought to provide evidence that self-reported work demands—monotonous work and working under time pressure—are associated with back trouble whereas evidence for the other aspects was not convincing. Work demand was not found to predict disability from back disorders in the one longitudinal study in which this was considered.[40] Poor social support was associated with back trouble in the only relevant longitudinal study[41] whereas the results of six cross-sectional studies were conflicting. In the longitudinal

215

study the outcome measure was claiming for injury, so it remains uncertain whether social support affected morbidity or injury reporting.

Individual risk factors

Height and weight

Evidence for a connection between body height and overweight and low back pain is contradictory. In three reviews six studies were cited which suggested that tall people have an increased risk of low back pain whereas 10 studies did not show the association.[10 11 13] Evidence that height is associated with sciatica and herniated disc is convincing; seven studies reported an association while one did not. Ergonomic disadvantage of tall people and nutritional disadvantage of a greater disc volume were the suggested explanation.[10] In the same reviews 11 studies were cited on the relationship between overweight and low back pain. An association was detected only in one cross-sectional study[42] but not in a 10-year follow-up of metal industry workers.[43] In an 11-year follow-up study obesity predicted admission to hospital for herniated lumbar intervertebral disc in men but not in women[44] whereas in a case-referent study no such association was present.[33]

Physical fitness

The association between physical fitness and back disorders was examined in 39 studies, assessment of fitness being based on the measurement of aerobic capacity, isometric strength, or endurance of the trunk muscles. Most of the studies were cross-sectional or of case series from which conclusions cannot be drawn about temporal order, and the results of six longitudinal studies were inconsistent. Poor aerobic capacity was not associated with low back pain in the Danish general population in a one-year follow-up,[45] but good endurance of back muscles prevented first-time occurrence of low back pain.[46] In a three-year follow-up, least fit fire fighters had most back injuries but age may have confounded the analysis.[47] In a 10-year follow-up of metal industry employees, trunk muscle strength did not predict the future occurrence of low back pain,[48] nor was there an association between back injury claims and trunk muscle strength or cardiorespiratory capacity in a three-year follow-up study in the aircraft industry.[49 50] Among six studies cited on low back pain and spinal mobility, correlation was found in four, and in a longitudinal study less mobility even seemed protective.[46]

Smoking

Four reviews presented evidence from 12 studies that smoking is associated with low back pain, sciatica, or herniated intervertebral disc, whereas three were negative.[10–13] Smoking habits vary across occupational groups, which may lead to confounding by occupational load. Indeed, Boshuizen *et al.* detected a correlation between smoking and back pain only in occupations that require physical exertion.[51] Pain in the extremities turned out to be more strongly related to smoking than back pain, which suggests a general influence of smoking on pain. According to Boshuizen *et al.* the evidence points to only a slight increase in back pain among smokers.[51] Nevertheless, an exposure-effect correlation has been reported in some studies.[42 52] Cigarette smoking was found to promote disc degeneration as assessed by magnetic resonance imaging in a study of identical twins discordant for this factor,[53] a finding that is biologically plausible as animal studies have shown that exposure to smoking impairs the nutrition of the disc.[34]

Personality characteristics and stress symptoms

In the review by Bongers *et al.* 18 studies were cited in which the following personality characteristics were considered in relation to low back disorders:[39] personality type defined by the Minnesota Multiphasic Personality Inventory (neuroticism, hysteria, anti-social), type A behaviour (competitiveness), extrovert personality, psychological dysfunctioning (depression), coping styles, attitude towards own health, low social class, low educational level, and a wide variety of stress symptoms. Personality traits and emotional problems were associated with back trouble not only in cross-sectional studies but also in one longitudinal study, although the results were not consistent.[41] The association between back trouble and stress symptoms reported in many cross-sectional studies was tentatively supported by a longitudinal study but there was no connection with job dissatisfaction.[54] In a 10-year follow-up of metal industry employees, depressive symptoms predicted future development of low back symptoms and clinical findings in men, but not vice versa.[55] The association of stress symptoms and back disorders on the contrary, was reciprocal. In women stress symptoms predicted future low back symptoms and findings but none of the other associations were significant. These differences have not been explained.

An association between low educational level and low social class independent of physical load was reported in two longitudinal studies.[56 57]

Psychosocial is a vague concept covering many different features related to individuals or to work. More vigorous investigations are needed to identify stages in the development of low back trouble at which different components of the psychosocial complex have their effects. It seems likely that these factors affect pain and illness behaviour more than they do underlying derangements or pathology.

Summary

Low back disorders are one of the most important health problems in the working population; there has been much epidemiological research but the current picture remains obscure. Most studies have been cross-sectional with inherent biases, and few risk factors have been established prospectively. Physically heavy work is associated with an increased risk of low back pain and also disc degeneration. Frequent lifting of heavy loads and lifting while twisting increase the risk of both pain and disc herniation, whereas prolonged sitting increases the risk of pain. Motor vehicle drivers are at higher than average risk. Psychosocial factors at work are also related to low back pain and reporting of back injuries. Smoking is associated with low back pain and disc degeneration, and mental stress with low back pain, whereas the evidence for tallness, physical fitness, trunk muscle performance, and mobility is less consistent. Overall, data are mainly qualitative and little is known about exposure-effect relationships.

Further cross-sectional studies have limited use and progress will depend on well designed longitudinal and case-referent surveys. The almost universal "exposures" and problems of everyday life must be filtered out, leaving sharper and more measurable data on clear cut deviations from the normal range. Precise classification of disabling symptoms by location, duration and severity, together with standardised clinical tests and imaging techniques can do the same for outcome. Finally such concepts as latency and induction time are required in the quantitative analyses of risk.

Osteoarthritis of the hip and knee

Osteoarthritis is a degenerative process in joints, the earliest sign of which is loss of cartilage, followed by joint space narrowing on radiography. Subsequent bony changes include sclerosis in the subchondral bone, osteophyte formation, and bone cysts. Clinical signs of osteoarthritis include pain and restricted range of joint movement. Radiographic criteria for diagnosis introduced by Kellgren and Lawrence have been commonly used but there has been variation in grading in different studies which hampers comparison of the results.[58] Osteoarthritis of the two large weight bearing joints, the hip and knee, is common in elderly people. These diseases cause pain, limit daily activities, and worsen the quality of life for many people and commonly lead to early retirement from work.

The effects of physical load at work on the development of hip and knee osteoarthritis have not been extensively studied, probably because prevalence increases only during the last two decades of the working life. Earlier studies were contradictory but more recent epidemiological evidence suggests that work-related physical factors contribute substantially to these diseases.

218

Table 10.4   Prevalence of hip osteoarthritis (%)

| Age | Mini-Finland Health Survey[a] | | 9 surveys combined[b] | | Northern England (Leigh)[c] | | HANES-I[d] |
	men (n = 3322)	women (n = 3895)	men	women	men (n = 173)	women (n = 207)	both sexes (n = 2358)
30–44	0·3	0·7					
45–54	1·9	2·8					
55–64	6·6	7·9	18	10	18·6	12·0	2·3
65–74	11·9	11·7					3·9
75–	16·4	21·2					
Total (age-adjusted)	4·6	5·5					

[a]Heliövaara et al. 1993;[8] symptom history and clinical examination [b]Felson 1988,[59]
[c]Kellgren and Lawrence 1958,[60] [d]Tepper and Hochberg 1993,[61] radiographic examination.

Occurrence and impact

Estimates of the prevalence of hip osteoarthritis vary considerably and comparable data are found only in the age-range 55 to 64 years (table 10.4). In radiographic studies the prevalence was about 18% in men and 10% in women but in one study (Health and Nutrition Examination Survey—HANES-I) it was only about 2%.[61] In the Mini-Finland Health Survey, in which osteoarthritis was defined on the basis of symptoms and clinical findings, prevalence in men aged 55–64 was 6·6% and in women 7·9%.[8] It was lower than the estimates from most of the radiographic studies, and increased steeply with age.

The prevalence of knee osteoarthritis also increases with age but unlike hip osteoarthritis it is much more common in women (table 10.5). Knee osteoarthritis was detected radiographically in 28% of men and in 40% of

Table 10.5   Prevalence of knee osteoarthritis (%)

| Age | Mini-Finland Health Survey[a] | | Northern England[b] | | HANES-I[c] | |
	men (n = 3322)	women (n = 3895)	men (n = 550)	women (n = 566)	men (n = 2428)	women (n = 2765)
30/35–44	0·3	1·6	5·5	4·0	1·2	1·2
45–54	4·0	9·7	8·2	13·1	2·2	3·6
55–64	9·0	24·2	28·1	40·0	5·1	7·5
65–74	12·8	33·0	26·4	49·1	9·0	20·3
75–	15·7	38·4				
Total (age-adjusted)	5·5	14·5				

[a] Heliövaara et al. 1993;[8] symptom history and clinical examination
[b] Lawrence et al. 1966,[62] [c]Anderson and Felson 1988;[63] radiographic examination

219

Table 10.6   Impact of clinically verified osteoarthritis in the Finnish population (age 30 years or more). (Adapted from Heliövaara et al. 1993.)[8]

	Hip	Knee	Any joint	No osteoarthritis	Population attributable fraction*
Impairment (%)					
at least slight	63·7	67·0	53·6	29·0	15·3
severe	7·4	11·5	2·2	2·6	18·2
Inability to work (%)					
at least slight	43·7	58·4	34·7	21·6	9·1
complete	15·2	23·1	5·6	8·0	6·6
Consultations with a doctor in past 12 months					
mean number	3·3	3·3	3·1	2·4	9·5
at least 10 times	8·4	8·7	7·1	4·1	10·5
In hospital for any reason in past 12 months (%)	19·5	18·3	15·5	15·4	2·1
Ever in hospital for osteoarthritis (%)	4·7	9·6	0·8	0·2	75·6
Operated for osteoarthritis (%)	2·9	6·9	0·4	0·1	82·3

* The proportion of the impact in the population attributable to the observed morbidity

women of age 55 to 64 years in Northern England,[62] compared with 9% and 24% in the Mini-Finland Health Survey. In the Finnish survey, two thirds of the people with hip or knee osteoarthritis were found to have some functional impairment on clinical examination.[8] This was severe in 7% of those with hip disease and 12% of those with knees affected (table 10.6). Of severe functional impairment in the population, 18% is attributable to osteoarthritis. Hip osteoarthritis caused complete inability to work in 15% of the cases, and knee disease in 23%. Osteoarthritis rarely requires admission to hospital and was responsible for only about 2% of all admissions; surgical procedures were more common for the knee than the hip.[8]

Risk factors for hip osteoarthritis

Work-related factors

In most studies only job title has been used as the measure of exposure to work-related loading factors but in a few more detailed assessment has been attempted, usually by questionnaire or interview, some of which have provided insight into possible exposure-effect relationships.

In the Mini-Finland Health Survey the prevalence of hip osteoarthritis was highest in agriculture and forestry both in men (6·9%) and in women (6·8%).[8] Among men the lowest prevalence was in technical and administrative work (2·2%) and among women in housewives (2·9%). With physical stress defined on a score from 0 to 5 the relative risk of both unilateral and bilateral hip disease increased linearly with increasing score. The odds ratios (95% confidence intervals) for scores 4 and 5 were 2·3 (1·2 to 4·3) and 2·9 (1·5 to 5·8), respectively.

In England a cross-sectional study was carried out in a random sample of 1231 men aged 60–76 selected from five rural general practices.[64] Subjects comprised current and retired farmers and those who reported having worked all their lives in offices. Pelvic radiographs were taken of all subjects who had not had hip replacements. Age-adjusted odds ratio for hip osteoarthritis (hip replacement or radiographically detected hip osteoarthritis) was 5·8 (1·1 to 31·5) in those who had farmed 1–9 years and 10·1 (2·2 to 45·9) in those who had farmed for 10 or more years. As the excess could not be attributed to any particular type of farming it was concluded that manual handling was the most likely explanation.

In a Swedish study hip osteoarthritis was assessed from radiographic examinations of colon or urinary tract in a population of 15 000 farmers and farmers' wives.[65] The reference population was from the city of Malmö where hip osteoarthritis had been assessed with the same methods. Male farmers in the age-range of 40–64 years had a 10-fold higher prevalence than the referents; no increase was found among the farmers' wives.

In a large register-based cohort study in Sweden blue-collar occupations were classified as having high or low exposure to dynamic and/or static forces on the lower extremities.[66] Data on osteoarthritis were obtained from the Hospital Discharge Register. The risk of admission to hospital for hip disease was two-fold greater among men with high than low exposure; high-risk occupations were farming, construction work, food processing, and fire fighting. Data for women were sparse but female mail carriers showed an excess risk.

Two case-referent studies have also shown increased risk of hip osteoarthritis among farmers. In a Swedish study the relative risk of hip operation for osteoarthritis was 3·2 (1·8 to 5·5) in those who had farmed more than 10 years but longer exposure did not result in greater risk.[67] Heavy work load and accidents were not related to hip disease. In a British study the cases were men aged 60–75 years who had had hip replacements or had severe narrowing of the hip joint space.[68] Severe osteoarthritis was related to farming for more than 10 years (odds ratio 2·0, 95% CI 0·9 to 4·4) and also to prolonged standing (at least two hours/day, 40 years or more) and manual lifting (lifting or moving loads over 25 kg for 20 years or more). In this study sports and obesity did not have a significant effect.

No difference was detected in the prevalence of hip osteoarthritis between Swedish shipyard labourers and white-collar workers in a cross-sectional study;[69] the possible effect of selection was not discussed. Retired professional dancers have a high prevalence of hip osteoarthritis;[70] dancers have increased joint laxity which can predispose to osteoarthritis and their joints are exposed to high forces and risk of injury.

Table 10.7   Relative risk and 95% confidence interval (95% CI) for developing hip osteoarthritis from medium or high exposure before the age of 49 years as compared to low exposure. (Adapted from Vingård et al. 1991.)[71]

	Medium exposure		High exposure	
	RR*	95% CI	RR*	95% CI
Static or dynamic	1·82	1·02–3·24	2·42	1·45 to 4·04
Static only	1·21	0·64–2·31	2·92	1·69 to 5·01
Dynamic only	1·92	1·11–3·32	2·17	1·27 to 3·73
Metric tonnes lifted	1·58	0·93–2·66	1·84	1·12 to 3·03
Number of lifts				
(>40 kg)	1·38	0·81–2·36	2·40	1·50 to 3·83
Number of jumps	1·83	1·06–3·14	1·52	0·91 to 2·53

* Adjusted for age, body mass index, smoking, and sports activities up to the age of 29 years.

In a further case-referent study detailed exposure assessments were made by interviewing all subjects.[71] Cases were all Swedish men aged 50–70 years who underwent hip replacement in four large hospitals between 1984 and 1988, and referents were sampled at random from the catchment population. Information on physical load was obtained up to the age of 49. Long-term exposure to both static and dynamic physical loads systematically increased the risk of severe hip osteoarthritis (table 10.7). Men with high exposure to dynamic or static work loads had a relative risk of 2·4 (95% CI 1·5 to 4·0) and those with high exposure to heavy lifting (>40 kg) between the ages of 30 to 49 years had the highest relative risk, 3·3 (95% CI 2·0 to 5·6). This study is an example of how accurate assessments of exposure improve the ability to detect significant associations.

Hereditary and congenital factors

The prevalence of hip osteoarthritis increases with increasing age and is similar in men and women (table 10.4).[59] [72] The risk factors for the two sexes may be somewhat different.[61] The disease is less common among non-white than among white people, which points to hereditary factors but may also reflect differences in life-style.[59] There is evidence that hereditary factors are associated with generalised osteoarthritis but these two forms of disease do not appear to be closely connected.[59] Congenital and developmental defects, such as congenital dislocation of the hip, slipped femoral epiphysis, and Legg-Calvé-Perthes disease (aseptic necrosis of the head of the femur) are predisposing factors for the development of hip osteoarthritis.[59] Congenital defects are certainly important in the development of unilateral hip osteoarthritis.[61]

Overweight

In his review Felson described the evidence of the association between overweight and hip osteoarthritis as conflicting but suggested that it might be a disease promoter in those with developmental predisposition.[59] Recent studies have shown that overweight is a stronger risk factor for bilateral than for unilateral hip osteoarthritis. In the Mini-Finland Health Survey[73] odds ratios (adjusted for age, sex, injuries, and physical stress at work) for body mass index (BMI) values 25·0–29·9, 30·0–34·9, and >35·0 with BMI <25 as the reference were 1·5 (95% CI 1·1 to 2·2), 1·6 (1·0 to 2·5), and 1·2 (0·5 to 3·0) for unilateral hip osteoarthritis and 1·4 (1·0 to 2·0), 2·3 (1·5 to 3·5), and 2·8 (1·4 to 5·7) for bilateral hip osteoarthritis, respectively. In the HANES-I survey the odds ratio for overweight (BMI >27·3 for women and BMI >27·8 for men) and unilateral hip osteoarthritis was 0·54 (0·26 to 1·16).[61] For bilateral hip osteoarthritis the odds ratio was 2·00 (0·97 to 4·15). Confounding effects of age, race, education, trauma, and skin fold thickness were controlled for. Both these studies were cross-sectional and do not allow causal inference, as the temporal sequence cannot be known.

In a case-referent study of people receiving hip prostheses, overweight at ages of 20, 30, 40 and 50 years was assessed retrospectively by interview.[74] Relative risk contrasted overweight (BMI >the mean BMI+1SD) and lean subjects (BMI <the mean BMI−1SD). Odds ratios for overweight at these ages were respectively 1·7 (0·9 to 3·0), 1·8 (1·0 to 3·2), 2·5 (1·4 to 4·5), and 2·3 (1·2 to 4·4). Adjustments were made for the confounding effects of age, smoking, and physical load at work. These findings show that overweight at younger age increases the risk of severe hip osteoarthritis.

Trauma

Major injuries entailing ligament tears or cartilaginous damage affecting the hip joint are rare.[59] Minor injuries, however, may occur in conjunction with injuries to the lower limb and if repeated, might conceivably promote the development of osteoarthritis. Severe injuries to the lower limb may change its biomechanical properties and thus lead to abnormal loading on the hip joint. This hypothesis is supported by two studies, HANES-I and the Mini-Finland Health Survey.[61 73] In the former, a history of hip trauma was associated with increased risk of unilateral osteoarthritis, odds ratio 13·7 (3·7 to 51·1), whereas no case of bilateral hip osteoarthritis with a history of hip trauma was detected.[61] Hip trauma was a significant risk factor for osteoarthritis in men, odds ratio 24·2 (3·8 to 15·3), but not in women, odds ratio 4·2 (0·5 to 34·7). In the latter study, a history of injury to the lower limb was associated more strongly with unilateral hip osteoarthritis, odds ratio 2·1 (1·4 to 3·1), than with bilateral disease, odds ratio 1·5 (0·9 to 2·3).[73]

Sports

Sports activities strengthen the musculoskeletal system but in many sports the tissues are also liable to be injured and sport can thus have both preventive and deleterious effects. It is difficult to draw definite conclusions from the contradictory results of most of the studies because the effects of selection and confounding have not been controlled and many studies lack proper reference groups.[59] In a controlled study of cumulative 21-year incidence of admission to hospital for osteoarthritis of the hip, knee, or ankle in former élite athletes the incidence of hip osteoarthritis was 5·3% in endurance sports athletes, 2·5% in mixed sports athletes, 3·5% in power sports athletes, and 1·4% in the control group.[75] In endurance athletes hospital admission occurred first in old age, but mixed and power sports athletes were at increased risk of premature osteoarthritis.

A case-referent study of hip prosthesis recipients by Vingård et al. showed a clear-cut association between sports and hip osteoarthritis.[76] In this study men with high exposure to sports (assessed as lifetime cumulated hours) had a relative risk of 4·5 (2·7 to 7·6) compared with those with low exposure. Track, field and racket sports seemed to be most hazardous. Furthermore, men who had been exposed to high physical load both from work and from sports had a relative risk of 8·5 (4·0 to 17·9) of severe disease as compared with those with low exposure in both activities. This study, in which the confounding effects of age, overweight, and smoking were controlled, provides strong evidence that excessive physical load plays an important part in the development of severe hip osteoarthritis. It is probable that minor and major injuries in sports are promoters of the degenerative process.

Risk factors for knee osteoarthritis

Work-related factors

According to many cross-sectional studies, workers in occupations with heavy physical demands have a higher prevalence of knee osteoarthritis than those in less demanding jobs. Some studies, however, have failed to show such a correlation perhaps because of differential health-based selection among workers. In England, Kellgren and Lawrence reported a higher prevalence of knee osteoarthritis at the age of 40 to 50 years in coal miners than in manual workers and office workers.[77] In a subsequent study no specific tasks in mining could be associated with the increased risk and it was concluded that knee injuries were the causal factor.[78] Dockers have been reported to have a higher prevalence of knee osteoarthritis than civil servants in sedentary work,[79] and shipyard workers than office workers and teachers.[80] Carpet and floor layers aged 25–49 years whose job requires frequent kneeling had an increased prevalence of radiographic patellar osteophytosis but not of other signs of osteoarthritis as compared with house painters.[81] At least three cross-sectional studies failed to confirm the correlation between heavy labour and knee osteoarthritis. Foundry workers were compared with a sample of a general population,[82] concrete reinforcement workers with house painters,[83] and lumberjacks with men in light physical work or office work.[84] None were found to be at increased risk.

In HANES-I, the associations between knee osteoarthritis and physical demands of jobs were examined.[63] After control for confounding by race, education level, and body mass index a significant relationship was found in the age-group 55–64 years for strength demands of job in women (OR 3·1, 95% CI 1·0 to 9·4 for an increase from low to moderate or from moderate to high) but not in men, and for knee-bending demands in women (OR 3·5, 95% CI 1·2 to 10·5) for an increase from no to some knee-bending, or from some to much knee-bending, and in men (OR 2·5, 95% CI 1·2 to 5·0). The attributable risk of knee osteoarthritis associated with job-related knee-bending was estimated as 0·32 in 55–64 year-old but in younger age groups the associations were not significant, tending to suggest that the disease develops only after a long period of repetitive occupational exposure.

In the Mini-Finland Health Survey the highest prevalence of knee osteoarthritis was among men and women in agriculture and forestry and lowest among professionals.[8] The odds ratios for both unilateral and bilateral knee disease increased with physical stress score of work from score 0 as a reference, to 2·1 (1·2 to 3·8) and 1·6 (1·0 to 2·6) at scores 4 and 5, respectively. In the Swedish register-based cohort study high risk occupations for admissions to hospital for knee osteoarthritis were firefighting (OR 2·9 compared with low-exposure blue-collar workers, adjusted for age, county, and degree of urbanisation), farming (OR 1·5), and construction work (OR 1·4) among men, and cleaning (OR 2·2) among women.[66]

Only one longitudinal study on knee osteoarthritis in relation to occupational physical demands has been reported.[85] In the Framingham cohort which has been followed for over 40 years, occupational status was assessed in 1948–51 through 1958–61 and osteoarthritis was assessed by weight-bearing radiographic examination of the knees in 1983–85 when the mean age of the subjects was 73 years. Each subject's job was characterised by its level of physical demand and knee bending. Men with knee-bending and at least moderate physical demands at work were at increased risk of later knee osteoarthritis (OR 2·2, 95% CI 1·2 to 3·6) as compared with those with neither. A small case-referent study also confirmed the association between knee osteoarthritis and heavy physical work.[86] Patients with severe osteoarthritis treated by total knee arthroplasty were two to three times more likely than community controls to have performed heavy work.

Hereditary and congenital factors and defects

The prevalence of knee osteoarthritis increases with age and is consistently higher in women than in men, particularly in older age groups (table 10.5).[8] The results from both the Mini-Finland Health Survey[8] and HANES-I[87] have indicated that the sex difference is stronger for bilateral than for unilateral knee osteoarthritis, which suggests that the underlying factors are hormonal or structural. HANES-I is the only study that has provided data on racial differences in the prevalence of knee osteoarthritis within one country.[63] The prevalence was higher in black women than in white women (OR 2·1, 95% CI 1·4 to 3·2, adjusted for age and weight) but no significant difference was found in men. The authors could give no explanation for these findings but proposed genetic factors. According to Felson, knee osteoarthritis fits into the generalised osteoarthritis syndrome which in its nodal form has a hereditary pattern.[59] Congenital defects appear to be of minor importance in this disease.[59]

Overweight

Several cross-sectional studies have indicated an association between knee osteoarthritis and overweight.[59] In the Mini-Finland Health Survey a linear trend in correlation was detected in both sexes with body mass index, especially in bilateral disease,[8] a finding reported earlier by Davis et al. from HANES-I.[87] Confirmation for a causal link with overweight was obtained from the results in a study which showed an association with high self-reported minimum adult weight, a proxy for long-term obesity.[63] In the Framingham Study, obesity also predicted the development of knee osteoarthritis 36 years later; for overweight women the age-adjusted relative risk was 2·1 (1·6 to 2·6) and for men 1·5 (1·1 to 1·9).[88] In women a decrease in body mass index of 2 units or more (approximately 5·1 kg) during the 10 years before examination was reported to reduce the odds of developing knee osteoarthritis by over 50%.[89] Cases of severe knee osteoarthritis were 3·5 times more likely than controls to have been obese at the age of 20 years.[86]

Trauma

Both in experimental animals and in humans major injury causes osteoarthritis.[59] Kellgren and Lawrence stated that injury is a more important cause of osteoarthritis in the knee than in any other joint.[60] Two large cross-sectional studies have shown that injury is associated more strongly with the risk of unilateral than of bilateral disease.[8 87] In the Mini-Finland Health Survey, 9% of knee osteoarthritis was attributable to injuries;[8] in the Framingham study knee injury also predicted knee osteoarthritis[90] and in a case-control survey severe cases of osteoarthritis were nearly five times more likely than controls to have had a significant knee injury.[86]

Sports

Evidence for an association with sports activities is not convincing even though many sports have a high risk of causing injury; however, adequate reference groups and control for confounding and selection factors are few.[59] In former male élite athletes the cumulative 21 year rate of admission to hospital for osteoarthritis of the knee was 2·5% in endurance athletes, 1·9% in mixed sports athletes, and 3·0% in power sports athletes compared with 1·3% in a control group.[75] In these athletes the odds ratio for admission to hospital for osteoarthritis of the hip, knee, or ankle (very few cases) was 2·4 (1·3 to 4·7) in endurance sports, 2·4 (1·3 to 4·2) in mixed sports and 2·7 (1·5 to 4·8) in power sports after adjustment for confounding by age, occupation, and body mass index. It was concluded from this study that as participation in sports may predispose to premature osteoarthritis proper treatment of injuries to the joints is important.

Summary

Far fewer epidemiological studies have been conducted of hip and knee osteoarthritis than of low back disorders. An advantage of studying osteoarthritis is that the outcome can be clearly defined both in cohort and in case-referent studies. Osteoarthritis develops insidiously, which makes it difficult to define the onset but radiographic diagnosis can be obtained independent of exposure, which in symptom-based definitions is usually not the case. Similar problems of exposure assessment are faced as in studies of low back disorders especially concerning heaviness of work. Specific loading factors of the lower limbs such as kneeling or knee bending can easily be assessed in qualitative terms but quantitatively it is difficult.

In the Mini-Finland Health Survey 50% of knee and 59% of hip osteoarthritis in people aged 30 years or more were attributable to three risk factors—overweight, injuries, and physical demands of work.[8] These figures indicate that a considerable proportion of these disabling diseases, so common in elderly people, could be prevented if these factors could be reduced. At the work site, prevention of accidents is of primary concern, but more is to be learned about acceptable physical demands; proper treatment of joint injuries is also important.

Upper limb disorders

Upper limb disorders and their connection with strenuous tasks at work is subject to considerable controversy in the field of work-related musculoskeletal disorders. Concepts such as cumulative trauma disorder, repetitive strain injury, and overuse syndrome have frequently been used for these complaints. Terms of this kind are nonspecific labels covering a variety of disorders and implying aetiology that has not always been convincingly ascertained.[91] An epidemic of repetitive strain injury in Australia in the early 1980s attained wide repute: mechanisation, automation of work, and the rapid introduction of personal computers were blamed for the epidemic, but it has also been suggested that a liberal labour insurance policy and loose diagnostic criteria played an important part.[92] Since then there has been concern about possible epidemics of this kind in other industrialised countries.[91 93] It has also been emphasised that the use of vague all-covering diagnostic labels should be discouraged. Accordingly, this review will be restricted to definable disorders of the hand, wrist, forearm, and elbow, including tenosynovitis, peritendinitis, carpal tunnel syndrome, and epicondylitis, albeit generally accepted criteria for these diagnoses have still to be established.[93 94]

Hand-wrist tendon syndromes

Tenosynovitis denotes inflammation of the tendon sheath whereas inflammation of the myotendinous junction is called peritendinitis. Tenosynovitis occurs where the tendon passes under the retinaculum at a joint, whereas the most common site of peritendinitis is in the distal part of the forearm. In epidemiological studies these two diseases are usually not differentiated and thus a collective term tendon syndrome is used here. These syndromes occur more commonly on the extensor than the flexor side of the wrist and forearm.

Occurrence

Few studies have reported the incidence of tendon syndromes. In the 1940s an incidence of 0·3/100 person years was noted among 12 000 English car factory workers.[95] In a Finnish cohort study the incidence of visits to a doctor's office for tendon syndrome was investigated in employees of a large meat-processing plant:[96] the incidence/100 person years was 12·5 in male meat cutters, 16·8 in female sausage makers, 25·3 in female packers and less than 1 among foremen and men and women in office workers. The dominant hand was affected in 72% of the cases and the median age was 35 years.

Work-related risk factors

Work-related risk factors possibly include repetitive movements of the hand and wrist, unaccustomed repetitive work, forceful movements, vibration, cold environment, excessive flexion or extension of the hand and wrist, pinch grip, direct blow, and direct pressure.[94 97] Prevalence ranges from 3% to 56% in exposed groups and from 1% to 14% in reference groups.[98] Part of the wide variation is probably attributable to differences in diagnostic criteria.

In a critical review of upper limb disorders criteria of validity were applied to evaluate the studies.[99] Only two cross-sectional studies of tendon syndromes met the criteria, one of which was by Silverstein *et al.* in industrial workers.[100] After an initial classification of jobs, four exposure groups were recognised based on repetitiveness and force demands of work. The prevalence of hand-wrist tendon syndrome was 0·6% in low force and low repetition jobs and 10·8% in high force and high repetition jobs; no association with vibration, postures, or other work factors was detected. In the other cross-sectional study, the prevalence of the tendon syndrome was 56% among female food packers and 14% among female shop clerks.[101] Here, criteria for repetitiveness were based on cycles/work day and video recording of joint positions and movements and for force on weight of packages lifted. In the first study,[100] the adjusted odds ratio contrasting high force and high repetition jobs with low force and low repetition jobs was 31·7 (95% CI 2·6 to 386·9) and in the second,[101] an unadjusted odds ratio between the exposed and the reference group was 8·1 (4·3 to 15·3).[99] The unadjusted common odds ratio based on meta-analysis was 9·1 (4·9 to 16·2); although based on only a few studies, this suggests a causal connection between repetitive, forceful work and the development of tendon syndrome.

In the cohort study among employees in a meat-processing plant by Kurppa *et al.* the incidence rate ratio for visits to a doctor's office with tendon syndrome in manually strenuous jobs was 12·0 for men and 30·5 for women.[96] These estimates may overestimate risk because affected workers in strenuous jobs are more likely to seek medical advice than other workers.

Individual risk factors

Tendon syndrome occurs at all ages, predominantly in women: among industrial workers the job-adjusted odds ratio was 4·3 for women as compared with men.[100] There is little evidence of an effect of hormonal or other personal factors; tenosynovitis can, however, also be caused by some systemic diseases and bacterial infections.

Carpal tunnel syndrome

Carpal tunnel syndrome is thought to result from impingement of the median nerve in the carpal canal. Impingement may be the result of congenital or post-traumatic narrowness of the canal or the pressure may be increased by thickening of other structures or frequent deviation of the wrist. Typical symptoms include pain, tingling, and numbness in the sensory distribution of the nerve (I-IV fingers) which may waken the subject at night. In more severe cases, signs of motor dysfunction appear, such as thenar muscle atrophy and weakness. Traditionally the diagnosis of carpal tunnel syndrome has been based on the characteristic symptoms and simple clinical tests (Tinel's sign and Phalen's test). Recently the combination of typical symptoms together with signs of impairment of median nerve conduction in neurophysiological examination has been proposed as the gold standard for carpal tunnel syndrome.[102] [103] The specificity and sensitivity of simple clinical tests are low in reference to the gold standard and no general agreement on the criteria for diagnosis has been reached.[102] In one study, industrial workers with symptoms of carpal tunnel syndrome had poorer results than industrial workers without symptoms in the neurophysiological measurement of median nerve function, and the latter were poorer than those of non-industrial referents.[104] The significance of impairment of nerve function in subjects without symptoms is not known.

Occurrence

The prevalence of carpal tunnel syndrome has been investigated in the general population in the Netherlands, the diagnosis being based on typical symptoms and abnormality in median nerve conductivity at the wrist.[105] The prevalence of undetected carpal tunnel syndrome in women was 5·8% (95% CI 3·5 to 8·1%) in adults (25–74 years); a further 3·4% (1·5 to 5·3%) had the syndrome diagnosed earlier. The prevalence in adult men was 0·6% (0·02 to 3·4%). The influence of diagnostic criteria on prevalence estimates is depicted in table 10.8 based on data from a study of workers in ski manufacture by Barnhart *et al.*[106] Both prevalence rates and prevalence ratios between exposed and unexposed groups differed considerably, depending on the criteria. Comparisons between different studies must therefore be made with caution.

In a comprehensive review of work-related carpal tunnel syndrome Hagberg and coworkers describe 15 cross-sectional studies with 32 different occupational or exposure groups.[107] In all studies carpal tunnel syndrome was defined by both symptoms and clinical tests and the

Table 10.8 Prevalence and prevalence ratio (PR) for carpal tunnel syndrome in repetitive and non-repetitive jobs according to diagnostic criteria. (Adapted from Barnhart et al. 1991.)[106]

Criteria	Repetitive (%)	Non-repetitive (%)	PR (95% CI)
Hand pain	87	68	1·27 (1·05 to 1·55)
Paraesthesia	85	70	1·21 (1·00 to 1·46)
Nocturnal hand pain	67	46	1·47 (1·07 to 2·03)
One or more symptoms	97	83	1·17 (1·03 to 1·33)
One or more signs (Tinel, Phalen)	45	21	2·17 (1·30 to 3·61)
Electrophysiological criteria only	34	19	1·79 (1·01 to 3·20)
Electrophysiological criteria and signs	15	3	4·92 (1·17 to 20·7)
Electrophysiological criteria and signs or symptoms	33	18	1·79 (0·94 to 3·39)

prevalence ranged from 1% to 61%. The lowest rate, based on the simple clinical tests, was found for slaughterhouse workers (mean age 31·8 years) and the highest, based on electrodiagnosis only, for grinders in a steel mill (age not reported).

Work-related risk factors

In a review, Stock concluded that there is strong evidence for a causal relationship between repetitive forceful work and development of carpal tunnel syndrome,[99] a view not shared by all.[103 108] The most rigorous study was by Silverstein et al. who found a 15-fold increase among workers with high repetition and high force requirements as compared with those with low repetition and low force requirements.[109] This estimate was based on a small number of cases, but the results were supported by a study of fish-processing workers in China.[110]

Wrist flexion and extension, particularly in combination with a pinch grip have been reported to be associated with increased risk of the syndrome, postures in which the pressure in the carpal tunnel is increased.[111] The effect of vibration is difficult to distinguish from that of force and repetitiveness because these exposures often occur together. Ill fitting gloves and low temperatures have been suggested as risk factors, both of which add to force demands.[111]

According to Hagberg et al. at least 50%, and possibly as many as 90%, of all cases in exposed populations are attributable to physical load factors at work.[107] These estimates need to be considered cautiously because of variation in the diagnostic criteria and often poor validity of the studies.

Individual risk factors

Carpal tunnel syndrome is more common in women than in men. In one study, however, there was no sex difference between men and women in the same jobs.[109] Based on clinical series, carpal tunnel syndrome is related to congenital narrowness of the carpal tunnel, some diseases (including diabetes, gout, amyloidosis, carpal ganglion, and hypothyroidism), obesity, pregnancy, and menopause. In studies of workers the effect of the individual factors has proved small. Evidence for a connection between the use of contraceptive pills and carpal tunnel syndrome among women is contradictory.[109 110]

Epicondylitis

Symptoms of epicondylitis include pain in the region of the lateral or medial epicondyle of the humerus provoked by exertion of the wrist and fingers. The diagnosis is based on typical symptoms, local tenderness on palpation, and pain on resisted flexion or extension of the wrist and fingers. There is controversy about the pathogenesis of this disease but the

231

most common view is that there are tears at the insertions of the muscles.[112]

Occurrence

In a sample of the Swedish general population with an age range of 31 to 74 years, the prevalence of lateral epicondylitis was 1%–3% in both sexes. The highest prevalence was 10% in women aged 40 to 50 years.[113] In occupational studies the prevalence of epicondylitis has ranged from 0·8% to 9% in exposed groups and from 0·8% to 2% in referent groups.[98]

Work-related risk factors

Overexertion of the wrist and fingers or blunt trauma are considered to be the main causes of epicondylitis but there are few controlled studies of the relation to work.[112] Meat cutters can overstrain the extensor and flexor muscles of the wrist and fingers, especially when cutting frozen meat. In a cross-sectional study, an age-adjusted rate ratio of 6·4 (95% CI 0·99 to 40·9) was found when meat cutters were contrasted to construction foremen.[114] In another study of female packers with repetitive work and female shop assistants with non-repetitive work no difference was found.[101] In the latter study, epicondylitis always occurred together with some other soft tissue disorder of the neck, shoulder or upper limb.

Among workers in engineering the prevalence of lateral epicondylitis was 7·4%.[115] Epicondylitis was not related to job category based on elbow stress but blue-collar workers tended to claim work as the cause for the affliction whereas white-collar workers claimed leisure activities, such as house repairs and gardening. Nearly all the symptoms were in the dominant arm.

In a longitudinal study in a meat-processing factory, the prevalence of epicondylitis was assessed clinically in three repeated cross-sectional surveys[116] and the incidence estimated in a 31-month follow-up.[96] The subjects represented both strenuous manual jobs (meat cutters, sausage makers, and packers) and non-strenuous jobs (supervisors, maintenance men, office workers). The prevalence of epicondylitis was 0·8% among workers in both categories, which does not suggest that strenuous manual tasks played a major part but the result may be biased by worker selection. In the follow up, people with epicondylitis being defined as those who had sought medical advice, the annual incidence was 1% in employees in non-strenuous jobs, 11·3% in female sausage makers, 7·0% in female packers, and 6·4% in male meat cutters. The authors' explanation for the discrepancy between prevalence and incidence was that workers in strenuous jobs were more troubled by their complaint and more prone to seek medical advice.

In a cross-sectional study of workers in a fish-processing industry, jobs were classified for their repetitiveness and forcefulness by observation.

Epicondylitis was not work-related but among workers with less than 12 months experience in their job, none in low repetitive and low force jobs had epicondylitis whereas the prevalence was 33% among those in high repetitive and high force jobs.[110]

Individual risk factors

Epicondylitis rarely occurs in people younger than 30 years. No clear evidence is available on the impact of other individual factors on the occurrence of the disease.

Summary

Evidence that repetitive forceful manual work is associated with an increased risk of hand-wrist tendon syndromes and carpal tunnel syndrome is quite consistent, but the relation of epicondylitis to work demands is in dispute. Tendon syndromes and epicondylitis are easy to diagnose in aetiological studies but controversy prevails about diagnostic criteria for carpal tunnel syndrome. Electrophysiological testing is recommended as the gold standard but as an invasive test its suitability to large population studies is doubtful. In addition to these well-defined disorders other pain syndromes or "repetitive strain injuries" of the upper limb are common in manually strenuous tasks. Without proper definition of these syndromes epidemiological research is difficult.

Accurate assessment of work-related exposure is a problem in upper limb disorders. Activity deviating from an acceptable range has to be defined and measured. Current knowledge of the correlation between work demands and upper limb disorders is only qualitative and little is known of exposure-effect connections, and so far no attention has been paid to induction or latency times. It seems possible that the induction time for tendon syndromes may be short (days or weeks), making assessment of exposure less demanding, whereas for carpal tunnel syndrome and epicondylitis the induction time may be longer. Discovery of the appropriate induction times for each disease is an important challenge for future research. With few exceptions, studies on upper limb disorders have been cross-sectional. Well-designed prospective and case-referent studies with rigorous exposure assessment are clearly needed.

1 Social Insurance Institution. *Statistical yearbook of the Social Insurance Institution.* Helsinki: SII; T1: **28**: 1993.
2 Spitzer WO, Leblanc FE, Dupuis M, *et al.* Scientific approach to the assessment and management of activity-related spinal disorders. A monograph for clinicians. Report of the Quebec Task Force on Spinal Disorders. *Spine* 1987; **12(7S)**.
3 Andersson GBJ, Pope MH, Frymoyer JF. Epidemiology. In: Pope MH, Frymoyer JF, Andersson G, eds. *Occupational low back pain.* New York: Praeger, 1984: 101–14.

4 Deyo RA, Tsui-Wu Y-J. Descriptive epidemiology of low-back pain and its related medical care in the United States. *Spine* 1987; **12**: 264–8.

5 Lawrence JS. Disc degeneration. Its frequency and relationship to symptoms. *Ann Rheum Dis* 1969; **28**: 121–38.

6 Powell MC, Wilson M, Szypryt P, Symonds EM, Worthington BS. Prevalence of lumbar disc degeneration observed by magnetic resonance in symptomless women. *Lancet* 1986; **i**: 1366–7.

7 Leino P, Berg M-A, Puska P. Is back pain increasing? Results from National surveys in Finland during 1978/9–1992. *Scand J Rheumatol* 1994; **23**: 269–76.

8 Heliövaara M, Mäkelä M, Sievers K. Tuki-ja liikuntaelinten sairaudet Suomessa. [*Musculoskeletal diseases in Finland*]. Helsinki: 1993; Publication of the Social Insurance Institution AL:35.

9 Frank A. Low back pain. *BMJ* 1993; **306**: 901–9.

10 Kelsey JL, Golden AL, Mundt DJ. Low back pain/prolapsed intervertebral disc. *Rheum Dis Clin North Am* 1990; **16**: 699–716.

11 Skovron ML. Epidemiology of low back pain. *Baillière's Clin Rheumatol* 1992; **6**: 559–73.

12 Garg A, Moore JS. Epidemiology of low-back pain in industry. *State of the Art Reviews in Occupational Medicine* 1992; **7**: 593–609.

13 Riihimäki H. Low-back pain, its origin and risk indicators. *Scand J Work Environ Health* 1991; **17**: 81–90.

14 Kelsey JL. An epidemiological study of the relationship between occupations and herniated lumbar intervertebral discs. *Int J Epidemiol* 1975; **4**: 197–205.

15 Heliövaara M. Occupation and risk of herniated lumbar intervertebral disc or sciatica leading to hospitalization. *J Chronic Dis* 1987; **40**: 259–64.

16 Heliövaara M, Mäkelä M, Knekt P, Impivaara O, Aromaa A. Determinants of sciatica and low-back pain. *Spine* 1991; **16**: 608–14.

17 Chaffin DB, Park KS. A longitudinal study of low-back pain as associated with occupational weight lifting factors. *Am Ind Hyg Assoc J* 1973; **34**: 513–25.

18 Punnett L, Fine LJ, Keyserling WM. Back disorders and non-neutral trunk positions of automobile assembly workers. *Scand J Work Environ Health* 1991; **17**: 337–46.

19 Frymoyer JW, Pope MH, Clements JH, Wilder DG, MacPherson B, Ashikaga T. Risk factors in low-back pain: An epidemiological survey. *J Bone Joint Surg Am* 1983; **65**: 213–8.

20 Kelsey JL, Githens PB, White AA III, Holford TR, Walter SD, O'Connor T. An epidemiological study of lifting and twisting on the job and risk for acute prolapsed intervertebral disc. *J Orthop Res* 1984; **2**: 61–6.

21 Mundt DJ, Kelsey JL, Golden AL, Pastides H, Berg AT, Sklar J. An epidemiological study of non-occupational lifting as a risk factor for herniated lumbar intervertebral disc. *Spine* 1993; **18**: 595–602.

22 National Institute for Occupational Safety and Health (NIOSH): *Work practices guide for manual lifting*. Cincinnati: Department of Health and Human Services, NIOSH 1981: Technical report no. 81–122.

23 Marras WS. Toward an understanding of dynamic variables in ergonomics. *State of the Art Reviews in Occupational Medicine* 1992; **7**: 655–77.

24 Burdorf A, Govaert G, Elders L. Postural load and back pain of workers in the manufacturing of prefabricated concrete elements. *Ergonomics* 1991; **34**: 909–18.

25 Burdorf A. Exposure assessment of risk factors for disorders of the back in occupational epidemiology. *Scand J Work Environ Health* 1992; **18**: 1–9.

26 Burdorf A. Sources of variance in exposure to postural load on the back in occupational groups. *Scand J Work Environ Health* 1992; **18**: 361–7.

27 Burdorf A. Bias in risk estimates from variability of exposure to postural load on the back in occupational groups. *Scand J Work Environ Health* 1993; **19**: 50–4.

28 Bongers PM, Boshuizen HC, Hulshof CTJ, Koemeester AP. Back disorders in crane operators exposed to whole-body vibration. *Int Arch Occup Environ Health* 1988; **60**: 129–37.

29 Boshuizen HC, Bongers PM, Hulshof CT. Self-reported back pain in tractor drivers exposed to whole-body vibration. *Int Arch Occup Environ Health* 1990; **62**: 109–15.

30 Bongers PM, Hulshof CTJ, Dijkstra L, Boshuizen HC, Groenhout HJM, Valken E.

Back pain and exposure to whole body vibration in helicopter pilots. *Ergonomics* 1990; **33**: 1007–26.

31 Pietri F, Leclerc A, Boitel L, Chastang J-F, Morcet J-F, Blondet M. Low-back pain in commercial travellers. *Scand J Work Environ Health* 1992; **18**: 52–8.

32 Kelsey JL, Hardy RJ. Driving of motor vehicles as a risk factor for acute herniated lumbar intervertebral disc. *Am J Epidemiol* 1975; **1**: 63–73.

33 Kelsey JL, Githens PB, O'Connor T, Weil U, Calogero JA, Holford TR. Acute prolapsed lumbar intervertebral disc. An epidemiologic study with special reference to driving automobiles and cigarette smoking. *Spine* 1984; **9**: 608–13.

34 Holm SH. Nutrition of the intervertebral disc. In: Weinstein JN, Wiesel SW, eds. *The Lumbar Spine*. Philadelphia: W. B. Saunders, 1990: 244–60.

35 Andersson GBJ, Chaffin DB, Pope MH. Occupational biomechanics of the lumbar spine. In: Pope MH, Frymoyer JW, Andersson G, eds. *Occupational low back pain*. New York: Preager, 1984: 39–70.

36 Holmström EB, Lindell J, Moritz U. Low back and neck/shoulder pain in construction workers; occupational work load and psychosocial risk factors. Part 1: relationship to low back pain. *Spine* 1992; **17**: 663–71.

37 Riihimäki H. Back pain and heavy physical work: a comparative study of concrete reinforcement workers and maintenance house painters. *Br J Ind Med* 1985; **42**: 226–32.

38 Riihimäki H, Tola S, Videman T, Hänninen K. Low-back pain and occupation. A cross-sectional questionnaire study of men in machine operating, dynamic physical work, and sedentary work. *Spine* 1989; **14**: 204–9.

39 Bongers PM, deWinter CR, Kompier MAJ, Hildebrandt VH. Psychosocial factors at work and musculoskeletal disease. *Scand J Work Environ Health* 1993; **19**: 297–312.

40 Åstrand N-E, Isacsson S-O. Back pain, back abnormalities, and competing medical, psychological, and social factors as predictors of sick leave, early retirement, unemployment, labour turnover and mortality: a 22 year follow up of male employees in a Swedish pulp and paper company. *Br J Ind Med* 1988; **45**: 387–95.

41 Bigos SJ, Battié MC, Spengler DM, Fisher LD, Fordyce WE, Hansson TH. A prospective study of work perceptions and psychosocial factors affecting the report of back injury. *Spine* 1991; **16**: 1–6.

42 Deyo RA, Bass JE. Lifestyle and low-back pain: The influence of smoking and obesity. *Spine* 1989; **14**: 501–6.

43 Aro S, Leino P. Overweight and musculoskeletal morbidity: a ten-year follow-up. *Int J Obes* 1985; **9**: 267–75.

44 Heliövaara M. Body height, obesity, and risk of herniated lumbar intervertebral disc. *Spine* 1987; **12**: 469–72.

45 Gyntelberg F. One year incidence of low back pain among male residents of Copenhagen aged 40–59. *Danish Medical Bulletin* 1974; **1**: 30–6.

46 Biering-Sorensen F. Physical measurements as risk indicators for low-back trouble over a one-year period. *Spine* 1984; **9**: 106–19.

47 Cady LD, Bishoff PD, O'Connell ER, Thomas PC, Allan JH. Strength and fitness and subsequent back injuries in fire fighters. *J Occup Med* 1979; **4**: 269–72.

48 Leino P, Aro S, Hasan J. Trunk muscle function and low back disorders: A ten-year follow-up study. *J Chronic Dis* 1987; **4**: 289–96.

49 Battié MC, Bigos SJ, Fisher LD, Hansson TH, Nachemson AL, Spengler DM. A prospective study of the role of cardiovascular risk factors and fitness in industrial back pain complaints. *Spine* 1989; **14**: 141–7.

50 Battié MC, Bigos SJ, Fisher LD, Hansson TH, Jones ME, Wortley MD. Isometric lifting strength as predictor of industrial back pain reports. *Spine* 1989; **14**: 851–6.

51 Boshuizen HC, Verbeek JHAM, Broersen JPJ, Weel ANH. Do smokers get more back pain? *Spine* 1993; **18**: 35–40.

52 Frymoyer JW, Pope MH, Costanza MC, Rosen JC, Wilder DG. Epidemiologic studies of low-back pain. *Spine* 1980; **5**: 419–23.

53 Battié MC, Videman T, Gill K, *et al.* Smoking and lumbar intervertebral disc degeneration: an MRI study of identical twins. *Spine* 1991; **16**: 1015–21.

54 Riihimäki H, Wickström G, Hänninen K, Luopajärvi T. Predictors of sciatic pain among

concrete reinforcement workers and house painters—a five-year follow-up. *Scand J Work Environ Health* 1989; **15**: 415–23.

55 Leino P, Magni G. Depressive and distress symptoms as predictors of low back pain, neck shoulder pain, and other musculoskeletal morbidity: a 10-year follow-up of metal industry employees. *Pain* 1993; **53**: 89–94.

56 Heliövaara M, Knekt P, Aromaa A. Incidence and risk factors of herniated lumbar intervertebral disc or sciatica leading to hospitalization. *J Chronic Dis* 1987; **40**: 251–8.

57 Viikari-Juntura E, Vuori J, Silverstein B, Kalimo R, Kuosma E, Videman T. A life-long prospective study on the role of psychosocial factors in neck-shoulder and low-back pain. *Spine* 1991; **16**: 1056–61.

58 Kellgren JH, Lawrence JS. Radiological assessment of osteo–arthrosis. *Ann Rheum Dis* 1957; **16**: 494–501.

59 Felson DT. Epidemiology of hip and knee osteoarthritis. *Epidemiol Rev* 1988; **10**: 1–28.

60 Kellgren JH, Lawrence JS. Osteo-arthrosis and disk degeneration in an urban population. *Ann Rheum Dis* 1958; **17**: 388–97.

61 Tepper S, Hochberg MC. Factors associated with hip osteoarthritis: Data from the First National Health and Nutrition Examination Survey (NHANES-I). *Am J Epidemiol* 1993; **137**: 1081–8.

62 Lawrence JS, Bremner JM, Bier F. Osteo-arthrosis. Prevalence in the population and relationship between symptoms and X-ray changes. *Ann Rheum Dis* 1966; **25**: 1–23.

63 Anderson JJ, Felson DT. Factors associated with osteoarthritis of the knee in the first national health and nutrition examination survey (HANES I). Evidence for an association with overweight, race, and physical demands of work. *Am J Epidemiol* 1988; **128**: 179–89.

64 Coggon D, Croft P, Cruddas M, Cooper C. Osteoarthritis of the hip in farmers. Book of abstracts. *9th International Symposium Epidemiology in Occupational Health.* Cincinnati Ohio 23–25 September 1992: 199.

65 Axmacher B, Lindberg H. Coxarthrosis in farmers. *Clin Orthop* 1993; **287**: 82–6.

66 Vingård E, Alfredsson L, Goldie I, Hogstedt C. Occupation and osteoarthrosis of the hip and knee: a register-based cohort study. *Int J Epidemiol* 1991; **20**: 1025–31.

67 Thelin A. Hip joint arthrosis: an occupational disorder among farmers. *Am J Ind Med* 1990; **18**: 339–43.

68 Croft P, Cooper C, Wickham C, Coggon D. Osteoarthritis of the hip and occupational activity. *Scand J Work Environ Health* 1992; **18**: 59–63.

69 Lindberg H, Danielsson L. The relation between labor and coxarthrosis. *Clin Orthop* 1984; **191**: 159–61.

70 Andersson S, Nilsson B, Hessel T, *et al.* Degenerative joint disease in ballet dancers. *Clin Orthop* 1989; **238**: 233–6.

71 Vingård E, Alfredsson L, Fellenius E, Goldie I, Hogstedt C, Köster M. Coxarthrosis and physical load from occupation. *Scand J Work Environ Health* 1991; **17**: 104–9.

72 Vingård E. *Work, sports, overweight and osteoarthrosis of the hip. Epidemiological studies.* Solna Sweden, Arbetsmiljöinstitutet. Arbete och hälsa 1991; 25 (doctoral thesis).

73 Heliövaara M, Mäkelä M, Impivaara O, Knekt P, Aromaa A, Sievers K. Association of overweight, trauma and work load with coxarthrosis. A health survey in 7217 persons. *Acta Orthop Scand* 1993; **64**: 613–8.

74 Vingård E. Overweight predisposes to coxarthrosis. Body mass index studied in 239 males with hip arthroplasty. *Acta Orthop Scand* 1991; **62**: 106–9.

75 Kujala UM, Kaprio J, Sarna S. Osteoarthritis of weight bearing joints of lower limbs in former élite male athletes. *BMJ* 1994; **308**: 231–4.

76 Vingård E, Alfredsson L, Goldie I, Hogstedt C. Sports and osteoarthrosis of the hip. *Am J Sports Med* 1993; **21**: 195–200.

77 Kellgren JH, Lawrence JS. Rheumatism in miners. Part II: X-ray study. *Br J Ind Med* 1952; **9**: 197–207.

78 Lawrence JS. Rheumatism in coal miners. Part III: Occupational factors. *Br J Ind Med* 1955; **12**: 249–51.

79 Partridge REH, Duthie JJR. Rheumatism in dockers and civil servants: a comparison of heavy manual and sedentary workers. *Ann Rheum Dis* 1968; **27**: 559–68.

80 Lindberg H, Montgomery F. Heavy labour and the occurrence of gonarthosis. *Clin Orthop* 1987; **214**: 235–6.
81 Kivimäki J, Riihimäki H, Hänninen K. Knee disorders in carpet and floor layers and painters. *Scand J Work Environ Health* 1992; **18**: 310–6.
82 Lawrence JS, Moyneux MK, Dingwall-Fordyce I. Rheumatism in foundry workers. *Br J Ind Med* 1966; **23**: 42–52.
83 Wickström G, Hänninen K, Mattsson T, Niskanen T, Riihimäki H, Waris P. Knee degeneration in concrete reinforcement workers. *Br J Ind Med* 1983; **40**: 216–9.
84 Sairanen E, Brushaber L, Kaskinen M. Felling work, low-back pain and osteoarthritis. *Scand J Work Environ Health* 1981; **7**: 18–30.
85 Felson DT, Hannan MT, Naimark A, Berkeley J, Gordon G, Wilson PW, Anderson J. Occupational physical demands, knee bending, and knee osteoarthritis: results from the Framingham Study. *J Rheumatol* 1991; **18**: 1587–92.
86 Kohatsu ND, Schurman DJ. Risk factors for the development of osteoarthritis of the knee. *Clin Orthop Rel Res* 1990; **261**: 242–6.
87 Davis MA, Ettinger WH, Neuhaus JM, Cho SA, Hauck WW. The association of knee injury and obesity with unilateral and bilateral osteoarthritis of the knee. *Am J Epidemiol* 1989; **130**: 278–88.
88 Felson DT, Anderson JJ, Naimark A, Walker AM, Meenan RF. Obesity and knee osteoarthritis: The Framingham Study. *Ann Intern Med* 1988; **109**: 18–24.
89 Felson DT, Zhang Y, Anthony JM, Naimark A, Anderson JJ. Weight loss reduces the risk for symptomatic knee osteoarthritis in women. *Ann Intern Med* 1992; **116**: 535–9.
90 Felson DT. The epidemiology of knee osteoarthritis: results from the Framingham Osteoarthritis Study. *Semin Arthritis Rheum* 1990; **20(Suppl 1)**; 42–50.
91 Hadler N. The roles of work and of working in disorders of the upper extremity. *Baillière's Clin Rheumatol* 1989; **3**: 121–41.
92 Miller MH, Topliss DJ. Chronic upper limb pain syndrome (repetitive strain injury) in the Australian workforce: a systematic cross sectional rheumatologic study of 229 patients. *J Rheumatol* 1988; **15**: 1705–12.
93 Barton N. Repetitive strain disorders. Often misdiagnosed and often not work related. *BMJ* 1989; **299**: 405–6.
94 Kurppa K, Waris P, Rokkanen P. Peritendinitis and tenosynovitis. *Scand J Work Environ Health* 1979; **5(Suppl 3)**: 19–24.
95 Thompson AR, Plewes LW, Shaw EG. Peritendinitis crepitans and simple tenosynovitis: a clinical study of 544 cases in industry. *Br J Ind Med* 1951; **8**: 150–60.
96 Kurppa K, Viikari-Juntura E, Kuosma E, Huuskonen M, Kivi P. Incidence of tenosynovitis or peritendinitis and epicondylitis in a meat-processing factory. *Scand J Work Environ Health* 1991; **17**: 32–7.
97 Armstrong TJ, Silverstein BA. Upper-extremity pain in the workplace—role of usage in causality. In Hadler N, ed. *Clinical concepts in regional musculoskeletal illness*. Orlando: Grune & Stratton 1987: 333–54.
98 Armstrong TJ, Buckle P, Fine LJ, Hagberg M, Jonsson B, Kilbom Å, et al. A conceptual model for work-related neck and upper-limb musculoskeletal disorders. *Scand J Work Environ Health* 1993; **19**: 73–84.
99 Stock S. Workplace ergonomic factors and the development of musculoskeletal disorders of the neck and upper limbs: A meta-analysis. *Am J Ind Med* 1991; **19**: 87–107.
100 Silverstein BA, Fine LJ, Armstrong TJ. Hand wrist cumulative trauma disorders in industry. *Br J Ind Med* 1986; **43**: 779–84.
101 Luopajärvi T, Kuorinka I, Virolainen M, Holmberg M. Prevalence of tenosynovitis and other injuries of the upper extremities in repetitive work. *Scand J Work Environ Health* 1979; **5 (Suppl 3)**: 48–55.
102 de Krom MCTFM, Knipschild PG, Kester ADM, Spaans F. Efficacy of provocative tests for diagnosis of carpal tunnel syndrome. *Lancet* 1990; **335**: 393–5.
103 Gerr F, Letz R, Landrigan PJ. Upper-extremity musculoskeletal disorders of occupational origin. *Annual Review of Public Health* 1991; **12**: 543–66.
104 Stetson DS, Silverstein BA, Keyserling WM, Wolfe PA, Albers JW. Median sensory distal amplitude and latency: Comparisons between nonexposed managerial/professional employees and industrial workers. *Am J Ind Med* 1993; **24**: 175–89.

237

105 de Krom MCTFM, Knipschild PG, Kester ADM, Thijs CT, Boekkooi PF, Spaans F. Carpal tunnel syndrome: Prevalence in the general population. *J Clin Epidemiol* 1992; 45: 373–6.

106 Barnhart S, Demers PA, Miller M, Longstreth WT Jr., Rosenstock L. Carpal tunnel syndrome among ski manufacturing workers. *Scand J Work Environ Health* 1991; 17: 46–52.

107 Hagberg M, Morgenstern H, Kelsh M. Impact of occupations and job tasks on the prevalence of carpal tunnel syndrome. *Scand J Work Environ Health* 1992; 18: 337–45.

108 Moore ST. Carpal tunnel syndrome. *Occupational Medicine: State of the Art Reviews* 1992; 7: 741–62.

109 Silverstein BA, Fine LJ, Armstrong TJ. Occupational factors and carpal tunnel syndrome. *Am J Ind Med* 1987; 11: 343–58.

110 Chiang H-C, Ko Y-C, Chen S-S, Yu H-S, Wu T-N, Chang P-Y. Prevalence of shoulder and upper-limb disorders among workers in the fish-processing industry. *Scand J Work Environ Health* 1993; 19: 126–31.

111 Silverstein BA, Fine LJ, Armstrong TJ. Carpal tunnel syndrome: causes and a preventive strategy. *Seminars in Occupational Medicine* 1986; 1: 213–21.

112 Kurppa K, Waris P, Rokkanen P. Lateral elbow pain syndrome. *Scand J Work Environ Health* 1979; 5 **(Suppl 3)**: 15–8.

113 Allander E. Prevalence, incidence and remission rates of some common rheumatic diseases and syndromes. *Scand J Rheumatol* 1974; 3: 145–53.

114 Roto P, Kivi P. Prevalence of epicondylitis and tenosynovitis among meat cutters. *Scand J Work Environ Health* 1984; 10: 203–5.

115 Dimberg L. The prevalence and causation of tennis elbow (lateral humeral epicondylitis) in a population of workers in an engineering industry. *Ergonomics* 1987; 30: 573–80.

116 Viikari-Juntura E, Kurppa K, Kuosma E, Huuskonen M, Kuorinka I, Ketola R. Prevalence of epicondylitis and elbow pain in the meat-processing industry. *Scand J Work Environ Health* 1991; 17: 38–45.

11 Work stress

STANISLAV KASL, BENJAMIN AMICK

Introduction

In this chapter we intend to use the perspective of occupational epidemiology to examine the evidence that links stress at work to a variety of outcomes, including specific diseases, biological risk factors, indicators of mental health and well being, and lifestyle factors. The evidence is considerable and many of the issues are complex. Accordingly, our primary aim is to provide the reader with a conceptual and methodological framework and with guidelines for organising and evaluating the vast research literature. Our secondary aim is to offer a selected review of the evidence, so that the reader may become familiar with some of the findings, as well as understand in more concrete terms the conceptual and methodological issues.

This chapter is somewhat of an anomaly in this volume: (1) it encompasses a variety of both work dimensions and health outcomes, rather than focusing on a particular exposure or a particular disease; (2) it concerns itself with specific methodological issues that are concrete applications of the points raised more generically in the methodology chapters; and (3) it offers a fairly heavy dose of the behavioural and social sciences where they impinge on medicine and epidemiology.

It is important for readers to appreciate from the outset the difference in issues and problems faced by investigators who are concerned with work stress and health (and by ourselves in summarising the evidence), compared with questions that fall within the traditional boundaries of occupational health and deal with work-related injuries and diseases. We offer two illustrations.

Payoff from traditional designs

The bread and butter paradigm in occupational epidemiology is the detection of disease differences by occupations or job titles and then tracing them to exposure to some environmental agent or hazard. This approach is generally too simple for strategies linking psychosocial aspects of the work environment to health and well-being. Consider the following contrast: angiosarcoma of the liver is so rare that just three or four cases were enough to alert health officials and start a search for agents.[1] The disease and its natural history are such that many problems are minimal: (a) differential diagnosis, pinning down its occupational origin; (b) relatively short latency between exposure and diagnosis or death; (c) absence of multiple risk factors; (d) lack of effective treatment, making it easier to track cases in retrospective cohort designs. Moreover, the search for agents produced quick convergence on polyvinyl chloride as the probable cause. Corroboration came in quickly from many manufacturing locations around the world. Finally—and this is something not available to investigators examining work stress and health—short term laboratory studies on animals provided confirmatory evidence. In short, a tight little package and a scientific success story.

Contrast this with the results obtained when the occupational epidemiology paradigm is applied to psychosocial aspects of work and psychological disorders. In a study entitled: "Job stress and psychiatric illness in the U.S. Navy",[2] the authors identified through case files all Navy men admitted to hospital with a psychiatric diagnosis in the years 1966–1968, and then calculated rates of first (in the Navy) admissions by occupation. Jobs that had high and low rates were designated as high and low risk jobs, but independent assessments of severity of working conditions failed to show any association with this classification. Job satisfaction data on a separate sample produced ambiguous results, showing both more boredom and more overall job satisfaction in the high risk jobs. In general, the jobs with higher rates tended to be more routine and those with lower rates, more technical. Data on individual characteristics showed that men in high risk jobs were older, of lower education, of lower social class of origin, more likely to be divorced or single, and so on. As these are all characteristics the men brought with them to the jobs, and as these characteristics have been found in innumerable studies to be associated with higher rates of treated (and untreated) mental illness, the conclusion is compelling that this approach failed to reveal anything about job stresses—in fact it failed to be a study of job stress at all.

Strategy of sentinel health events

It was suggested by Rutsein *et al.* that to develop a list of Sentinel Health Events is a useful strategy in occupational health.[3] Such events represent a disease, disability, or untimely death that is related to occupation and the occurrence of which signals the need for epidemiological or industrial hygiene studies and preventive intervention. The list of occupational diseases proposed by the authors included predominantly conditions that are not intrinsically occupational, for example, malignant neoplasm of the bladder; rather, such conditions are recognised to be occupational as a result of investigation in which the industry or occupation and the agent need to be considered. Such a reconstruction of aetiology is relatively easy, say, for injuries on the job, or some skin disease, but is next to impossible for outcomes with complex aetiologies, such as clinical depression or coronary heart disease. We simply do not have a way of taking the paradigm for occupational bladder cancer and applying it to "occupational depression" or "occupational low self-esteem." The issue cannot be refined through measurement approaches, as this raises the danger that in attempting to measure, say "occupational depression," we would be asking the respondent not only to describe symptoms, but also to provide causal attribution or explanation for such symptoms. This is highly suspect; and to try to ask about symptoms only at work is also an unwarranted strategy.

Work stress as a hazardous exposure

Two assertions need to be valid to proceed with this chapter: first, that work stress represents a distinct and definable set of work dimensions or exposures (specifically, what work stress is and is not); secondly, that these dimensions can be measured satisfactorily with reasonable consensus among investigators. In actuality, neither of these assertions can be justified. We therefore proceed by abandoning the concept of stress as a scientific concept and retain it as a lay term, which denotes an approximate area of research interest and which carries with it a certain broad, intuitive "theory." However, a brief discussion of why the concept of stress is troublesome is still useful, as other more specific concepts that can be substituted run into some of the same difficulties.

If we attempt to identify work stress by a process of exclusion, we would suggest that work hazards that are physical, chemical, or biological are outside the domain of work stress. Stated somewhat differently, we could propose that stress is not involved when these hazards cause disease and that psychosocial variables do not affect the underlying biomedical-aetiological process. However, it should be apparent that a precise definition by exclusion is not possible as it may not be clear how narrowly we can define a hazardous but non-stressful exposure. For example: (a) industrial noise can be seen both as a physical and a psychological stimulus;[4-6] (b) ergonomic issues are not easily separated into physical and psychological;[7 8] (c) exposure to carcinogens and toxic materials may have a psychological impact, depending upon information and awareness;[9 10] (d) symptom checklists pose particular difficulties for separating physical and psychological disorders, for example, the increased reporting of eye strain among female office workers who use video display terminals (VDT).[11]

If we attempt to define work stress directly, and not by exclusion, we run into the well-documented problem that agreement has not been reached on the unique defining characteristics of environmental conditions thought of as "stressors" in the workplace.[12-15] Various authors have proposed different lists of work dimensions, which they have nominated for inclusion, but the underlying criteria are either not spelt out or they are not the same for different authors. At best one can derive an approximate definition of environmental stress: excess demand on a person's resources to cope with the demands. Incidentally, this definition by itself does not rule out purely physical or biological stressors.

It should be realised that our attempts to identify work stress by the process of exclusion are limited to excluding hazards that are physical, chemical, or biological. There is additional difficulty in separating work stress from other psychosocial influences. This leaves open the question whether or not all psychosocial hazards in the work place can be subsumed under the concept of work stress. Given the difficulty noted in the previous paragraph, we can see that deciding on whether or not a particular work is stressful will not carry wide consensus. Our solution in this chapter is to examine a number of dimensions widely investigated and ask for each: does exposure have negative health consequences? If it does, we would not object to that exposure being called a work stressor. However, since this presents circular reasoning—if it has adverse consequences, it is a stressor, and if it doesn't, it isn't—we must acknowledge that we have thereby rendered meaningless the broad question: "Does work stress affect health?" Hence our retreat from stress as a scientific construct to stress as a lay term and useful label only.

Conceptual dilemmas and methodological difficulties

As the work stress research domain is part of the more general stress and health literature, it is worth noting that some of the conceptual and terminological confusion and disagreement characterising the stress field in general also applies to occupational stress. Above all, it is important to realise that the term stress is used in several fundamentally different ways:

- Stress is an environmental condition, susceptible to an objective definition and measurement. The term "stressor" is often used in this context. Clearly, this meaning of stress is closely aligned with general occupational epidemiology.
- Stress is a subjective perception or appraisal of an objective environmental condition. This definition embraces the notion that stress is subjective and reflects a psychological tradition.
- Stress is a particular response or reaction. Included here would be a variety of proximal and distal outcomes, including dysphoric mood, psychophysiological symptoms of tension, biological variables such as neuroendocrine levels, as well as incidence of specific disease states.
- Stress is a particular relational term linking environmental character-istics and personal characteristics, in particular, the excess of environmental demand beyond the person's capacity. The theoretical formulation known as the "Person-Environment Fit" is an example of this relational approach to concepts.[16]
- Stress is a process that includes other important components such as appraisal, coping, and re-appraisal, and cannot be reduced to any simple stimulus-response or cause-effect formulation.

This multiplicity of meanings entails various difficulties, some of which are resolved more easily than others. For example, there is ample reason for rejecting stress as a response: the emphasis in occupational epidemiology is on identifying harmful exposures, that is to say, the focus is on the stimulus side of the stimulus-response equation. Moreover, there are no unique stress reactions or stress diseases (such as elevated cortisol levels or ulcers) that would automatically denote the presence of a stressor. Stress as a relational term may also be seen as an unwise departure from the scientific strategy that even complex processes are best studied as an interplay of "simple" (unidimensional) variables. The creation of complex study variables is likely to represent premature closure on a problem and will make it difficult to isolate crucial processes, such as might be needed for designing effective interventions. At the same time, the relational use of stress is a justified reminder that it is rarely proper to study exposure to a work stressor without simultaneously considering selected characteristics of the person exposed.

A much more difficult issue to resolve centres on the alternatives posed by the first as against the second use of the term stress. For example, if the impact of an objective hazard is completely mediated by a person's subjective perceptions and reactions, then the second definition becomes much more appropriate than the first. If, on the other hand, the primary pathway of causation is from objective exposure to disease outcome and the subjective perceptions are more or less irrelevant epiphenomena, then the objective measurement of exposure must be our focus. This is a dilemma that is likely to be resolved differently, depending upon the particular dimension of interest. For example, it is likely that the impact of machine-paced repetitive work can be studied reasonably well without subjective perceptions,[17][18] while the impact of lack of control over job decision-making may work primarily through subjective perceptions.[19]

The choice between an objective and a subjective approach to the assessment of work stressors is not just linked to theoretical considerations or some preliminary evidence about a particular stressor. There are also many difficult methodological and practical issues which bear on this choice, and which are altered, depending on research design (prospective or cross-sectional) and the outcome of interest (depression or serum cholesterol).[15][20] Below is a skeletal presentation of some of the important concerns and issues.

The most serious concern about subjective measures of exposure centres on the confounding or contamination that may affect the measurement of both the exposure and the outcome variables and create spurious or spuriously high associations:

- *Overlap in content.* Exposure may be measured by asking "How often are you bothered by . . ." (for example, ignorance of supervisor's expectations, as a reflection of role ambiguity) and outcome may be measured by asking "How often are you bothered by . . ." (for example, headache, as an indication of distress-tension).
- *Influence of a personal trait*: people who are highly neurotic, for example, may evaluate their work environment negatively and may also experience symptoms of distress or dysphoria. This would create a spurious association even if the two measures were independent in actual content.
- *Influence of a shared response.* Stable response tendencies (particularly to complain to or give socially desirable replies) may influence both the measure of subjective exposure and of some outcome indicators of mental health or well-being.

When the outcome of interest is measured by procedures that are separate and distinct from self-reports that are the basis for assessing the hazard, then confounding in measurement is not an issue. For example, serological data or electrocardiographic findings are completely distinct from any subjective self report. However, reverse causation still may be a serious concern: in a cross-sectional or retrospective design, the presence of a disease of the heart for example may influence perceptions of work, such as how demanding the job is. This could be a true effect, in the sense that for the ill, demands of the job are objectively more challenging, or it could represent an impact of illness on perceptions alone, in the sense that judging the job as excessively demanding becomes part of an explanation of the origins of the respondent's state of health. In any case, objective measurement of work hazard would not reveal any association. In short, distinct measurement procedures, separating the independent and the dependent variables, do not protect against reverse causation, or ambiguity of direction of effects. What does protect is either a prospective study design or a "silent" dependent variable. The latter means that the variable, such as some biochemical ratio, has no side effects and that the respondent is unaware of his or her level.

Strong study designs are helpful but do not eliminate all problems. Thus in a fully prospective study of coronary heart disease, which includes baseline data on cardiovascular risk factors, a particular subjective perception of work conditions ("my job is hectic") may relate to the incidence of coronary heart disease, and it does so independently of cardiovascular risk factors. Because of the design and distinct measurement procedures, there is a strong basis for inferring that such a perception is an independent risk factor for coronary heart disease. However, we still need to know what kind of a variable it is, how strongly is it determined by specific objectively assessed work conditions, and what characteristics of the individual and his or her social environment (ranging from cardiovascular fitness and lifestyle habits to neuroticism and spousal social support) also influence it. From an occupational health perspective, we want to understand the potential for intervention—above all, what specific modifications of the work setting or the work-person interface, would be beneficial.

This discussion leads to the conclusion that the objective assessment of work stressors is a necessary starting point for work stress and health studies. A complete substitution of subjective exposure data for objective information, however minimal (job titles for example), is unlikely to be a useful strategy. At the same time, subjective perceptions and related processes, have an important part to play. This role is best seen by analogy to that of molecular and other biomarkers, in general epidemiological research.[21] [22] They can help with the measurement of internal exposure, including the "psychologically effective" dose, they can identify an early state of response to the exposure, and they can identify individual susceptibilities and effect-modifying host characteristics.

We must close with an explicit recognition of several points. First, measures of occupational exposures based on self-reports are extremely convenient and are a tempting substitute for objective assessments. Secondly, the theoretically driven need to measure subjective perceptions of the work setting, with their strong evaluation and reactive components, is separable from the use of self reports as convenient approximations of objective exposures. Self-reports are likely to be reasonable approximations for simple dimensions, such as number of hours worked or the number of persons for whom the respondent works, but not for complex concepts such as role ambiguity.[23] Thirdly, objective measurement of work hazards and conditions is usually difficult, cumbersome, and potentially complicated,[24–27] whereas easily collected data may be only peripherally useful. Fourthly, objective measurement of work hazards will not solve all our major methodological problems. For example, self-selection into exposure conditions, influenced by prior personal characteristics, can confound the apparent impact. Prospective designs in which the cohort is identified before exposure, and of course disease as well, allows much better control of the self-selection issue, while objective measurements do not address this concern.

Aspects of work with likely impact on health

In this section, we shall discuss aspects of the work setting that are worthy of our attention because of their possible effects on health. As the relevant studies are so numerous, an integrated overview is difficult and a precise evaluation of the evidence would be a lengthy undertaking. Our strategy is therefore to pay attention to reports that address a variety of outcomes, such as job satisfaction, psychological strain, and specific diseases, and which need not reflect only the stress perspective. From these publications, we derive a list of dimensions which have been implicated to some extent: that is, the evidence is rarely definitive or conclusive, and the criteria of impact may be rather narrow (for example, job satisfaction and turnover, but not physical health symptoms or biomedical outcomes). Thus our list is only suggestive and probably overly inclusive. In later sections we deal with selected evidence in greater depth.

This section is based on an earlier review[28] and on some more recent general publications and overviews.[19 29–37] We suggest that the following dimensions of the work setting be provisionally considered as having an impact on health and well-being.

Physical conditions at work

These include:

- those related to comfort, such as heat, cold, and humidity
- hazardous exposures to radiation, chemicals, and pollutants
- those related to symptoms or annoyance, such as dust and fumes
- noise
- dangerous machinery.

The presumption is that apart from direct effects, which presumably bypass cognitive or emotional processing, such as radiation and cancer, indirect effects are likely, either because awareness of exposure to hazards may have its own consequences or because the physical conditions interact with psychosocial variables.[38]

Ergonomic aspects of the job

These include bad machine design, physical constraints on movement, discomfort, vibrations, heavy physical demand, and pacing by or breakdown of machinery.

Temporal aspects of work day and tasks

Examples are:
- shift work, particularly rotating shifts
- overtime, unwanted or "excessive" hours
- two jobs
- piecework compared with hourly pay (pay mechanisms influencing pace)
- fast pace of work, particularly with demands for high vigilance
- not enough time to complete work, deadlines
- scheduling of work and rest cycles
- variation in work load
- interruptions.

Work content (other than temporal aspects)

Examples are:
- fractionated, repetitive, monotonous work, low skill requirement
- autonomy, independence, influence, control
- use of existing skills
- opportunity to learn new skills
- mental alertness and concentration
- unclear and conflicting tasks or demands
- insufficient resources (such as skills, machinery, and organisational structure), for given work demands or responsibilities.

Interpersonal—work group

This covers:
- opportunity to interact with co-workers during work, during breaks, and after work
- size and cohesiveness of primary work group
- recognition for work performance
- social support
- instrumental support
- equitable work load.

Interpersonal—supervision

This covers:

- participation in decision making
- receiving feedback and recognition from supervisor
- providing supervisor with feedback
- closeness of supervision
- social support
- instrumental support
- unclear or conflicting demands.

Financial and economic aspects

Such as:

- pay and basic wages
- additional compensation (overtime, shiftwork, bonuses)
- retirement benefits
- other benefits (for example, health care)
- equity and predictability of compensation.

Organisational aspects

Including:

- size
- structure (for example, "flat" structure with relatively few levels in the organisation)
- having a staff position compared with a line position
- working on the boundary of the organisation
- relative prestige of the job
- unclear organisational structure (lines of responsibility, organisational basis for role conflict and ambiguity)
- organisational administrative red tape, and cumbersome or irrational procedures
- discriminatory policies (in hiring or promotion, for example).

Actual or threatened changes

Many of the dimensions listed above can undergo change and such changes may also be worthy of attention because of their possible impact on health. The kinds of changes that are likely to be important are often more global than dimensional: promotion, demotion, loss of job, full-time to part-time transition, increased job insecurity, various organisational changes, and so on. The interest in changes at work and their possible impact on health goes beyond the simple idea that some changes may lead to a higher level of chronic exposure to a stressor, such as overload or deadline pressures. The additional notion is that change may be stressful in itself and that adapting to the new circumstances creates new temporary demands that must be met as well.

In addition to the above listing of the specific aspects of the work setting, it is prudent to consider, however tentatively, the broader context of work. For example, community perceptions of certain jobs, and of the company itself, may translate into issues of status, prestige, and respect which affect the community (non-work) life of the job occupant. However, most considerations of the interface between work and non-work have involved the roles of spouse and parent[29][30][39][40] and of the family setting with its own stresses and dynamics.[41]

We have noted that this list of work dimensions is unevenly supported by empirical evidence; furthermore, the evidence may be in support of impact on some indicators of health and well-being and non-existent or negative for other indicators. For example, aspects of mental health are more likely to be affected by jobs that are insufficiently challenging (boring, repetitive, monotonous, fractionated), while physical health outcomes are more likely to be linked to jobs that are excessively challenging (qualitative and quantitative overload, time pressures).

The list also represents a fragmentation of the evidence and we need some framework to put it back together into a coherent picture. The next two paragraphs represent steps in this direction; the first is more pertinent to mental health and well-being and the second to biological health.

On the basis of a review of studies of determinants of job satisfaction, Locke characterised desirable conditions at work as follows:[42] (a) work represents mental challenge with which the worker can cope successfully and leads to involvement and personal interest; (b) work is not physically too tiring; (c) rewards for performance are just, informative, and in line with aspirations; (d) working conditions are compatible with physical needs and they facilitate work goals; (e) work leads to high self-esteem; and (f) agents in the work place help with the attainment of job values.

In an earlier statement, we tried to outline some possible components of a pathogenic process that may eventually lead to clinical events:[43] (a) the work condition tends to be chronic rather than intermittent or self-limiting; (b) habituation or adaptation to the chronic condition is difficult; (c) disengagement is not possible and instead, some form of vigilance or arousal must be maintained; (d) failure to meet the demands of the work setting has serious consequences (for example, high level of responsibility for outcomes such as the lives of others or equipment or profits); and (e) there is a spillover of the effects of the work role into other areas of functioning (such as family and leisure), so that the daily impact of the demanding job becomes cumulative and health-threatening, rather than being daily defused or erased, thereby having little long-term impact on health. The last point is the most speculative and in need of most additional documentation. It may also be the one where the characteristics of the job incumbent, in addition to the job itself, are most influential.

Range of study designs and types of evidence

An ideal non-experimental observational study of occupational stress would have the following characteristics:

- The cohort is identified before exposure
- The environmental condition (exposure) is objectively defined and measured
- Self-selection into exposure conditions is minimised by exploiting opportunities for natural experiments, with changes in the work setting that lead to comparable groups of exposed and unexposed employees
- Potential confounding variables, primarily biological risk factors and initial health status, are assessed and their influence monitored in analysis
- Period of follow-up is adequate to take the cohort through crucial periods of adaptation and disease causation
- Mediating processes are studied and vulnerability factors that interact with exposure are included.

This ideal is seldom attained; in fact, even relatively barren longitudinal designs are a distinct rarity.[44] However, when such a design is approximated, the payoff in terms of clear results can be rewarding. An example of this design is a study of coronary disease in bank clerks in Belgium.[45][46] Two banks were involved and both were initially similar. One remained a semi-public savings bank and the bank clerks continued in relatively non-demanding jobs; the other became a private commercial bank in which the jobs were more competitive and the clerks invested clients' money in somewhat risky enterprises. Baseline risk factor information was obtained. After 10 years of follow up, the clerks in the commercial bank had a 50% higher rate of events (sudden death, fatal and non-fatal infarctions), after adjustment for baseline risk. Interestingly, the excess risk associated with the type of bank was seen only among those relatively high on baseline risk factors. Finally, stress measured subjectively showed no significant change.[47]

Broad studies of many occupations

The research literature on work stress includes a great variety of designs and approaches. A preliminary and indirect approach is the examination of occupational differences in mortality and morbidity. For example, Fletcher has presented British mortality data for selected occupations.[48] High standardised mortality ratios (SMRs) in men for diseases of the circulatory system were noted in electrical engineers, and bricklayers and labourers (3·42 and 2·39, respectively) and low SMRs in university teachers and engineering foremen (0·47 and 0·51, respectively). While the low ratios in teachers have been repeatedly noted (see earlier review by

Kasl,[13]) the other data are not easily interpretable. Also puzzling is the fact that the mortality in women, classified by husband's occupation, showed a pattern of high and low SMRs similar to that in men. This tends to undermine the interpretation that the occupational classification says something about work exposures, whether or not they specifically involved stress. German morbidity data for myocardial infarction were examined separately for blue and white collar workers.[49] For the former, high rates were observed in metal polishers, annealers, and galvanisers, and for sawyers and wood-working machinists; low rates were found in farmers, gardeners, and unskilled construction workers. For white collar jobs, high rates were seen in technical assistants (biological, physical, and chemical) and low rates in teachers, clergymen, members of parliament, and administrators. Again, the results are a mixture of the familiar (farmers, teachers) and puzzling (technical assistants). Even if one could carry out some indirect adjustments for social class differences and associated lifestyle habits such as smoking, these occupational differences are at best tenuous leads.

An American study of occupational differences in one year prevalence of major depressive disorder showed high odds ratios in lawyers (3·6), other teachers and counsellors (not college) (2·8), and secretaries (1·9).[50] These results were adjusted for sociodemographic factors, were based on diagnostic interviews (not symptom checklists), and include both treated and untreated disorders, an improvement over previous reports.[51] In spite of these strengths, there are puzzles and problems. For example, in contrast to the above group of teachers and counsellors, the group called teachers (secondary school) had extremely low rates; this suggests that self-selection may be an alternative explanation to effect of the work environment. A similar puzzle is that in contrast to the high rates among lawyers, former lawyers had low rates. The distinction between former and current also made a big difference among production inspectors, testers, and samplers: the rates were low for current workers and high for former workers. This suggests that selective mobility may confound or obscure some of these prevalence estimates.

Intensive studies of single occupations

In contrast to the broad examination of many occupations, with the attendant inability to control for even major confounders, there are studies which concentrate on a single or few occupations, to study work stress in depth. Again, there is a great variety of approaches. One approach is to seek the special sources of stress in a particular occupation, such as ministers of religion,[52] seafarers,[53] prison officers,[54] policemen,[55] and health care personnel.[56] This approach has several limitations: (a) it leads to development of measures unique to a particular job and makes it difficult to carry out cross-occupation comparative studies; (b) the initial step entails no linkage to health outcomes, or only to relatively weak outcomes such as job satisfaction;[57] (c) it represents a strong commitment to a psychological (experiential, phenomenological) approach to stress and neglects the possibility that adverse health outcomes may be the consequence of other work exposures not consciously identified in this manner. For example, it is somewhat of a surprise to find that policemen complain most about administrative issues and contacts with the court system,[58] and air traffic controllers complain about having little to do during off-peak hours;[59] the possibility that denial and distortion influence these perceptions certainly cannot be ruled out.

The study of a single occupation (or occupational group) is a research strategy that is not easy to evaluate. For example, the interest in prison personnel is relatively new[60] and the evidence is just beginning to accumulate.[61 62] Thus it is not clear what evidence will eventually emerge that may add to our knowledge about the impact of work stress on health. Two occupations, air traffic controllers and bus drivers, will be discussed to explore this issue further.

The interest in air traffic controllers can be traced to an early report, which showed a higher incidence of hypertension particularly among those working in regions with high air traffic volumes.[63] A major study was undertaken as a result.[64] In many ways this was a superbly designed longitudinal investigation of a single occupation over three years. A rich variety of measurements were obtained to monitor daily fluctuations in work load and outcomes, as well as to detect longer term effects. Nevertheless, the results failed to provide support that air traffic controllers were indeed at greater risk of hypertension: hypertension was defined as being above a cutoff on more than one reading, even if the last measurements were within normotensive range. Aspects of work such as work load were not clearly related to longer term health outcomes, though daily fluctuations in load were associated with some outcomes (for example, fluctuations in cortisol levels), particularly among workers who were highly involved in their work. In general, stable personal characteristics, such as amicability and type A personality, proved to be relatively important,[65] and life change distress measures predicted illness rates and injuries equally well if they were or were not work-related.[66] More recent data have cast doubt on the possibility that blood pressure levels among air traffic controllers are actually higher than expected.[67 68] An additional complicating factor is that air traffic controllers move out of their jobs at a relatively young age and it is possible that the length of exposure is not sufficient for their work to have had an irreversible impact on blood pressure.

The initial interest in occupational stress among bus drivers may date back to Rosenman's and Friedman's reinterpretation of the high rates of coronary heart disease among drivers of double-decker London buses,[69] compared with rates among the more physically active conductors.[70] They suggested that bus drivers experienced more stress than conductors. In support of this interpretation they showed that in the peripheral areas of London (with their lower density of traffic) bus drivers had disease rates which were somewhat lower than conductors, and that the originally observed excess applied only to the central city. More recent data have confirmed the excess of cardiovascular disease and gastrointestinal illnesses (as well as musculoskeletal problems) among bus drivers.[71–73] A study was undertaken in California which showed higher prevalence of hypertension among bus drivers.[74] In a companion publication, the authors described the development of a measure of self-reported stressors, based on several different aspects of work, such as rule violations, accidents, physical danger, passengers, and so on.[75] Surprisingly, high stress was found to be related to lower prevalence of hypertension, and lower mean blood pressure among normotensives. It is difficult to interpret this finding; it is possible that the "stress" arises as a result of being a careful and vigilant bus driver who maintains tight control over the work so that the various stressors do not even arise. Of course, this is a completely *post hoc* interpretation. In any case what remains true is that objectively defined exposures, such as driving in heavy traffic, are associated with excess risk.[71]

These studies of air traffic controllers and bus drivers raise some doubts about the research strategy of identifying a particular occupation that has high rates of some disease (compared with many other occupations), and then concentrating on that occupation to investigate the impact of a suspected work stressor in depth and in detail. In principle this works well if the difference in level of exposure to some hazard that describes the difference across occupations can be made even bigger or clearer or more precise by studying only individuals within the high risk occupation. Such may be the case for rare carcinogens to which only a small subset of workers within the high risk occupation is exposed. But it may not work well if the levels of exposure in the high risk occupation are relatively homogeneous and if, in addition, we don't exactly know what the hazard is and tend to fall back on subjective measures of exposure. We may end up identifying personal characteristics that explain variations in outcome within the single group, but are no longer explaining the overall higher rates found in this group.[65 76]

Cross-sectional studies of subjective stressors and self-reported outcomes

A design that is too common is the cross-sectional survey in which interview or questionnaire-based data are collected on a number of job stressors, such as role conflict and role ambiguity, quantitative and qualitative overload, job monotony, closeness of supervision, and so on.

Data on "job strains" are collected in the same manner: job satisfaction, depression, anxiety, irritation, self-esteem, psychophysiological symptoms, smoking, alcohol consumption, and so on.[77] Objective data on aspects of the work setting are not obtained; even differences across different occupations or job titles go unexamined. The primary purpose of analysis is to show the link between job stressors and job strains, thereby suggesting cause-effect correlations. The analysis may be reasonably sophisticated, including multivariate adjustments for such factors as age, education, income, and gender, and testing complex causal models. Good national samples can provide useful descriptive information of wide generalisability.[78]

The main question is: what do we learn about the impact of work stressors on health and well being? The answer has to be: very little. We simply do not know the extent to which various measurement problems (discussed earlier), together with the cross-sectional nature of the design, have created associations that are spurious or spuriously inflated. The magnitude of associations between stressors and outcomes tends to form a reasonably replicable pattern characterised by:

- fairly high correlations with such outcomes as job satisfaction, life satisfaction, and global measures of happiness
- moderate correlations with symptom checklists reflecting dysphoria
- low correlations with somatic symptoms
- negligible correlations with lifestyle factors such as cigarette smoking and alcohol and drug use.

However, as noted already, this pattern is a reflection of both true effects as well as methodological artifacts, making interpretation difficult. For example, when measurement of mental health variables shifts from symptom checklists to specific psychiatric diagnoses, the linkages to work environment variables tend to weaken considerably.[79] Against this uncertainty, only zero correlations (no association) are informative.

It needs to be emphasised that this pessimistic conclusion applies to interpreting the association between the two sets of variables. However, such measures are far from useless. For example, descriptive data for a particular occupation or job title may show high levels of stressors or strains, thus justifying closer attention to that occupation. Similarly, such measures used in stronger designs and with a variety of outcome measures will provide more interpretable findings.

Cross-sectional designs that include biological variables

Studies of subjective stressors that include biological variables have at least two advantages: first, they measure outcomes in a way, which is quite distinct from the measurement of the putative independent variable, and secondly, they collect data on variables which may be thought of as describing potential pathways between stressors and distal disease outcomes. However, it must be noted that two somewhat different classes of biological variables have been used: (a) established risk factors for a specific disease, such as blood pressure or serum cholesterol, and (b) biological indicators of stress reactivity, such as corticosteroids and catecholamines. While the former have a reasonable chance of indicating increased risk for specific disease outcomes (if reflecting chronic levels), the latter have a much more tenuous connection with disease outcomes. They cannot even describe adequately the full stress-reactivity-adaptation process.[80]

Broad cross-sectional surveys of samples that combine many occupational groups tend to produce few significant correlations between a great variety of subjective job stressors on the one hand, and biological indicators of coronary disease risk, on the other.[16 77 81] There may be two reasons why this kind of a broad research strategy is insensitive to detecting associations, if they exist. First, the meaning of a subjective stressor may change when one goes from one occupation to another. Consider the item "Is your job hectic?" When asked of blue-collar workers in various assembly-line and machine-paced jobs it could reflect a specific aspect of pacing, plus some elements of quality control, and allowances for taking breaks. However, when the occupations also include managers, teachers, farmers, doctors, and others, then high-low scores on the total study population are difficult to interpret. It is not implausible to suggest that those scoring high, but coming from a wide variety of jobs, are more likely to share common personal characteristics than common work characteristics. Secondly, the cross-sectional design will not be sensitive to processes that reflect mostly acute dynamics, but not long-term chronic effects, nor to processes that make their impact early on in the tenure on a job, but with later adaptations (including leaving the job), which hide any early effects.

When the research strategy becomes more focused in terms of the selection of target occupations, the use of theory to guide selection of work stressors, and a careful choice of outcome variables, we may expect greater payoff in terms of linkages between subjective stressors and biological outcomes. In a study entitled "Atherogenic risk in men suffering from occupational stress," the authors studied blue collar workers in steel and metal plants, some of which were reducing their work force.[82] They assessed both objective indicators (job instability and shift work) and subjective indicators, such as perceived job insecurity and perceived increase in workload. Atherogenic risk was defined as the ratio of low and high density lipoproteins, and this was adjusted for potential confounders, such as body weight, smoking, and alcohol consumption. The results showed that increased atherogenic risk was associated with an interaction of objective and subjective stressors, such as job instability and perceived job insecurity. A later report, which measured high risk of coronary heart disease by adding hypertension to the atherogenic risk indicator,[83] noted the associations with additional variables such as low promotion prospects at work, competitiveness at work, and feelings of sustained anger. A study of work stress and blood pressure incorporated a careful selection of occupational settings, rigorous adjustment for many variables (including family history of hypertension and severe noise-induced hearing loss), and a careful selection of work stressor measures.[84] Men with raised diastolic blood pressure reported having little opportunity for promotion and for participation in decisions at work, an uncertain job future, unsupportive coworkers and foremen, and overall dissatisfaction with their job. In short, different work environments are associated with different levels of blood pressure after adjusting for currently recognized risk factors, and we are beginning to identify some of the subjective work stressors that may explain the differences.[85]

Designs that describe changes in biological variables over time

Studies of work stress that include repeat measurements of some biological variable are typically of two kinds. First, there are investigations of long term trends or changes. Here the interest is to see if baseline assessments of work stressors will predict future changes in a biological risk factor, adjusting for covariates and for baseline levels of the risk factor. Obviously, this is a variation on the classical prospective design in epidemiology, but the outcome is not disease, but change in risk factor. There are two drawbacks to this strategy. The more important is that not much will be learned if the impact of the stressors is already fully played out and manifest in the baseline (cross-sectional) associations. Thus, it is most useful when the exposures to stressors are of recent origin or, even better, if the cohort is identified before a new exposure. The other problem is that levels of risk factors are reversible and continued monitoring of outcomes may change the picture and the conclusions.

Secondly, there are investigations of short term trends. Here the interest is more in acute reactivity and the designs include 24 hour monitoring, changes during the working day, and comparisons of working and non-working occasions, for example before work day begins, after work day ends, and during vacation. Depending on the specific design used, the assumptions behind the chosen strategy differ somewhat. Some of the assumptions are as follows:

- fluctuations during the working day will identify work stressors which have acute effects; if such stressors recur frequently, repeated occasions of acute reactivity translate into irreversible changes and/or into greater incidence of clinical outcomes
- increases in risk factors beyond the end of the working day result from

slow unwinding from work, rather than a stressful non-work situation, and such slow unwinding is a long term risk

• decline in a variable during the working day reflects low stress, not the fact that anticipation before the start of the working day created higher levels. Clearly, then, repeat measurements of a biological variable enrich the study design but do not guarantee an improvement over simple cross-sectional data collection.

Studies of long term changes in risk factors in relation to work stress are not common and possibly their value is not substantial. In a five year follow-up study of blood pressure among Finnish white-collar and blue-collar workers, the main predictors of future blood pressure levels (above baseline) were change in weight and "frequency of mild intoxication."[86] Work-related variables such as monotony, discomfort from noise, and "holding one's tongue in the working place" did not contribute to the prediction. A five-year blood pressure study of Australian government employees examined five aspects of perceived work stress:[87] qualitative and quantitative demands, job control, future control, and work support. For men, none of the scales contributed significantly to the prediction of future blood pressure levels; for women, significant associations were obtained only in specific age strata such as the association of low future control stress with lower blood pressure in women over 50 years of age. The paucity of findings is disappointing. The design of a Canadian study suggests that enriched study designs may be needed; namely, the study should include change in a job stressor, not just baseline effects, and should include stable personal traits as possible moderators.[88]

The monitoring of acute effects of work stressors on biological variables is a research strategy that is rising in popularity. A simple approach is to measure the increase in some biological indicator from the start to the end of a work day and to relate the magnitude of the increase to type of job and work conditions. The presumption is that larger increases will be observed in more stressful working conditions. For example, in a study of blood pressure in a prison setting work-related increases among guards were greater in maximum security than minimum security prisons.[89] Among other correctional personnel, those involved in treatment had higher increases than service and clerical workers, particularly for women. Sometimes the blood pressure effect is seen only among those with a family history of hypertension.[90]

The comparison of levels of an indicator at work and at home after work has been useful in identifying jobs and work conditions that show a spillover effect or delayed unwinding after work. For example, Rissler found delayed recovery from high arousal levels among female workers who were given unwanted overtime, as indexed by adrenaline excretion rates.[91] A similar effect was demonstrated for sawmill workers, whose

257

work is repetitive, machine paced, and highly constricting,[92] and for video display unit operators.[93] A recent review has led to the suggestion that it is repetitive monotony rather than uneventful monotony that is pathogenic; work on assembly line or clerical data entry work is an example of the former, while supervisory monitoring of automated technical processes exemplifies the latter.[94] Among white collar employees, grouped by gender and clerical versus middle management level, women may be at greatest risk of slower unwinding.[95]

New technology for ambulatory monitoring can only enrich our study designs, although it may also overwhelm us with too much data to digest comfortably. For example, a study of British firemen, using an index of ventricular cardiac strain shown by ambulatory electrocardiogram (ECG) monitoring, showed that higher strain scores were recorded for station officers and those working on busy stations, especially if they were also on medication.[96] A Swedish study of some seven different occupations also used 24-hour ECG monitoring to investigate the role of work place social support.[97] People who reported low social support had higher systolic blood pressure and higher heart rate. Interestingly, the effect on heart rate was also observed during leisure and rest, suggesting chronic autonomic arousal. In this study the impact of social support on the spillover phenomenon was stronger than the effect of stressors, such as job demands and decision latitude.

Studies of acute reactivity and of long term changes in biological risk factors cannot substitute for studies that target specific disease outcomes for documenting the impact of work stress. In the next section, we will examine the evidence with respect to cardiovascular disease and focus on the job strain model or formulation.[33 36] We do this because most of the evidence regarding work stress and physical health deals with heart disease, and because the job strain model has become influential in guiding a fair amount of recent research.

Work stress and cardiovascular disease

There is long-standing interest in the possible role of stress in the aetiology of cardiovascular disease.[14 32 98] The extension of this interest to work stress was a natural development and has stimulated a large body of research.[32 36 99] There is no single theoretical framework or perspective which can bring this diverse research evidence together and do justice to the complexity of findings. Specifically, we find the following:

- True inconsistencies across findings from different studies.
- Opportunistic analyses of longitudinal data, originally obtained for another purpose, which contribute valuable evidence but do not allow

for precise comparisons of risk factors across studies or examination of goodness of fit for a particular theoretical formulation.

- Varying degrees to which confounding risk factors, such as physical inactivity, cigarette smoking, and dietary intake, have been examined and controlled in different reports.
- Unclear role of stable personal characteristics, non-work stress exposures and social environmental influences. These variables probably act both as confounders of work stress and as moderators of such effects. These other classes of psychosocial influences on cardiovascular disease have their own confusing and hard-to-integrate research evidence.

A highly influential formulation is the Karasek job demands-control or "job strain" model.[33] There are two dimensions of the work environment that are emphasised: (1) psychological work load demands ("My job requires working very fast."), and (2) job decision latitude, which itself has two components: decision authority ("My job allows me to make a lot of decisions on my own") and skill utilisation ("My job requires a high level of skill.") The pathogenic work environment is represented by the combination of high demands and low decision latitude; such a combination is referred to as high "job strain." This formulation brings together two separate traditions in work stress research on cardiovascular disease: the role of high demands and the role of control.[19]

Two additional comments are in order. One is that it is not clear whether or not the model specifically asserts an interactive correlation, implying that high levels of demand lead to cardiovascular disease only in the presence of low decision latitude. A less restrictive formulation would simply assert that these are two important dimensions that may act additively or interactively. Unfortunately, many of the recent studies create a single variable of job strain as the overall risk factor; this prevents an examination of any interaction—the novel feature of this whole formulation—and obscures even the issue of whether one or other or both the component dimensions influence the risk of cardiovascular disease. The second comment is that most occupations form a pattern so that high demands are correlated with high decision latitude. Thus the high job strain combination picks up somewhat anomalous jobs that deviate from the overall trend of positive association.[100]

The job strain model is not the only relevant formulation. For example, the British tradition emphasises social class differences.[101] In this approach, social class is a central concept, which influences both biomedical risk factors for cardiovascular disease as well as psychosocial working conditions.[102] In that sense, work stress and the concept of job strain become part of the explanatory dynamics linking social class and cardiovascular disease. The medical sociology tradition also seems to favour an emphasis on social class and social-structural variables; for example, Siegrist *et al.* emphasised the social inequalities in work-related stressors and socioemotional supports and what they call "impaired control over social status."[103][104] It is a fair criticism to assert that the Karasek job strain model pays insufficient attention to the broader issues of social inequality.

A review of the evidence on job strain and cardiovascular disease suggests that there is reasonable support for the model,[36] though some major studies have yielded negative evidence.[105][106] The incorporation of the dimension of social support appears to be a valuable modification of the model, but it also tends to undermine the original formulation.[107] The support appears better when the outcomes are risk factors for cardiovascular disease, notably blood pressure, than when they are clinical disease or mortality. The use of an imputation strategy, in which actual jobs become proxies for scores on the dimensions of demands and latitudes, is useful in that it draws our attention to selected specific jobs, but makes the task of evaluating and integrating the overall evidence more difficult.[108]

A disturbing aspect in the overall evidence is that job strain has been measured differently in the different studies and that it is difficult to pin down the precise pathogenic dimensions that are involved. For example, some of the Swedish case-control and hospital studies rather consistently found that jobs that were both "hectic" and characterised by "few possibilities to learn" were those with highest risk for cardiovascular disease.[109] It is difficult to know what "hectic" means in terms of physical demands and physical activity, as opposed to psychological components such as deadline pressures, multiple simultaneous demands, and the constant need to maintain vigilance. Physical demands and levels of physical activity at work influence the development of cardiovascular disease on their own and their clear separation from other dimensions that might be relevant is highly desirable.[110–112] Similarly, "few possibilities to learn" cannot distinguish repetitive from uneventful monotony[94] and may cover a variety of job conditions, only some of which might be involved in cardiovascular disease risk. It is also interesting to note that the Swedish studies, as well as other evidence, have implicated shift work as a condition associated with higher risk of cardiovascular disease;[99][113] it appears to be an independent risk factor not interacting with other variables such as dimensions in the job strain model. It is likely that aspects of the work environment that relate to cardiovascular disease such as shiftwork and overtime are not incorporated into the job strain model. The model should not be viewed as a comprehensive statement of stressful work conditions.

Finally, it should be noted that the epidemiological model of disease causation postulated by the job strain and cardiovascular disease studies is ambiguous. In studies in which the outcome is morbidity or mortality from cardiovascular disease, the research reports adjust for standard risk factors before examining the role of job strain. This suggests a model in which job strain is believed to be a risk factor independent of and not operating through the other established risk factors. However, studies in which the outcome is one of the usual risk factors for cardiovascular disease, the model being tested is that job strain affects cardiovascular disease risk factors, which then mediate the impact on cardiovascular disease. The two models are not compatible. If the latter is the proper one, then the strategy of adjusting for known risk factors before testing the impact of job strain on cardiovascular disease is incorrect: one does not adjust in a causal model for the impact of variables that mediate the risk-disease association. This point is generic for much of the general work stress and health literature: we need more explicit causal and conceptual models to guide analyses. Work stress may influence disease directly, or through risk factors, or both. But it is not sufficient to adjust automatically for known risk factors if they are available.

Overview

In this chapter we have tried to examine the topic of work stress and health from an occupational health perspective rather than a psychological one. We noted the many difficulties one encounters in trying to investigate this complex topic. These difficulties are both conceptual and methodological. The former include uncertainties about how the concept of stress, and the surrounding theory, should be formulated. The latter include both issues of measurement of the relevant exposure variables and of the related processes, as well as research design issues, as strong prospective designs are often needed to establish a causal connection between work stress and disease outcome.

We next offered a rather long list of work dimensions that are potential indicators of specific components of work stress. The list is backed up unevenly by research evidence and only in a minority by studies of clinical-biomedical outcomes. But it serves to translate an unmanageable concept, stress, into specific measurable dimensions and alerts us to the breadth of possibilities of risk factors that may be involved. In the next section we discussed the types of research strategies and study designs used and tried to show what one can learn from them. The order of presentation of these designs was intended to describe increasingly more direct strategies for examining the work stress-health linkage. Finally, the last section was the most focused look at the evidence: we concentrated on a specific model of work stress and examined a specific dimension of health, cardiovascular disease.

1 Creech L, Johnson M. Angiosarcoma of liver in the manufacture of polyvinyl chloride. *J Occup Med* 1974; **16**: 150–1.

2 Schuckit MA, Gunderson EKE. Job stress and psychiatric illness in the U.S. Navy. *J Occup Med* 1973; **15**: 884–7.

3 Rutsein D, Mullan RJ, Frazier TM, Halperin WE, Melius JM, Sestito JP. Sentinel health events (occupational): a basis for physician recognition and public health surveillance. *Am J Public Health* 1983; **73**: 1054–62.

4 Evans GW, ed. *Environmental Stress*. New York: Cambridge University Press, 1982.

5 Jones DM, Chapman AJ. *Noise and Society*. Chichester: Wiley, 1984.

6 Kryter KD. Non-auditory effects of environmental noise. *Am J Public Health* 1972; **62**: 389–98.

7 Corlett EN, Richardson J. *Stress, Work Design, and Productivity*. Chichester: Wiley, 1981.

8 Shepard RJ. *Men at Work*. Springfield, Ill.: Thomas, 1974.

9 Houts PS, McDougall V. Effects of informing workers of their health risks from exposure to toxic materials. *Am J Ind Med* 1988; **13**: 271–9.

10 Schottenfeld RS, Cullen MR. Occupation-induced post-traumatic stress disorders. *Am J Ind Med* 1985; **142**: 198–202.

11 Haynes SG, LaCroix AZ, Lippin T. The effect of high job demands and low control on the health of employed women. In: Eds, Quick JC, Bhagat RS, Dalton JE, Quick JD *Work Stress*. New York: Praeger, 1987: 93–110.

12 Cooper CL, Payne R, eds. *Causes, coping and consequences of stress at work*. Chichester: Wiley, 1988.

13 Kasl SV. *Epidemiological contributions to the study of work stress*. In: Cooper CL, Page R, eds. *Stress at Work*. Chichester: Wiley, 1978: 3–48.

14 Kasl SV. Stress and health. *Am J Public Health* 1984; **5**: 319–41.

15 Kasl SV, Cooper CL (eds). *Stress and Health: Issues in Research Methodology*. Chichester: Wiley, 1987.

16 French JRP Jr, Caplan RD, Harrison R. *The Mechanisms of Job Stress and Strain*. Chichester: Wiley, 1982.

17 Cox T. Repetitive work. Occupational stress and health. In: Cooper CL, Smith MJ, eds. *Job stress and blue collar work*. Chichester: Wiley, 1985: 85–112.

18 Smith MJ. Machine-paced work and stress. In: Cooper CL, Smith MJ eds. *Job stress and blue collar work*. Chichester: Wiley, 1985: 51–64.

19 Sauter SL, Hurrell JJ Jr, Cooper CL, eds. *Job control and worker health*. Chichester: Wiley, 1989.

20 Frese M, Zapf D. Methodological issues in the study of work stress: objective vs subjective measurement of work stress and the question of longitudinal studies. In: Cooper CL, Payne R, eds. *Causes, coping, and consequences of stress at work*. Chichester: Wiley, 1988, 375–411.

21 Hulka BS, Wilcosky TC, Griffith JD. *Biological markers in epidemiology*. New York: Oxford University Press, 1990.

22 McMichael AJ. Invited commentary—"molecular epidemiology:". New pathways or new travelling companion? *Am J Epidemiol* 1994; **140**: 1–11.

23 Spector PE, Dwyer DJ, Jex SM. Relation of job stressors to affective, health, and performance outcomes: A comparison of multiple data sources. *J Appl Psychol* 1988; **73**: 11–9.

24 Hacker W. Objective work environment: Analysis and evaluation of objective work characteristics. In: *A healthier work environment: basic concepts and methods of measurement*. Copenhagen: WHO Regional Office for Europe, 1993: 42–57.

25 Hackman JR, Oldham GR. Development of the Job Diagnostic Survey. *J Appl Psychol* 1975; **60**: 159–70.

26 House JS. *Occupational stress and mental and physical health of factory workers*. Ann Arbor: ISR Research Report, 1980.

27 Jenkins GD, Nadler DA, Lawler EE III, Cammann C. Standardized observation: An approach to measuring the nature of jobs. *J Appl Psychol* 1975; **60**: 171–81.

28 Kasl SV. Assessing health risks in the work setting. In: Hobfoll S, ed. *New directions in health psychology assessment*. Washington, D.C.: Hemisphere Publishing Corporation, 1990: 95–125.

29 Barling J, ed. *Employment, stress, and family functioning*. Chichester: Wiley, 1990.

30 Eckenrode J, Gore S, eds. *Stress between work and family*. New York: Plenum Press, 1990.
31 Evans GW, Johansson G, and Carrere S. Psychosocial factors and the physical environment: interrelations in the workplace. In: Cooper CL, Robertson IT, eds. *International review of industrial and organizational psychology*. London, Wiley, 1994: 1–29.
32 Fletcher BC. *Work, stress, disease, and life expectancy*. Chichester: Wiley, 1991.
33 Karasek R, Theorell T. *Healthy work. Stress, productivity and the reconstruction of working life*. New York: Basic Books, 1990.
34 Keita GP, Sauter SL, eds. *Work and well-being*. Washington, D.C.: American Psychological Association, 1992.
35 Landy F, Quick JC, Kasl SV. Work, stress, and well-being. *International Journal of Stress Management* 1994; 1: 33–73.
36 Schnall PL, Landsbergis PA, Baker D. Job strain and cardiovascular disease. *Annu Rev Public Health* 1994; 15: 381–411.
37 WHO. *A healthier work environment. Basic concepts and methods of measurement.* Copenhagen: WHO Regional Office for Europe, 1993.
38 Kasl SV, Chisholm RF, Eskenazi B. The impact of the accident at Three Mile Island on the behavior and well-being of nuclear workers. *Am J Public Health* 1981; 71: 472–83 & 484–95.
39 Gutek BA, Repetti RL, Silver DL. Nonwork roles and stress at work. In: Cooper CL, Payne R, eds. *Causes, coping and consequences of stress at work*. Chichester: Wiley, 1988: 141–74.
40 Repetti RL. Linkages between work and family roles. In: Oskamp S, ed. *Applied social psychology annual: vol. 7. Family processes and problems*. Beverly Hills: Sage, 1987: 98–127.
41 Pearlin LI, Turner HA. The family as a context of the stress process. In: Kasl SV, Cooper CL, eds. *Stress and health: issues in research methodology*. Chichester: Wiley, 1987: 143–65.
42 Locke EA. The nature and causes of job satisfaction. In: Dunnette MD, ed. *Handbook of industrial and organizational psychology*. Chicago: Rand McNally, 1976: 1297–349.
43 Kasl SV. The challenge of studying the disease effects of stressful work conditions. *Am J Public Health* 1981; 71: 682–4.
44 House JS. Chronic stress and chronic disease in life and work: conceptual and methodological issues. *Work and Stress* 1987; 1: 129–34.
45 Kittel F, Kornitzer M, Dramaix M. Coronary heart disease and job stress in two cohorts of bank clerks. *Psychotherapy and Psychosomatics* 1980; 34: 110–23.
46 Kornitzer MD, Dramaix M, Gheyssens H. Incidence of ischemic heart disease in two Belgian cohorts followed during 10 years. *European Journal of Cardiology* 1979; 9: 455–72.
47 Kornitzer MD, Kittel F, Dramaix M, De Backer G. Job stress and coronary heart disease. *Adv Cardiol* 1982; 29: 56–61.
48 Fletcher BC. The epidemiology of occupational stress. In: Cooper CL, Payne R, eds. *Causes, coping and consequences of stress at work*. Chichester: Wiley, 1988: 3–50.
49 Bolm-Audorff U, Siegrist J. Occupational morbidity data in myocardial infarction. *J Occup Med* 1983; 25: 367–71.
50 Eaton WW, Anthony JC, Mandel W, Garrison R. Occupations and the prevalence of major depressive disorder. *J Occup Med* 1990; 32: 1079–87.
51 Colligan MJ, Smith MJ, Hurrell JJ Jr. Occupational incidence rates of mental health disorders. *Journal of Human Stress* 1977; 3: 34–9.
52 Dewe PJ. New Zealand ministers of religion: identifying sources of stress and coping strategies. *Work and Stress* 1987; 1: 351–363.
53 Élo A-L. Health and stress of seafarers. *Scand J Work Environ Health* 1985; 11: 427–32.
54 Rutter DR, Fielding PJ. Sources of occupational stress: an examination of British prison officers. *Work Stress* 1988; 2: 291–9.
55 Cooper CL, Davidson MJ, Robinson P. Stress in the police service. *J Occup Med* 1982; 24: 31–6.
56 Leppanen RA, Olkinuora MA. Psychological stress experienced by health care personnel. *Scand J Work Environ Health* 1987; 13: 1–8.

57 McLaney MA, Hurrell JJ Jr. Control, stress, and job satisfaction in Canadian nurses. *Work and Stress* 1988; 2: 217–24.

58 Kroes WH, Margolis BL, Hurrell JJ. Job stress in policemen. *Journal of Police Science and Administration* 1974; 2: 145–55.

59 Crump JH. Review of stress in air traffic control: Its measurement and effects. *Aviat Space Environ Med* 1979; 50: 243–8.

60 Kalimo R. Stress in work: conceptual analysis and study on prison personnel. *Scand J Work, Environ Health* 1980; 6: 1–148.

61 Harenstam A, Palm U-B, Theorell T. Stress, health, and the working environment of Swedish prison staff. *Work and Stress* 1988; 2: 281–90.

62 Smith T. Cardiac measures of stress in British prison officers. *Work and Stress* 1988; 2: 301–8.

63 Cobb S, Rose RM. Hypertension, peptic ulcer, and diabetes in air traffic controllers. *JAMA* 1973; 224: 489–92.

64 Rose RM, Jenkins CD, Hurst MW. *Air traffic controller health change study.* Boston: Boston University School of Medicine, 1978. (A report to the FAA, Contract No. DOT-FA72WA-3211.)

65 Lee DJ, Niemcryk SJ, Jenkins CD, Rose RM. Type A, amicability, and injury: a prospective study of air traffic controllers. *J Psychosom Res* 1989; 33: 177–86.

66 Niemcryk SJ, Jenkins CD, Rose RM, Hurst MW. The prospective impact of psychosocial variables on rates of illness and injury in professional employees. *J Occup Med* 1987; 29: 645–52.

67 Booze CF Jr, Simcox LS. Blood pressure levels of active pilots compared to those of air traffic controllers. *Aviat Space Environ Med* 1985; 56: 1092–6.

68 Maxwell VB, Crump JH, Thorp J. The measurement of risk indicators for coronary heart disease in air traffic control officers: A screening study in a healthy population. *Aviat Space Environ Med* 1983; 54: 246–9.

69 Rosenman RH, Friedman M. The possible relationship of occupational stress to clinical coronary heart disease. *California Medicine* 1958; 89: 169–74.

70 Morris JN, Heady JA, Raffle PAB, Roberts CG, Parks JW. Coronary heart disease and physical activity of work. *Lancet* 1953; 2: 1111–3.

71 Netterstrom B, Juel K. Impact of work-related and psychosocial factors on the development of ischemic heart disease among urban bus drivers in Denmark. *Scand J Work Environ Health* 1988; 14: 231–38.

72 Netterstrom B, Juel K. Peptic ulcer among urban bus drivers in Denmark. *Scand J Soc Med* 1990; 18: 97–102.

73 Winkleby NA, Ragland OR, Fisher JM, Syme SL. Excess risk of sickness and disease in bus drivers: A review and synthesis of epidemiological studies. *Int J Epidemiol* 1988; 17: 255–62.

74 Ragland DR, Winkleby MA, Schwalbe J, Holman BL, Morse L, Syme SL, *et al.* Prevalence of hypertension in bus drivers. *Int J Epidemiol* 1987; 16: 208–14.

75 Winkleby MA, Ragland DR, Syme SL. Self-reported stressors and hypertension: evidence of an inverse association. *Am J Epidemiol* 1988; 127: 124–34.

76 Bartone PT. Predictors of stress-related illness in city bus drivers. *J Occup Med* 1989; 31: 657–63.

77 Caplan RD, Cobb S, French FRP Jr, Harrison RV, Pinneau SR Jr. *Job demands and worker health.* Washington, DC: PHEW Publication No (NIOSH) 75–160, 1975.

78 Quinn RP, Shepard LJ. *The 1972–73 quality of employment survey.* Ann Arbor: Institute for Social Research. 1974.

79 Bromet EJ, Parkinson DK, Curtis EC, Schulberg HC, Blane H, Dunn LO, *et al.* Epidemiology of depression and alcohol abuse/dependence in a managerial and professional work force. *J Occup Med* 1990; 32: 989–95.

80 Rose RM. Endocrine responses to stressful psychological events. *Psychiatr Clin North Am* 1980; 3: 251–76.

81 Sorensen G, Pirie P, Folsom A, Luepker R, Jacobs O, Gillum R. Sex differences in the relationship between work and health: The Minnesota Heart Survey. *J Health Soc Behav* 1985; 26: 379–94.

82 Siegrist J, Matschinger H, Cremer P, Siedel D. Atherogenic risk in men suffering from occupational stress. *Atherosclerosis* 1988; **69**: 211–8.
83 Siegrist J, Peter R, Georg W, Cremer P, Seidel D. Psychosocial and biobehavioral characteristics of hypertensive men with elevated atherogenic lipids. *Atherosclerosis* 1991; **86**: 211–8.
84 Matthews KA, Cottington EM, Talbott E, Kuller LH, Siegel JM. Stressful work conditions and diastolic blood pressure among blue collar factory workers. *Am J Epidemiol* 1987; **126**: 280–91.
85 Schlussel YR, Schnall PL, Zimbler M, Warren K, Pickering TG. The effect of work environments on blood pressure: evidence from seven New York organizations. *J Hypertension* 1990; **8**: 679–85.
86 Aro S. Occupational stress, health-related behavior, and blood pressure: A 5-year follow-up. *Prev Med* 1984; **13**: 333–48.
87 Chapman A, Mandryk JA, Frommer MS, Edye BV, Ferguson DA. Chronic perceived work stress and blood pressure among Australian government employees. *Scand J Work Environ Health* 1990; **16**: 258–69.
88 Howard JH, Cunningham DA, Rechnitzer PA. Personality (hardiness) as a moderator of job stress and coronary risk in Type A individuals: A longitudinal study. *J Behav Med* 1986; **9**: 229–44.
89 Ostfeld AM, Kasl SV, D'Atri DA, Fitzgerald EF. *Stress, crowding and blood pressure in prison.* Hillsdale, New Jersey: L Erlbaum Associates, 1987.
90 Theorell T. Family history of hypertension—an individual trait interacting with spontaneously occurring job stressors. *Scand J Work Environ Health* 1990; **16 (Suppl 1)**: 74–9.
91 Rissler A. Stress reactions at work and after work during a period of quantitative overload. *Ergonomics* 1977; **20**: 13–6.
92 Johansson G, Aronsson G, Lindstrom BP. Social psychological and neuroendocrine stress reactions in highly mechanized work. *Ergonomics* 1978; **21**: 583–99.
93 Frankenhaeuser M, Johansson G. Stress at work: psychobiological and psychosocial aspects. *International Review of Applied Psychology* 1986; **35**: 287–99.
94 Johansson G. Job demands and stress reactions in repetitive and uneventful monotony at work. *Int J Health Serv* 1989; **19**: 365–77.
95 Frankenhaeuser M, Lundberg U, Fredrikson M, Melin B, Tuomisto M, Myrsten A-L. Stress on and off the job as related to sex and occupational status in white-collar workers. *Journal of Organizational Behavior* 1989; **10**: 321–46.
96 Douglas RB, Blanks R, Crowther A, Scott G. A study of stress in West Midlands firemen, using ambulatory electrocardiograms. *Work and Stress* 1988; **2**: 309–18.
97 Unden A-L, Orth-Gomer K, Elofsson S. Cardiovascular effects of social support in the work place: Twenty-four-hour monitoring of men and women. *Psychosomatic Medicine* 1991; **53**: 50–60.
98 Dorian B, Taylor CB. Stress factors in the development of coronary artery disease. *J Occup Med* 1984; **26**: 747–56.
99 Kristensen TS. Cardiovascular disease and the work environment. *Scand Work Environ Health* 1989; **15**: 165–79.
100 Karasek PA, Theorell T, Schwartz JE, Schnall PL, Pieper CF, Michela JL. Job characteristics in relation to the prevalence of myocardial infarction in the US Health Examination Survey (HES) and the Health and Nutrition Examination Survey (HANES). *Am J Public Health* 1988; **78**: 910–8.
101 Pocock SJ, Shaper AG, Cook DG, Phillips AN, Walker M. Social class differences in ischaemic heart disease in British men. *Lancet* 1987; **II**: 197–201.
102 Marmot M, Theorell T. Social class and cardiovascular disease: The contribution of work. *Int J Health Serv* 1988; **18**: 659–74.
103 Siegrist J, Peter R, Junge A, Cremer P, Siedel D. Low status control, high effort at work, and ischemic heart disease: Prospective evidence from blue-collar men. *Social Science and Medicine* 1990; **31**: 1127–34.
104 Siegrist J, Siegrist K, Weber J. Sociological concepts in the etiology of chronic disease: The case of ischemic heart disease. *Social Science and Medicine* 1986; **22**: 247–53.

265

105 Alterman T, Shekelle RB, Vernon SW, Brau KD. Decision latitude, job strain, and coronary heart disease in the Western Electric Study. *Am J Epidemiol* 1994; **139**: 620–7.

106 Reed DM, LaCroix AZ, Karasek RA, Miller D, MacLean CA. Occupational strain and the incidence of coronary heart disease. *Am J Epidemiol* 1989; **129**: 495–502.

107 Johnson JV, Hall EM, Theorell T. Combined effects of job strain and social isolation on cardiovascular disease morbidity and mortality in a random sample of the Swedish male working population. *Scand J Work Environ Health* 1989; **15**: 271–9.

108 Pieper C, LaCroix AZ, Karasek RA. The relation of psychosocial dimensions of work with coronary heart disease risk factors: A meta-analysis of five United States data bases. *Am J Epidemiol* 1989; **129**: 483–94.

109 Kasl SV. An epidemiological perspective on the role of control in health. In: Sauter SL, Hurrell JJ Jr, Cooper CL, eds. *Job control and worker health*. Chichester: Wiley, 1989: 161–89.

110 Haan MN. Job strain and ischaemic heart disease: an epidemiologic study of metal workers. *Annals of Clinical Research* 1988; **20**: 143–5.

111 Kannel WB, Bélanger A, D'Agostino R, Israel T. Physical activity and physical demand on the job and risk of cardiovascular disease and death: The Framingham Study. *Am Heart J* 1986; **112**: 821–5.

112 Menotti A, Seccareccia F. Physical activity at work and job responsibility as risk factors for fatal coronary heart disease and other causes of death. *J Epidemiol Community Health* 1985; **39**: 325–9.

113 Akerstedt T, Knutsson A, Alfredsson L, Theorell T. Shift work and cardiovascular disease. *Scand J Work Environ Health* 1984; **10**: 409–14.

12 Work in agriculture

JAMES MERCHANT, STEPHEN REYNOLDS,
CRAIG ZWERLING

Introduction

Assessment of disease and injury among agricultural workers is a substantial challenge to the epidemiologist. The definition of the population at risk is highly variable by country and region. In developing countries, as many as 80% of the population may be engaged in largely subsistence agriculture. In highly developed countries in Western Europe and North America, the proportion of the work force engaged in agricultural production is now less than 2% and continues to contract as agriculture adopts industrial techniques of vertically integrated production. While three million Americans are fully engaged in agricultural production, as many as an additional nine million are exposed to agricultural risks as seasonal workers, part-time farmers, and farm family members who often contribute substantially to farm work.[1] In addition, lack of a uniform definition of agricultural work makes interpretation of epidemiological data difficult. In the United States, the Department of Labor combines agriculture, forestry and fishing in its definition of the agricultural sector. The United States Department of Agriculture and United States census require a minimum farm income of $1000 a year to define a farm.[2] As a result, measures of agriculturally-related disease using these definitions often grossly underestimate and inappropriately define the agricultural workforce at risk of disease and injury.

A second important methodological challenge facing the epidemiologist studying work in agriculture is the diversity and complexity of the agricultural environment. It is important to recognise the agricultural workforce as a subset of the rural population, which is itself at increased risk of disease and injury. Typically rural populations are poor and have less access to high quality health care.[3] Rural residents who are not engaged in agriculture are more often employed in small industries in which occupational risks are less often recognised and controlled. Rural residents are also at higher risk of a variety of preventable injuries, in part because of increased exposure to hazards and in part because of poorer access to trauma care.[4][5] Finally, the agricultural environment itself is highly variable and diverse.

Agricultural workers are exposed to a vast array of naturally occurring and synthetic chemical toxins, to substantial mechanical risks, and to multiple physical agents indigenous to their working and living environment. While agriculture is becoming more specialised, agricultural workers continue to be generalists with work-related exposures dictated by commodity, climate, season, and soil conditions. These multiple factors need to be understood by the epidemiologist in designing studies of the agricultural workforce.

The agricultural environment

The modern agricultural environment presents the potential for occupational exposure to a large number of hazardous agents—chemical, biological, and physical. Exposures vary depending on the type of crops and livestock produced, and the level of industrialisation of the particular region. Technological advances and socioeconomic forces have brought about dramatic changes in agriculture, resulting in significant changes in working conditions. In some cases these changes have proved beneficial, in others exposures have become intensified. Vertical integration of livestock production has led to an increase in specialisation, and workers devote more time to fewer tasks. In general, agricultural workers continue to work long hours under adverse climatic conditions while doing a wide variety of jobs. The population of workers also tends to be different from most occupational cohorts, including as it does a large proportion older than 65 years and younger than 16 years. The independence, mobility, and isolation of agricultural workers present considerable challenges for assessment and control of occupational exposures.

Livestock

The efficiency of livestock production has increased significantly in recent decades, through technological advances including the use of enclosed and controlled environments.[6] By monitoring and adjusting feed quality, temperature, and other factors, the amount of time and materials required to bring livestock to market can be substantially reduced. Enclosed facilities are now commonly used for swine, chickens, turkeys, and dairy cattle. As industrialisation of livestock production continues, the size of each operation continues to grow. Modern facilities may have capacities ranging from several hundred animals in one building in some swine and dairy barns, to more than 50 000 chickens in some poultry facilities. Many of the larger operations have hundreds of buildings. Some swine operations now have 30 000 sows capable of producing 600 000 pigs a year (compared with the 2000 pigs a year produced by a typical family farm). These produce a human waste equivalent of a metropolitan city of one million (one pig = biological oxygen demand of 2·5 people).

Environmental agents measured in poultry, swine, and dairy buildings include a complex mixture of irritant gases, microorganisms, and organic dusts. Dusts are biologically active and contain plant material (feed and bedding), animal-derived particles (skin, hair, feathers, droppings, urine), bacteria and fungi, microbial toxins (endotoxin, glucans, mycotoxins), mites and other arthropods and insects, feed additives and pesticides. Irritant gases include ammonia, hydrogen sulphide, methane, nitrogen oxides, and other gases produced by microbial action in manure and feed.[7–9] Air sampling studies have found total dust concentrations ranging from about 1 to 40 milligrams/m^3 of air (mg/m^3); respirable dust levels are much lower, in the range of 0·5 to 5 mg/m^3. Daily time-weighted average dust concentrations often exceed current occupational health standards for nuisance particulates, as well as proposed health guidelines of 2·5 mg/m^3 for total dust and 0·23 mg/m^3 for respirable dusts (based on respiratory studies of swine producers).[10–12]

Endotoxins (lipopolysaccharide fractions of the cell wall of Gram-negative bacteria) have been measured at concentrations ranging from 10 to 10 000 endotoxin units/m^3 of air (EU/m^3), often in excess of the suggested health guidelines (90 EU/m^3).[8 13–15] Airborne concentrations of bacteria have been found to range from 10^4 to 10^7 colony forming units/m^3 of air (CFU/m^3).[8 15–16] Bacteria recovered from livestock facilities have included various species of *Staphylococcus, Pseudomonas, Acinetobacter, E. coli, Enterobacter* and other genera.[8 17] Genera of fungi include *Aspergillus, Penicillium, Fusarium, Mucor, Cladosporium, Alternaria* and others.[16] Airborne concentrations of fungi tend to be several orders of magnitude lower, although some activities, such as bedding, and chopping and pitchforking of hay, produce levels of fungi and thermophilic bacteria as

269

high as 10^{10} CFU/m^3.[16] Measurements of total microorganisms (culturable and non-culturable) indicate that up to 95% of total airborne organisms may be non-culturable.[16] Airborne levels of mycotoxins have usually been extremely low, but deoxynivalenol (vomitoxin) and fumonisin B-1 have been detected in dairy barns at 1 to 5 micrograms/m^3 of air (μg/m^3).[16] Storage and predator mites (*Lepidoglyphus*, *Acarus*, *Tyrophagus*, *Caloglyphus*, *Chortoglyphus*, *Glycophagus*, and *Euroglyphus*) have been recovered from samples of dairy barn dust. Airborne levels of *L. destructor* reactivity as high as 12 μg/m^3 have been found using RAST-inhibition assays.[16 18]

Hydrogen sulphide, a potent respiratory irritant and toxin having a characteristic odour of rotten eggs, is produced by anaerobic bacterial activity in manure pits. If manure is undisturbed, airborne levels of hydrogen sulphide typically remain below a few parts per million (ppm). However, when liquid manure is agitated in swine facilities, hydrogen sulphide can be released at levels high enough to kill animals and humans (700 to 2000 ppm).[7] Ammonia, a highly reactive and alkaline irritant gas is also produced from microbial degradation of urea and uric acid.[19 20] Time-weighted average concentrations of ammonia greater than 100 ppm have been reported in turkey barns, far in excess of the current Occupational Safety and Health Administration permissible exposure limit of 25 ppm.[8] Levels in swine and chicken facilities also often exceed the level of 7 ppm suggested as a guideline based on studies of lung function changes in swine production workers.[7 11] A substantial proportion (15% to 25%) of ammonia is associated with particles, which may increase retention time in the respiratory system. During silo filling, nitrogen oxides are formed by enzymatic degradation of plant nitrates producing NO, NO$_2$, and N$_2$O$_4$.[16] For days after filling the silo, nitrogen dioxide often exceeds the permissible exposure limit of 3 ppm, and may reach levels as high as 2000 ppm. Farmers may also be exposed in confined areas to carbon monoxide and other combustion products from power washers, heaters, and other devices that use gas or diesel fuels.

Airborne concentrations of gases, dusts, and microorganisms are highest during activities such as tilling of bedding, agitation of manure, and during animal handling.[8] Season may also have a substantial effect in northern climates, exposure levels being much higher during the winter when buildings are closed to preserve heat.[8] Other exposures that are common to both traditional range production and confined production include injuries by the animals.

Crops

Production of crops exemplifies the variety of practices and exposures found in agriculture. Occupational exposures depend on the type of crop (grains, vegetables, fruits), and the size of the operation. On smaller farms, workers may be involved in the whole production cycle including soil preparation, planting, maintenance, harvest, storage, and transport. On larger units, jobs are often more specialised. Preparation of soil for planting involves tilling fields, discing, ploughing, and other activities requiring physical labour and the use of heavy machines. In addition to continued use of machinery during planting and growing of crops, workers may mix and apply fertilisers, insecticides, herbicides, fungicides, and other agricultural chemicals. Harvest involves manual labour (primarily for vegetables and fruits often provided by seasonal or migrant workers), or the use of combines, corn-pickers and other heavy machines. Workers performing these tasks are exposed to ultraviolet radiation from the sun, extremes of temperature and humidity, noise, ergonomic stresses, mechanical hazards, organic and inorganic dusts, and agricultural chemicals.

Additional activities include maintenance and repair of equipment, buildings, and fences. These may involve the use of power tools, and operations such as welding. This results in potential exposure to welding fumes, electrical hazards, solvents, and potential physical injury from tools.

Machines and equipment

The workhorse of the farm is the tractor. In addition to pulling equipment such as discs, harrows, planters, ploughs, balers, mowers, and other devices, tractors may provide the power to run machines such as elevator augers and feed grinders through power take-off connections. Although changes in tractor design have contributed significantly to improved safety, a large number of older tractors are still used for some of the most dangerous jobs. The narrow wheel base, and travel over sloping unstable ground contribute to tractor roll overs, responsible for about half of the traumatic fatalities in agriculture.[21] The lack of enclosed cabs on older vehicles, and extra riders who are often children, are also factors in tractor fatalities. Unguarded, rotating power take-offs are capable of catching clothing and wrapping arms, legs, or hair rapidly around moving parts.[6 22] This can result in extreme injuries including broken bones, "degloving" (the skin is pulled off the underlying muscles) and scalping injuries. Newer tractors tend to be larger and more stable with a wider wheel base, enclosed cabs, and shields or guards designed to enclose moving parts. Machines such as mowers, combines, corn pickers, and hay balers present the opportunity for crushing and cutting injuries from moving parts and blades.[6 22] Rotating parts on manure spreaders, feed grinders, and elevator augers also present the opportunity for entrapment of clothing and body parts on to the rotating shafts.[22] Newer machines with guards and other safety devices are less hazardous.

All terrain vehicles, snowmobiles, and motorcycles are unstable and are

271

often used in some areas for farm work. In addition to capsizes, workers using skid loaders have had limbs crushed between the moving parts. The use of slow moving farm vehicles on local roads has also contributed to automobile crashes. Noise is an important hazard from farm machines, especially tractors.[23][24] The use of leaded paint on farm equipment and leaded fuels has contributed to a potential for lead exposure among farmers, and the fuel stored in tanks above or below ground presents a fire hazard, as well as contributing to occupational exposure and contamination of wells and ground water.

In addition to mobile equipment, farmers are exposed to physical hazards from fixed machines such as grain dryers, which produce noise and the potential for injury from moving parts. Repair of equipment and buildings includes tasks such as welding and brazing, use of power tools, and exposure to a wide variety of paints and solvents used in maintenance of farm equipment.

Agricultural chemicals

Since the 1940s there has been explosive growth in the number of chemicals used in agriculture. On modern farms these include fertilisers, herbicides, crop insecticides, animal insecticides, fumigants, fungicides, antibiotics, vaccines, disinfectants, and other compounds. There are more than 50 000 kinds of registered pesticides alone. The number of pesticides applied has decreased in recent years as a result of production of more potent and efficient chemicals and the institution of integrated pest management and other conservation practices. The development of less toxic materials in packages requiring less handling has substantially reduced the risk of exposure, but acute chemical poisoning and chronic health effects, such as cancer, remain a concern.[25-27]

Pesticides are used in a variety of formulations consisting of active ingredients, carriers such as organic solvents or water, surface active ingredients (stickers, spreaders), stabilisers, dyes, and other chemicals.[28] The physical form may be solid, liquid solution, liquid emulsion, or vapour. Pesticides may be applied by tractors and sprayers, fixed pumping systems, aeroplanes, and helicopters. Individual backpack sprayers and other more labour intensive methods are also used. Potential exposures to dusts, aerosols, fogs, fumes, smokes, spray droplets, or vapours can occur during mixing, application, entry into fields, transport, or storage.[6] Dermal absorption is the most important route of exposure for many pesticides.[29] Factors affecting the efficiency of dermal absorption include the specific pesticide used (chemical structure, molecular size, solubility), location on the body, body moisture, temperature, and the use of protective clothing.

Veterinary medicines present opportunities for exposure during preparation and use. Antibiotics are often added to feed or water. Mixing of antibiotics is often done in rooms with little or no ventilation, and substantial levels of airborne dust can be generated. Vaccines may be given by injection, either by hand or with powered injection devices; in both there is potential for needle stick injuries. Necrosis of tissue is not uncommon following accidental injection of vaccines into workers. Backpack sprayers are used in some poultry facilities to aerosolise attenuated or killed viruses. Although there are few data on this practice, exposed workers have complained of respiratory symptoms.

Livestock facilities are cleaned and disinfected using a variety of chemicals and soaps.[8] Disinfectant solutions may be applied by power washers, low pressure sprays, fogging machines, or direct liquid application. Although the less hazardous quaternary ammonium compounds are gaining in popularity, phenols and formaldehyde solutions are still used. A unique exposure is from a commercial device that emits ozone, ostensibly to reduce airborne particles.

Exposure assessment and control

Exposure assessment of agricultural workers can be particularly difficult given the diversity of contaminants, seasonal patterns, the variety of tasks performed, and the mobility of workers. Sampling and analytical methods have been developed for most of the contaminants. Strategies for sample collection and the interpretation of data, however, have proved more intransigent.

Air monitoring

Air sampling has been used particularly to characterise exposures inside enclosed livestock facilities. Although the data are of limited value in determining health risks, they are useful for engineering control purposes. Personal breathing zone sampling is more appropriate for estimation of individual exposures, taking into account the effects of different tasks and locations over time. The sampling period may consist of the whole work shift, eight hours or more, or may be limited to shorter time periods that reflect the duration of specific tasks. Variables most commonly measured are dust, gases, microorganisms, endotoxins, and pesticides.

Airborne dust is collected on preweighed non-hygroscopic filters in 37 mm plastic cassettes, using sampling pumps at flow rates of one to two litres a minute.[8 10 11] Filters that have been used include PVC, Teflon, glass fibre, and polycarbonate. Cellulose acetate performs poorly because it gains weight from absorption of moisture. The change in mass is measured gravimetrically and the airborne mass concentration is calculated. In enclosed livestock environments, open-faced filter cassettes have been found to undersample compared with close-faced. Data on particle size distributions have been gathered with the use of cascade impactors, inspirable mass samplers, and respirable cyclones. Care must be taken to operate these devices at prescribed flow rates to ensure that performance characteristics related to particle collection efficiencies are met.[8] Standard validated sampling procedures published by the National Institute of Occupational Safety and Health are available for dust sampling, and are applicable to agricultural environments.

There is no accepted standard method of sampling and analysis of endotoxins. Endotoxins can be collected on a variety of filters using 37 mm cassettes at flow rates of about one to two litres per minute. Filter materials that have been used include glass fibre, polycarbonate, Teflon, and cellulose acetate.[14 30 31] Endotoxin is currently extracted from filters by one of three different methods: (1) agitation in sterile pyrogen free water at room temperature for two hours; (2) heating in pyrogen free water at 37 °C for 30 minutes; or (3) agitation in a buffer solution for one hour at 20 °C. Although gas chromatograph-mass spectrometry and high pressure liquid chromatography are capable of measuring chemical components, endotoxin is usually assayed using methods based on activation of an enzyme from horseshoe crabs, the Limulus Amoebocyte Lysate (LAL) test. LAL assays now use an endpoint chromogenic method and a kinetic chromogenic method. The optimum filter type, extraction method, and analytical procedure have not yet been identified, and it appears that the performance of different methods varies depending on the type of environment (swine, poultry, grain handling).[30]

Measurement of bioaerosols is accomplished by either microbial cascade impactors (Andersen microbial samplers) with selective media, or the All-Glass Impingers-30.[8 32] The Andersen microbial sampler is easily overwhelmed at the high bioaerosol concentrations associated with enclosed livestock buildings, silo unloading, and other operations. The All-Glass Impingers-30 offer advantages in that serial dilutions can be prepared from one sample and plated onto a number of selective media. Trypticase soy agar or blood agar are commonly used for culturing of total bacteria, while MacConkey's or eosin methylene blue agar have been used for Gram-negative bacteria. Use of MacConkey's agar may result in undersampling compared to the more nutrient-rich eosin methylene blue.[8] Collection of bioaerosols on polycarbonate filters with subsequent fluorescent microscopic analysis can be used to calculate total cultural and non-culturable bacteria and fungi.[32] Immunological components of bacteria, such as dander and mites, have been sampled using high volume samplers with glass fibre or Gortex filters, and analysed by RAST-inhibition assays.[18]

Gases such as carbon dioxide, ammonia, and sulphur compounds have been measured by a variety of published methods including colorimetric detector tubes, passive dosimeters, solid sorbent tubes with the gas chromatograph and gas chromatograph-mass spectrometer analysis, gas bags or bottles, and impingers with liquid solutions.[7] Ammonia is usually sampled by impingers containing dilute sulphuric acid, and analysed by specific ion electrode, wet chemistry, or ion chromatography.[19] The physicochemical interactions of reactive gases with particles and other airborne constituents present a difficult exposure assessment problem. Annular denuders and impingers with prefilters have been used to study the distribution of ammonia between gas and particle absorbed phases. The intermittent generation of gases such as hydrogen sulphide also presents an important problem for sampling.

Direct reading instruments have been used to measure noise, heat and humidity, dust, and gases including ammonia and carbon monoxide. Problems can be encountered with direct reading instruments that are affected by extreme temperatures and high dust levels. For example, although portable infrared detectors (MIRAN) can collect much data on many gases, they are not robust and can be damaged by high dust and ammonia concentrations. Ventilation in enclosed livestock buildings can also be evaluated by measuring air flow speeds and volumes with velometers and anemometers.[8] The large number of openings, the contribution of natural ventilation, and the tendency for fans to turn on and off automatically make precise measurement difficult.

Dermal assessment

Dermal contact is the most common route of exposure to pesticides.[29] Gauze pads or patches containing charcoal can be attached to the forearms, chest, back, and other body surfaces to collect material for subsequent analysis by high pressure liquid chromatography and other chemical methods.[29] Limitations of this approach include potential lack of uniformity between deposition on different body parts, and that absorption characteristics of the pads may be different from human skin. Addition of fluorescent tracer dyes to pesticides while being mixed or applied has allowed visualisation of deposition on workers' bodies.[33] Although quantification of deposition using an image sensing system and computer is under development, this remains primarily a research tool.

Task-based questionnaires

Supplementary information on exposure can be obtained by questionnaires concerning the types and duration of tasks that workers perform.

Biological monitoring

Biological monitoring can be used to measure the absorbed dose or biological effects of some agents. Measurement of cholinesterase in

275

workers exposed to organophosphate or carbamate pesticides is one of the few examples of biological monitoring in agriculture.[28]

Exposure control

Control of occupational exposures in agriculture is difficult primarily because of the isolation, mobility, and social environment of the workers.[6] Personal protective equipment, including dust masks, air purifying respirators, safety shoes, and protective clothing that should be used to minimise personal exposure, is sometimes difficult to obtain and is not readily accepted by workers. Engineering controls and changes in work practises are generally more effective in reducing exposure. Reduction of airborne agents in enclosed livestock facilities has been achieved by advances in ventilation, more frequent removal of manure, and addition of compounds such as fatty oils to animal feed.[8 20] Advances in farm equipment design have led to the introduction of shields for moving parts such as power take-offs, roll-over protection on tractors, and safety interlocks on skid loaders. Although health and safety regulations may help to reduce exposure, implementation and enforcement of regulations is difficult. As agriculture becomes more industrialised, and workers specialised, implementation of safety programmes similar to those that have been successful in manufacturing industries may become more feasible. Education remains an important component of exposure control strategies for the agricultural community.

Agricultural injuries

The rural context

In the United States, the epidemic of agricultural injuries is just part of the larger risk of accidental injuries in rural communities.[22] Epidemiological data show that the risk of death from unintentional injury is significantly higher in rural than in urban areas. In an analysis of United States deaths from unintentional injuries in the years 1980–1986, Baker found that the mortality in rural remote areas (population at risk, 4·0 million) was 66/100 000; for rural, non-remote areas (population at risk, 51·6 million) 53/100 000; but for large cities, only 39/100 000.[5] Rural communities have a disproportionate share of the injury mortality from both motor vehicle fatalities and other unintentional injuries. The ratio of rural to urban fatality rates was 2:1 or greater for a wide variety of injuries including drownings, motor vehicle crashes, unintentional firearm injuries, electrocutions, and house fires. In 1992, the United States National Safety Council (1993) found that 25 900—almost two thirds of the 40 300 motor vehicle fatalities—occurred in rural areas. Analysis of the United States National Highway Traffic Administration's fatal accident reporting system data for the years 1979–1981 showed that mortality was inversely correlated with population density.[4] This increased mortality was attributed to a number of causes including higher speeds in rural areas, poorer roads and infrastructure, less use of seat belts, greater prevalence of high risk trucks and utility vehicles, and poorer access to trauma care.

Some of this increased injury mortality might be attributed to the large number of poor people living in rural communities. Of the 45 million non-elderly rural residents, almost one fifth (8·3 million) have incomes below the poverty line of $11 600 for a family of four.[3] Rural communities account for one third of America's poor, and there is good evidence that poor people have higher unintentional injury rates.[5] However, Baker has shown that rural counties have the highest unintentional injury mortality rates regardless of average income.[5]

Mortality studies

It is widely agreed that workers in agriculture have a high risk of occupational injury, but measuring the risk is not easy. In the United States, two systems of data collection are useful: one maintained by the National Institute of Occupational Safety and Health and the other by the National Safety Council. Since 1980, the National Institute of Occupational Safety and Health has maintained the National Traumatic Occupational Fatality Register to track occupational fatalities in the United States. The system is based on data from death certificates and includes all deaths of people 16 years old or older from an external cause (International Classification of Diseases, Ninth Revision, E800–E999), certified as caused by an "injury at work." Because the certifiers do not code all occupational fatalities appropriately, this system is likely to underreport agricultural fatalities, especially among older workers.[34] In addition, the Register excludes all fatalities among farm children under 16 years of age. Even given these caveats, over the decade 1980–1989, the register indicated that agriculture (including forestry and fishing) was one of the four most dangerous industries in the United States, the occupational fatality rate being 18·33/100 000 workers. Only mining, construction, and transportation had higher mortality rates.

The National Safety Council database begins with the National Center for Health Statistics death certificate database, but adjusts it to account for missing or incomplete information using a set of assumptions known as the three-way split.[35] This database includes work-related deaths among all workers aged 14 years and older. Using these methods, the National Safety Council (1993) found that agriculture was the most dangerous industry in the United States with an occupational injury fatality rate of 37/100 000 compared with an all industry average of 7/100 000. The National Safety Council data suggest that agriculture has been the most dangerous industry in the United States for most of the past decade, followed closely by mining, and then by construction and transportation. While relative positions have been stable over the past decade, the absolute rates of occupational injury fatalities have decreased. In 1983, agriculture had 52 injury fatalities/100 000—41% higher than in 1992. A similar reduction was seen in most other industries. Studies in several states have found similar patterns.[36] [37]

Machine-related fatalities (6·28/100 000) and motor vehicle fatalities (2·88/100 000) together accounted for more than half the deaths. Using the National Traumatic Occupational Fatality Register for 1980–1985, Etherton et al. studied all machine-related fatal occupational injuries.[21] Of the 5061 machine-related fatalities, agricultural machines accounted for 2216 deaths—369 per year. Of the fatalities from agricultural machinery, 69% involved tractors. Of the tractor-related fatalities 52% were rollovers, emphasising the continued importance of this preventable injury. In another 16% the victim was run over, often after falling from the tractor, and about 7% were power takeoff injuries. This pattern is similar to that noted in Wisconsin from 1961–1975.

Farm fatalities are a special problem among two age groups: the old and the young. The National Traumatic Occupational Fatality Register data show that agricultural fatality rates increase with age[38]: 18·9/100 000 among 20–24 years old to 26·5/100 000 among 55–64 years old, and 52·3/100 000 among those 65 years old and older (see also Myers).[39] This dramatically increased fatality rate among farmers 65 years old and older is particularly impressive when we recall the previously mentioned evidence suggesting underreporting of work-related fatalities in that age group.[34]

Farms present lethal risks not only for the farmer, but also for the farm family and in particular for farm children. Using death certificates for Kentucky for the years 1979–1985, Stallones showed that 30·2% of the unintentional injury fatalities among boys and 38·5% among girls were caused by farm machinery.[40] Using national statistics for the years 1979–1981, Rivara found 286 fatal farm injuries/year among those 19 years of age and younger, and 51/year among those less than four years old.[41] Seven eighths of these deaths were machine-related and again, tractors were the machines most often responsible.

Morbidity studies

Until recently, most investigations of non-fatal agricultural injuries were simple case studies.[42] Such numerator data without any denominator for comparison were of little use in identifying the most important risk factors. Recently, however, a number of cohort studies and population based studies have begun to explore this territory.

Several recent studies have focused on dairy farms. In New York state, Pratt et al. followed a cohort of 600 farmers on 201 dairy farms for two years.[43] Monthly telephone calls ascertained any injuries among the cohort. The overall injury rate was 16·6/100 farmers/year. The rate was 19·5% among men, compared with 6·9% among women. This increased relative risk among men remained even when corrected for hours worked. Injury rates were slightly higher for older farmers, but did not show the dramatic increase among those over 65 years of age that the mortality data showed. Almost 60% of the injuries occurred in the barn. Although machinery was associated with 35% of the injuries, animals were also important, and caused 32% of the injuries. A Vermont study found that livestock were involved in 38% of the dairy farmer injuries and that these resulted in longer periods of disability than the injuries not caused by livestock.[44] In Ontario, Canada, a one year prospective study followed dairy and beef farmers monthly. The overall injury rate was only 7·0/100 farmer-years. Farmers older than 60 years had 2·6 times the risk of injury as those aged 20–39 years. Beef farmers had a relative injury risk of 2·3 compared with dairy farmers.

Using a population-based random sample in Alabama, Zhou and Roseman[45] interviewed 718 farmers with a response rate of 86·2%.[45] The cumulative one-year incidence of injuries was 9·9%. Machinery (28·6%), falls (23·2%), and animals (12·5%) caused the largest number of injuries. Forestry and dairy farms were the riskiest. In contrast to the findings in New York and Ontario, in Alabama farmers older than 64 years had only 38% of the risk of injury of farmers 25–44 years old. Alcohol consumption was associated with injury rates and showed a clear dose response pattern; however, the 95% confidence intervals at each level of consumption barely included one. As alcohol use has been clearly associated with a number of other unintentional injuries, this association with farm injuries is not unexpected, but had not been reported previously. Finally, the presence of residual impairment from a previous injury was a cause of a repeat injury (odds ratio, 3·71).

Analysing five years (1986–1990) of data from the National Health Interview Survey, investigators from the National Institute of Occupational Safety and Health calculated the prevalence of impairment and chronic disease among United States farmers.[46] Compared with other currently employed workers, farmers had an age-adjusted prevalence risk ratio of 2·8 for amputations. The excess risk persisted even when farmers were compared with blue collar workers. Farmers had evidence of impairment not only from acute but also from chronic trauma; for example, their age-adjusted prevalence risk ratio for arthritis was 1·4. The increased risk of arthritis was most evident at an earlier age, with a prevalence risk ratio of 2·2 among farmers aged 35–49 years. These results are consistent with the work of Thelin who, in a case-control study, found that operations for hip joint arthritis were more common among those with at least 10 years in farming (odds ratio, 3·2).[47]

Methodological issues

Even so straightforward a task as counting the number of agricultural fatalities is laden with methodological difficulties. In part, these are related to the means used to collect the data, but in part they are tied to conceptual difficulties of defining an agricultural injury. In the United States, three systems have been used to count occupational fatalities. The Bureau of Labor Statistics estimates injury rates with an annual survey of about 250 000 establishments. Unfortunately, United States law exempts employers with 10 or fewer employees from regulation and thus they are excluded from the survey—effectively excluding 89% of American farmers.

The National Safety Council estimates start with death certificates and then apportion injuries to work, home, or public, based on external cause and age. This strategy can be criticised as arbitrary and may have special difficulties with unusual industries such as agriculture in which occupation is often not defined or recorded. Finally, the National Institute of Occupational Safety and Health's National Traumatic Occupational Fatality Register system is limited by its dependence on the death certificate category "work-related" which may often be miscoded, especially in agriculture. The National Traumatic Occupational Fatality Register also assumes that the usual industry noted on the death certificates is the industry at which the deceased was working when the fatal injury occurred.

A study in the state of Pennsylvania compared information from the National Traumatic Occupational Fatality Register with data from a news clipping service and found that the register undercounted the agricultural deaths by 20%.[48] The recent creation of a new database, the Bureau of Labor Statistics' Census of Fatal Occupational Injuries may improve the situation. This new system uses a collaborative federal-state approach based on a variety of sources including death certificates, workers' compensation records, Occupational Safety and Health Administration reports, medical examiner reports, and police motor vehicle crash records.[49] In 1992, the Census of Fatal Occupational Injuries recorded 24 agricultural deaths/100 000 compared with the National Safety Council estimate of 37/100 000.

In part, these continuing difficulties may be related to differences in the definition of an agricultural injury. Because farms are often residences as well as workplaces, the work-relatedness of an injury is not always clear. For example, it is work-related when a farmer is injured using a farm tool for something other than farm production (using a tractor to give the children a hay ride)? Or when a child is injured falling from a tractor that she was riding while her dad worked? Or when a repairmen is injured fixing farm machinery on the farm? Or when the farmer is injured during a leisure activity on the farm such as swimming or shooting? Or when work is interrupted, such as when a farmer stops to help a stranded motorist and is injured? Murphy has proposed a classification code for farm injuries to account for the complexity of the agricultural environment, but it has not yet been generally accepted.[50]

Diseases

Respiratory

Agricultural respiratory exposures may be classified into four broad categories each of which contains a large number of specific agents (table 12.1).[1] By far the most common exposure leading to agricultural respiratory disease is to organic dust. While nearly all agricultural workers are exposed to some organic dust, workers who process textile fibres and grain often have high exposures, resulting in substantial risk of acute and chronic airway disease. Microbial components of organic dusts are increasingly recognised as important aetiological agents in acute febrile syndromes, airway inflammation and pulmonary hypersensitivity. Naturally occurring inhaled foreign proteins, including animal proteins,

Table 12.1 *Agricultural exposures and respiratory health effects*

Exposure	Health effects
Vegetable dusts: grain, cotton, flax, hemp, tobacco, coffee, tea, herbal tea, castor bean, soya bean, spices, pollens, and others	rhinitis asthma chronic bronchitis airways obstruction
Microorganisms: fungi and bacteria, including the thermophilic bacteria	febrile syndromes (mill fever, grain fever, mycotoxicosis, atypical farmer's lung, silo unloaders syndrome) hypersensitivity pneumonitis (farmer's lung, maple bark stripper's lung, bagassosis, among others)
Animal danders, proteins	rhinitis asthma hypersensitivity pneumonitis
Insects: mites, weevils, and others	rhinitis asthma hypersensitivity pneumonitis
Chemicals: ammonia hydrogen sulphide oxides of nitrogen fumigants fungicides herbicides insecticides rodenticides	rhinitis asthma bronchitis/bronchiolitis airways obstruction pulmonary oedema

mites and other insects, are now recognised as important sensitisers in allergic rhinitis and asthma.[18] Agricultural chemicals, indigenous to modern agriculture, provide additional sensitisers, irritants, and sometimes agents of pulmonary fibrosis.

An acute febrile response to high exposures to mouldy vegetable textile fibres, as occurs in the retting of flax, or in work with mouldy grain, hay, or silage, is now recognised as the organic dust toxic syndrome.[51] This syndrome is characterised by cough, fever, chills, weakness, myalgias, arthralgias, headache, extreme fatigue, and often anorexia and intolerance of smoking. The organic dust toxic syndrome may occur in epidemic form with high attack rates among exposed workers. Symptoms typically begin six to ten hours after exposure and may be severe enough to require admission to hospital and respiratory support. Bronchoalveolar lavage in affected workers has shown massive airway inflammation and evidence of bacterial and fungal contamination, both of which may persist for weeks.[52] In a prevalence survey of Wisconsin dairy farmers, nearly a quarter reported episodic febrile symptoms were consistent with this syndrome. Many dairy farmers report multiple episodes, which typically resolve spontaneously without medical attention. There is limited evidence that increasing numbers of episodes of the syndrome may progressively reduce lung function.[53]

Airway inflammation and obstruction from exposure to organic dusts, endotoxins and mycotoxins, mites, animal proteins, and some chemical agents are now well documented among agricultural workers. The airway diseases arising from these exposures include allergic rhinitis, asthma, bronchitis, and bronchiolitis.[1] Multiple cross-sectional studies of agricultural workers processing cotton, flax, hemp, and grain have documented dose-related increases in bronchitis and decreased expiratory flow rates during a working shift.[54 55] Workers exposed to these organic dusts over time have chronic airways obstruction attributable to respirable dust exposure, smoking being a second powerful risk factor. The World Health Organisation has recommended permissible exposure limits for vegetable textile dusts based on dose-related prevalence of byssinosis.[56] Similar recommendations have not been made for grain dusts.

Occupational asthma arising from exposures to grain dust, irritant gases (including ammonia and oxides of nitrogen) and from organophosphate pesticides is now well documented.[57] Measurements of airway hyperresponsiveness by methacholine or histamine challenge are increasingly used in epidemiological studies to assess airway response objectively. Agricultural workers who come into the workforce with airway hyperresponsiveness or who develop it as the result of exposure frequently select themselves out of agricultural jobs.[1] Cross-sectional studies therefore underestimate the asthma risk from agricultural work. As previously found with exposures to Western red cedar and cotton dust, prospective studies of workers with swine in confined spaces have shown an increased risk of progressive loss of lung function among workers, and acute, cross-shift reductions in lung function.[57–59] Management of occupational asthma in farmers who cannot or will not leave farming, which is often the case, is dependent on avoidance of exposure and respiratory protection, both of which are difficult to achieve in the agricultural environment.

Farmers face increased risks of fatal chemical pneumonitis and pulmonary oedema from high exposures to ammonia and hydrogen sulphide in confined animal houses, and to oxides of nitrogen from silos.[1] Dangerously high levels of anhydrous ammonia from spills from storage tanks, and spills of several irritant pesticides may also result in chemical pneumonitis, bronchiolitis, and pulmonary fibrosis. Paraquat is especially dangerous, when accidentally ingested or inhaled, and is a potent cause of pulmonary fibrosis.[60] Whereas these agriculturally related lung diseases are well recognised as a result of numerous case studies, because they are relatively uncommon they have not been systematically evaluated in population-based studies.

Hypersensitivity pneumonitis, or allergic alveolitis in the form of farmer's lung, have been well documented by epidemiological studies in Scotland, France, Sweden, Finland, Canada and the United States. Definitions vary: some investigators define farmer's lung to include exposure-related dyspnea together with serological evidence of antibodies to one or more antigens commonly found in mouldy hay or silage. Modern ELISA assays, which have replaced the traditional double immunodiffusion precipitin test, now show that a substantially higher proportion of farmers have antibodies to these farmer's lung antigens.[61] Epidemiological investigation of Wisconsin dairy farmers found the prevalence of farmer's lung to be less than 1%, but airway obstruction and bronchitis to be common, as among other farmers.[62] Merchant et al. in a nested case-control study of Wisconsin dairy farmers, found no evidence that farmers with antibodies to farmer's lung antigens had increased airway hyperresponsiveness or poorer lung function.[63]

Cancer

Epidemiological studies of agricultural cohorts have shown excess risks of cancer of the lip, stomach, brain, prostate, connective tissues, and the lymphatic and haematopoietic system among male farmers.[64–66] These associations have not been found in all studies.[67] Some studies have linked exposures with increased rates of certain cancers among farm women— ovarian cancer with triazine herbicides, breast cancer with some insecticides,[68 69] and various pesticides with multiple myeloma and non-Hodgkin's lymphoma.[70 71] In the United States, these excesses appear despite evidence that people on farms smoke less and have consistently lower mortality from all causes, heart disease, and many other cancers. As a result, the excess organ-specific cancer rates observed among farm workers are not likely to be occurring by chance.

The strongest link between agricultural chemical exposure and cancer has been found for the haematopoietic and lymphatic systems. Non-Hodgkin's lymphoma has been linked to phenoxyacetic acid herbicides in many studies, but not in all.[72–74] Non-Hodgkin's lymphoma has also been found to be more prevalent among grain millers exposed to fumigants, including phosphine and other insecticides,[75] and among forest and soil conservationists.[76] Insecticides and fungicides have been associated with increased rates among farmers of non-Hodgkin's lymphoma,[74] leukae-mia,[64] and multiple myeloma,[77] and a trend has been observed between leukaemia and duration of exposure among agricultural extension agents.[78] These studies are clearly important to our understanding of the aetiology and prevention of these cancers, but they also have important implications for those who are exposed to these agents from applications to lawns, gardens, parks, golf courses, aerial spraying in residential areas, and indoor application to plants in the home. While these cancer risks are difficult to calculate in non-occupationally exposed populations (because of low dose and poor exposure characterisation) studies of large cohorts of farmers and farm family members may overcome these difficulties.[66]

Renal

Acute and chronic renal diseases occur in agricultural populations. Nephrotoxicity has been associated with both organophosphates and chlorinated hydrocarbons.[79] Acute tubular necrosis, azotaemia, and chronic interstitial nephritis may follow acute poisoning by arsenic-containing insecticides,[80] and a number of adverse renal effects follow exposures to hexachlorobenzene, 2,4,5-T, and TCDD.[81] Several studies have shown increased risks of acute and chronic renal disease following exposure to organic solvents,[79 82] but no case–control study has evaluated the risk from their use as carriers of pesticides. Cohort studies of pesticide manufacturers and applicators have not adequately considered the risk of death from renal disease, but the cohorts have been small, renal disease is usually underreported on death certificates, and agricultural work is often misclassified and underreported. An association between cadmium polluted soil, increased levels of urinary cadmium, and poor renal function has been reported,[83] suggesting a potentially important environmental risk of renal disease in regions where cadmium from smelters or contaminated fertiliser pollute the soil.

Neurological

Acute neurotoxicity of pesticides, particularly from exposures to organophosphates, is well established. In addition, it has now become clear that persistent neurotoxic effects may result from acute pesticide poisoning.[84] Chronic exposures to pesticides have been linked to a number of clinical outcomes including reduced nerve conduction velocity, decreased sensory acuity, poorer neurobehavioural performance using standard test batteries, and non-specific symptoms including insomnia, mood alterations, and cognitive impairment. While epidemiological findings are still unclear, pesticides have also been proposed as causes of neurodegenerative diseases, including Alzheimer's disease, Parkinson's disease, and amyotrophic lateral sclerosis.[85–87] Rosenstock et al. published evidence that these conditions are more often observed in developing countries where more toxic pesticides are used, where exposures are often higher, and where environmental controls are less often available or used.[84] Large cohort studies of chronically exposed agricultural workers with linkage to neurodegenerative disease registries are an important priority for agricultural chemical research.

Reproductive

Adverse reproductive and developmental outcomes have been linked to agricultural chemical exposures. These have included menstrual cycle impairment from oestrogenic properties of organochlorine and organophosphate pesticides,[88] increased rates of spontaneous abortion among pesticide-exposed women,[89] and an association with increased risk of stillbirths.[90] Data regarding low birth weight and prematurity are unclear. There are some animal data suggesting that some pesticides retard fetal development, but good epidemiological data are not yet available.[88] Isacson and Munger observed low birth weights among women living in proximity to, and drinking water from, a reservoir that was heavily contaminated with agricultural chemicals.[27]

Other evidence of potential adverse developmental effects of pesticides come from studies of lactating women. An inverse correlation between duration of lactation and concentration of DEE (a stable degradation product of DDT) has been observed among North Carolina women.[91] Further evidence of a possible linkage to pesticide exposure and lactation dysfunction has been reported among Bedouin women who had seasonal lactation failure.[92] These findings are additionally important because of the role lactation plays in population control and in providing immunity to infants from endemic infectious diseases.

Dermatoses and zoonoses

Agricultural workers are exposed to a host of irritant and sensitising plants, and a large number of irritant agricultural chemicals, some of which are skin sensisers, arthropod bites and stings, in addition to heat, cold, and ultraviolet radiation. It is therefore not surprising that a review of a representative random sample of 280 000 private employers through the United States Bureau of Labor Statistics Annual Survey of Occupational Injuries and Illnesses, for the years 1973 through 1984, found the agricultural sector consistently to have the highest incidence of occupational dermatoses.[93] Skin disease was found to account for almost two thirds of all occupational illness in the agricultural sector.

A series of studies of California agricultural workers by O'Malley et al. established that agricultural workers are at high risk of occupational dermatoses. An assessment of over 14 000 workers' compensation cases of skin disease found agriculture to have the highest rate of any industrial sector, crop and livestock production ranking highest.[94] An assessment of 2722 claims for skin conditions causing time lost from work between 1978 and 1983, found causes most often attributed to plants (52·1%), chemical exposures (20·4%), and food products (12·5%). Forestry had the highest rate attributed to plants, horticulture the highest rate attributed to chemical exposure, and vegetable and melon subdivision the highest rate attributed to food products.

The California Pesticide Illness Surveillance Program provides further information regarding agricultural dermatoses. Eight active chemical ingredients or mixtures accounted for over half the cases, propargylate and sulphur preparations being by far the most common.[95] Crop service workers, especially ground applicators, and field workers were both found to be at high risk of pesticide related skin disease. This surveillance system has provided useful information, but the authors caution that the data suffer from underreporting and from limited sensitivity and specificity. A further methodological problem is that contact dermatitis, often reported as arising from an agricultural chemical exposure, is commonly confounded by exposures to numerous naturally occurring sensitisers.

Few targeted epidemiological studies of agricultural dermatoses have been undertaken. Cross-sectional studies have shown that okra cultivation commonly results in both contact and irritant dermatitis,[96] and that grape workers are more likely to have contact dermatitis and lichenified hand dermatitis than citrus or tomato workers. Despite the high prevalence of agriculturally related skin disease, evaluations of intervention schemes have not been reported and the use of personal protective equipment among farm workers is uncommon.

In addition to the common agricultural dermatoses, there are numerous dermatological zoonoses arising from exposure to dermatophytes, viruses, and bacteria transmitted from an infected animal or a contaminated object, such as a brush used on an infected animal.[97] The most common dermatophytes in farm animals arise from *Trichophyton* and *Microsporum* species and include *T. mentagrophytes, T. verrucosum, T. equinum,* and *M. canis.* The hosts for these fungi are cattle, dogs, and horses, but may include other livestock and wild animals. The dermatitis is characterised by pustular folliculitis with loss of hair, and may result in scarring. Direct contact with infected hosts is not necessary as the fungal hyphae may remain viable on contaminated objects for years. Prevention of these infections includes the use of gloves, changing of contaminated clothing, and hand washing with antifungal soap.

Pox viruses in cattle may be transmitted to man directly or by contaminated objects and cause milker's nodule and orf.[97][98] These dermatoses are clinically indistinguishable and present as reddish blue papules that mature into haemorrhagic pustules. Prevention is by sanitation, use of personal protective gloves and clothing, and vaccination of infected animals. Bacterial zoonotic skin infections transmitted from farm or wild animals include anthrax, brucellosis, erysipelas, tularaemia, and staphylococcal dermatitis.[97][98] Agriculturally related zoonotic diseases are relatively rare, have not been the subject of epidemiological research, and can be prevented by using protective gloves and hand washing, with special attention to minor skin injuries.

Hearing loss

Studies of noise exposure in agriculture show that most tractors emit noise in excess of 90 dB, nearly all tractors without cabs producing noise in excess of 85 dB.[23][24] Enclosed cabs substantially reduce, but do not always eliminate, hazardous noise levels. Other mechanised equipment, including combines, corn pickers, elevators, dryers, mixers, power saws, hammer mills, and blowers, also emit noise at levels associated with hearing loss if exposure is prolonged. Chain saws are important sources of hazardous noise levels. Farm animals may also produce noise in excess of 100 dB.

Relatively few epidemiological studies of noise-induced hearing loss among farmers and family members have been reported. Several studies have shown an increased prevalence of noise-induced hearing loss among farmers compared with controls in the 2000 to 8000 Hz range.[99–101] Higher rates of hearing loss have often been observed among older farmers; however, hearing loss has also been reported among young farmers in the 20–29 year range and among teen-aged farm children.[24][102] Few studies of agricultural workers have been population-based, but the study of May et al. assessed hearing loss in a random sample of New York dairy farmers.[100] Odds ratios of 4·1 in farm workers and significantly poorer hearing in the left ear were observed, but no significant effect of power tools, guns, motor cycles, snowmobiles, or headphones was found.[100] Protective cabs for tractors and the use of ear plugs and muffs are effective, but the efficacy of such prevention strategies has not been evaluated among agricultural workers.

1 Merchant JA. Agricultural respiratory diseases. *Seminars in Respiratory Medicine*. 1986; 7: 211–24.
2 Goudy W, Burke SC. *Iowa's counties: selected population trends. Vital statistics and*

socioeconomic data. Census Services, Department of Sociology, Iowa State University, 1991.

3 Rowland D, Lyons B. Triple jeopardy: rural, poor and uninsured. *Health Serv Res* 1989; **23**: 975–1004.

4 Baker SP, Whitfield MA, O'Neill B. Geographic variations in mortality from motor vehicle crashes. *N Engl J Med* 1987; **316**: 1384–7.

5 Baker SP, O'Neill B, Ginsburg MJ, Lee G. *The injury fact book*, 2nd edition. New York: Oxford University Press, 1992.

6 Reynolds SJ and Merchant JA. Hazards for farm workers. In: Eblen R, Eblen W, eds. *The Encyclopedia of the Environment.* 1992. Houghton Mifflin Co. (In press, 1994).

7 Donham KJ, Popendorf WJ. Ambient levels of selected gases inside swine confinement buildings. *Am Ind Hyg Assoc J* 1985; **46**: 658–61.

8 Reynolds SJ, Parker D, Vesley D, Janni K, McJilton C. Occupational exposure to organic dusts and gases in the turkey growing industry. *Appl Occup Environ Hyg* 1994b; **9**: 493–502.

9 Holness DL, O'Blenis EL, Sass-Kortsak A, Pilger C and Nethercott JR. Respiratory effects and dust exposures in hog confinement farming. *Am J Ind Med* 1987; **11**: 571–80.

10 Donham KJ, Haglind P, Peterson Y, Rylander R, Belin L. Environmental and health studies of farm workers in Swedish confinement buildings. *Br J Ind Med* 1989; **46**: 31–7.

11 Donham KJ, Reynolds SJ, Whitten P, Merchant JA, Burmeister L, Popendorf W. Respiratory dysfunction associated with enclosed swine facilities: dose-response of pulmonary function to environmental exposures. Accepted in *Am J Ind Med* 1995; 27(3): 425–38.

12 Report. *Threshold limit values for chemical substances and physical agents and biological exposure indices.* Cincinnati, American Conference of Governmental Industrial Hygienists, 1991–92.

13 Hagmar L, Schutz A, Hallberg T, Sjoholm A. Health effects of exposures to endotoxins and organic dust in poultry slaughterhouse workers. *Int Arch Occup Environ Health* 1990; **62**: 159–64.

14 Olenchock SA, May JJ, Pratt DS, Morey PR. Occupational Exposure to Airborne Endotoxins in Agriculture: In: *Detection of bacterial endotoxins with the limulus amoebocyte lysate test.* SW Watson, ed. New York: Alan R Liss, 1987: 475–87.

15 Donham KJ. Health hazards of pork producers in livestock confinement buildings: from recognition to control. *Proceedings from the Third International Symposium: Issues in health, safety and agriculture.* May 10–15, 1992, Saskatoon, Saskatchewan, Canada. CRC Press (in press, 1995).

16 Merchant JA, Thorne PS, Reynolds SJ. Biological Factors—Animal Exposures. In: Rosenstock L, Cullen M, eds. *Textbook of clinical occupational and environmental medicine,* Orlando: WB Saunders, 1994: 688–92.

17 Sauter EA, Peterson CF, Steele EE, Stroh RC, Dixon JE, Parkinson JF. The airborne microflora of poultry houses. *Poult Sci* 1981; **60**: 569–74.

18 Marx JJ Jr, Twiggs JT, Ault BJ, Merchant JA, Fernandez-Caldas E. Inhaled aeroallergen and storage mite reactivity in a Wisconsin farmer nested case-control study. *Am Rev Respir Dis* 1993; **147**: 354–8.

19 Manninen A. Analysis of airborne ammonia: comparison of field methods. *Ann Occup Hyg* 1988; **32**: 399–404.

20 Manninen A, Kangas J, Linnainmaa M, Savolainen H. Ammonia in Finnish poultry houses: effects of litter on ammonia levels and their reduction by technical binding agents. *Am Ind Hyg Assoc J* 1989; **50**: 210–5.

21 Etherton JR, Myers JR, Jensen RC, Russell JC, Braddee RW. Agricultural machine-related deaths. *Am J Public Health* 1991; **81**: 766–8.

22 Merchant JA. Agricultural injuries. *Occupational Medicine: State of the Art Reviews* 1991; **6**: 529–39.

23 Karlovich RS, Wiley TL, Tweed T, Jensen DV. Hearing sensitivity in farmers. *Public Health Rep* 1988; **103**: 61–71.

24 Broste SK, Hansen DA, Strand RL, Stueland DT. Hearing loss among high school farm students. *Am J Public Health* 1989; **79**: 619–22.

25 Blair A, Zahm SH. Methodologic issues in exposure assessment for case control studies of cancer and herbicides. *Am J Ind Med* 1990; **18**(3): 285–94.

26 Kross BC, Selim MI, Hallberg GH, Bruner DR, Cherryholmes K. Pesticide contamination of private well-water: a growing rural health concern. *Environment International* 1992; **18**: 231–41.

27 Munger R, Isacson P, Kramer M, Hanson J, Burns T, Cherryholmes K, *et al*. Birth defects and pesticide-contaminated water supplies in Iowa. In: Abstracts of papers presented at the twenty-fifth annual meeting. *Am J Epidemiol* 1992; **136**: 959.

28 Morgan DP. *Recognition and management of pesticide poisonings*. Fourth Edition. Washington, DC: US Environmental Protection Agency, 1989.

29 Popendorf WJ, Leffingwell JT. Regulating OP pesticide residues for farmworker protection. *Residue Reviews* 1982; **82**: 125–201.

30 Reynolds SJ, Milton DK. Comparing methods for analysis of airborne endotoxin. *Applied Occupational Environmental Hygiene* 1993; **8**: 761–7.

31 Milton DK, Feldman JA, Newberg DS, Bruckner RJ, Greaves IA. Environmental endotoxin measurement: the kinetic limulus assay with resistant-parallel-line estimation. *Environ Res* 1992; **57**: 212–30.

32 Thorne PS, Kiekhaefer MS, Whitten P, Donham KJ. Comparing bioaerosol sampling methods in barns housing swine. *Appl Environ Microbiol* 1992; **58**: 2543–51.

33 Fenske RA, Wong SM, Leffingwell JT, Spear RT. A video imaging technique for assessing dermal exposure. II. Fluorescent Tracer Testing. *Am Ind Hyg Assoc J* 1986; **47**: 771–5.

34 Kraus JF, Macurda J, Sahl J, Anderson C. Work-related fatal injuries in older California workers 1979–1988. *J Occup Acc* 1990; **12**: 223–35.

35 Brand S, Hoskin AF. *Allocation factor investigation*. Itasca: National Safety Council, 1993.

36 Stubbs HA, Harris J, Spear RC. A proportionate mortality analysis of California agricultural workers, 1978–1979. *Am J Ind Med* 1985; **6**: 305–20.

37 Stallones L. Surveillance of fatal and non-fatal farm injuries in Kentucky. *Am J Ind Med* 1990; **18**: 223–34.

38 NIOSH. *Fatal injuries to workers in the United States, 1980–1989: a decade of surveillance*. Washington, DC: US Dept of Health and Human Services, 1993: 15.

39 Myers JR. National surveillance of occupational fatalities in agriculture. *Am J Ind Med* 1990; **18**: 163–8.

40 Stallones L. Fatal unintentional injuries among Kentucky's farm children: 1979 to 1985. *Journal of Rural Health* 1989; **5**: 246–56.

41 Rivara FP. Fatal and nonfatal farm injuries to children and adolescents in the United States. *Pediatrics* 1985; **76**: 567–73.

42 Layde PM. Beyond surveillance: methodologic considerations in analytic studies of agricultural injuries. *Am J Ind Med* 1990; **18**: 193–200.

43 Pratt DS, Marvel LH, Darrow D, Stallones L, May JJ, Jenkins P. The dangers of dairy farming: The injury experience of 600 workers followed for two years. *Am J Ind Med* 1992; **21**: 637–50.

44 Waller JA. Injuries to farmers and farm families in a dairy state. *J Occup Med* 1992; **34**: 414–21.

45 Zhou C, Roseman JM. Agricultural injuries among a population-based sample of farm operators in Alabama. *Am J Ind Med* 1994; **25**: 385–402.

46 Brackbill RM, Cameron LL, Behrens V. Prevalence of chronic diseases and impairments among US farmers, 1986–1990. *Am J Epidemiol* 1994; **139**: 1055–65.

47 Thelin A. Hip joint arthrosis: an occupational disorder among farmers. *Am J Ind Med* 1990; **18**: 339–43.

48 Murphy DJ, Seltzer BL, Yesalis CE. Comparison of two methodologies to measure agricultural occupational fatalities. *Am J Public Health* 1990; **80**: 198–200.

49 Toscano G, Windau J. Fatal work injuries: results from the 1992 national census. *Monthly Labor Review* 1993; **116**: 39–48.

50 Murphy DJ, Purschwitz M, Mahoney BS, Hoskin AF. A proposed classification code for farm and agricultural injuries. *Am J Public Health* 1993; **83**: 736–8.

51 do Pico GA. Workgroup report: guidelines for evaluation of clinical cases. *Am J Ind Med* 1990; **17**: 132–5.

52 Emanuel DA, Marx JJ, Ault B, Roberts RC, Kryda MJ, Trehaft MW. Organic dust toxic syndrome (pulmonary mycotoxicosis)—A review of the experience in central Wisconsin. In: Dosman JA, Cockcroft DW, eds. *Principles of health and safety in agriculture.* Boca Raton, CRC Press, 1988: 72–5.

53 Guernsey JR. The prognostic significance of farmer's lung disease antibodies relative to measures of respiratory disease in a Wisconsin dairy farming population. Merchant JA thesis advisor, PhD, University of Iowa, 1985.

54 Merchant JA. Biological factors—Plants and vegetable exposures. In: Rosenstock L, Cullen M, eds. *Textbook of clinical occupational and environmental medicine,* Orlando: WB Saunders Company, 1994: 693–8.

55 Broder I. Overview of adverse pulmonary effects of grain dust. In: Dosman JA, Cockroft DW, eds. *Principles of health and safety in agriculture.* Boca Raton, CRC Press. 1989: 97–103.

56 WHO: *Report of a WHO Study Group. Recommended health-based occupational exposure limits for selected vegetable dusts. Technical Report Series 684,* Geneva, World Health Organisation, 1983.

57 Chan-Yeung M, Malo JL. Natural history of occupational asthma. In: Bernstein IL, Chan-Yeung M, Malo JL, Bernstein DI, eds. *Asthma in the workplace.* New York, Marcel Dekker, 1993: 299–322.

58 Glindmeyer HW, Lefante JJ, Jones RN, Rando RJ, Abdel Kader HM, Weill H. Exposure-related declines in the lung function of cotton textile workers. Relationship to current workplace standards. *Am Rev Respir Dis* 1991; **144**: 675–83.

59 Schwartz DA, Landas SK, Lassise DG, Burmeister LF, Hunninghake GW, Merchant JA. Airway injury in swine confinement workers. *Ann Intern Med* 1992; **116**: 630–5.

60 Smith LL. Paraquat toxicity. *Philosophical transactions of the Royal Society of London. Series B: Biological Sciences* 1985; **311**: 647–57.

61 Marx JJ Jr, Gray RL. Comparison of the enzyme-linked immunosorbent assay and double immunodiffusion test for the detection and quantification of antibodies in farmer's lung disease. *J Allergy Clin Immunol* 1982; **70**: 109–13.

62 Gruchow HW, Hoffman RG, Marx JJ, Emanuel DA, Rimm AA. Precipitating antibodies to farmer's lung antigens in a Wisconsin farming population. *Am Rev Respir Dis* 1981; **124**: 411–5.

63 Merchant JA, Miller E, Campbell J, Twiggs J, Marx J, Ault B et al. Case–control assessment of lung function among dairy farmers. *Am Rev Respir Dis* 1991; **143**: Suppl (part 2 of 2): A101.

64 Brown LM, Blair A, Gibson R, Everett GD, Cantor KP, Schuman LM, et al. Pesticide exposures and other agricultural risk factors for leukaemia among men in Iowa and Minnesota. *Cancer Res* 1990; **50**: 6585–91.

65 Burmeister LF. Cancer in Iowa farmers: recent results. *Am J Ind Med* 1990; **18**: 295–301.

66 Blair A, Dosemeci M, Heineman EF. Cancer and other causes of death among male and female farmers from twenty-three states. *Am J Ind Med* 1993; **23**: 729–42.

67 Blair A, Zahm SH. Cancer Among Farmers. In: Cordes DH, Rea DF, eds. *Occupational medicine: state of the art reviews.* Philadelphia, PA: Hanley and Belfus, 1991: 335–54.

68 Falck F, River A, Wolff MS, Gobolds S. Pesticides and polychlorinated biphenyl residues in human breast lipids and their relationship to breast cancer. *Arch Environ Health* 1992; **47**: 143–6.

69 Wolfe JS, Toniolo PG, Lee LW, Rivera M, Dubin H. Blood levels of organochlorine residues and risk of breast cancer. *J Natl Cancer Inst* 1993; **85**: 648–52.

70 Zahm SH, Babbitt PA. The role of agricultural pesticide use in the development of non-Hodgkin's lymphoma in women. *Arch Environ Health.* 1993; **48**(5): 353–8.

71 Zahm SH, Weisenburger DD, Saal RC, Vaught JB, Babbitt PA, Blair A. Pesticides and multiple myeloma in men and women in Nebraska. In: *Supplement to agricultural health and safety: workplace environment, sustainability.* HH McDuffie, JA Dosman, KM Senechok, SA Ohenchock, A Sentnilselson, eds. University of Saskatchewan Press, 1984: 75–81.

72 Hoar SK, Blair A, Holmes FF, Boysen CD, Robel RJ, Hoover R, et al. Agricultural herbicide use and risk of lymphoma and soft-tissue sarcoma. *JAMA* 1986; **256**: 1141–7.

73 Wigle DT, Semenciw RM, Wilkins K, Riedel D, Ritter L, Morrison HI, et al. Mortality study of Canadian male farm operators: non-Hodgkin's lymphoma mortality and agricultural practices in Saskatchewan. *J Natl Cancer Inst* 1990; **82**: 575–82.

74 Zahm SH, Weisenburger DD, Babbitt PA, Saal RC, Vaught JB, Cantor KP, et al. A case-control study of non-Hodgkin's lymphoma and the herbicide 2,4-Dichlorophenoxyacetic acid (2,4-D) in eastern Nebraska. *Epidemiology* 1990; **1**: 349–56.

75 Alavanja MCR, Blair A, Masters MN. Cancer mortality in the US flour industry. *J Natl Cancer Inst* 1990; **82**: 840–8.

76 Alavanja MCR, Blair A, Merkle S, Teske J, Eaton B, Reed B. Mortality among forest conservationists. *Arch Environ Health* 1989; **44**: 94–101.

77 Boffetta P, Stellman SD, Garfinkel L. A case-control study of multiple myeloma nested in the American Cancer Society prospective study. *Int J Cancer* 1989; **43**: 554–9.

78 Alavanja MCR, Blair A, Merkle S, Teske J, Eaton B. Mortality among agricultural extension agents. *Am J Ind Med* 1988; **14**: 167–76.

79 Finn WF. Environmental toxins and renal disease. *J Clin Pharmacol* 1983; **23**: 461–72.

80 Fowler BA, Weissberg JB. Arsine poisoning. *N Engl J Med* 1974; **291**: 1171–4.

81 Yarbrough JD, Chambers JE, Robinson KM. Alterations in liver structure and function resulting from chronic insecticide exposure. In: *Effects of Chronic Exposures to Pesticides on Animal Systems*. JE Chambers, JD Yarborough, eds. New York: Raven Press, 1982: 25–9.

82 Sandler DP, Smith JC. Chronic Renal Disease Risk Associated with Employment in Industries with Potential Solvent Exposure. In: Bach PH, Gregg NJ, Wilks MF, Delacruz L, eds. *Nephrotoxicity: mechanisms, early diagnosis, and therapeutic management*. New York: Marcel Dekker, 1991: 247–52.

83 Staessen JA, Lauwerys RR, Geert I, Roels HA, Vyncke G, Amery A. Renal function and historical environmental cadmium pollution from zinc smelters. *Lancet* 1994; **343**: 1523–7.

84 Rosenstock L, Keifer M, Daniell WE, McConnell R, Claypoole K. Chronic central nervous system effects of acute organophosphate pesticide intoxication. *Lancet* 1991; **330**: 223–7.

85 Tanner CM, Langston JW. Do environmental toxins cause Parkinson's disease? A critical review. *Neurology* 1990; **40**: 17–30.

86 Deapen EM, Henderson BE. A case-control study of amyotrophic lateral sclerosis. *Am J Epidemiol* 1986; **123**: 790–9.

87 Gunnarsson LG, Bodin L, Soderfeldt B, Axelson O. A case-control study of motor neurone disease—Its relation to heritability, and occupational exposures, particularly to solvents. *Br J Ind Med* 1992; **49**: 791–8.

88 Mattison DR, Bogumil RJ, Chapin R, Hatch M, Hendricks A, Jarrell J, et al. Reproductive effects of pesticides. In: Baker SR, Wilkinson CF, eds. *Advances in modern environmental toxicology: the effects of pesticides on human health*. Princeton, Princeton Scientific Publishing Co., 1990: 297–389.

89 Rupa DS, Reddy PP, Reddi OS. Reproductive performance in population exposed to pesticides in cotton fields in India. *Environ Res* 1991; **55**: 123–8.

90 McDonald AD, McDonald JC, Armstrong B, Cherry NM, Côté R, Lavoie J, et al. Congenital defects and work in pregnancy. *Br J Ind Med* 1988; **45**: 581–8.

91 Rogan WR, Gladen BC, McKinney JD, Carreras N, Hardy P, Thullen JD, et al. PCBs and DDE in human milk: effects on growth, morbidity, and duration of lactation. *Am J Public Health* 1987; **7**: 1294–7.

92 Forman MR, Lewando-Hunt G, Graubard BI, Chang D, Sarov B, Naggan L, et al. Factors influencing milk insufficiency and its long-term health effects: the Bedouin infant feeding study. *Int J Epidemiol* 1992; **21**: 53–8.

93 Mathias CGT, Morrison JH. Occupational skin diseases, United States results from the Bureau of Labor Statistics Annual Survey of occupational injuries and illnesses, 1973–1984. *Arch Dermatol* 1988; **124**: 1519–24.

94 O'Malley M, Thun M, Morrison J, Mathias CG, Halperin WE. Surveillance of

occupational skin disease in the Supplementary Data System. *Am J Ind Med* 1988; **13**: 291–9.

95 O'Malley MA, Mathias CG. Distribution of lost-work-time claims for skin disease in California agriculture: 1978–1983. *Am J Ind Med* 1989; **14**: 715–20.

96 Matsushita T, Aoyama Km Manda F, Ueda A, Yoshida M, Okamura J. Occupational dermatoses in farmers growing okra (Hibiscus esculentus L.) *Contact Dermatitis* 1989; **21**: 321–5.

97 Abrams K, Hogan D, Maibach HI. Pesticide-related dermatoses in agricultural workers. *Occupational Medicine: State of the Art Reviews* 1991; **6**: 463–92.

98 Armstrong KR, Post K. The role of farm animals in the control of zoonotic skin diseases in man. In: Dosman JA, Cockcroft DW, eds. *Principles of health and safety in agriculture*. Boca Raton; CRC Press, 1989: 288–91.

99 Plakke DL, Dare E. Occupational hearing loss in farmers. *Public Health Rep* 1992; **107**: 188–92.

100 May JJ, Marvel M, Regan M, Marvel LH, Pratt DS. Noise-induced hearing loss in randomly selected New York dairy farmers. *Am J Ind Med* 1990; **18**: 333–7.

101 Crutchfield CD, Sparks ST. Effects of noise and vibration on farm workers. *Occupational Medicine: State of the Art Reviews* 1991; **6**: 355–69.

102 Ejercio VS, Hansen DA, Pierce WE. Prevention of hearing loss among farmers. In: *Principles of Health and Safety in Agriculture*. Dosman JA, Cockcroft DW, eds. Boca Raton, CRC Press, 1989, 327–328.

13 Work and pregnancy

ALISON McDONALD

Introduction—women's work

The past century has seen enormous improvements in women's political, social, and economic status. Employment of women, which is an integral part of this process, has increased everywhere, but to an extent that has varied with culture, religion, political system and economic development.[1] Remarkable changes took place in the former Union of Soviet Socialist Republics (USSR) between 1917 and 1991; in 1922 women comprised 25% of the workforce and in the 1980s, 51%. Other countries of eastern Europe evolved in a similar way. The objective of equality for women was nowhere achieved, however, as their work tended to be inferior in pay and status to that of men. In Scandinavian countries, which have come nearest to this goal, women comprise a high proportion of the work force, for example reaching 48% in Finland in 1985.

In contrast, in the countries of the Middle East and North Africa, the work force has the lowest proportion of women, for example in the 1980s, in Iran and Algeria around 10%, in Syria and Iraq between 10% and 20%, in Egypt and Tunisia 21%, and in Morocco and Turkey 35%.[2] Overall numbers of the economically active include those in part-time employment which is much commoner among women than among men. Part-time work helps to compensate for the fact that in most countries women continue to bear the main burden of work in housekeeping and child-rearing. Table 13.1 shows for nine countries, varying in degree of industrialisation and economic level and in political and cultural pattern, the proportion of women who are working and their distribution by industrial sector.[2] There is much variation but in developing countries from 25–60% of economically active women work in either agriculture or manufacturing, with reproductive hazards in both.

Reproductive hazards in the workplace

Workplace hazards are described briefly here: more detailed information can be found in comprehensive texts such as that by Rom.[3]

Physical

Extremes of temperature

Some industrial environments, including work in tropical climates, are extremely warm. If deep body temperature exceeds 38°C the fetus may be affected.[4] In guinea-pigs, raising of core body temperature causes first a reduction in cell proliferation and finally death.[4] Microencephaly and other central nervous defects have been caused in guinea-pigs and sheep by intermittent elevation of body temperature by 2·5°C. Excessive cold is less often encountered but may occur in work involving refrigeration.

Noise and vibration

Loud noise is common in industry especially in manufacturing sectors where sound levels often reach 90 decibels or more. Sound waves can be transmitted across the uterine wall, but only high levels reach the fetus. However, they are not received by the fetal auditory apparatus in early pregnancy because it is filled with fluid which acts as a buffer.[5] Auditory brain responses have been detected from 26 weeks and vibro-acoustic stimulation with an artificial larynx causes diminution of gross body and breathing movements. Strong vibration may be experienced by a small proportion of women in manufacturing and occasionally in other types of work. Because the fetus receives sound and vibration only late in pregnancy, neither is likely to cause spontaneous abortion.

Non-ionising radiation

The number and variety of devices in the workplace that emit radio frequency waves (300 kHz–300 MHz) or microwaves (300 MHz to

294

Table 13.1 Distribution (%) of economically active women by industrial sector in selected countries (1988–91)[2]

	Iran (10%)*	Brazil (32%)	Indonesia (42%)	Kenya (45%)	Australia (50%)	Germany (FR) (54%)	China (60%)	USA (64%)	USSR (90%)
Agriculture, fishing	28·0	14·7	56·4	20·9	3·9	4·0	8·4	1·3	18·5
Mining	–	–	0·3	0·3	0·3	0·1	4·7	0·2	–
Manufacture	23·0	11·7	11·9	6·9	9·8	23·3	38·4	12·5	28·9
Electricity, gas, water	0·2	0·5	< 0·1	1·0	0·4	0·4	1·2	0·6	–
Construction	1·0	0·5	0·2	1·3	2·1	1·8	3·6	1·1	10·1
Trade	1·6	11·7	19·6	6·0	28·2	21·2	12·3	21·2	7·9
Transport, storage, commerce	0·9	0·9	0·2	3·4	3·7	3·7	4·3	3·8	8·3
Financing	1·1	5·6	0·4	4·7	13·3	9·5	1·4	13·4	0·7
Services	44·1	54·4	10·9	55·6	38·4	36·0	25·4	45·7	25·6

* Proportion of women in paid employment in parenthesis.

295

300 GHz) has greatly increased in the past two decades. Visual display terminals emit the former and microwave equipment is used in many industries for drying, gluing and plastic processing. Less common sources are microwave transmitters, radar and diathermy. Michaelson reviewed the health implications of radio-frequency and microwave energies and found that in animal experiments any effect could be explained by heating.[6]

Ionising radiation

Soon after the discovery of x rays cancers were observed and teratogenic potential was reported in the 1920s.[7] Radiologists, radiographers, dentists and dental attendants, nurses and nursing attendants may be at risk. Nuclear workers and some industrial workers such as those who manufacture cathode ray tubes may also be exposed.

Chemical

Organic solvents

Organic solvents are extensively employed in industrial processes and are commonly mixed. They are used as diluents in paints and glues, dyes and printing inks, for degreasing and cleaning, in plastics, agricultural products, and pharmaceuticals and as fuels. They are toxic to the nervous system, can have acute effects and may, with prolonged exposure, cause mental deterioration or peripheral neuropathy. Some special uses are tetrachloroethylene in dry-cleaning, carbon disulphide in rayon manufacture and toluene and xylene in painting.

Pesticides

Many pesticides and insecticides are used in agriculture and horticulture; all are capable of having toxic effects; when they do, it is often as a result of an accident. In pesticide production and in crop spraying, especially in greenhouses, exposure may be high. Tests of teratogenicity in animals have been negative with malathion, but occasionally positive with carbaryl and lindane.

Heavy metals

These are toxic and can pass the placenta and are capable of damaging the embryo or fetus. Lead is widely used in the manufacture of batteries, rubber, glass, and enamels. In the British pottery industry at the turn of the century women were thought to be at substantial risk of stillbirth and miscarriage and in 1913 regulations stipulated that no women of childbearing age should work with lead. Inorganic mercury is extensively used in the manufacture of sodium hydroxide and in mercury vapour lamps, and various electric and electronic components. Conversion of inorganic to organic mercury in industrial effluents and contamination of fish has caused serious nervous disease in children.[8] Other metals commonly used are cadmium in low melting point alloys and solders, pigments, and batteries, and manganese for dry cell batteries and in the chemical industry.

Anaesthetic gases

Nitrous oxide and three halogenated compounds—halothane, enflurane and isoflurane are in common use, either singly or in combination. Anaesthetists, nurses, and attendants are mainly exposed. Since scavenging was introduced and has become widely used, concentrations in air have fallen.

Drugs

In the pharmaceutical industry workers may be exposed to hormones, cytotoxic drugs and solvents, all potentially fetotoxic or teratogenic. The preparation and administration of cytotoxic drugs may also expose pharmacists and nurses, although exhaust hoods have reduced exposure.

Biological

Protozoa, bacteria, and viruses are found wherever there are humans or animals. Febrile illness in early pregnancy, presumably caused by infection, has been associated with spontaneous abortion.[9 10] Three infective agents are known to cause congenital defects: rubella virus, cytomegalovirus and *Toxoplasma gondii*.[8] The risk of exposure is greatest where opportunities for spread of infection are high, such as in day care centres. Toxoplasmosis is found in small mammals especially cats, and by infecting a pregnant woman may cause neonatal disease and later mental retardation in her offspring. Veterinarians and keepers of pet stores are at risk.

Ergonomic

Heavy weight lifting is required in some occupations, particularly in factory, sales, and service work. Nurses and other medical personnel have often to lift patients, sometimes in awkward positions. It is commonly thought that strenuous exertion may lead to spontaneous abortion or preterm birth, and there have been suspicions about standing or working for long hours, as is often required in service jobs, sales and factory work, and about shift work, which may disturb circadian rhythm.

General epidemiology of pregnancy outcome

Fetal death

Prevalence

Once an ovum is fertilised and a zygote formed, its failure to survive and develop into an embryo constitutes a pregnancy loss. In a small prospective study of volunteers, 25% of 171 biochemically detected pregnancies ended within six weeks of the last menstrual period.[11] Little is known about this early phase of pregnancy and it is unsure whether such early losses have the same causes as recognised spontaneous abortions that occur later. Without biochemical or histological detection of pregnancy, ascertainment of the prevalence of abortions is inevitably incomplete. If a woman thinks that she has had an abortion she may see a physician or seek hospital treatment, especially if bleeding continues. Physicians or hospital records may be used to record abortions; otherwise, information must be obtained from the women themselves. Miscarriages are well remembered, early losses less well.[12]

The measured frequency of spontaneous abortion varies with the method of ascertainment. From physician records in a prepaid medical plan, a rate of 13·3% of all pregnancies was found.[13] In Finland, from computerised hospital discharge records, 7·5% of total pregnancies ended in abortions,[14] but when polyclinic records were added a rate of 10% was obtained.[15] Although this figure omitted some early abortions, it was estimated that it included nearly 85% of those that were recognised.

In a large survey in Montreal past pregnancies were studied; this was because spontaneous abortions treated in hospital (estimated at 7% of pregnancies) omitted many that occurred early and the figure was unrepresentative. The rate of spontaneous abortions in past pregnancies was reported to be 22·2%,[16] the high figure resulting from the fact that the history of past pregnancies was taken just after a delivery. Women who abort repeatedly may keep trying until they reproduce successfully. Thus the true prevalence of abortion is best obtained from women who have completed their families.

Epidemiology

The epidemiology of fetal death was studied in 1962 by Shapiro and Denson using medical records of women enrolled in the prepaid Health Insurance Plan of New York.[13] In a total of 6844 pregnancies in one year there were 970 fetal deaths—62 (0·1%) stillbirths and 908 (13·3%) spontaneous abortions. Whereas stillbirths were likely to be fully recorded, spontaneous abortions were recorded only for women who consulted a doctor. The frequency of spontaneous abortion rose with maternal age; at 35 years it was double that under 20 years. A direct correlation was found between gravidity and total fetal mortality. Women with a history of previous fetal death had about twice the risk of those who reported only live births.

Roman analysed data on all pregnancies reported by 2836 women doctors of average age 38·4 years,[17] many whose reproductive histories were complete.[18] Out of a total of 6439 pregnancies, there were 973 fetal deaths (13·1%). When all women and pregnancies were combined, the fetal death rate by gravidity followed a J-shaped curve, lowest in second pregnancies. Within gravidity groups fetal death rates remained fairly constant until the last parity order of the group, when they fell. After a fetal loss, women apparently tended to become pregnant again and move into a higher gravidity group. Within parity orders, women were subject to different rates of fetal loss indicating heterogeneity of risk. Thus the J-shaped curve of fetal loss rates often reported by gravidity may be an artefact. The important risk factors for fetal death were increasing age, and (in women who had had at least one previous pregnancy) number of previous spontaneous abortions. This heterogeneity of risk has been confirmed.[19] Cigarette smoking adds a small increase in risk.[19] Maternal age and number of previous spontaneous abortions may be confounding factors.

Prematurity

Prematurity is measured by birth weight and length of gestation. The standard definition of prematurity in the past was a birth weight of less than 2500 g, now simply termed low birth weight. The maturity of an infant has been recognised to be of greater importance than its weight and is measured by gestational age calculated from the first day of the last menstrual period or estimated by ultrasound scan. A preterm birth is defined as one of less than 37 weeks gestation. In industrialised countries the rates of low birth weight and preterm birth are similar (4–8%); in developing countries, however, from 10–45% are of low birth weight, although the proportion pre-term remains relatively constant.[20] When less than 10% of births are of low birth weight, most are also preterm, but as the percentage rises an increasing proportion are of more than 37 weeks gestation. Whereas babies of low birth weight who are mature in terms of gestational age are small but usually healthy, preterm birth is the most important cause of perinatal mortality and disability in surviving children.[21] There are racial variations in gestation length and weight at birth. In the United States this partly explains the higher frequency of low birth weight in blacks than whites but this is also attributed to the lower average socioeconomic status of blacks.[22] Because of its greater significance and more constant rate, preterm birth has become the outcome measure of choice in occupational reproductive studies.

In the First British Perinatal Mortality Survey of 16 994 singleton births in one week in March 1958, 283 (1·7%), women who went into

Table 13.2   Studies of maternal factors associated with preterm birth

	Odds ratios*		
	Fedrick *et al.* 1976[23]	Kaltreider *et al.* 1980[24]	McDonald *et al.* 1992[25]
Age < 20 years	1·3	1·7	1·5
Previous spontaneous abortion	1·2	1·7	1·3
Previous preterm or LBW	up to ten fold	3·0	3·4
Low prepregnancy weight	1·5		1·3
Low social class	1·5	2·0	1·4
Unmarried	1·5	1·9	
Cigarette smoker	2·0		1·4

* $p < 0.01$

spontaneous labour before 37 weeks and were delivered of a live or stillborn infant weighing < 2500 g without major defect, were compared with the remaining women[23]; see first column of table 13.2. Associations were found with low maternal age, low maternal weight, maternal smoking, low social class, illegitimacy, and previous perinatal death or preterm birth. In the United States the Obstetric Statistical Cooperative analysed 404 474 deliveries, 1970–76, in 16 hospitals,[24] see second column of table 13.2. Risks of low birth weight and preterm birth were reported for maternal age, social class (ward versus private patient), marital status, and previous abortion.

In the large survey of births in Montreal, Canada in 1982–84 (see p 303), the association between cigarette, alcohol, and coffee consumption and prematurity was studied in 40 000 women who had a spontaneous labour, excluding those who had an induced labour or certain prenatal complications, chronic or acute disease, or multiple pregnancy see third column in table 13.2. Thus these three studies gave similar results.[25]

Longitudinal analyses of data from the Norwegian Medical Registry of Births, in which preterm birth was defined as a gestation of less than 36 weeks and a birth weight of less than 2500 g, were undertaken of a large series of women who had three consecutive singleton births from 1967 to 1976.[21] If the first birth was not preterm, 4·4% of second births were preterm compared with 17·7% if the first was preterm, and 28% if the first two were preterm. This longitudinal study showed that the lower proportion of preterm births found in second births in cross-sectional studies was an artefact and that the proportion of preterm births decreases steadily as parity increases; it also showed that some women have a strong tendency toward preterm birth.

Table 13.2 shows that the risk of preterm birth is raised in pregnancy the very young, in women who are unmarried, of low socioeconomic status, low educational attainment, low prepregnancy weight, and in cigarette smokers. These characteristics are unlikely to be evenly distributed among occupational groups and in consequence are potentially serious confounding factors in occupational research. Bleeding or threatened abortion, *abruptio placentae*, *placenta praevia*, multiple birth, congenital defect and abnormalities of fetal position were also risk factors, but are less likely to be associated with type of occupation.

Congenital defect

The variety of congenital defects is vast, but many are of relatively minor importance. Some 15% of infants have some abnormality, but lethal or serious defects, sometimes referred to as "major" defects affect only about 3%, of which 20–25% are genetic in origin.[8] In many others, multiple genes play an important part, leaving perhaps 10% that are probably the result of environmental influences.[26] The agents concerned may cause chromosomal damage before conception or distort embryonic development; either could cause a defect. About 40% of spontaneously aborted fetuses have a chromosomal abnormality, some with a recognisable defect such as Down's syndrome.[27] As ova are present from birth, chromosomal abnormalities from environmental agents could arise at any time in a woman's life up to fertilisation. Occasionally aberrant chromosomes are transmitted from a parent and are therefore genetically determined. Because it may well be that each specific type of congenital defect is of unique aetiology, total rates of congenital defect are of limited epidemiological value.

Most individual types of serious defect are rare and difficult to investigate. For one of the commoner groups, however, (anencephaly and spina bifida) some risk factors are known. The occurrence of these defects is correlated with socioeconomic status and varies with ethnic and religious group and geographic area, all factors capable of confounding occupational studies.[28]

Occupational epidemiology

Characteristics of employed women

A report in 1955 suggested that prematurity was more common in employed women than in those who were not employed[29] but since then the reverse has been found.[30][31] A study by Savitz *et al.* based on the United States Natality Survey gave useful information on employed women in the United States.[31] The connection between reproductive risk factors and employment was examined by calculating prevalence ratios for each factor in relation to work. Working women were more often of optimal reproductive age, more highly educated, had a higher family income, began prenatal care earlier and gained more weight during pregnancy. Employed women had many fewer previous births and, controlling for gravidity, more stillbirths and abortions—spontaneous and induced. By employment sector, professional women had the most favourable demographic and behavioural characteristics and women employed as operatives and service workers the least.

Longitudinal studies

A cohort of female employees can be defined and pregnancy outcome analysed according to degree of exposure. This approach is seldom feasible for investigating fetal death or congenital defect, but has been used for preterm birth. In studies of physical activity, ergonomic factors and preterm birth, questionnaires have been completed during pregnancy and outcome obtained from hospital records. Fetal death and congenital defect have been investigated in Scandinavian countries by linking census, employer, or union lists of employed women with hospital discharge registries. By this means those who had a delivery (International Classification of Diseases codes 650–652 [8th revision] or abortion, (spontaneous 643, other 645 and induced 640–642), were identified.[14] Exposures were obtained from occupational titles or by questionnaire from the workplace or the employee herself.

In many countries, social security numbers are available for employed persons and can theoretically be linked to obstetrical and gynaecological records but do not appear to have been used except in a study of women in the United States Army. Social security numbers served to identify hospital deliveries, but many errors were found which prevented the matching of records.[32]

In a study which used recorded information, details of employed people in Finland were taken from the census. The occupations of the women and their husbands were classified by an industrial hygienist into seven exposure categories. Relative risks of spontaneous abortion were estimated by logistic regression after adjustment for age, parity, and marital status. Another longitudinal study in which chemical exposures and spontaneous abortion were investigated was carried out in Denmark (see p 315).[33 34] Both questionnaire and hospital records were used to determine pregnancy outcome. Women who worked a month or more in one of 12 occupations (six with chemical exposure and six with little chemical exposure) during the period 1972–80 were taken from employer and union lists. A postal questionnaire was used which included pregnancy and employment history and detailed information on chemical exposure.

Case-control studies

Pregnancies with adverse outcome and controls from the same population comparable in important respects are selected; their exposures are investigated and compared. For example a study was made in Montreal of 301 women who gave birth to babies with congenital defect with a control for each case was matched for age, educational level, hospital, and date.[35] Chemical exposures were assessed in detail by industrial hygienists, unaware of the case-control status of each subject. Relative risks were obtained by analysis of the matched pairs discordant for one of nine groups of chemicals.

Several case-control analyses have used longitudinal record linkage. For example, information about women employed in eight pharmaceutical factories in Finland was obtained from employers and spontaneous abortions were extracted from the hospital discharge registry supplemented by polyclinic records (see p 314).[36] In Finland a register of congenital defects has been maintained since 1963 and a continuing case-control study of selected defects since 1967.[37] Defects are compulsorily noted by the maternity hospital. At the maternity clinic the birth immediately before the case is taken as control and both mothers are interviewed by midwives about all occupational and leisure time activities.

Cross-sectional or prevalence studies

In these, occupation (exposure) and outcome are ascertained at the same time. There have been three large studies of this kind.

In France, a national survey of births in 1981 investigated the correlation between arduous working conditions and preterm birth.[30] A two-stage random sample of births was selected by geographical area. A total of 5508 women were interviewed within six days of birth using a standard questionnaire. Information was obtained on obstetrical history, prenatal care, course of pregnancy and, for the 2955 women who had done some paid work during pregnancy, detailed occupational information. Data on confinement and the child's health at birth were obtained from medical records. The findings are described on page 318.

In the United States, a national sample of 9941 live births in 1980 was selected from birth certificates, low birth weight infants being over-sampled in a four to one ratio. Information was obtained from hospitals, other health care providers, and from mothers. Questionnaires concerning employment and certain characteristics were sent to 7825 married mothers. Eighty percent of the eligible sample responded. Two studies based on this survey are described later.[31 38]

In Montreal, over a two-year period, May 1982 to May 1984, 56 067 women were interviewed in 11 maternity units in which about 90% of the city's births take place.[39] The women were questioned soon after delivery or abortion about their just completed pregnancy and all previous pregnancies (104 000 in all) and personal, social, and detailed occupational factors. Occupations were coded according to the Standard Occupational and Industrial Classifications with employment subdivided into 60 classes in six main industrial sectors. Abortions induced for personal or health reasons were distinguished; those induced because of a defective fetus were included in the analysis of defects. Details of the outcome of current pregnancies were extracted from obstetric and paediatric records and for previous pregnancies from the mothers themselves. Analyses of prematurity were based on current pregnancies[40] and of fetal death on previous pregnancies[16] to include the many cases not treated in hospital. Logistic regression was used to allow for up to eight confounding variables in comparisons of adverse outcomes expected in an occupational group with the numbers observed.

Pros and cons

Longitudinal (cohort) and case-control studies generally give more reliable findings than those that are cross-sectional. It is important nevertheless that the cohorts and case series should be representative in terms of occupation and exposure under study. Thus, a cohort defined from union lists will exclude non-union employees and cohorts of pregnant women attending antenatal clinics exclude women who do not attend. In record linkage studies much laborious work can be avoided. A combination of pregnancy outcomes identified from hospital discharge data, and from the woman herself is better than using either source alone. For example, in a study of anaesthetic gas exposure exposed women responded and reported all their abortions that were recorded in the hospital files whereas among those who were not exposed and did not respond to the questionnaire some had had abortions recorded in hospital files.[41]

A cross-sectional survey such as that in Montreal had the merit of size and relative efficiency but, even so, rare exposures and outcomes could not be usefully investigated. The main problem in this approach is the risk of recall bias, especially when the outcome is seriously distressing.

Risks in specific occupations

Operating rooms

In 1967, an increased risk of abortion in female anaesthetists in the USSR was reported: 110 women had 31 pregnancies of which 15 ended in abortion.[41] This report led to studies elsewhere; anaesthetic gases were suspected of being fetotoxic, although in the original publication heavy work was mentioned as an additional factor. By 1982 there had been eight records of an increased number of miscarriages among anaesthetists or operating room personnel compared with control groups. There were, however, two that showed no association, one of which was of women doctors who were asked to complete a questionnaire on operating room exposure and pregnancy history.[41] Of the 670 who were exposed, 13·8% had abortions—the same rate as for the 6377 who did not work in an operating room.[18]

In the other negative study, a postal questionnaire was completed by nurses about operating room exposure and pregnancy history; pregnancies were also retrieved from the hospital discharge registry.[41] By verifying self-reported abortions against hospital records it was found that all the exposed women who had abortions responded, whereas those who did not reply to the questionnaire and were not exposed included some who had had abortions that were recorded in the registry. In the self-reported abortions, a significant excess was found in women exposed, but not after addition of those found in the registry. This suggests that the positive findings in the eight other questionnaire studies could have resulted from a similar bias.

In a study reported in 1985 that was based on registered information of outcome, data on exposure for both abortions and controls were obtained from head nurses not informed of the case-control status.[42] A small increased risk was found, but this was not significant (relative risk 1·2, 95% CI 0·3 to 4·6). In the Montreal survey of 46 operating room nurses, there was no excess of abortions at less than 16 weeks (the usual time), but between 16 and 28 weeks there were 4 abortions compared with 1·4 expected (p < 0·05).[16] Overall it seems doubtful whether exposure to anaesthetic gases is related to risk of miscarriage although, as the authors of the 1967 report suggested, heavy work in the operating room may present some hazard.

Laboratory work

In 1978, a small study in Sweden found an association between abortion and hospital laboratory work.[43] In the following year, it was reported that eight major defects were found in 245 progeny of women who worked in a university laboratory; two were oesophageal atresia and two anal atresia.[44] This unusual finding was further investigated in a study of all 200 cases of gastrointestinal atresia reported to the Swedish congenital malformation registry; seven cases were in laboratory workers compared with 2·5 expected.[45]

Heidam in Denmark found no association between laboratory work and abortion, nor a suggestion of exposure to any particular chemical.[33] Axelsson et al. reported an association (but not significant) with solvent exposure[46] and in another laboratory an excess of abortions in one time period but not another.[47] No risk was found in the Montreal survey;[16] two other studies reported positive findings but both had weak designs.[14 48] Thus, neither for abortion nor for any particular defect is there strong evidence for a link with laboratory work.

Physiotherapy

A study was carried out in Finland in which the personal identification numbers of all registered female physiotherapists listed in the Central

Register of Health Care Personnel were linked with the hospital discharge register and the register of congenital malformations.[49] In the period 1973–1983, 204 women who had an abortion were each matched for age with three referent mothers who had a normal delivery. In addition, 46 women who had a child with a malformation were matched with five referents. Postal questionnaires were sent enquiring about use of therapeutic equipment (ultrasound, deep heat therapy, electrical treatments) and lifting of patients. In addition, information about pregnancy history, personal habits, chronic diseases and febrile illnesses during the first trimester were sought. The response rates were 92% for cases and 89% for referents.

Exposure to ultrasound and to short wave diathermy gave odds ratios of about three for spontaneous abortion after 10 weeks gestation, but when allowance was made for potentially confounding variables neither was significant. Both ultrasound and short waves were significantly associated with congenital defects, but with low exposure only. In this study, heavy lifting was significantly associated with spontaneous abortion and febrile illness in early pregnancy with unspecified congenital malformations. In the Montreal survey, 75 women who worked in physiotherapy had fewer abortions than expected (eight observed, 13 expected).[16] Both the Finnish study and the Montreal survey suggest that currently used physiotherapy equipment is not a hazard for abortion. In Denmark, where the national file of physiotherapists was linked to the congenital malformation registry, 54 mothers of cases and 247 referent mothers were interviewed.[50] No association was found between malformations and exposure to electromagnetic radiation.

Nursing

Nursing exposes many young women of child-bearing age to various hazards, both ergonomic and chemical. In a study of pregnancy outcome in hospital personnel, nursing and ancillary staff reported more uterine contractions between the fourth and seventh months of pregnancy than other staff and had more preterm births and low birth weight infants.[51]

Administration of antineoplastic drugs has been investigated because many are mutagens, carcinogens, and teratogens. In Finland no association with abortion was found but a relative risk of 4·7 (based on eight cases) for congenital defects.[42] In Montreal there was also an association with defects (eight cases observed, four expected)[52] but not with abortion.[16] Of the eight congenital defects in Finland two were of the ear, face and neck, and four of the limbs; in Montreal, the excess defects were musculoskeletal (three babies with club foot, one with congenital dislocation of the hip and two with hernias). Thus, neither in Finland nor in Montreal did the defects suggest a specific teratogenic effect. Abortion received further attention in Finland,[53] and in France[54] where, in studies

306

by questionnaire, women who gave cytotoxic drugs had an increased risk, but this was not seen in Montreal. Because the data were collected retrospectively the possibility that biased recall may explain the positive findings cannot be excluded.

Child minding

With the rise in employment of women, day care centres have increased in number and the age of the children reduced. As noted on page 297, child minders are exposed to many infectious agents which could affect the outcome of pregnancy. Attention has recently been paid to the increasing public health problem of cytomegalovirus infection in day care workers,[55] because this infection in pregnant women can cause deafness and mental retardation in the fetus. In a study of six day care centres in Iowa, 62% of day care providers were seronegative on entry. Seroconversion occurred in two centres, which had higher rates of oral excretion and acquisition than the other four.[56] A few child minders (not only in day care centres) were studied in the Montreal survey and no increase in abortion or defect was observed.

Leather work

In a large case-control study of perinatal deaths in Leicestershire, medical records were reviewed and mothers interviewed.[57] Offspring of leather workers were at increased risk of perinatal death and particularly of malformed or macerated stillbirths. The malformations included three cases of trisomy 18—a rare chromosomal defect. The Montreal survey was of insufficient size to test this hypothesis. Leather work was significantly associated with stillbirth without defect but, again, the numbers were small.[58] Toluene is a solvent commonly used in shoe manufacture and some indication of an increased abortion risk has been reported.[59]

Risks associated with specific factors

Physical

Non-ionising radiation

The introduction of visual display terminals (VDTs) into offices and their use especially by young women led to questions about any hazard to pregnancy. Anxiety was first aroused by reports in 1978–80, mainly in North America, of unusually high rates of miscarriage in a small number of large office blocks. All but one of these clusters of miscarriages and birth defects were reported in the non-scientific press. The exception was a cluster in Dallas, Texas, observed in 1980 by an occupational physician and investigated by the National Institute of Occupational Safety and Health.[60] A questionnaire given to 69 current employees in an accounting department with 29 VDTs identified six abortions in 19 consecutive pregnancies in a three-year period. The investigators compared this number with 1·5 abortions expected, based on the age-parity rates of fetal death found in the survey described on page 298.[13] Nevertheless the authors concluded that, given the numbers of women of child-bearing age working with VDTs and the frequency of abortion and birth defect, this cluster was probably a chance occurrence. In a later review of eight similar clusters including this one, it was concluded that they could all have occurred by chance.[61] Because of the importance of the question, however, a considerable number of planned epidemiological studies have now been reported (see table 13.3).

Using information for cases and controls from the Finnish congenital defect registry (see p 303), occupations were classified according to probability of work with VDTs.[37] Definite use was recorded for 51 cases and 60 controls, giving an odds ratio of 0·9.[62] In Sweden, groups of women of similar socioeconomic status were selected from census records whose occupations carried a high, medium, or low probability of VDT use. The three groups were linked by personal identity numbers with the birth defect registry and the inpatient registry containing information on admission to hospital for pregnancy. Two periods were studied: 1976–7 (5130 pregnancies) and 1980–1 (4875 pregnancies). No significant differences were found between the high, medium, and low exposure groups in spontaneous abortion, stillbirth, early neonatal death, low birth weight, or certain malformations.[63] Also in Sweden, a list of female clerks at social security offices was linked to hospital registries of abortion and defect.[66] For 4117 pregnancies, exposure was graded jointly by union representatives and employers into five grades of VDT use ranging from none to extensive (but not more than 15 hours a week). The authors concluded that the groups did not differ significantly in frequency of fetal death or congenital defect.

In the remaining studies where information on exposure or outcome or both was obtained from the women themselves there were varying results. Based on the registry study described above,[63] a case-control study was carried out in which new exposure information was obtained by postal questionnaire.[64] This gave an increased odds ratio for defects. In a study of case-control design, pregnancies were ascertained from the records of a prepaid medical plan.[67] Women were sent questionnaires on VDT use long after the pregnancies were completed; the odds ratio for abortion for those who used a VDT more than 20 hours a week was 1·8 ($p < 0.05$). In the Montreal survey (see p 303), women were questioned on hours of exposure; the risk of abortion in previous pregnancies was for no use 1·0, less than 15 hours a week 0·95 and 15 or more hours a week 1·00.[68] In current pregnancies the relative risks for the same groupings were 0·96, 1·14, 1·23, respectively. For stillbirth, congenital defect, preterm birth,

Table 13.3 Odds ratios for use of visual display terminal and abnormal pregnancy outcomes.

		Spontaneous abortion Use of VDT		Stillbirth	Congenital defect	Preterm birth	Low birth weight
		Any	Extensive				
Kurppa et al. 1985[62]		1·0	1·1		0·9		
Ericson et al. 1986[63]		1·1	1·2		1·1		
Ericson et al. 1986[64]		1·0	1·2		1·6*		
Butler et al. 1986[65]		1·1					
Westerholm et al. 1987[66]		1·2		0·5	0·9		
Goldhaber et al. 1988[67]		1·19*	1·8* (≥20 hrs)		1·4		
McDonald et al. 1988[68]	current	0·97	1·23* (≥15 hrs)	0·82	0·94	1·08	
	previous		1·00 (≥15 hrs)		0·71	1·12	1·03
Bryant et al. 1989[69]		0·98					
Neilson et al. 1990[70]		0·94					
Schnorr et al. 1991[71]		0·93	1·00 (≥25 hrs)				
Lindbohm et al. 1992[72]		1·1					

* p < 0·05

and low birth weight no difference was found in current or previous pregnancies between users and non-users. There were reasons to suspect that information given on exposure in current pregnancies might have been affected by recall and other sources of bias. This interpretation was supported by further analyses of abortion rates by occupation which showed no association with frequency of VDT use.

In a recent study designed to test the hypothesis that electromagnetic fields emitted by VDTs were associated with spontaneous abortion, two groups of telephone operators were compared, one of whom used VDTs and the other whose tasks were similar did not.[71] Hours of use were obtained from company records and electromagnetic fields were measured at both types of work station. Abortions were ascertained by telephone interview and verified in hospital records. Among 2430 women interviewed there were 882 pregnancies; the relative risk for 1–25 hours use was 1·04 (95% CI 0·61 to 1·79) and for more than 25 hours use, 1·00 (95% CI 0·61 to 1·74). This was a convincing study, and since earlier positive findings could be attributable to recall bias, it can probably be concluded that the use of a VDT does not entail a risk of spontaneous abortion. Further assurance has been provided by a meta-analysis of reports to 1991.[73] In a recent Finnish study however, in which abortions were ascertained from records and VDT use by questionnaire, the relative risk was 1·1 (95% CI 0·7 to 1·6) but in a sub-group (25% of the total of 87 operators) who worked with machines which gave high intensity very low frequency fields; the relative risk was 3·4.[72] This finding will need confirmation before concerns are raised afresh.

Ionising radiation

Reproductive risks of occupational exposure to ionising radiation have been estimated from many sources and protection standards gradually made more strict.[74] The main source of information on fetal risk has been exposure of pregnant women to the atomic bombs dropped at Hiroshima and Nagasaki. Exposures were well-documented and surviving children thoroughly examined and followed to middle age. The defects found were microcephaly, eye malformations, and mental retardation; dose-response has been periodically revised. Before the atomic bombs were dropped, the results of in-utero exposure to therapeutic ovarian irradiation were reported.[7] Of 53 live and stillborn infants, 14 were microcephalic (see also chapter 3).

A report that maternal abdominal diagnostic x ray examinations resulted in an increase of leukaemia and childhood cancers[75] has been criticised although other findings have tended to support it.[74] These suggest that in-utero exposure to only a few mSV might be damaging. A study of the doses received by Canadian radiology technicians over an 11-year period (1977–88) showed that the mean annual doses received were, in diagnostic radiology, 0·2 mSV, in nuclear medicine, 1·8 mSV, and in radiotherapy, 1·1 mSV.[76] These levels are well below the limit set.

There is little epidemiological information on pregnancy outcome in radiographers. In Finland a case-control study of abortions recorded in hospital files was negative[42] and in the Montreal survey an increased risk of abortions was found after 16 weeks but not earlier.[16] This might have been due to ergonomic factors rather than radiation; recall bias also cannot be eliminated.

Temperature, noise, vibration

There is no direct evidence of human fetal damage from these factors.

Chemical

A serious difficulty in the epidemiological investigation of occupational exposures is that they are rarely to single substances. In a search for substances hazardous to the fetus, occupations of a national sample of women in Finland were classified into seven categories of presumed exposure: solvents, automobile exhaust fumes, polycyclic aromatic hydrocarbons, other chemicals, metals, textile dust, and animal microorganisms.[14] None of the women in these exposure groups had significantly higher incidences of spontaneous abortion. The authors commented that in interpreting the findings three possible sources of distortion needed to be considered: failure to include possible confounding factors such as smoking and alcohol consumption, variation in the frequency of induced abortions between groups, and ascertainment of abortions only from hospital records. In table 13.4 are listed reports of studies of spontaneous abortion in which attempts have been made to identify exposures to specific types of chemical; table 13.5 lists case-control studies of congenital defects.

Hexachlorophene used for hand-washing in hospitals was suspected of causing congenital defects,[83] but this hypothesis was not supported.[42 84] The possibility that occupational exposures may cause chromosomal abnormalities was investigated in a major cytogenetic study of consecutive hospital cases of spontaneous abortion in New York.[27] Mothers of cases and of referents of the same gestational age from a prenatal clinic were interviewed. Reported occupational exposures were equally common in karyotypically normal and abnormal aborted fetuses, thus not suggesting an occupational cause of chromosomal abnormalities.

Organic solvents

In a survey listed in table 13.4[33 34] and described on p 302 six occupational groups selected for chemical exposure were: hospital laboratories, industrial laboratories, dental assistants, gardeners, painters, and factory workers. They were compared with six groups with less

Table 13.4 Studies of spontaneous abortion with information about chemical exposure

	Occupation	Number of pregnancies	Type of exposure and evidence of risk	Odds ratio (95% CI or p value)
Hemminki et al. 1982[77]	Sterilising staff	1443	545 exposed to ethylene chloride: abortion rate 15·1% (<0·01) 605 not exposed to ethylene chloride: abortion rate 4·6%	
Axelsson et al. 1984[46]	Laboratory	1160	489 exposed to solvents: abortion rate 10·6% 488 not exposed to solvents: abortion rate 10·1%	1·3 (0·9 to 1·9)
Heidam 1984[33]	Laboratory—industry Laboratory—university	91 115	Compared with other occupations	1·2 (0·6 to 2·5) 0·7 (0·3 to 1·5)
Heidam 1984[34]	Factory Painting Gardening Dental assistant	357 38 102 259		1·7 (1·0 to 2·9) 2·9 (1·0 to 8·8) 0·9 1·0
Hemminki et al. 1985[42]	Nurses	*169/469	Exposure to anaesthetic gases: 55 cases, 36 controls Exposure to hexachlorophene: 31 cases, 82 controls Exposure to cytostatic drugs: 12 cases, 41 controls	1·2 1·1 0·8
McDonald et al. 1988[16]	Manufacturing	3142	504 exposed to solvents: stillbirth abortion	2·8 (<0·01) 1·2 (<0·01)
Taskinen et al. 1986[36]	Pharmaceutical manufacture	*44/132	Exposure to methylene chloride: 38 cases, 119 controls Exposure to oestrogens: 39 cases, 121 controls	2·3 (=0·06) 4·2 (<0·03)
Kyyronen et al. 1989[78]	Dry cleaning	*130/289	High exposure to tetrachloroethylene: 9 cases, 6 controls	3·6 (<0·05)
Lindbohm et al. 1990[59]	Monitored for solvent exposure	*73/167	Exposure to any solvent: Exposure to aliphatic hydrocarbons (high): 8 cases, 5 controls Exposure to toluene in shoe work: 5 cases, 2 controls	2·2 (1·2 to 4·1) 3·9 (1·1 to 14·2) 9·3 (1·0 to 84·7)

* Numbers of cases and controls

Table 13.5 Case-control studies of congenital defects and chemical exposures

	Type of defect	Cases-controls	Type of exposure and evidence of risk	Odds ratio
Holmberg et al. 1980[79]	Central nervous system	120/120	Organic solvents:	6·0 (p < 0·01)
Holmberg et al. 1982[80]	Oral clefts	388/388	Organic solvents:	3·5 (p < 0·05)
Hemminki et al. 1985[42]	Miscellaneous	38/99	Anaesthetic gases:	1·2
			Hexachlorophene:	0·2
			Cytostatic drugs:	4·7 (p = 0·02)
McDonald et al. 1987[35]	Miscellaneous	301/301	Aromatic solvents: associated with mainly renal-urinary defects	
Tikkanen et al. 1988[81]	Heart defects	160/160	No association found	
Cordier et al. 1990[82]	Miscellaneous	325/325	Solvents: oral clefts:	3·5

chemical exposure, including office workers, technical assistants and designers, occupational therapists, and physiotherapists. An increased risk of abortion was found in factory workers and painters, both of whom were exposed to organic solvents, but in none of the six groups was exposure to a single chemical associated with a significantly increased risk. In the study of pharmaceutical factory workers (see table 13.4) a total of 1795 pregnancies were reported, including 1179 deliveries and 142 abortions.[36] The abortion rate during employment was 10·9% compared with 10·6% before or after employment, and 8·5% in the corresponding hospital districts. A case-control analysis was based on 44 women who aborted while employed and three age-matched controls for each. Information on exposures was obtained from occupational physicians and nurses who were unaware of case-control status. Significant associations were found with exposure to the organic solvent methylene chloride and to oestrogens.

In the Montreal survey exposures of occupational groups to chemicals were classified by two industrial hygienists. In manufacturing jobs entailing solvent exposure, risks of stillbirth (OR 2·8) and to a lesser extent of abortion (OR 1·2) were found.[16] In Finland a study of dry-cleaning and laundry workers suggested that tetrachloroethylene exposure specifically might be implicated.[78] Another informative study in Finland, although not large, was undertaken of women who were monitored biochemically for organic solvents in the course of occupational surveillance.[59] Exposures were classified on the basis of job descriptions, stated use of solvents and biochemical measurements. The odds ratio adjusted for potential confounding was 2·2 for solvents in general; for aliphatic hydrocarbons it was 3·9, for exposed graphic workers 5·2 and for toluene-exposed shoe workers (only two cases) 9·3.

For congenital defects (table 13.5), organic solvents were associated in the Finnish case-control study with defects of the central nervous system[79] and oral clefts[80] but not with cardiovascular defects.[81] In other studies,[82 85 86] oral clefts and sacral agenesis were associated with solvent exposure and with printing where exposure to solvents occurs. In a case-control study of congenital defects in the Montreal survey a detailed investigation was undertaken of maternal workplace exposures for 301 cases and matched controls.[35] Chemical exposures were classified into nine groups: aliphatic solvents, aromatic solvents, plasticisers, metals, oils, bactericides and pesticides, detergents, gases, and miscellaneous substances. Only aromatic solvents showed an important excess association with congenital defects, which were predominantly renal or urinary. Toluene was the commonest aromatic solvent implicated.

Pesticides

The information on pesticide exposure is scanty. No risk of abortion was found in gardeners in Denmark, but only some 10% were significantly exposed.[34] In the Montreal survey, in 65 pregnancies in agricultural and horticultural workers there was some excess of abortions at 16–28 weeks, but none earlier.[16] In California, an excess of limb defects was found when either parent was an agricultural worker.[87]

Metals

Mercury exposure in dentistry was unrelated to risk of abortion in Montreal or in Denmark[16 34] and the same was true of low level lead exposure in Finland.[88] A risk of abortion has been reported in women who worked in a Swedish smelter[89] and in both Finland[90] and Montreal[16] with the manufacture of metal and electrical products. However the information on metal exposure in these studies was imprecise.

Plastics

In Finland a significantly increased risk of abortion was reported in women who worked in a plant where polyurethane was manufactured.[91] In Montreal too few women worked in the production of polyurethane to test this hypothesis but an association with polystyrene was found.[92] Work in Finland with reinforced plastics was not associated with adverse effects and[93] in Montreal this could not be tested as there was insufficient information on this type of exposure.

Biological

No information has been published on the reproductive effects of work entailing biological exposures, but it can be inferred that there may well be risks.

Ergonomic

Physical exertion

There is no consensus on whether physical exertion, perhaps because it may entail differing aspects, has adverse effects in pregnancy: some studies have been positive[94] and some negative.[95 96] Physical fitness is generally considered to be an asset in labour, recovery, and coping with a newborn baby, but there may be degrees of physical exertion that are harmful. An analysis of pregnancies in women on active service in the United States Army was informative.[32] Between 1981 and 1982, 22 450 women were known to have given birth. Social security numbers were available for ascertaining pregnancy outcome in army hospitals. On enroling they had been tested for physical capacity and allocated to one of five categories of job, which ranged from low physical demand to heavy work. Many characteristics were recorded and nine potentially confounding factors were included in the analysis. Unfortunately many work records were not

315

successfully matched with obstetric records and the analysis was restricted to 6674 singleton births. There were 604 preterm births (9%), a proportion which rose with increasing physical work demands (6·1%, 8·5%, 8·4%, 9·8%, 10·1%). However, although the findings were consistent with a correlation between physical effort and preterm birth, the large amount of missing data requires that interpretation be cautious.

In the United States Natality Survey[31, 38], the occupational classification used contained detailed descriptions of physical activities and environmental factors for 12 000 distinct occupations at more than 75 000 sites. This permitted a comprehensive analysis of physical activities and environmental factors for 2711 white married women. The only significant association was between a long working week of 40 or more hours and low birth weight.[38] For reasons given on page 299, low birth weight is an unsatisfactory index because it is affected by many confounding variables. However, a negative result is not surprising in a study that was not large and in which ergonomic factors were derived from an occupational classification.

Answers to questions about physical and other work requirements in the Montreal survey showed that lifting heavy weights 15 or more times a day was associated with an increased risk of fetal death (table 13.6). Questions about lifting heavy weights were asked in a few other surveys and the activity was found to be associated with abortion in three,[36 49 78] but not in two.[46 59] An increased risk of preterm birth was found with heavy lifting in the Montreal survey but not in Sweden.[98]

Shift work

Shift work has not been consistently defined in studies of reproductive performance. In the Montreal survey women were asked whether they worked in the day, evening, day and evening, night, rotating shift or other schedule. In the analysis, rotating shift was combined with other schedules and termed "changing shift." This group had a significantly increased risk of spontaneous abortion (relative risk 1·45, 95% CI 1·0 to 1·9). In Sweden, in a study of laboratory personnel, a relative risk of 3·2 (95% CI 1·36 to 7·47) was found in shift workers.[46] The same authors subsequently studied the schedules of hospital personnel who do more shift work than any other occupational group. Official Swedish statistics indicated that in 1982, 32·5% of all working women worked irregular or inconvenient hours. Inconvenient hours were defined as work before or after 06.45–17.45; irregular hours as work outside this period and not beginning or ending at the same time each day. In a questionnaire study of 807 women employed at a hospital from 1980 to 1984, women were divided into six work-schedule groups.[97] Those who worked irregular hours or rotating shifts had a slight but not significantly increased rate of abortion (odds ratio, 1·44, 95% CI 0·83 to 2·51) compared with those who did day work.

Table 13.6 *Ergonomic factors and pregnancy outcome (odds ratios (95% confidence interval or p value))*

	Fetal death		Preterm birth	
	Montreal survey[16]	Other studies	Montreal survey[40]	Other studies
Lifting heavy weights ≥15×daily	1·5 (<0·01)	Axelsson et al. 1984[46] 1·4 (0·9–2·02) Taskinen et al. 1986[36] 3·6 (1·0–13·7) Kyyronen et al. 1989[78] 1·9 (1·0–2·8) Taskinen et al. 1990[49] 3·5 (1·1–9·0) Lindbohm et al. 1990[59] about 1	1·3 (<0·01)	Ahlborg et al. 1990[98] 1·71 (0·85 to 3·44)
Other physical effort	1·4 (<0·01)			
Standing	1·2 (<0·01)			Teitelman et al. 1990[99] 2·7 (1·24 to 5·95) Klebanoff et al. 1990[96] 1·28 (0·02 to 1·61) Launer et al. 1990[100] 1·56 (1·04 to 2·6)
Long work week	1·2 (<0·01)			
Changing shift	1·3 (<0·01)	Axelsson et al. 1984[46] 3·2 (1·36–7·47) Axelsson et al. 1989[97] 1·4 (0·83–2·51)	1·3 (<0·05)	

However, they were also found to have had more children of low birth weight than day workers; this might suggest that the women who worked these hours differed from day workers in other ways.

Fatigue

In the survey of working conditions and preterm birth in France,[31] it was found that manual, service, and shop workers had higher preterm delivery rates than professional, administrative, or clerical workers. Physically tiring working conditions, standing, carrying heavy loads, assembly line work, and considerable physical effort were related to a higher rate of preterm birth and low birth weight. In this survey, 35% of employees stood most of the time, 15% had to carry heavy loads, 7% were assembly line workers, and 23% were considered to have a physically demanding job. These work requirements were strongly related to type of occupation. Assembly line work was carried out by production workers, standing was common in all occupations except clerical, carrying heavy loads and physical effort were most common in production, shop, and service workers. No significant link was found with low birth weight, but women with three or four of these work demands had a higher preterm delivery rate than other women. In 1977–8, Mamelle et al. studied working conditions in detail in women who gave birth in two maternity units—one in a large city and one in a small town.[101] By scoring numerically five aspects of occupational fatigue, they constructed an index. The components included standing, work on conveyer belt or industrial machine, physical effort, mental stress from routine work, a noisy, cold, or wet atmosphere, and manipulation of chemicals. The score correlated closely with the risk of preterm birth.

In Montreal, an approximate replica of the Mamelle index was also correlated with pre-term birth, but more weakly.[40] As preterm birth is associated with poor socioeconomic conditions and work with a high fatigue index tends to be done by under-privileged women, this may be the explanation rather than that fatigue causes preterm birth. It is noteworthy that in Montreal only two work characteristics—standing and a long work week—were associated with preterm birth or fetal death and that these risks were seen only in women who stopped work before the 28th week of pregnancy. The highest levels of all the specific ergonomic factors were significantly associated with abortion. Because the data were obtained retrospectively an additional grouped analysis was undertaken to reduce the possibility of recall bias, which could well have occurred in view of the distressing nature of miscarriage.[16] Lifting, physical effort and standing remained correlated at a 5% level of significance, consistent with a causal explanation.

Conclusions

Epidemiological studies, which have been carried out only in industrialised countries, suggest that employment during pregnancy carries a small excess risk of fetal death but little if any risk of preterm birth. By applying the frequency of job requirements from the Montreal survey to the estimated numbers of pregnant women who were employed in the Province of Quebec a total excess of 1% of fetal deaths was estimated to be attributable to occupation. For preterm births the excess was lower still (0.2%), and for congenital defects too low to calculate.[102] The following groups were estimated to have a 3% excess of fetal death: nurses, waitresses, cleaners, laundry and dry-cleaning workers, and women in certain manufacturing jobs. Teachers, health workers other than nurses, saleswomen, and some manufacturing jobs had about a 1% increase in risk. Administrative and clerical workers were at virtually no risk.

With regard to specific risk factors, physical exertion and ergonomic requirements and probably exposure to solvents are apparently associated with some increased risk of fetal death. For congenital defects, there remains insufficient evidence of an association of any particular chemical, with the possible exception of solvents, to imply causation. This is hardly surprising as extensive epidemiological research has failed to incriminate any environmental agents, apart from ionising radiation, rubella virus, cytomegalovirus and *toxoplasma gondii*.

It is by no means certain that the risks that have been identified are real because, although the possibility of confounding can be greatly reduced, it cannot be eliminated. Even the increased risks in manufacturing industries that have been repeatedly noted in this review could be attributable to the characteristics of industrial workers and their less privileged lifestyle. If the risks are real, however, there remains the question of how they can be prevented because removal from exposure once pregnancy is recognised is probably too late.[102] In the absence of better information, the only prudent course is to ensure that so far as possible women of childbearing age are not required to undertake potentially hazardous work.

1 Kahne H, Giele LZ. *Women's work and women's lives*. Oxford: Westview Press, 1992.
2 International Labour Office. *Yearbook of Labour Statistics*. Geneva: International Labour Organisation, 1992.
3 Rom NN, ed. *Environmental and occupational medicine*. Boston: Little Brown, 1983.
4 Miller MW, Ziskin MC. Biological consequences of hyperthermia. *Ultrasound Med Biol* 1989; 15: 707–22.
5 Creasy RK, Resnik R. *Maternal-fetal medicine*. 2nd Ed, Philadelphia: WB Saunders, 1989.
6 Michaelson SM. Health implications of exposure to radio frequency/microwave energies. *Br J Ind Med* 1982; 39: 105–19.
7 Murphy DP. Ovarian irradiation; its effect on the health of subsequent children. *Surg Gynec Obstet* 1928; 47: 201–15.

8 Kalter H, Warkany J. Congenital malformations; etiologic factors and their role in prevention. *N Engl J Med* 1983; **308**: 424–31, 491–7.
9 McDonald AD. Maternal health and congenital defect—a prospective investigation. *N Engl J Med* 1958; **258**: 767–73.
10 Kline J, Stein Z, Susser M, Warburton D. Fever during pregnancy and spontaneous abortion. *Am J Epidemiol* 1985; **121**: 832–42.
11 Wilcox AJ, Weinberg CR, Baird DD. Risk factors for early pregnancy loss. *Epidemiology* 1990; **1**: 382–5.
12 Wilcox AJ, Horney LF. Accuracy of spontaneous abortion recall. *Am J Epidemiol* 1984; **120**: 727–33.
13 Shapiro S, Jones EW, Densen PM. Life table of pregnancy terminations and correlates of fetal loss. *Millbank Memorial Fund Quarterly* 1962; **40**: 7–32.
14 Lindbohm M-L, Hemminki K, Kyyronen P. Parental occupational exposure and spontaneous abortions in Finland. *Am J Epidemiol* 1984; **120**: 370–8.
15 Lindbohm M-L, Hemminki K. Nationwide data base on medically diagnosed spontaneous abortions. *Int J Epidemiol* 1988; **17**: 568–73.
16 McDonald AD, McDonald JC, Armstrong B, Cherry NM, Côté R, Lavoie J, et al. Foetal death and work in pregnancy. *Br J Ind Med* 1988; **45**: 148–57.
17 Roman E. Fetal loss rates and their relation to pregnancy order. *J Epidemiol Community Health* 1984; **38**: 29–35.
18 Pharoah POD, Alberman E, Doyle P, Chamberlain G. Outcome of pregnancy among women in anaesthetic practice. *Lancet* 1977; 1: 34–6.
19 Risch HA, Weiss NS, Clarke A, Miller AB. Risk factors for spontaneous abortion and its recurrence. *Am J Epidemiol* 1988; **128**: 420–30.
20 Villar J, Belizan JM. The relative contribution of prematurity and fetal growth retardation to low birth weight in developing and developed societies. *Am J Obstet Gynecol* 1982; **143**: 793–8.
21 Bakketeig LS. The risk of preterm or low birth weight delivery. In: Reed DM, Stanley FJ, eds. *The epidemiology of prematurity*. Baltimore-Munich: Urban and Schwartzenberg, 1977; 231–41.
22 Garn SM, Shaw HA, McCabe KD. Effect of socio-economic status on weight-defined and gestational prematurity in the United-States. In: Reed DM, Stanley FJ, eds. *The epidemiology of prematurity*, Baltimore-Munich: Urban and Schwartzenberg, 1977, 127–43.
23 Fedrick J, Anderson ABM. Factors associated with spontaneous preterm birth. *Br J Obstet Gynaecol* 1976; **83**: 342–50.
24 Kaltreider DF, Kohl S. Epidemiology of preterm delivery. *Clin Obstet Gynecol* 1980; **23**: 17–30.
25 McDonald AD, Armstrong BG, Sloan M. Cigarette, alcohol, and coffee consumption and prematurity. *Am J Public Health* 1992; **82**: 87–90.
26 Brent RL. Environmental teratogens. *Bull N Y Acad Med* 1990; **66**: 123–63.
27 Warburton D. Effects of common environmental exposures on spontaneous abortion of defined karyotype. In: *Prevention of Physical and Mental Defects Part C*, New York, Alan R Liss Inc 1985; 31–6.
28 Horowitz I, McDonald AD. Anencephaly and spina bifida in the Province of Quebec. *Can Med Assoc J* 1969; **100**: 1–8.
29 Stewart A. A note on the obstetric effects of work during pregnancy. *British Journal of Preventive and Social Medicine* 1955; **9**: 159–61.
30 Saurel-Cubizolles MJ, Kaminski M. Pregnant women's working conditions and their changes during pregnancy: a national study in France. *Br J Ind Med* 1987; **44**: 236–43.
31 Savitz DA, Whelan EA, Rowland AS, Kleckner RC. Maternal employment and reproductive risk factors. *Am J Epidemiol* 1990; **132**: 933–45.
32 Ramirez G, Grimes RM, Annegers JF, Davis BR, Slater CH. Occupational physical activity and other risk factors among US army primigravidas. *Am J Public Health* 1990; **80**: 728–30.
33 Heidam LZ. Spontaneous abortions among laboratory workers; a follow-up study. *J Epidemiol Community Health* 1984; **38**: 36–41.
34 Heidam LZ. Spontaneous abortions among dental assistants factory workers, painters

and gardening workers: a follow-up study. *J Epidemiol Community Health* 1984; 38: 149–55.

35 McDonald JC, Lavoie J, Côté R, McDonald AD. Chemical exposures at work in early pregnancy and congenital defect: a case-referent study. *Br J Ind Med* 1987; 44: 527–33.

36 Taskinen H, Lindbohm M-L, Hemminki K. Spontaneous abortions among women working in the pharmaceutical industry. *Br J Ind Med* 1986; 43: 199–205.

37 Hemminki K, Mutanen P, Luoma K, Salionemi I. Congenital malformations by the parental occupation in Finland. *Int Arch Occup Environ Health* 1980; 46: 93–8.

38 Peoples-Sheps MD, Siegel E, Suchindran CM, Origasa H, Ware A, Barakat A. Characteristics of maternal employment during pregnancy: effects on low birth weight. *Am J Public Health* 1991; 81: 1007–12.

39 McDonald AD, McDonald JC, Armstrong BG, Cherry NM, Delorme C, Nolin AD, Robert D. Occupation and pregnancy outcome. *Br J Ind Med* 1987; 44: 521–6.

40 McDonald AD, McDonald JC, Armstrong BG, Cherry NM, Nolin AD, Robert D. Prematurity and work in pregnancy. *Br J Ind Med* 1988; 45: 56–62.

41 Axelsson G, Rylander R. Exposure to anaesthetic gases and spontaneous abortion: response bias in a postal questionnaire study. *Int J Epidemiol* 1982; 11: 250–6.

42 Hemminki K, Kyyronen P, Lindbohm M-L. Spontaneous abortions and malformations in the offspring of nurses exposed to anaesthetic gases, cytostatic drugs and other potential hazards in hospitals based on registered information of outcome. *Br J Ind Med* 1985; 39: 141–7.

43 Strandberg M, Sandback K, Axelson O, Sundell L. Spontaneous abortions among women in a hospital laboratory. *Lancet* 1978; i: 384–5.

44 Meirik O, Kallen B, Gauffin U, Ericson A. Major malformations in infants born of women who worked in laboratories while pregnant. *Lancet* 1979; ii: 91.

45 Ericson A, Pol M, Källen B, Meirik O, Westerholm P. Gastrointestinal atresia and maternal occupation during pregnancy. *J Occup Med* 1982; 27: 515–8.

46 Axelsson G, Lütz C, Rylander R. Exposure to solvents and outcome of pregnancy in university laboratory employees. *Br J Ind Med* 1984; 41: 305–12.

47 Axelsson G, Rylander R. Outcome of pregnancy in women engaged in laboratory work in a petrochemical plant. *Am J Ind Med* 1989; 16: 539–45.

48 Vaughan TL, Daling JR, Starzyk PM. Fetal death and maternal occupation. An analysis of birth records in the State of Washington. *J Occup Med* 1984; 26: 676–8.

49 Taskinen H, Kyyronen P, Hemminki K. Effects of ultrasound, short waves and physical exertion on pregnancy outcome in physiotherapists. *J Epidemiol Community Health* 1990; 44: 196–201.

50 Larsen AI. Congenital malformations and exposure to high frequency electro-magnetic radiation among Danish physiotherapists. *Scand J Work Environ Health* 1991; 17: 318–23.

51 Saurel-Cubizolles MJ, Kaminski M, Llado-Archipoff J, Du Mazautrin C, Estryn-Behar M, Berthier C *et al*. Pregnancy and its outcome among hospital personnel according to occupation and working conditions. *J Epidemiol Community Health* 1985; 39: 129–34.

52 McDonald AD, McDonald JC, Armstrong BG, Cherry NM, Côté R, Lavoie J, Nolin AD, Robert D. Congenital defects and work in pregnancy. *Br J Ind Med* 1988; 45: 581–8.

53 Selevan SG, Lindbohm M-L, Hornung RW, Hemminki K. A study of occupational exposure to antineoplastic drugs and fetal loss in nurses. *N Engl J Med* 1985; 313: 1173–8.

54 Stücker I, Caillard J-F, Collin R, Grout M, Poyen D, Hémon D. Risk of spontaneous abortion among nurses handling antineoplastic drugs. *Scand J Work Environ Health* 1990; 16: 102–7.

55 Demmler GJ. Summary of a workshop on surveillance for congenital cytomegalovirus disease. *Reviews of infectious disease* 1991; 13: 315–29.

56 Murph JR, Baron JC, Kice Brown C, Ebelhack CL, Bale JF. The occupational risk of cytomegalovirus infection among day care providers. *JAMA* 1991; 265: 603–8.

57 Clarke M, Mason ES. Leatherwork: a possible hazard to reproduction. *BMJ* 1985; 290: 1235–7.

58 McDonald AD, McDonald JC. Outcome of pregnancy in leatherworkers. *BMJ* 1986; **292**: 979–81.

59 Lindbohm M-L, Taskinen H, Markku S, Hemminki K. Spontaneous abortion among women exposed to organic solvents. *Am J Ind Med* 1990; **17**: 449–63.

60 Landrigan PJ, Melius JM, Rosenberg MJ, Coye MJ, Binkin NJ. Reproductive hazards in the workplace—development of epidemiologic research. *Scand J Work Environ Health* 1983; **33**: 83–8.

61 Purdham J. Adverse pregnancy outcome amongst VDT operators—the cluster phenomenon. In: Pearce BG, ed. *Allegations of reproductive hazards from VDUs.* Nottingham: Humane Technology, 1984: 27–40.

62 Kurppa K, Holmberg PC, Rantala K, Nurminen T, Saxen L. Birth defects and exposure to video-display terminals during pregnancy. *Scand J Work Environ Health* 1985; **11**: 353–6.

63 Ericson A, Källen B. An epidemiological study of work with video screens and pregnancy outcome: I. A registry study. *Am J Ind Med* 1986; **9**: 447–57.

64 Ericson A, Källen B. An epidemiological study of work with video screens and pregnancy outcome: II A case-control study. *Am J Ind Med* 1986; **9**: 459–75.

65 Butler WJ, Brix KA. Video display terminal work and pregnancy outcome in Michigan clerical workers. In: Pearce BG, ed. *Allegations of reproductive hazards from VDUs.* Nottingham: Humane Technology 1986: 67–91.

66 Westerholm P, Ericson A. Pregnancy outcome and VDU work in a cohort of insurance clerks. In: Knave B, Wideback PG eds. *Work with display units.* Stockholm: Elsevier, 1987: 104–10.

67 Goldhaber MK, Polen MR, Hiatt RA. The risk of miscarriage and birth defects among women who use visual display terminals during pregnancy. *Am J Ind Med* 1988; **13**: 695–706.

68 McDonald AD, McDonald JC, Armstrong BG, Cherry NM, Nolin AD. Work with visual display units in pregnancy. *Br J Ind Med* 1988; **45**: 509–15.

69 Bryant HE, Love EJ. Video display terminal use and spontaneous abortion risk. *Int J Epidemiol* 1989; **18**: 132–8.

70 Neilson CV, Brandt LPA. Spontaneous abortion among women using video-display terminals. *Scand J Work Environ Health* 1990; **16**: 323–8.

71 Schnorr TM, Grajewski BA, Hornung RW, Thun MJ, Egelund GM, Murray WE *et al.* Video-display terminals and the risk of spontaneous abortion. *N Engl J Med* 1991; **324**: 727–33.

72 Lindbohm M-L, Hietanen M, Kyyronen P, Sallmen M, von Nandelstadth P, Taskinen H *et al.* Magnetic fields of video-display terminals and spontaneous abortion. *Am J Epidemiol* 1992; **136**: 1041–51.

73 Parazzini F, Luchini L, LaVecchia C, Giorgio-Crosignani P. Video display terminal use during pregnancy and reproductive outcome—a meta analysis. *J Epidemiol Community Health* 1993; **47**: 265–8.

74 Upton AC, Shore RE, Harley NH. The health effects of low level ionising radiation. *Am Rev Publ Health* 1992; **13**: 127–50.

75 Stewart AM, Webb J, Giles D, Hewitt D. Preliminary communication: malignant disease in childhood and diagnostic irradiation in utero. *Lancet* 1956; **ii**: 447–8.

76 Huda W, Bews J, Gordon K, Sutherland JB, Sont WN, Ashmore JP. Doses and population irradiation factors for Canadian radiation technologists (1978–88). *Can Assoc Radiol J* 1991; **42**: 247–60.

77 Hemminki K, Mutanen P, Saloniemi I, Niemi M-L. Spontaneous abortion in hospital staff engaged in sterilising instruments with chemical agents. *BMJ* 1982; **285**: 1461–3.

78 Kyyronen P, Taskinen H, Lindbohm M-L, Hemminki K, Heinonen OP. Spontaneous abortions and congenital malformations among women exposed to tetrachloroethylene in dry cleaning. *J Epidemiol Community Health* 1989; **43**: 346–51.

79 Holmberg PC, Nurminen M. Congenital defects of the central nervous system and occupational factors during pregnancy. A case-referent study. *Am J Ind Med* 1980; **1**: 167–76.

80 Holmberg PC, Hernberg S, Kurppa K, Raita R, Rantala K. Oral clefts and organic solvent exposure during pregnancy. *Int Arch Occup Environ Health* 1982; **50**: 371–6.

81 Tikkanen J, Heinonen OP. Cardiovascular malformation and organic solvent exposure during pregnancy in Finland. *Am J Ind Med* 1988; **14**: 1–8.

82 Cordier S, Ha M-C, Ayme S, Goujard J. Maternal occupational exposure and congenital malformations. *Scand J Work Environ Health* 1992; **18**: 11–17.

83 Halling H. Suspected link between exposure to hexachlorophene and malformed infants. *Ann NY Acad Sci* 1979; **320**: 426–435.

84 Baltzar B, Ericson A, Kallen B. Delivery outcome in women employee in medical occupations in Sweden. *J Occup Med* 1979; **21**: 543–8.

85 Erickson JD, Cochran WM, Anderson CE. Parental occupation and birth defects. *Contributions to Epidemiology and Biostatistics* 1979; **1**: 107–17.

86 Kucera J. Exposure to fat solvents. A possible cause of sacral agenesis in man. *J Pediatr* 1986; **72**: 857–9.

87 Schwartz DA, Newsum LA, Heifetz RM. Parental occupation and birth outcome in an agricultural community. *Scand J Work Environ Health* 1986; **12**: 51–4.

88 Taskinen H. Spontaneous abortion among women occupationally exposed to lead. In: Hogstedt C, Reuterwall C, eds. *Progress in occupational epidemiology*. New York: Elsevier 1988: 197–200.

89 Nordstrom S, Beckman L, Nordenson I. Occupational and environmental risks in and around a smelter in northern Sweden. V Spontaneous abortions among female employees and decreased birth weight in their offspring. *Hereditas* 1979; **90**: 291–6.

90 Hemminki K, Niemi M-L, Koskinen K, Vainio H. Spontaneous abortions among women employed in the metal industry in Finland. *Int Arch Occup Environ Health* 1980; **47**: 53–60.

91 Lindbohm M-L, Hemminki K, Kyyronen P. Spontaneous abortion among women employed in the plastics industry. *Am J Ind Med* 1985; **8**: 579–86.

92 McDonald AD, Lavoie J, Côté R, McDonald JC. Spontaneous abortion in women employed in plastic manufacture. *Am J Ind Med* 1988; **13**: 1–6.

93 Harkonen H, Holmberg PC. Obstetric histories of women occupationally exposed to styrene. *Scand J Work Environ Health* 1982; **8**: 74–7.

94 Homer CJ, Beresford SAA, James SA, Siegel E, Wilcox S. Work-related physical exertion and risk of preterm low birth weight delivery. *Paediatr Perinat Epidemiol* 1990; **4**: 161–74.

95 Berkowitz GS, Kelsey JL, Holford TR. Physical activity and the risk of spontaneous preterm delivery. *J Reprod Med* 1983; **28**: 581–8.

96 Klebanoff M, Shiono P, Carey J. The effects of physical activity during pregnancy on preterm delivery and birth weight. *Am J Obstet Gynecol* 1990; **163**: 1450–6.

97 Axelsson G, Rylander R, Molin I. Outcome of pregnancy in relation to irregular and inconvenient work schedules. *Br J Ind Med* 1989; **46**: 393–8.

98 Ahlborg G, Bodin L, Hogstedt C. Heavy lifting during pregnancy—a hazard to the foetus: a prospective study. *Int J Epidemiol* 1990; **19**: 90–7.

99 Teitelman AM, Welch LS, Hellenbrand KG, Bracken MB. Effect of maternal work activity on preterm birth and low birth weight. *Am J Epidemiol* 1990; **131**: 104–13.

100 Launer LJ, Villar J, Kestler E, De Onis M. The effect of maternal work on fetal growth and duration of pregnancy: a prospective study. *Br J Obstet Gynaecol* 1990; **97**: 67–70.

101 Mamelle N, Laumon B, Lazar P. Prematurity and occupational activity during pregnancy. *Am J Epidemiol* 1984; **119**: 309–22.

102 McDonald AD. The retrait préventif: an evaluation. *Can J Public Health* 1994; **85**: 136–9.

METHODOLOGY

14 Study design

CORBETT McDONALD

Introduction

It is not the purpose of this chapter to add yet another summary of epidimiological theory to the many already available. The focus instead will be on aspects of design in studies that have had some success in achieving their objective. The first dozen chapters of this book have presented the current state of epidemiological knowledge on important work-related diseases; this review will draw most of its examples from the same material.

Occupational epidemiology has a clear purpose, to identify, evaluate, and quantify factors in the workplace which impair health and shorten life so as to be able to control them. There are also questions of productivity and work satisfaction but these are not the main concern. It is against the primary objective that research designs are to be judged, rather than on purely scientific criteria, although obviously these cannot be ignored. A good design is one that works, that produces the required information reliably and efficiently. As ever, Voltaire's admonition, "le mieux est l'ennemi du bien" is applicable. Although perfectionism can hinder progress, the wrong answer can certainly do so; some information is better than none provided that it is essentially correct. Thus health policies and priorities can be soundly based on surveillance schemes that provide relative but not absolute data; safe environmental conditions can be achieved with only approximate information on exposure response, and the effectiveness of preventive measures may have to be assessed without controlled trials. To demand complete knowledge can too easily lead to inaction, or action taken in ignorance, than which, to paraphrase von Clausewitz "nothing is more terrifying."

Basic principles

Plans and hypotheses

It is unwise to conduct even a simple epidemiological study without a plan, including a clear statement of purpose and an unambiguous definition of the hypothesis to be tested. In practice, most studies are descriptive, and more concerned with identifying likely hypotheses than with testing them. A common problem is that the population available is the only one of its kind with no other easily available on which to test any associations that are found. In these circumstances the investigator would be wise to define and test one or perhaps two best bets from the outset.

Design strategies

It is often recommended that before embarking on an observational study the researcher should consider the design of a controlled experiment and get as close to that as possible. The converse is also true: an investigator concerned with the feasibility of an experimental design for evaluation should perhaps consider the best observational alternative. There is a narrow but important line that separates the two main approaches—the experiment in which treated and untreated are allocated by a random procedure and the observational study in which the groups are selected or self-selected. However, even the first approach does not guarantee comparability nor that its findings can be generalised, and the second, although potentially generalisable, may be subject to serious bias. Between the two are the quasi-experimental designs which may entail a degree of randomisation, of circumstances but not of subjects, which can achieve considerable validity and generalisability but have so far been little used in occupational health.

The various possible approaches to evaluation have some parallels with the range of designs available for aetiological research. Aside from the few occasions when experimental studies of human exposure are useful and ethically possible, for example, challenge tests in asthma and some clinical experimentation with solvents, the investigator is presented with the choice of three designs rather simplistically classified as cross-sectional

326

(prevalence), case-referent (case-control) and longitudinal (cohort). These three designs have more in common than might at first appear. They differ only in the method of sampling the sick (cases) and the healthy (referents) from an appropriately defined "base population". It is important to appreciate that all study populations are selected in time and space and usually in many other ways, and can never be considered with certainty as wholly representative of the universe. To achieve fair and valid comparisons, cases and the populations from which they come must be closely similar to those in which are found the non-cases (or controls). Whatever the study design, the test of comparability lies in the question: Would this "control" have been included for analysis if in fact it had been a "case"? This simple but fundamental question is applicable in all designs.

Cohort studies

In essence, subjects are selected in some defined manner, usually in the past, and their morbidity or mortality observed over a given period of time. Quite separately the relevant occupational exposures of the cohort, as a group or individually, are recorded. Comparisons are then made between mortality or morbidity rates in the study group and those in some non-exposed population or (a) within the cohort in sub-cohorts defined by level of exposure or (b) within the cohort by comparing the exposure of cases against non-cases. Let us now consider the problems. First, no cohort is ever a random sample of all men or women even at a given time and place. Innumerable socioeconomic and biological factors determine in part the characteristics of those included for study and, similarly, their duration and severity of occupational exposure. Second, a cohort defined before exposure, for example, at time of first employment, or even at birth, may differ importantly from one recruited from persons in employment at a given date, who are to that extent survivors. Third, uneven standards of health care and diagnosis can cause systematic bias in disease ascertainment; for example medical surveillance may be directed at those most heavily exposed: necropsies tend to be more common if compensation is an issue. For these reasons comparisons against any external reference are liable to considerable bias, compounded if the cohort is defined cross-sectionally. The most reliable approach is for the cohort to be assembled before exposure or at first employment and probably for the comparisons to be made internally. This requires adequate data on the level of exposure for each cohort member and, as this may be difficult to obtain for everyone, it may well be best to concentrate on cases and a limited number of controls (non-cases).

Case-referent studies

The cohort design just outlined can also be regarded as a method of identifying cases and non-cases in a defined population for possible case-referent analysis. This approach may not be feasible especially for uncommon diseases. It may then be best to ascertain by a standard procedure all incident (new) cases within an identifiable population for a defined period of time. Controls can then be selected from similar but "healthy" people in the same population who would have been diagnosed as cases had they had the same type of disease. Should this approach also be considered too difficult or expensive the investigator may be forced back on an easier but less reliable strategy, namely the use of some available case series and the more difficult and uncertain task of finding appropriate controls.

These three examples with increasing relaxation of requirements for case selection are part of a continuum with implications of two kinds. The less that cases and controls can be related to a birth cohort the more difficult will it be (a) to obtain estimates of absolute and attributable as opposed to relative risk and (b) to be confident of the validity of the exposure comparisons. The latter is obviously the more important issue because apart from the inherent uncertainties related to selection and self-selection in any observational study many other types of bias may occur when cases and controls do not reflect the same base population.

Cross-sectional studies

Although often derided as inferior to the prospective and retrospective designs just reviewed, this view is not entirely justified. In some circumstances, a cross-sectional survey can achieve reasonably good ascertainment of cases and controls within an identifiable population, as was outlined in the second option for case-control studies. Of course, assumptions have to be made concerning the connection between prevalent disorders and their earlier incidence, and proper consideration must be given to the extent of potential bias resulting from the loss, perhaps because of illness, of employees who properly formed part of the base cohort before the cross-sectional phase of ascertainment. Both these problems can usually be dealt with if the effort is made to do so.

Bias and confounding

No topic is given more space in Last's *Dictionary of epidemiology* than bias; the main cause of which is "selection" in its various guises. Bias results from systematic error in collection, recording, analysis, or interpretation of data. It is serious when it leads to faulty conclusions especially on questions of cause and effect. Even with great care it is difficult to be sure that all possibility of bias has been eliminated from an epidemiological investigation; it is largely for this reason that the principles of study design have been developed. As important as the avoidance of bias is the necessity to ensure that a study is capable of coping with it. The double-blind randomised controlled trial is perhaps the best example of absolute priority being given to this objective–but at the price of generalisability.

To attribute some index disease incidence to a particular exposure requires (a) knowledge of what would have happened without it and (b) the absence of any important coincidental (confounding) factor capable of explaining the presence or absence of the association. Age, sex, and a wide range of socioeconomic and personal factors are common confounders, but so too are systematic errors (or bias) in observation, recording, and analysis if related to both the disease and the exposure of interest. A special aspect of confounding, known as interaction, (also termed effect modification) is recognised when the association between exposure and disease varies with level of exposure to some other factor. Such interactions may vary in degree and may or may not be biological; if the latter we are dealing with a causal cofactor and not confounding.

Biased observation need not necessarily bias the results of a study. For example, radiologists undoubtedly overestimate disease progression when chest x ray films are presented in known temporal order, but readings made in this way are considerably more sensitive to change than when based on films presented in random order. Provided, however, that the readers are blind to the exposure hypothesis under test, the conclusions may well be correct, even though derived from potentially biased readings.

The main types of bias in epidemiological studies result from the following: (a) instrumental or observer error ("measurement bias"); (b) errors in case definition, detection, recall, response, or reporting ("information bias"); (c) an unrepresentative sampling frame or non-random selection ("selection bias"); (d) failure to record or allow for confounding factors coincidentally related to the causal hypothesis ("confounding bias"). While confounding can thus be a cause of bias, bias can also result in confounding and even in a statistical but not biological interaction.

Study size

As discussed in chapter 18, concepts of chance, probability, and power are of considerable importance in the interpretation of survey findings and so must also be considered in study design. As a result of innumerable unknown factors, random variation must be expected in the distribution of health, human susceptibility, and environmental factors in any large population. When sampling from the universe of events remarkable but meaningless associations between occupation and disease will be found. Yates' comment that, "the one in a million chance occurs exactly one in a million times no matter how unlikely it seems when it happens to you" poses a special problem in epidemiology. The fundamental need is to separate chance associations from those that reflect cause and effect. No observational study or surveillance scheme, undertaken without a limited number of well-defined hypotheses can ever do more than raise suspicions which, strictly speaking, have then to be tested in another population. Of course the suspicion may be so strong or have such dire consequences that any further study cannot be justified. This type of quandary is not rare in occupational epidemiology and can be resolved only in terms of cost and benefit, and the unavoidable questions: for whom.

In circumstances where there is a sufficiently important hypothesis to be tested, it follows that the investigation should be designed to do so as convincingly as possible. Low level risks present great difficulty because they require very large studies that are particularly susceptible to error because of countless unforeseen and unidentifiable factors. Thus it is seldom wise to attempt the direct estimation of marginal risks, usually from low level exposures but instead, to estimate risks at low levels by intelligent extrapolation from exposure-response data and the use of all other available information. On the other hand when the risks are large quite small studies can be extremely informative. Even when the number of workers at risk is limited, the investigator should not be unduly deterred by statistical estimates of low power. Given a well designed study a probability even as low as 0·2 may be critically important. It is unlikely that any granting agency today would have funded the classic cohort study by Doll in the 1950s of only 111 asbestos textile workers[1] much less the daily treatment with two oranges and one lemon of two out of 12 sailors with scurvy by Lind in 1747.[2] Even so, occupational epidemiologists need to consider the power of their study quite seriously when planning an investigation. In practice we want to be sure that if the risk is large our study will detect it but if small there is less need for the same degree of confidence. Before seeking statistical advice on study size we must therefore be clear what we mean by magnitude and seriousness of risk and levels of confidence. This obviously depends on the nature of the disease and of the exposure in question. As these problems are complex and quantification difficult, power calculations require much more than the application of a simple statistical formula. These issues are discussed well in Rothman's text.[3]

Designs for a purpose

Work-related epidemiological studies are roughly classifiable under five main headings: search and surveillance, hypothesis testing, assessment of confounding and interaction, quantification of exposure-response, and evaluation of control measures. The objectives under these headings are not mutually exclusive and others could be added. Evaluation is the subject of chapter 17 and need not be discussed further here. Some of the three basic study designs mentioned earlier are better suited to one purpose than another, but their success or failure in practice is mainly determined by the detailed protocol and how competently it is implemented. In the preceding chapters, findings from many studies have been cited; only some will be discussed here, selected as far as possible for their lessons in methodology.

Above all, epidemiology is the science of causation in medicine, and directly or indirectly, most epidemiologists are mainly concerned with some aspect of cause and effect. The discrimination of causal associations between occupational factors and disease from those resulting from chance or coincidence, is often a lengthy process requiring the accumulation of many and varied kinds of evidence. From first suspicion to general acceptance of the nature, circumstances, and severity of a given risk inevitably takes time and, as the forgoing chapters of this book have shown, there are remarkably few occupational diseases in which all the time honoured criteria of Bradford Hill have been satisfied. Until they are, there will always remain some uncertainty about the extent to which potential hazards have been adequately controlled. The unmet need for sufficient epidemiological study in the workplace is apparent everywhere, regrettably because its importance is not sufficiently appreciated by funding bodies or by industry.

It is against this background that study designs should be considered. Ideally the growth of epidemiological knowledge should approximate to some sort of rational sequence through stages in which different types of question are answered. With some notable exceptions, such as the strategic planning for the carcinogenic risks of asbestos[4] and synthetic mineral fibres[5] this has seldom been the case. Even so, the suggested priorities have all too often been ignored by investigators who, with their sponsors, remained stuck in the early crude phase of hypothesis testing rather than move to the more difficult but much more important problems that still require an answer.

These preliminary comments are to emphasise the overriding need for epidemiological investigators to select carefully the questions their studies are to address, having regard for the present state of knowledge. Only then, in relation to the resources and opportunities available, can the most appropriate and efficient study design be selected. Sometimes diseases that may possibly be related to work have no known cause, in some the causal factors are suspected but untested, and in others the cause is clear enough but more information is needed about the nature of the agent and the role of additional factors. There remains the issue of exposure-response, important in relation to causation and essential for rational policies of control. Finally, and to complete the circle, is the requirement for surveillance, to monitor the impact of occupational disease and trauma as a guide to the direction of health services and further epidemiological research. When faced with "God is the answer," it was the wise epidemiologist who added "But what is the question?"

Detection of possible causes

The early detection of work-related disease and of the factors responsible has an important place in occupational health practice which calls for constant vigilance, surveillance and inquiry. The problem can be approached either by examining the occurrence of diseases that might be caused or aggravated by the working environment or by studying the health of workers exposed to specific hazards. The latter option is really an hypothesis testing exercise for which appropriate study designs are discussed below. The other question, whether a given disease might be causally related to work, can be addressed in three main ways. These include statistical analyses of routinely available national or regional data on mortality or morbidity, surveillance and reporting schemes backed by additional case-control studies, and specific case-control studies perhaps preceded by a cross-sectional survey for case ascertainment. Longitudinal (cohort) surveys are not indicated in the search for hypotheses.

Statistical analyses

Mortality statistics have been of limited value even in Britain where information on occupation is obtained by correlating death certificates and the census. These data have provided a broad general picture of mortality by geographical region and social class but are seldom sufficiently specific on type or duration of employment to be informative on occupational risks. In some European countries, including Britain, more useful analyses have been made by linking mortality to occupation as recorded at successive censuses. The potential utility of this approach has been discussed by Fox[6]; a recent example is provided in a Danish study by Hansen who showed that furnace workers were at increased risk of lung cancer as compared with men in other occupations selected by the same procedure.[7] Analyses of lung cancer mortality by county in the USA using census populations have identified regions at high risk and raised questions about the possible contribution of local industry.[8] Or again, geographical analyses of mesothelioma deaths in Western Europe in 1976 showed high rates in certain shipyard cities, suggesting the aetiological role of crocidolite used in naval insulation.[9]

Of greater promise was the use made by Milham of mortality in men aged 20 years or more in Washington State, 1950-1979.[10] Proportional mortality ratios were calculated for 438 100 deaths coded to 158 causes of death groups and 218 occupational classes. Among the important findings from this analysis was the first indication that leukaemia might be causally related to electromagnetic fields (see also chapter 4). Although laborious, this approach, which does not require the use of population denominators, deserves a wider trial. Apart from mortality, many countries have increasingly reliable cancer registries. Some use has been made of these in cohort studies, for example of man-made mineral fibre workers,[11] but little or none for the generation of hypotheses on occupational cancers. The calculation of proportional morbidity ratios might also be informative.

Disease surveillance

Past requirements in many countries for the notification by medical practitioners of infections and industrial diseases acquired a bad image. For the doctors the task was of minimal interest and unrewarding; there was no feedback and it was unclear that much use was made of the data collected. As a result the requirement to notify was poorly observed and the results were of even more dubious value. In recent years, however, there has been some revival in interest in the surveillance of occupational disease, by government in Finland and the USA, and by physicians themselves in the United Kingdom.[12] For agencies with responsibility for prevention and control any information on disease incidence is important, but perhaps of more relevance epidemiologically are the physician–based schemes in Britain. The way in which these have developed and their potential for the early detection of unrecognised hazards in the workplace are worth consideration.

It has long been apparent that credit for the discovery of new causes of environmental disease belongs not to epidemiology but to the perspicacity of astute clinicians and pathologists.[13] What is needed is a framework whereby clinical suspicions can be freely expressed and small scale epidemiological studies rapidly undertaken to identify hypotheses requiring fuller investigation. It was largely in this spirit that a number of clinically based reporting schemes were recently set up in the UK, the largest of which are the SWORD (Surveillance of Work-related and Occupational Respiratory Disease) project for work-related respiratory diseases[14] and EPIDERM, for occupational skin diseases.[15] Both schemes are cost effective in that each relies on specialist physicians' voluntary participation and a small coordinating group. Also important is the fact that the driving force for their continuation is the need felt by participants for informal contact with exchange of experience and access to advice and information.

The main features of the SWORD scheme, to which EPIDERM is similar, include strict confidentiality, a high level of participation (over 80% of all thoracic physicians and a larger number of occupational physicians), monthly reporting of *incident* cases with diagnosis, suspected cause, age, sex and place of residence and a rapid analysis with brief commentary returned to all participants. In 1992, after three years' operation, a change was made: a core group of about 30 chest physicians with major interest in occupational respiratory diseases continue to report monthly and the rest (about 400), in 12 random samples, for one month of the year only. This strategy has proved successful and is now being extended to the occupational physicians. As a result the annual number of new cases of work-related respiratory disease reported is estimated at about 3500, 28% attributed to occupational asthma, 20% to mesothelioma, 14% to pneumoconiosis and lung cancer, and 8% to inhalation accidents.[16] The annual incidence of occupational dermatoses, almost all due to irritant or allergic diseases, may well be higher but cannot yet be reliably estimated.

The value of these schemes for hypothesis generation after simple epidemiological screening is increasingly clear. A controlled retrospective study, based on cases of occupational asthma in chemical and pharmaceutical workers, estimated risk in relation to time from first exposure, smoking habit, and a history of asthma in childhood.[17] A detailed analysis of over 1000 cases reported in 1989–90, against population denominators, allowed incidence rates to be calculated by age, sex and occupation.[18] The follow up of reported cases of asthma and inhalation accidents is providing estimates of the frequency and nature of serious long term medical and employment effects. A more sophisticated case-control study still in progress is showing the feasibility of estimating the pattern of exposure-response for asthma resulting from exposure to isocyanates.

Prevalence surveys

Cross-sectional studies are seldom the ideal method for testing hypotheses but they can be useful for generating them, especially if they are based on fairly large, well-defined, and broadly representative populations. If these requirements are not met, associations based either on small numbers or in special circumstances provide poorly based hypotheses. Because of inherent uncertainty over the time dimension and selective losses, causal associations can be lost or underestimated. On the other hand, as disease and exposure status may both be known to subject and observer, recall bias and biased observation may create associations that do not truly exist. Despite these problems, prevalence surveys are relatively easy and inexpensive and the results are seldom seriously incorrect. Thus for categories of disease in which epidemiological knowledge is limited but for which an occupational component is more than likely, this approach has a useful place. Several diseases in this book are in that category, for example, the adverse outcomes of pregnancy and the highly prevalent and varied back and limb disorders.

An investigation of work in pregnancy conducted by McDonald and her colleagues in Montreal in 1982 and 1983, was large and comprehensive.[19] The results have been the subject of many reports,[20] several aspects of which are discussed in chapter 13. This survey was designed to explore all possible associations between a wide range of factors in the working environment and the occurrence of fetal death, prematurity and the many types of congenital defect while, at the same time, taking account of eight or more important confounders. Thus, although many associations inevitably carried odds ratios which, as judged by their confidence intervals, were potentially important, it was not difficult to identify those that deserved to be tested as specific hypotheses. For example, association of exposure to solvents, aromatic in particular, was a recurrent finding with spontaneous abortion, stillbirth, and several types of congenital defect. Equally strong were the associations between various kinds of ergonomic stress and abortion and, perhaps, preterm birth. On the other hand it was also clear that most other aspects of women's work, especially those in non-industrial jobs, did not at present warrant further epidemiological research. This survey, although effective in the exploration of possible hypotheses, was extremely expensive and well beyond the resources of most investigators. However, some of its features are desirable even in smaller studies. In particular, the survey was based on a well defined general population over an adequate period and all possible confounders were recorded and used. With more limited resources the number of outcomes studied could also be limited to reduce errors associated with small unrepresentative populations and insufficient allowance for confounders. A similar study in France of work in pregnancy by Mamelle *et al.* met these requirements by focusing the study on ergonomic factors and premature birth.[21]

The musculoskeletal diseases provide similar evidence of the value of prevalence surveys. Those that were large and comprehensive led to hypotheses that were later confirmed and those that were small and in special populations often inconsistent. In the former category were data obtained incidentally from the Framingham Heart Study[22] and several large surveys in Scandinavia.[23] The results obtained from smaller studies were sometimes confusing, perhaps because they were based on highly selected groups such as patients after orthopaedic operations. A number of investigations designed to test hypotheses generated by these surveys are discussed below.

Hypothesis testing

To establish cause and effect requires more than the testing of a defined null hypothesis, even several times; in particular there are questions about possible confounders, appropriate latency and most important, the quantitative correlation between exposure and response. Although the strength of the evidence afforded by any study is dependent on all these aspects it is not essential that each one be fully evaluated from the start. Should this become necessary more demanding investigations may be required, as discussed below. The earlier chapters of this book suggest that almost all studies used at the initial phase of hypothesis testing were case-referent in type. These fell into three categories differing in the nature of the population base from which cases and referents were sampled. First are the studies in which the cases were selected from various kinds of geographically-related medical register, second, from a specified population base and, third, from a fully defined cohort. In addition, there were a few cohort studies set up and analysed *a priori* for the specific purpose of hypothesis testing. There have also been case-referent studies based on poorly defined populations with results less often discussed in this book. The main features of all four main study designs are described below in sequence.

Registered cases

Several important investigations have used this approach, for example, two concerned with osteoarthritis of the hip and workload,[22] [23] two with malignant disease and mineral dusts,[24] [25] and two with brain damage and solvents.[26] [27] In the first pair, cases were from hospital registers over a 4–5 year period, in one from outpatients under investigation for prostatic symptoms,[22] (some of whom had a hip joint replacement) and in the other from men who had received hip joint replacement.[23] Referents in the first study were selected from the outpatients who had no radiographic evidence of hip osteoarthritis and in the second at random from the general population. In both studies the occupational history and workload, together with information on such possible confounders as sports and hobbies, were obtained by interview and questionnaire, in one study blind. Designs of this type are clearly feasible and although subject to recall bias can give useful information. However, the use of population controls and the possibility of observer bias in one of the studies cited are potential problems and, in both studies, results based on men with prostheses cannot be applied confidently to osteoarthritis of the hip generally.

The methods of case and referent selection in the two investigations of malignant disease also had strengths and weaknesses. In one study, patients with fatal malignant mesothelial tumours diagnosed at necropsy or biopsy were ascertained from pathologists throughout North America in 1972 and in Canada over a longer period.[24] From the same pathology records, deaths from non-pulmonary cancer, but with pulmonary metastases, matched for sex, age, and year of death, were chosen as controls. Next of kin were interviewed in detail about occupational dust exposure, asbestos in particular, by a public health nurse, blind as to case-referent status. The data were also coded blind. In the other study, of lung cancer among male residents of a pottery town in central Italy, cases were, identified from the death register during a 16 year period and referents of similar age and date of death in men who had died from other causes, excluding pneumoconiosis and chronic bronchitis.[25] Public health nurses, who were blinded to study hypothesis and causes of death, obtained detailed work histories by interview with next of kin, later coded as to the probability of silica exposure. These designs seem valid in that the cancer deaths selected for study reflect all cases of interest diagnosed by a defined method in an identifiable population. However, the diagnosis of mesothelioma even at necropsy could conceivably have been biased by the pathologists' knowledge of the work history and the causes of death accepted (or excluded) and both referent series may or may not have been comparable in terms of opportunity for employment in exposed jobs. The exclusion of pneumoconiosis and chronic bronchitis from the referent series in the Italian study made some difference to the result and although justified by the investigators[28] was questioned by others.[29]

The studies of solvent exposure provide an interesting contrast. In the Swedish investigation cases and referents were selected from a regional pension fund register, as skilled but disabled workers with and without specified mental disorders; their sex was not specified.[26] Work histories, taken from the register, allowed the identification, with duration of employment, of those who had worked in painting, varnishing or carpet laying—jobs assumed to have entailed exposure to solvents. In concept the design is simple enough but there remain questions about the type of people who work in the three categories of exposed employment and about whether these categories provide a sufficiently sensitive, specific, or indeed valid measure of solvent exposure. A similar hypothesis was investigated rather differently and on a larger scale in Canada some years later.[27] Two series of cases were selected from male patients, one with a wide range of psychiatric disorders and the other with diagnoses of pre-senile dementia, admitted for five days or more to specified mental hospitals in Montreal and elsewhere in Quebec. Two series of age and sex matched controls were selected (a) from admissions to general hospitals and (b) from neighbourhood residents. Lifetime occupational histories were obtained by telephone and jobs classified for intensity and duration of exposure to solvents by three different procedures. Information on seven important confounding factors was also recorded. While this design was careful to take account of many sources of error its weakness lay in the comparability of response to detailed questions put to patients with mental illness and to referents. However, any resulting bias was probably against finding a difference.

Population based studies

In this category can be considered five case-control investigations, three of diseases allegedly related to non-ionising radiation and two on the possible association between childhood leukaemia and lymphoma and paternal exposure to radiation in the nuclear industry. The advantage of having all cases within a given population is that the method of ascertainment is free of the kinds of selection bias associated with hospital admission or other hospital services, characteristic of the designs dependent on case registration. Provided that the ascertainment method is satisfactory, referents (non-cases) can be selected in much the same way. Although all five studies to be considered claimed to be population based, none achieved this objective completely. The extent of the deficiency was small and probably unimportant in a Finnish investigation of the association between visual display terminals (VDT) and spontaneous abortion.[30] The cases and controls were identified from the national hospital discharge register and polyclinic records, from which it was said that 94% of all births and 80–90% of all recognised spontaneous abortions could be identified, together with the women's place of employment. Cases and controls were selected from women on the register who worked in banks and offices and a record of VDT use and various ergonomic conditions was obtained by questionnaire from the women themselves. Weaknesses in this study were the relatively low questionnaire response rates (74% and 76%) and the real possibility of recall bias in records obtained after the pregnancy outcome was known.

Two other surveys relied on the reliability and completeness of death certification in two fairly uncommon malignancies—breast cancer in men[31] and brain tumour, also in men.[32] In both studies the aim was to assess the correlation between these tumours and work that entailed exposure to electromagnetic fields. These exposures were recognised from work histories obtained by interview with the subjects or their next of kin. The validity of studies of this kind depend (a) on whether the likelihood of diagnosis of such tumours is independent of social factors related to occupational opportunities and (b) as in all retrospective inquiries, on the magnitude of any possible recall bias.

Finally, there are the two studies of leukaemia and lymphoma in young persons reported recently from Britain.[33][34] In both these inquiries a considerable effort was put into the discovery of cases from all possible sources over a defined period of years, 1958–90 in the Scottish study[33] and 1950–85 in West Cumbria.[34] On the assumption that this near complete ascertainment was achieved the investigators felt justified in taking controls matched for sex, age and place of residence from the same birth registers. In the Cumbrian study, information on exposure to ionising radiation, particularly of fathers before the conception, but also on many other factors, was obtained by questionnaire from parents. In the Scottish investigation information of this kind was obtained by detailed study of employment and other records concerning the fathers. As the procedures used for ascertainment and case and control selection in these two important studies were so similar, the disparate conclusions reached suggest that the explanation may lie in differing methods of estimation of exposure. One was certainly subject to recall bias and the other perhaps to lower sensitivity.

Nested designs

An obvious way of maximising the probability of equal ascertainment of cases and non-cases and for achieving comparable information on exposure for both is to do so within a longitudinal cohort study. In principle all cohort members are subject to the same standards of observation and disease diagnosis and records of exposure are established before the disease outcome is known. This is an idealised concept; in practice, the more heavily exposed, perhaps because of questions of compensation, are often studied more thoroughly than others. Even so, internal analyses within a cohort are generally considered more reliable and robust that any other. The laborious task of conducting a cohort survey purely to identify cases and controls to test a causal hypothesis is not easily justified, however, unless exposures can then be estimated from available work histories, thus avoiding the potential bias of questionnaires. Two examples may illustrate this.

A cohort of over 13 000 workers of a factory in Britain producing friction materials was traced to the end of 1979, by which time there had been 149 deaths from lung cancer and 10 from mesothelioma.[35] Except for two short periods when crocidolite was required for a specific contract in a well-defined area of one workshop, only chrysotile was used. To test the association between mesothelioma and fibre type a nested case-control study was undertaken based on the 10 cases and four controls for each, matched for sex, age, date of start, and duration of employment during the crocidolite period of workers who had survived the case. For these 50 subjects work histories were analysed for their participation in or proximity to the crocidolite process. Eight of the 10 with mesothelioma had worked on the crocidolite contract compared with three of the 40 controls. This study would have been impossible had it not been within a cohort.

More recently, the study of an enormous cohort of some 68 000 dust-exposed workers from 29 mines and factories from five provinces in China allowed the identification of 319 deaths in men from lung cancer.[36] To assess their association with silica exposure a nested case-control study was made. Where possible four controls for each case were selected at random from men who had been born in the same decade, worked in the same mine or factory and survived the case. From work histories and industrial hygiene records exposures to silica were estimated for 316 of the 319 cases and 1352 of the 1358 controls. In the basic analysis, odds ratios were then calculated at various levels of cumulative dust and silica exposure by type of industry. Once again this cost effective analysis was possible only after having identified and traced the initial cohort.

Full cohort studies

With the growing appreciation that well-designed case-referent studies can be reliable when based on effective ascertainment within a defined population—cross-sectional or longitudinal—the fully fledged cohort survey is less often used or needed purely for the purpose of testing a causal hypothesis. A distinction must here be made between this objective and the definition of quantitative exposure-response correlations when the question of causation has been adequately settled, as will be discussed below. It goes without saying that if the detailed assessment of exposure is of critical importance and cannot be obtained without serious risk of recall or other bias a cohort-like design is virtually essential. Even so, there remains the efficient strategy of case-control nesting. Nevertheless, as full studies are still undertaken without any attempt at any such short cut, the circumstances where this has been thought necessary are worth examination. Five fairly recent examples will be briefly considered, three concerned with the effects of ionising[37 38] or non-ionising radiation,[39] one with man-made mineral fibres,[40] and one with diatomaceous earth.[41] All these have in common that the exact nature of the exposure was critically important and neither this nor the identification of cases with this information were obtainable outside a cohort.

In neither of the studies of radiation effects is the explanation hard to find. Gardner *et al.* had access, with some difficulty, to the birth records of 1068 children probably born in the parish of Seascale, Cumbria, where it was suspected that an apparent excess of childhood leukaemia might be related to the presence of a large nuclear reprocessing plant.[37] By tracing through National Health Service records it was found that after excluding 43 emigrations, five of a total of 27 deaths were from leukaemia, whereas only 0·53 would have been expected at national rates. No other cause of death was in excess. Thus the link between leukaemia and birth in Seascale was confirmed but, as this had been previously observed, it was not strictly an independent test of the hypothesis nor, of course, that the cases were related to the nuclear plant. The other study of ionising radiation by Checkoway *et al.* sought to test the possibility that excess cancer risk might be related to low level exposure (< 50 rads).[38] A cohort of over 8000 employees of a radiation research establishment whose cumulative exposure had been individually recorded, were followed and 92% were traced. Of 966 deaths, 194 were from cancer, an SMR of only 0·78. However, prostatic cancer and leukaemia both showed a low but not significant excess. In their attempt to assess the cancer-inducing effect of electromagnetic radiation, Thériault *et al.* were faced with a similar problem (see also chapter 4).[39] Only by selecting a cohort of hydroelectric employees could they have any reasonable possibility of ascertaining the occurrence of malignant disease (in their study from cancer registries) and accomplishing the difficult task of measuring their exposure to electromagnetic fields.

The two remaining studies of lung cancer and exposure to mineral dusts faced other difficulties. It was not expected that any risk associated with man-made mineral fibres (MMMF) would be as great as from asbestos and yet almost all occupational exposures to the former were potentially confounded by the latter. Only in the manufacture of MMMF could it be assumed that the exposures were reasonably pure, albeit low. It was therefore evident that unless MMMF exposure could be measured with precision, as was later explored using lung burden analyses,[42] a case-referent approach was not feasible. The only alternative was to undertake cohort studies of MMMF production workers, such as that by Enterline *et al.*, and because of low exposure and great economic importance, this had to be on a large scale (see also chapter 5).[40] The evaluation of the carcinogenicity of crystalline silica has similar problems. Occupational exposures are extremely widespread but frequently confounded by other carcinogens such as radon, arsenic and asbestos, usually to an unknown degree. For this reason, the case-control design was not appropriate, except perhaps in small communities with a major silica-using industry. An example that met these requirements by the use of registered cases was discussed above.[11] The alternative taken by Checkoway *et al.* and by a few others (see chapter 5) was to undertake cohort surveys in industries entailing exposure to silica but no other important carcinogens.[41] The diatomaceous earth industry of California provided this opportunity; the investigators could have opted for a nested case-control analysis but because of additional objectives decided against doing so.

Confounding and interaction

Several references have been made to the complicating effect of confounders on correlations between cause and effect, but without further clarification or consideration of its relevance to study design. The nature of confounding and of the related phenomenon of interaction needs to be understood so that due allowance can be made for them while keeping the questions they raise in reasonable perspective. Because of the infinite complexities of life it is always possible to find an alternative explanation for even the most obvious causal relationship. No industrial exposure is pure and several agents conceivably responsible for the disease of interest may occur together. Man has learned to deal with this problem by a process of progressive refinement. Consider the diseases associated with asbestos, a collective term for a variety of mineral fibre silicates regardless of their physical and chemical characteristics, which are usually encountered occupationally in mixtures. In early studies no distinction was made in defining exposure, but later it became clear that the main types of fibre differed considerably in their pathogenicity. Much research is now being directed at the extent to which diseases attributed to the most common fibre type (chrysotile) are the result of exposure to the previously unrecognised presence at low concentration of yet another fibrous silicate (tremolite). We have here an example of confounding progressively recognised at three stages.

Even had these possibilities been suspected many years ago, which they were,[43] it would have been difficult to design studies to deal with them. However, let us first consider another potential confounder in asbestos disease correlations, namely cigarette smoking. Once again, a series of questions arise. First, is the association with asbestos entirely explained by smoking? Although not explicitly investigated, it would be remarkable if asbestos workers differed systematically in this respect from other workers. Secondly, is the occupational risk confined to smokers? Some initial evidence from American insulation workers suggested that this might be so[44] but a later study of the same cohort reported that whereas the risk relative to the non-smoking non-exposed was fivefold for non-smoking asbestos workers and 10 fold for unexposed smokers, it was 50 fold for asbestos workers who smoked—suggesting a simple multiplication of risks.[45] However, in five other cohorts where a similar analysis was made the general pattern varied but was on average less than multiplicative, the interactive risk becoming less as the level of either variable increased.[46] Thus despite the existence of over 50 cohort studies of lung cancer in asbestos workers—possibly the most extensively studied correlation in all epidemiology—there were only six studies in which the analysis of this interaction was possible, and the results did not agree! The question then is: Does it matter? It has been argued that the information might be useful for deciding the public health priority of controlling asbestos exposure or reducing cigarette consumption—not, in practice, a very relevant issue. More realistically it has been argued that the information has a bearing on our understanding of carcinogenic mechanisms; in which case, perhaps the question should be framed and studied quite specifically. The evidence of a similar type of interaction between solvent exposure and alcohol consumption in relation to pre-senile dementia has been mentioned; if confirmed this would also throw light on certain pathogenic mechanisms.

Other examples of joint action of more than one factor in the causation of occupational disease are provided by a longitudinal study of noise-induced hearing loss in Finland[47] and both cross-sectional[48-50] and longitudinal studies[51] of work-related asthma in the UK. In the Finnish investigation chain saw noise measured objectively was more hazardous in lumberjacks with than in those without vibration-induced white finger, after allowance for the confounding effects of age, duration of exposure, and ear muff usage. The authors speculated that vibration might act on both disorders through a common mechanism affecting sympathetic nervous system activity. Similarly, in the studies of asthma, evidence was obtained that atopy and smoking independently increased the probability of sensitisation and, in two groups, of respiratory symptoms in employees

342

exposed to either laboratory animals,[48] tetrachloranhydride,[49] or platinum.[51]

Returning to the more general question of confounders, of which interaction is a special kind, it is important to consider the possibility in study design. If the investigator has reason to believe that there are variables, related to both exposure and the disease(s) of interest, which could seriously bias the result in either direction, appropriate steps must be taken. One possibility is to neutralise the effect of a confounder by matching either cases and referents or exposed and unexposed subjects for that particular variable. However, it is seldom feasible to do this for more than two variables, of which age, sex, location, and time usually have some priority. Alternatively, if the study is large enough it may be possible to deal with the problem during analysis either by stratification or by some regression method (see chapter 18). The concept of matching has obvious appeal but can readily lead to overmatching with serious loss of study power. The reason for this lies in the complex webs of correlation which directly and indirectly link any one human characteristic with many others. It is not difficult to see that even age and sex are related to most aspects of work and the associated exposures. Some advice in Manson's text, listing four criteria which should be met before matching is attempted, is worth noting[52]:

- There should be no interest in evaluating the association between the disease and the factor to be matched.
- There should be a reasonable likelihood that, if matching is not done, the factor will be confounding.
- There should be a reasonable likelihood that the amount of confounding introduced is more than trivial.
- There should be no possibility that the factor is part of the causal pathway linking the exposure and disease under study.

Axelson added another dimension to the assessment of confounding: "It is reasonable, also, to require that evidence (from outside the study) with regard to causality for a suggested confounding factor is of about the same firmness as the evidence for accepting a connection between exposure and outcome in a particular study."[53]

There remain occasions, nevertheless, in which the evidence for the effect of confounding factors (from outside the study) is considerably better than for the occupational factors under test. In pregnancy studies, for example, there are some ten confounders that cannot be ignored in any consideration of fetal death, prematurity and certain congenital defects. In the large survey in Montreal of work and pregnancy these were recorded and used to correct the expected figures for abnormal outcomes.[19] Except for a subsidiary case-control study of chemical exposures and congenital defect in which matching on four basic variables was used,[54] the larger number of confounders in most analyses were mainly dealt with by logistic regression.

The main conclusion from this review is that in designing any study the possibility of confounding and interactive factors should be carefully considered and provision made to record any that appear potentially important. Except perhaps for age and sex, matching for such variables is probably unwise as this will preclude their evaluation in the final analysis.

Exposure-response

It is sometimes claimed that the assessment of quantitative correlations between amounts of exposure and risk of specific adverse effects is the high point in occupational epidemiology. It is primarily a descriptive task, however, mainly required for control rather than scientific purposes and then only in certain circumstances. It is usually assumed that the underlying causal hypotheses have been adequately tested, and the nature of important interactions reasonably well understood. Measures of confidence in the descriptive function are therefore more relevant than arbitrary levels of statistical significance. On occasion, however, the final product, which will be expressed in statistical terms, may need to be tested against hypotheses related to thresholds and linearity. As it is risk that is being assessed, measures of disease incidence, not prevalence, are required. This is less of a problem when the response is immediate or at least closely related in time to first exposure. Unfortunately, it is when the disease in question occurs after many years latency, is often insidious in onset, and both progressive and disabling, that the need for information on exposure-response is most pressing. As a result, considerable difficulties are inevitably encountered in deciding how best to deal with (a) the temporal and intensity aspects of exposure (data on the latter are usually of poor quality), (b) the availability of data on prevalence rather than incidence and (c) selective removal from view of subjects at varying stages of disease severity. In all these problems, study design has considerable relevance.

Measurements of response

This aspect is fully discussed in chapter 16, but not specifically in the present context. The ascertainment of disease incidence inevitably requires a longitudinal study design, ideally initiated before first exposure. With the exception of fatalities and accidental injuries, when historical recording may be feasible, the first occurrence of most other diseases requires serial observation at fairly short intervals. This is a laborious procedure and cohort members may easily be lost from view. In a recently completed longitudinal study of asthma-related changes in a cohort of nearly 800 workers exposed to flour or laboratory animals, observations were made six-monthly over a five year period (see chapter

6). Even so, only 77% were present at the second visit and an average of 9% were lost on each subsequent occasion, leaving only 32% of the original cohort still employed at the end of the study.

In view of the importance of environmental dust control there have been many surveys of exposure-response in workers at risk from coal, silica, asbestos, cotton, and other potentially noxious dusts. Some have entailed single or serial cross-sectional observations, usually at routine periodic medical examinations, information being obtained by questionnaire, chest radiography, and pulmonary function tests. In all these studies there have been serious problems and agreement on their findings has been limited. In addition to the matter of exposure assessment it is difficult to standardise observations of this kind within and between studies, especially over time. The solution may lie in attempting to find reliable and acceptable criteria for the identification of critical events in the disease process so that incidence rather than prevalence rates can be estimated. To minimise bias from selective losses from the study group these events should ideally be at a stage before there are important symptoms or disability. It would remain necessary to relate these events to the natural history of the disease in question, probably best in studies divorced from the occupational environment. In any chronic and progressive disease which calls for the estimation of exposure-response this kind of approach is needed but examples of its use are hard to find.

It is hardly surprising, therefore, that somewhat less controversial data on quantitative risk assessment have been obtained from studies of mortality. Although straightforward in principle their validity depends on whether deaths provide an adequate reflection of the disease in question. This will not be so when case fatality is low or long delayed, and outcome is affected by treatment and social factors. It might also be unreliable if the cause of death is difficult to discover or is influenced by such potential biases as compensation or the certifying physician's aetiological prejudices. For example, the diagnosis of pneumoconiosis, mesothelioma, and other occupationally related cancer could be strongly affected by the doctor's knowledge of the past work history. This kind of bias is extremely difficult to detect, much less correct, even when the possibility is recognised.

Estimation of exposure

In all but diseases of fairly short latency the nature and intensity of exposure constitute the most difficult part of any epidemiological survey. This problem, in principle and in practice, is reviewed in chapter 15; here consideration is limited to the effect on study design. The concept of exposure has three main components: identification of the agent(s), estimates of intensity, and appropriate measures of duration and timing. The last two aspects are sometimes dealt with by some kind of cumulative index. When the purpose of the study is the quantitative description of the correlation between exposure and its effects it is reasonable to expect that an acceptable definition of the three components has been reached before the study is designed.

The agent—The data on exposure must be reasonably specific about this. Various surrogates ranging from type of industry, through department or process, to job descriptions, although often adequate for hypothesis generation and testing, are not so for the present purpose. On the other hand, the search for complete specificity may even introduce bias, and it may well be sufficient to settle for an index believed to provide a reliable reflection of the important ingredient. Thus, respirable dust measurements *in defined circumstances* can be used as an adequate surrogate for asbestos fibres, crystalline silica and possibly coal, cotton, and certain agents associated with asthma. The estimation of exposure-response is not an academic exercise but one designed to produce information necessary for control; the measure of exposure used in the study must therefore meet this requirement. It follows that until cause and effect is established the study of quantitative correlations may be premature.

Intensity—This unfortunately is the critical variable as it is always the basis of hygiene standards. Even contemporary measures are difficult but estimates for the past are almost impossible, quite apart from questions of the equivalence of area sampling and personal sampling methods. The latter issue can be resolved only by arbitrary decisions unrelated to epidemiology, the former by educated guesswork. The way ahead is undoubtedly by some form of cumulative biological assessment such as measurement of tissue retention.

Time-related factors—Of these, duration of employment is a crude measure but usually obtainable. As compared with other variables payroll records provide a reliable record of tasks performed with precise dates. It is a matter of judgement depending on the nature of the agent and its effects to decide the way in which gaps in exposure should be treated. It may often be best to consider them at periods of minimal exposure. More difficult is the question of variations in level of exposure—often gross and entailing short high peaks interspersed with relatively long troughs. In the absence of epidemiological data to the contrary the answer to this problem is arbitrary as is the way it is dealt with in control regulations.

Examples

Despite the extensive list of hygiene standards recommended by governmental and other agencies few are based on the results of epidemiological research. This is no criticism of the standards themselves but testimony to the magnitude of the problem, the reasons for which have been outlined. Three occupational hazards—ionising radiation, noise, and asbestos—provide examples of methods, limitations, and achievements.

Radiation—I consider two studies, that of Kneale *et al.* in 1984[55][56] and Beral *et al.* in 1985.[57][58] Objective measurements of intensity and duration of exposure for each subject were available in both studies and the possibility of a linear non-threshold relationship was not an issue. In the latter study, the methods of which were described by Fraser *et al.*,[57] great care was taken to ensure that the cohort finally selected for study was complete, with best possible work histories and records of exposure and fully traced. Of 49 456 male and female employees in several plants, 9542 were excluded because early records had been destroyed, plus a further 368 for whom essential information was missing, leaving 39 546 of whom 2477 (6%) had died. Despite great care taken in all aspects of the investigation, the results were less than conclusive. Partly this was because radiation records were available for only 20 382 (52%) of the final cohort, partly because even after correcting for social class and region of residence the SMRs were low (76 overall) and partly because despite great size the cohort had limited power at low exposure levels. Of these problems perhaps the most difficult were the low SMRs, presumably because of healthy worker or other selective effects for which no allowance could be made. Much the same uncertainties were encountered in the analyses of Kneale *et al.* compounded by less clearly described methods for the collection and validation of data or details of study design.

Noise—From the stand-point of study design, investigations into the quantitative connection between noise exposure and hearing loss leave much to be desired (see chapter 9). However, a recent study from China of dose-response of noise–induced hypertension illustrates the achievements of a simple but well designed inquiry.[59] The subjects were 1101 female workers in a Beijing textile mill. The study was cross-sectional in that blood pressures and sound pressure levels at the workplace were measured in a standard manner over a two month period, with records for each subject of age, years worked, salt intake, smoking and drinking habits, current pregnancy, and use of anti-hypertensive drugs. As there was good reason to believe that noise levels had remained the same over many years and that there was little likelihood of bias from selection into or out of employment this cross-sectional design was both valid and efficient. The results were equally clear-cut.

Asbestos—Of the 50 or more cohort mortality studies of lung cancer risk and asbestos exposure only about a dozen have attempted to quantify exposure-response (see chapter 5). All these studies encountered four major difficulties: (1) measurements of exposure were almost wholly lacking for relevant periods in the more distant past, (2) any measurements that were available were of dust particle and not fibre concentrations and there was no reliable or accepted method of conversion, (3) information on fibre type, dimensions and other important characteristics of exposure were crude and almost unusable and (4) while the two major components

347

of exposure—duration and intensity—were usually combined as a cumulative index, there is no biological justification for this. Some attempts have been made to deal with this problem by more complicated methods of analysis[60] but the other three seem insuperable without an entirely different approach to exposure estimation. So far as mineral fibres are concerned the most promising alternative is the use of lung burden analyses which, although still at an exploratory stage, have provided considerable insight into the differing risks of lung cancer in miners and textile workers[61] and into fibre type-specific risks of mesothelioma.[62 63] The epidemiological potential of lung burden analyses has been reviewed[64] and the use of biological methods of exposure estimation is discussed further in chapter 15. The impact of these methods on study design will be considerable.

Conclusions

Several conclusions can be drawn from this review and a few underlying principles of study design identified. Among the latter, the necessity for a well-defined question and the importance of comparing like with like are paramount. Whatever the type of investigation, valid comparisons depend on a proper appreciation of the base population from which cases of special interest are sampled and on an assurance that the methods of ascertainment and exposure estimation are free from bias. Wherever possible, cases should be defined in terms of incidence and not prevalence, preferably at an early stage in the disease before symptoms or disability have had an important selective effect on employment.

For the early detection of work-related diseases and of clues to their cause, prevalence surveys in fairly large and representative populations have been effective whereas studies of small series and in narrow occupational groups are susceptible to unsuspected confounders. It is possible that large scale surveillance schemes that are clinically based and appropriately designed may prove to be an effective and cost effective method of identifying new and uncontrolled occupational diseases.

For hypothesis testing, there seems little doubt that case-referent studies based on reasonably complete ascertainment within a defined population over time or, in certain circumstances, cross-sectionally are usually the best approach. In these surveys the need to ensure the unbiased collection of data on exposure is obviously important and, if possible, that quantitative estimates are made. Questions of confounding and synergism need to be carefully considered and steps taken to record factors of possible importance. However, except in circumstances where the number of cases and referents is strictly limited, confounding is better better dealt with during analysis than by matching.

Finally there is the vexing and difficult problem of establishing quantitative relationships between exposure and response. So long as the emphasis remains on attempts to estimate past levels of intensity in the workplace of agents, the pathogenic characteristics of which are poorly understood, no real solution seems likely. The future, at least for chemical and physical agents, must lie in the development of biological markers able to provide for exposed workers an integrated measure of total "dose." In the meantime epidemiologists, hygienists, and control agencies must recognise and cope as best they can with the assumptions and approximations that have to be made.

1 Doll R. Mortality from lung cancer in asbestos workers. *Br J Ind Med* 1955; **12**: 81–6.
2 Lilienfeld AM, Lilienfeld DE. *Foundations of Epidemiology* (2nd ed). New York: Oxford University Press, 1980, 30–7.
3 Rothman KJ. *Modern epidemiology*. Boston: Little, Brown, 1986, 79–82.
4 Working Group on Asbestos and Cancer. Report and recommendations. *Arch Environ Health* 1965; **11**: 221–9.
5 Gilson JC. Aims of the conference. In: *Biological effects of man-made mineral fibres. Vol 1.* Copenhagen: WHO/EURO, 1984. 1–3.
6 Fox AJ. Linkage methods in occupational mortality. JC McDonald, ed. In: *Recent advances in occupational health I.* Edinburgh: Churchill Livingstone, 1981. 107–17.
7 Hansen ES. A mortality study of Danish stokers. *Br J Ind Med* 1992; **49**: 48–52.
8 Blot WJ, Fraument JF. Changing patterns of lung cancer in the United States. *Am J Epidemiol* 1982; **115**: 664–73.
9 McDonald JC, McDonald AD. Epidemiology of mesothelioma from estimated incidence. *Prev Med* 1977; **6**: 426–46.
10 Milham S. Mortality from leukaemia in workers exposed to electric and magnetic fields. *N Engl J Med* 1982; **307**: 249.
11 Simonato L, Fletcher AC, Cherrie JW, Andersen A, Bertazzi P, Charnay N et al. The International Agency for Research on Cancer historical cohort study of MMMF production workers in seven European countries: extension of follow-up. *Ann Occup Hyg* 1987; **31**: 603–23.
12 Meredith SK, McDonald JC. Surveillance systems for occupational disease. *Ann Occup Hyg* 1995; 1995; **39**: 257–60.
13 McDonald JC, Harrington JM. Early detection of occupational hazards. *J Soc Occup Med* 1981; **31**: 93–8.
14 Meredith SK, Taylor VM, McDonald JC. Occupational respiratory disease in the United Kingdom: a report to the British Thoracic Society and the Society of Occupational Medicine by the SWORD project group. *Br J Ind Med* 1991; **48**: 292–8.
15 Cherry NM, Beck MH, Owen-Smith V. Surveillance of occupational skin disease in the United Kingdom: the Occ-Derm project. Proceedings of the 9th International Symposium on Epidemiology in Occupational Health, Cincinnati, DHHS (NIOSH), Publication No 94-112, 1994: 608–9.
16 Sallie BA, Meredith SK, Ross DJ, McDonald JC. SWORD '93. Surveillance of work-related and occupational respiratory disease in the UK. *Occup Med* 1994; **44**: 177–82.
17 Meredith SK, McDonald JC (on behalf of the SWORD project group). Occupational asthma in chemical, pharmaceutical, and plastics processors and manufacturers in the United Kingdom. *Ann Occup Hyg* 1994; **38** Suppl 1: 833–7.
18 Meredith SK. Reported incidence of occupational asthma in the United Kingdom, 1989–90. *J Epidemiol Community Health* 1993; **47**: 459–63.
19 McDonald AD, McDonald JC, Armstrong B, Cherry NM, Delorme C, Nolin AD, et al. Occupation and pregnancy outcome. *Br J Ind Med* 1987; **44**: 521–6.
20 McDonald AD. Work and pregnancy. *Br J Ind Med* 1988; **45**: 577–80.
21 Mamelle N, Laumon B, Lazar P. Prematurity and occupational activity during pregnancy. *Am J Epidemiol* 1984; **119**: 309–22.

22 Croft P, Cooper C, Wickham C, Coggon D. Osteoarthritis of the hip and occupational activity. *Scand J Work Environ Health* 1992; **18**: 59–63.
23 Vingärd E, Hogstedt C, AJfredsson L, Felienius E, Goldie I, Köster M. Coxarthrosis and physical load from occupation. *Scand J Work Environ Health* 1991; **17**: 104–9.
24 McDonald AD, McDonald JC. Malignant mesothelioma in North America. *Cancer* 1980; **46**: 1650–6.
25 Forestiere F, Lagorio S, Michelozzi P, Cavariani F, Arca M, Borgia P *et al*. Silica, silicosis and lung cancer among ceramic workers: a case-referent study. *Am J Ind Med* 1986; **10**: 363–70.
26 Axelson O, Mane M, Hogstedt C. A case-referent study on neuropsychiatric disorders among workers exposed to solvents. *Scand J Work Environ Health* 1976; **2**: 14–20.
27 Cherry NM, Labrèche FP, McDonald JC. Organic brain damage and occupational solvent exposure. *Br J Ind Med*. 1992; **49**: 776–81.
28 Forestiere F, Lagorio S, Michelozzi P, Perucci CA, Axelson O. Letter to Editor. *Am J Ind Med* 1987; **12**: 221–2.
29 Hessel PA, Sluis-Cremer GK. Letter to Editor. *Am J Ind Med* 1987; **12**: 219–20.
30 Lindbolm ML, Hietanen M, Kyyrönen P, Sailmén M, von Nandelstadh P, Taskinen H *et al*. Magnetic fields of video-display terminals and spontaneous abortion. *Am J Epidemiol* 1992; **136**: 1041–51.
31 Demers PA, Thomas DB, Rosenblatt KA, Jimenez LM, McTiernan A, Stalsberg H *et al*. Occupational exposure to electromagnetic radiation and breast cancer in males. *Am J Epidemiol* 1991; **134**: 340–7.
32 Thomas TL, Stolley PD, Steinhagen A, Fontham ETH, Bleeker ML, Stewart PA *et al*. Brain tumour mortality among men with electrical and electronics jobs: a case-control study. *J Natl Cancer Inst* 1987; **79**: 233–8.
33 Kinlen LJ, Clarke K, Balkwill A. Paternal preconceptional radiation exposure in the nuclear industry and leukaemia and non-Hodgkins lymphoma in young people in Scotland. *BMJ* 1993; **306**: 1153–8.
34 Gardner MJ, Snee MP, Hall AJ, Powell CA, Downes S, Terrell JD. Results of case-control study of leukaemia and lymphoma among young people near Sellafield nuclear plant in West Cumbria. *BMJ* 1990; **300**: 423–9.
35 Berry G, Newhouse ML. Mortality of workers manufacturing friction materials using asbestos. *Br J Ind Med* 1983; **40**: 1–7.
36 McLaughlin JK, Chen J-Q, Dosemeci M, Chen R-A, Rexing SH, Wu Z *et al*. A nested case-control study of lung cancer among silica exposed workers in China. *Br J Ind Med* 1992; **49**: 167–71.
37 Gardner MJ, Hall AJ, Downes S, Tenell JD. Follow-up study of children born to mothers resident at Seascale, West Cumbria. *BMJ* 1987; **295**: 822–7.
38 Checkoway H, Mathew RM, Shy CM, Watson JE, Tankersley WG, Wolf SH *et al*. Radiation, work experience, and cause specific mortality among workers at an energy research laboratory. *Br J Ind Med* 1985, **42**: 525–33.
39 Thériault G, Goldberg M, Miller AB, Armstrong B, Guénel P, Deadman J *et al*. Cancer risks associated with occupational exposure to magnetic fields among electric utility workers in Ontario and Quebec, Canada, and France: 1970–1989. *Am J Epidemiol* 1994; **139**: 550–72.
40 Enterline PE, Marsh GM, Henderson V, Callahan C. Mortality update of a cohort of US man-made mineral fibres workers. *Ann Occup Hyg* 1987; **31**: 625–56.
41 Checkoway H, Heyer NJ, Demers PA, Breslow NE. Mortality among workers in the diatomaceous earth industry. *Br J Ind Med* 1993; **50**: 586–97.
42 McDonald JC, Case BW, Enterline PE, Henderson V, McDonald AD, Plourde M, *et al*. Lung dust analysis in the assessment of past exposure of man-made mineral fibre workers. *Ann Occup Hyg* 1990; **34**: 427–41.
43 Wagner JC, Sleggs CA, Marchand P. Diffuse pleural mesothelioma and asbestos exposure in the North Western Cape Province. *Br J Ind Med* 1960; **17**: 260–71.
44 Selikoff IJ, Hammond EC, Churg J. Asbestos exposure, smoking and neoplasm. *JAMA* 1968; **204**: 104–10.
45 Hammond EC, Selikoff IJ, Seidman H. Asbestos exposure, smoking and death rates. *Ann NY Acad Sci* 1979; **330**: 473–90.

46 Berry G, Newhouse ML, Antonis P. Combined effects of asbestos exposure and smoking on mortality from lung cancer and mesothelioma in factory workers. *Br Jl Ind Med* 1985; **42**: 12–8.

47 Pyykkö I, Starck J, Färkkilä M, Hoikkala M, Korhonen O, Nurminen M. Hand-arm vibration in the aetiology of hearing loss in lumberjacks. *Br J Ind Med* 1981; **38**: 281–9.

48 Venables K, Upton JL, Hawkins ER, Tee RD, Longbottom JL, Newman Taylor AJ. Smoking, atopy and laboratory animal allergy. *Br J Ind Med* 1988; **45**: 667–71.

49 Venables K, Topping MD, Howe W, Luczynska CM, Hawkins ER, Newman Taylor AJ. Interaction of smoking and atopy in producing specific IgE antibody against a hapten protein conjugate. *BMJ* 1985; **290**: 201–4.

50 Venables K, Tee RD, Hawkins ER, Gordon DJ, Wate CJ, Farrer NM *et al*. Laboratory animal allergy in a pharmaceutical company. *Br J Ind Med* 1988, **45**: 660–6.

51 Venables K, Dally MB, Nunn AJ, Stevens JF, Stephens R, Farrer N *et al*. Smoking and occupational allergy in workers in a platinum refinery. *BMJ* 1989; **299**: 939–42.

52 Monson RR. *Occupational epidemiology, 2nd Edition*. Boca Raton, CRC Press, 1990, 41.

53 Axelson O. Case-control studies, with a note on proportional mortality evaluation. Karvonen M, Mikheev MI, eds. In: *Epidemiology of occupational health*. Copenhagen, WHO Regional Publications, European Series No 20, 1986, 194.

54 McDonald JC, Lavoie J, Côté R, McDonald AD. Chemical exposures at work in early pregnancy and congenital defect: a case-referent study. *Br J Ind Med* 1987; **44**: 527–33.

55 Kneale GW, Mancuso TF, Stewart A. Job-related mortality risks of Hanford workers and their relation to cancer effects of measured doses of external radiation. *Br J Ind Med* 1984; **41**: 6–8.

56 Kneale GW, Mancuso TF, Stewart A. Job-related mortality risks of Hanford workers and their relation to cancer effects of measured doses of external radiation. *Br J Ind Med* 1984; **41**: 9–14.

57 Fraser P, Booth M, Beral V, Inskip H, Firsht S, Speak S. Collection and validation of data in the United Kingdom Atomic Energy Authority mortality study. *BMJ* 1985; **291**: 435–9.

58 Beral V, Inskip H, Fraser P, Booth M, Coleman D, Rose G. Mortality of employees in the United Kingdom Atomic Energy Authority, 1946–1979. *BMJ* 1985; **291**: 440–7.

59 Yiming Z, Shuzheng Z, Selvin S, Spear R. A dose-response relation for noise induced hypertension. *Br J Ind Med* 1991; **48**: 179–84.

60 Vacek PM, McDonald JC. Risk assessment using exposure intensity: an application to vermiculite mining. *Br J Ind Med* 1991; **48**: 543–7.

61 Sébastien P, McDonald JC, McDonald AD, Case B, Harley R. Respiratory cancer in chrysotile textile and mining industries exposure inferences from lung analysis. *Br J Ind Med* 1989; **46**: 180–7.

62 McDonald JC, Armstrong B, Case B, Doell D, McCaughey WTE, McDonald AD, Sébastien P. Mesothelioma and asbestos fibre type: evidence from lung tissue analysis. *Cancer* 1989; **63**: 1544–7.

63 Rogers AJ, Leigh J, Berry G, Fergusson DA, Mulder HB, Ackad M. Relationship between lung asbestos fibre type and concentration and relative risk of mesothelioma. *Cancer* 1991; **67**: 1912–20.

64 McDonald JC. Epidemiological significance of mineral fiber persistence in human lung tissue. *Environ Health Perspect* 1994; **102**(S5), 221–4.

15 Assessment of exposure

BRUCE CASE

Introduction

Occupational epidemiology attempts to identify and quantify causal relationships between health events and one or more exposure variables encountered in the workplace. The definition of health events is usually straightforward (including pathological changes, radiological abnormalities, and death certificate diagnoses). The definition of exposure varies from historical estimates based on recollection of working conditions to precise measurement of actual physical or chemical agents at or near the target organ in the individual worker in real time. Exposure assessment can be the Achilles heel of occupational epidemiology, both because of the practical difficulties involved and because of theoretical problems of interpretation introduced by uncertainty. This weakness extends into the areas of prevention and control and of quantitative risk assessment. Imprecision in exposure assessment leads to wider confidence intervals and often greater disagreement as to "safe levels" within and beyond the workplace.

Exposure assessment is a multidisciplinary field combining principles and practices from epidemiology, biostatistics, industrial hygiene, engineering, and biomedical science. Other disciplines such as psychology and economics also contribute. Given this complexity, there are few comprehensive discussions of the topic available. Only one excellent recent text covers all of the principles from an epidemiological standpoint.[1] Summary discussions are available elsewhere.[2-8]

This chapter presents general principles of exposure assessment. Individual examples from a variety of studies are used to illustrate concepts. I have a biological orientation and bias, and other perspectives having more direct epidemiological roots should be consulted for a balanced view.[1-11] Many examples come from the assessment of exposure to mineral particles, although examples are included of other chemical and physical exposures. No attempt is made to review the different kinds of assessment of "exposure" for ergonomically related diseases, stress, or work accidents. This chapter is an outline, and many topics of interest such as questionnaire and interview design and validation, statistical modelling of measurement error, and detailed biokinetic approaches cannot be adequately developed in a short summary.

Exposure assessment includes a spectrum of activities from traditional techniques such as direct observation of the workplace and questionnaire completion by workers, to the contemporary use of total exposure assessment methodology and biological markers. Between these approaches lies the vast area of environmental or "external" exposure measurement, which provides the bulk of current information on past and present exposures. Other issues related to exposure assessment, including variability of exposure, the role of confounding and interaction in exposure assessment, selected statistical considerations for exposure, and validation of exposure will be discussed. The latter category receives special attention as it is of increasing importance.

Historical context

Assessment of exposure begins with an understanding of the history of methods, techniques, and principles learned through a century of experience. A good beginning is a classical textbook of occupational medicine such as Hunter's *Diseases of Occupations*,[12] coupled with a detailed history of methods obtained from primary industrial hygiene sources for the workplace in question. The historical approach is necessary not only for its instructional value, but also because many studies in occupational epidemiology involve exposure which occurred in the remote past. For example, one of the largest and most complete studies—a source of more than 100 methodological and other papers—is the cohort study of more than 11 000 Quebec chrysotile asbestos miners and millers by McDonald *et al.*[13][14] This cohort comprised exclusively workers born between 1891 and 1920, more than 7000 of whom had died, and most relevant exposure having been accumulated before age 55. Exposures contributing to death and disease were thus concentrated in time many decades ago, beginning as early as 1904 and culminating in 1975. Despite this disadvantage, and the relative lack of environmental exposure measures in the earliest periods, the conclusions reached concerning asbestos and disease were conclusive. Backwards extrapolation of workplace exposure measurements obtained in more recent periods, information on job titles obtained from company records, and information on confounders such as smoking obtained directly from workers were combined. The results, outlined in chapter 5, are instructional for occupational epidemiology and for its extension to industrial control and risk assessment.

Exposure and dose

Precise definitions are limiting. For example, should the term *exposure* apply to materials present in the ambient air (or other media), as is traditionally the case, or should it be confined to the material that ultimately enters the body? The latter definition may seem more applicable to the term *dose*, but at what time do ambient levels become exposures, and when does exposure become dose?

In fact, *exposure* does not exist in the abstract, and for the purposes of occupational epidemiology can be defined as the interaction between the concentration of a substance in air or other media and one or more human workers. Exposure is proximate to dose. If *biologically effective exposure*— which requires a human receptor—is the concern, there is a considerable overlap, and the argument that *biologically effective dose* is a more appropriate term has merit. Whatever the semantic difference, it is the biologically effective exposure or dose—in humans—that will increasingly form our main concern.

Dose is modified in many ways once it is present within the body, so perhaps this term should be applied to the concentration of material present at the site at which it exerts its effects—the target organ, receptor, subcellular component, or molecule. This presupposes that the target— and therefore the mechanism—is known, which it most often is not.

Biological relevance

The first decision to be made is which exposure(s) to measure. This decision, akin to hazard identification in risk assessment, requires some understanding of both toxicology and biochemistry, as we must choose exposures that are likely to have a biological effect. Current approaches give equal weight to animal studies and to previous human epidemiological work, and neither should be ignored. We must also know how exposure triggers disease. It is possible to argue that a detailed knowledge or theory of mechanism(s) of action is necessary before any relevant exposure can be assessed with competence. Similarly, assessment of exposure without a biologically rational aetiologic hypothesis is likely to be part of a fishing expedition: it is analogous to ecological study as an epidemiological method. The more tightly focused the hypothesis, the more necessary understanding of mechanisms becomes. Regrettably, basic science has been slow to provide knowledge of mechanisms, and such knowledge is rarely available in the quantitative terms that would best suit epidemiological analysis. It has been argued that empirical evidence of association of exposure and disease is more important than biological rationale in the discovery of causal relationships. This has without doubt been true up to now, but largely where exposures are single and at extremely high concentration. It is likely that the different temperament and approach of epidemiologists and basic scientists will increasingly need to be overcome in multidisciplinary efforts.[15]

A model of occupational exposure

A simple model for occupational disease is depicted in figure 15.1. In this ideal schema there is a single mechanism, which is operated by a single exposure. The mechanism is known in quantitative terms, and prospective, reliable, and valid measurements of the exposure which triggers it have been available to industrial hygienists for the lifetime of the industry. The health end point under study is also single. In this ideal model it is always triggered by the mechanism at a constant rate and in a linear fashion, with a well-established threshold (which may or may not be located at zero exposure). There are no confounders of either exposure or disease, no sources of biased information on exposure (which is always direct), and no disease misclassification.

A more complex theoretical model is provided in figure 15.2. Here it is evident that mechanisms are unknown and probably include several "black boxes". For each mechanistic box, more than one exposure may be operative in more than one way. In this figure, exposure B is nearest to the (unknown) mechanism that most heavily influences disease production. This exposure can be derived from another exposure A, and modified by exposure C. The modification can be subtractive, additive, multiplicative,

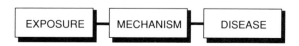

Figure 15.1   An idealised conception of the exposure-disease relationship

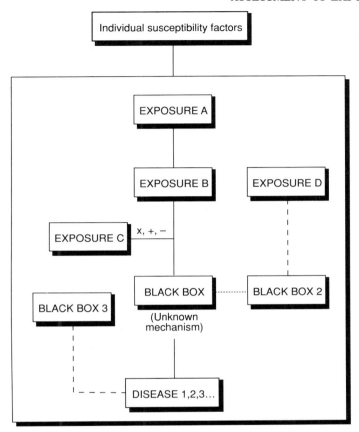

Figure 15.2   A more complex exposure-disease scheme

or take virtually any quantitative form. A fourth exposure type, D, may operate independently on the same mechanistic black boxes, again in any number of quantitative ways. The connection between exposure(s) and disease, mediated by the mechanism(s), may be linear as in figure 15.1, but it may instead be curvilinear or even sigmoidal or bell-shaped. Disease(s) caused by the exposure(s) may be well understood and easily diagnosed, or they may be poorly understood (for example, Hodgkin's disease), or often misdiagnosed (for example, malignant mesothelioma). It may be a single, well-classified cause of morbidity or mortality (for example, carcinoma of bronchial origin), or a poorly classified, loosely connected group of lesions (for example, non-Hodgkin's lymphomas).

Each of these types of error and uncertainty can complicate or render useless exposure assessment. Finally, external factors such as lifestyle (smoking, socioeconomic status, access to health care, diet) and susceptibility factors such as genetic make up may influence any part of the exposure-mechanism-disease chain. Given the complexity of the problem it is amazing that occupational epidemiology has been so successful in the identification of hazardous exposures. The problems are likely to increase in complexity as our knowledge of mechanisms expands and the nature of exposure changes over time.

Essential elements

Definition of a single exposure implicated in a single health outcome should include the following elements for assessment purposes:

- assurance that the single exposure chosen has biological relevance/rationale
- latency, age and time of first exposure
- complete chemical and physical characterisation of the exposure
- concentration or intensity of the exposure
- frequency distribution of the exposure
- total (net) duration of the exposure through the worker's job history
- degree of confidence that exposure has occurred at all

All of the above may also vary over time, which must form an additional part of any operational definition of exposure. This is true even for biological relevance: an exposure that is thought to be causative today may prove to be incidental in the future. Similarly, exposures not known, or not known to have biological effects, may later be seen to have been present in the workplace or to be possible causes of observed disease. Put another way, it is necessary to be sure that the proper exposure is being studied. Studies of asbestos exposure in the asbestos textile industry, for example, have consistently shown much higher lung cancer rates than those in the mining and milling of the same materials.[13 14 16 17] This is the case even though exposure to fibres, and deposition of fibres in lung tissue, is much higher in mining and milling, and study of workplace and deposited fibres shows chemical and physical measurements to be similar.[18] Other exposures such as mineral oil used as a dust suppressant in the textile industry have been suggested,[18] but to date the evidence for this is unconvincing.[17] The relevant exposure, or perhaps the relevant detail of a known exposure such as asbestos fibre length, remains to be confirmed. Exposure assessment may have missed the biologically relevant material altogether, or inadequately characterised some aspect of the known exposures such as chrysotile or tremolite asbestos fibre.

Latency, the interval between the appearance of symptoms or diagnosis of disease and first exposure, is another time-related variable, which signals the importance of accurate assessment of past exposures. For mesothelioma, for example, latency has been estimated at a mean of about 35 years, and longer for some fibre types.[19] The connection can be more complex, as is seen in the fact that mesothelioma incidence appears to be related to the third or fourth power of time since first exposure,[14 19 20] leading to decreasing lifetime risk with increasing age at first exposure.

Additional information on exposures may become available such that past exposures are seen to have had variable chemical or physical make up over time. An example is given by tyre and other workers heavily exposed to industrial talc used as a lubricant. It is now clear that such workers may have been exposed to different materials present within the talc depending on its source, including both asbestiform and non-asbestiform tremolite and other asbestos fibre types. Rarely, low-grade commercial varieties of talc have comprised more true fibrous tremolite than talc,[21] and pneumoconiosis has been an occasional result,[21 22] although other health effects of this material remain controversial.[22-25] Shipping records can be useful in identifying sources of raw materials and can therefore (in association with expert consultation) contribute to accurate exposure assessment. This is only part of the picture: the tyre and rubber industry is an extensively studied work environment with a wide variety of exposures. This has resulted in the production of a great deal of data using a variety of approaches for multiple exposures and multiple diseases.[10]

Concentration or intensity of exposure will be principally affected by production volume and by the introduction of major control measures. These include ventilation, dust suppression, isolation of work processes, institution and proper use of personal protection, and substitution of production processes that result in lower concentration. In a few industries, such as the man-made mineral fibre (MMMF) production process,[26-32] these factors have been well worked out over the history of the industry. Often it is necessary to form qualitative categories of exposure era, based on production and control changes, and to combine these with job title data. Concentration is defined by measurement, which may be either by personal sampling (sampler worn by the worker during the work shift) or by area sampling. The latter category may use fixed samplers, and while theoretically less useful in that individual exposure is not ascertained, such measurements are extremely useful for measuring trends of exposure over time. Personal and fixed or area measurements are sometimes defined as direct and indirect, respectively. These terms are too general, have vague common usage, and have different meanings in other areas of exposure assessment.

Exposure frequency within a given production era is a function of a worker's duties, so it becomes important to know the movements for each man or woman on the job in relation to each point source.

Duration of exposure can be expressed simply in terms of total gross time worked, but this will lack precision. Ideally, an index of cumulative exposure can be constructed from information on exposure concentration, frequency, and job titles, if concentration and frequency are known with confidence for each title. Absences from the job for extended leave or sick leave should also be accounted for. Sometimes work shift may also be of importance in the calculation of concentration and frequency, particularly in relation to production rates.

All of the above depends on confidence in our estimates of actual working conditions and production processes. We must first rate confidence in the probability that exposure has occurred at all, and then obtain quantitative, or at a minimum qualitative, indices of exposure concentration and frequency. Source documents and databases such as standard industrial and chemical classifications, job lists, and research databases in toxicology may be helpful,[33-36] and government, industry or labour compilations may be specific to the industry in one country[33 36] or internationally. The wider the classification net, the wider the confidence interval is likely to be on actual exposure.

Current limitations

Having fulfilled the conditions for a comprehensive definition of exposure for assessment purposes, we must acknowledge that our concepts of exposure are changing. Exposure assessment in the past has been one-dimensional, documenting single sources, single media, and usually single compounds. Good results have nevertheless been obtained in many studies as a result of the massive, single-media exposures to particular toxins in the remote past. As the magnitude of concentration of workplace contaminants decreases and complex work environments increase, more attention will need to be given to multiple exposures and their interaction and to exposure from multiple routes. A new concept of measurement, total exposure assessment methodology (TEAM) has emerged,[6 37-39] together with a variety of modelling schemes, to account for these and other variables. Because these methods are best suited to studies of low-dose exposure, they have arisen in the context of environmental rather than occupational epidemiology. Their application to the latter is evident and will become important. An example of their importance is provided by the observation that inhalation of volatile organic compounds (such as tri- and tetrachloroethylene) in houses is greater from showers and areas where water collects than from water ingestion. Tetrachloroethylene concentrations are elevated in the air of dry-cleaning establishments and in the houses of people receiving dry cleaned clothes,[40] and in breath measurements of both workers and customers.

The use of time-activity diaries in environmental exposure assessment using TEAM concepts also accounts well for the temporal variable of exposure, and within- and across-shift exposure variation should make use of these concepts. Again, these approaches have been used principally in environmental epidemiology. Time-activity diaries provide a measure of where subjects spend parts of their day in relation to exposure point sources, and data on factors such as exertion, which may affect dose rates. In occupational epidemiology, time-activity records could also account for individual within- and across-shift exposure variation which might not be ascertained by conventional sampling.

Economic and social factors also change the nature of the task of exposure assessment. Already, much of industrialised society has been transformed from manufacturing and resource-based economies to those based on service industries. Further, there is an increasing trend to smaller workplaces. Finally, there has been—partly as an outcome of occupational epidemiology—a general downward trend in permissible exposures, sometimes to levels below which it may be difficult to detect them. While the latter condition may be desirable it will make exposure assessment more complex and more expensive, and pressure will be applied not to measure some exposures at all. The shrinking workplace and reduced government and industry resources will further reduce the means available, at a time when the change to a service economy is changing the work environment and the exposures that it entails.

Biological path and exposure route

Occupational exposure can occur directly through the respiratory, gastrointestinal, and integumentary systems. The dermal route of exposure is important because it is common and results in a high percentage of lost workdays: in Quebec in some years more than 40% of occupational diseases reported to the workmen's compensation board were skin disorders. For the most part, however, these diseases are less severe than those produced by exposures through other routes. Identification of the responsible exposures is more direct for skin diseases than for the gastrointestinal and respiratory routes of exposure. This is because contact dermatitis constitutes more than 90% of these diseases, and most of the latter have a direct irritant rather than an allergic aetiology. It is thus a simpler matter to detect the responsible chemical or other substance. This is particularly true for materials such as strong acids, which produce skin irritation and lesions almost immediately. Even substances having an allergic mechanism, such as poison ivy or oak in agricultural and other outdoor workers, are likely to do so within days of first exposure, and within hours on re-exposure. The long lag time or latency observed for some diseases with primarily inhaled or ingested toxins is thus not an important factor, and the causative exposures are more likely to be correctly identified. This may be less true in complex chemical work environments.

Gastrointestinal exposures may be primary, such as ingestion of toxins, or secondary as, for example, when dusts or fibres cleared from the lung by mucociliary action are then swallowed. This type of exposure cannot be directly measured. A concise list of possible types of gastrointestinal exposure from food, water, and soil was offered by Lioy.[41] Factors such as

361

solubility of the material and its contact rate (for ingestion, with the gastrointestinal tract) are added to the basic concepts of concentration and frequency.

It should be noted that true gastrointestinal exposures include only those which ultimately both enter the body through the alimentary canal and exert their effects on the cells of the tract. Examples include chemical gastritis as an acute effect and carcinoma of the colorectal epithelium as a chronic effect. Exposures to and diseases of the liver, pancreas, and other solid organs are not gastrointestinal tract exposures or lesions, although they are often mistakenly grouped together.

Exposure by inhalation occurs with gases, mists, vapours, fumes and dusts. Principles in this area are well-established and have been reviewed in detail elsewhere.[42 43] Gases may be irritant or non-irritant, the latter being more difficult to detect and therefore to measure retrospectively. Generally, irritant gases are more soluble than non-irritant gases and hence produce more immediate effects in the upper airways. Non-irritant gases such as nitrogen dioxide can penetrate deeply into the lung before their detection. The small particle size of fumes (by definition, $0 \cdot 1$ μm to $1 \cdot 0$ μm particle diameter) may similarly make them difficult to detect. Dusts, if their concentration is sufficient, may have been visible in air and as settled dusts in the workplace, and overall dustiness is one of the workplace conditions that can be well assessed by worker recall. The physical make up of dusts, of course, may not have been known to workers, and there is always a risk of confusion between nuisance dusts and those of more biological interest.

Some inhaled substances are sequestered within the lung and it is therefore in that organ that most of their effects are seen. Typical examples are asbestos (for fibrous dusts) and free silica (as quartz, for non-fibrous dusts). The important aspects of inhaled particulate exposures may be summarised by the 5 ds:

- Dose (and the exposure, frequency, and concentration that produce it)
- Diameter (which determines the respirability and deposition mechanism, which is principally:
  (1) impaction in the nasal passages and upper airways for large particles,
  (2) settling under the force of gravity or sedimentation for the bulk of respirable non-fibrous particles under $2 \cdot 0$ μm diameter,
  (3) brownian motion or diffusion at low (less than $0 \cdot 1$ μm) particle diameters,
  (4) interception, the mechanism by which particles may accumulate at branch points in the bronchial tree, is mainly dictated by particle length rather than diameter and is therefore most applicable to fibrous particles.

- Deposition (especially in the alveoli)
- Durability (or biopersistence, which reflects retained dose and thus has particular importance for chronic disease such as pneumoconiosis and cancer: chemical and physical make up are principal contributors to this characteristic).
- Dissolution and clearance mechanisms, which vary in relative importance from one exposure to another, again based largely on chemical and physical make up.

Translocation is the movement of a substance between one compartment of the organism and another. Elaborate schemes and diagrams are available to describe this phenomenon, together with biotransformation, metabolism, concentration, storage, and elimination. Any such scheme renders the appearance of what happens to internal doses extremely complex while at the same time oversimplifying the principles involved. We are constantly gaining new knowledge of mechanisms of translocation, biotransformation, concentration, and elimination. These vary for different exposures and circumstances, and between individual subjects (and species). Much of the data are derived from animal experiments, but increasingly biological movement of exposures is assessed in exposed human populations. To take one recent example, a variety of chlorophenols in urine were found to be related to airborne monochlorobenzene in dye intermediate production workers.[44] Urine concentrations were seen to vary as a function of exposure over the work shift with some lag time, but measurement at the end of the work shift was proportional to daily average exposure. Another example is a recent study of exposure to nitrogen dioxide.[45] NO_2 is absorbed at a rate of 80% to 90% in humans following inhalation, but it does not cross the alveolar barrier into blood. Instead, nitric acid is formed and then dissociated to form free radicals: NO_2^- ions. These enter the blood and form methaemoglobin and nitrosylhaemoglobin, but the mechanisms and quantitative reactions have not been fully worked out. Unlike NO_2, most nitrogen oxide (NO) is absorbed directly into the blood. Although the high affinity of NO for oxygen would suggest rapid transformation to nitrosylhaemoglobin and methaemoglobin these reactions appear to be much smaller *in vivo* than predicted.

In general, the most important translocations are those that occur between the respiratory compartment and blood[42 43] and between the blood and other compartments. These include the liver (where most biotransformation occurs) and the kidney (where most concentration of toxin occurs before elimination). Some biological tissues, such as adipose tissue, may also act as storage depots for certain chemicals and their metabolites: dioxin is one example. Translocation also occurs within compartments of the same organ, such as the movement of particles from the alveolar compartment into the pulmonary interstitium, where it may

363

produce a fibrotic reaction (pneumoconiosis). The movement of particles such as asbestos fibres from initial deposition at airway bifurcations to ultimate translocation into interstitial compartments has been well worked out in animal inhalation experiments followed by morphometric examination.[46 47]

Biotransformation and metabolism are complex topics beyond the scope of this chapter. It is sufficient to note here that materials that are not toxic may become so through biochemical mechanisms, usually in the liver and usually involving chemical reactions either of conjugation (combination of a material with a normal body element, usually a protein), or of chemical degradation (oxidation, by far the most common reaction; reduction, or hydrolysis). All mechanisms usually result in a less toxic product, but too much conjugation can reduce the concentration of the conjugating protein unacceptably. Oxidation can produce toxic intermediates, a good example of which is the cancer-causing epoxide produced following exposure to vinyl chloride.[48] This epoxide, 2-chloroethylene oxide, alkylates DNA and is the probable direct cause of angiosarcoma in exposed workers.[49] Physical agents such as dusts may also cause intermediate reactions that result in disease. Asbestos fibres and other dusts stimulate the production of oxygen radicals by inflammatory cells,[50] and there is increasing evidence that these free radicals or their products, such as hydrogen peroxide, are involved in the pathogenesis of lung fibrosis and possibly of neoplasia.[51]

Concentration in the kidney and elimination in the urine are further potential sources of increased exposure to toxins within these organs. Blood flow to the kidney for the purpose of glomerular filtration is high, and part of the function of the renal structure is to concentrate the urine and its constituents.[9] The result can be an amplified acute or chronic effect of toxins. Others, such as heavy metals, may directly damage renal tubular cells. Once a toxin is concentrated in the urine it may also spend a long time in contact with the epithelium of the ureters and bladder, the latter being most affected. The effect of aromatic amines on the development of bladder cancer is one example.

Strategies of exposure assessment

Ascertainment of job titles

Regardless of the types of environmental or biological measurement available, or the ways in which they are used, most studies in occupational epidemiology depend on the accuracy of the job titles assigned to workers. These may be available as lists of task or pay-oriented job titles provided by an employer, or can be constructed from duties recalled by workers. Often all that is available is description of duties recalled by workers or employers or a description of the production process by company personnel. Standardised job titles may be used in some industries in some countries, and if so descriptions of the duties involved, including activity levels and some environmental information, may be available.[35]

Ideally, a list of relevant job-title-derived exposure categories should be constructed by experts for each epidemiological study. In practice, this has been possible for studies with large numbers[7 8 13 14 52] but has prohibitive costs in smaller studies.

It is equally important to translate the list of job titles into accurate time and concentration-corrected exposure estimates. Job titles may or may not correspond well to the duties performed and in some instances may prove of little use in exposure assessment. Electrical workers, for example, have highly variable exposure to electromagnetic fields, yet are often grouped together.[52 53] Even within a single job category within one industry exposures may be heterogeneous over time, as a result of changes in production processes and means of control.[7]

Job exposure matrices

A job exposure matrix (JEM) is the logical outcome of the application of lists of job titles to potential exposures for each. Job titles, however arrived at, are examined by expert raters to calculate the exposures that may have occurred. The matrix may be viewed in two dimensions—sequentially held job titles on one axis and one or more individual chemicals on the other—or in three, with quantitative measurements for each exposure added.

JEMs have been called a "fixed set of rules for translating any job into a list of exposures"[7] and as such involve numerous strategies. Studies of exposure to man-made mineral fibres[30–32] present the simplest type of JEM in that a single class of substances is examined with the exposures being estimated for each of a large number of job categories over several technological eras of exposure intensity defined by evolutionary steps in control technology.[26–32]

Similarly, in a study of occupational solvent exposure and organic brain damage, Cherry *et al.* made job category assessments according to a standard occupational code assigned by a panel of experts.[54] Job descriptions were provided by cases (or proxy) and referents as a list of all recalled lifetime employment. In addition an exposure checklist was used to provide subjective impressions of exposure to the solvent and to potential confounders such as pesticides or alcohol. Exposure to solvents was then rated by the same experts on a four-point scale (over 50% of threshold limit value, 30 to 50% of threshold limit value; less than 30% threshold limit value but more than the average citizen, and not more than the average citizen). Individual ratings of exposure made on the same scale by one person using uncategorised job descriptions produced risk estimates similar to those produced by the experts.

365

For more general occupational studies or new population-based studies, job exposure matrices have been constructed to be uniformly applied to different industries (and referents). Hoar *et al.* have produced a job exposure matrix in the United States which consist of over 500 categories and 376 exposures known or suspected to be toxic or carcinogenic,[55] and similar but somewhat smaller schemes have been constructed elsewhere.[56] The application of such a large matrix is unwieldy, particularly for a study which is focused on one or a few exposures.[7] In addition, despite its apparently comprehensive nature, such a scheme is not applicable to job titles where exposures exist that have not previously been suspected of causing disease, and may not even include job titles that are applicable to the industry under investigation.

Subject by subject exposure assessment

An exposure assessment scheme may combine a categorisation of probability of exposure (or expert confidence that exposure has occurred), frequency, and intensity to produce an overall semi-quantitative impression of exposure.[7 8] This can then be combined with duration figures and related to disease in case-control or other studies. An index of exposure can be constructed by experts for each subject based on his job history, exposures ascertained from multiple sources, and concentration and frequency data. This approach has considerable advantages when numerous exposures (or diseases) are being explored at the same time, as in hypothesis-generating designs and case-control designs where disease is known before the study but exposures are not. Any type of information may be used, including worker recall of past conditions, but there is ultimate reliance on expert coding of individual job histories by people trained in industrial hygiene or related technical fields. The approach has some of the difficulties inherent in job exposure matrix designs, and indeed could be regarded as a multi-dimensional matrix.[7] The argument has been made that this approach is more cost effective than the earlier job-exposure matrix design in that the matrix, although complex and expensive to generate, may be constructed for one group of workers (and referents) at a time, and as such represents value for money.[7 57]

Instruments of exposure measurement

Company records

In practice, our knowledge of actual exposure is often confined to lists of workers' past job titles. Sometimes no such records exist, in which case we will be dependent on workers' and others' recall. In either case, an important limitation on our ability to estimate exposure is introduced: our information is on the kind of work done, rather than what the workers were exposed to. If we know with confidence that the type of work was invariably associated with a given exposure, have some knowledge of the frequency and concentration of that exposure, and are sure that no other exposures or confounding factors were present in the workplace, we can proceed to extrapolate to exposure using one of the strategies described above. This is rarely the case: exposures are more likely to be multiple, interrelated, and variable in both frequency and intensity in the workplace. In addition, the company records or worker recall are themselves subject to error.

As an example, consider three women with mesothelioma who worked in the Quebec chrysotile asbestos mining region. All were believed to have develped their disease from environmental or domestic exposure, as none were listed as employees of the asbestos companies in the comprehensive records available.[13][14] The cases would be important for risk assessment purposes. However, occupations other than mining in the area involved asbestos exposure: in this case the three women worked in a 10- to 15-person unventilated shop which repaired jute bags that had held asbestos, including imported amphiboles which were demonstrable in lung tissue analysis.[58] Similarly, 17 of 23 asbestos miners and millers employed in another Quebec chrysotile district were found to have been exposed to varying concentrations of crocidolite or amosite by lung tissue analysis, possibly from undocumented work in a local factory employing 300.[59]

External measurement of exposure

The most common measurement of exposure is by sampling of materials in the workplace, usually in air. As indicated previously, such assessment may be either of individual exposure by personal sampling or of so-called indirect exposure by fixed or area sampling. The applied science of industrial hygiene is most directly concerned with this type of assessment of exposure, and measurements designed by hygienists are those upon which most exposure assessment schemes rely. Most measurements are not obtained for the purposes of epidemiological study, but for control purposes. As such they may be aimed more at deciding whether certain limits are exceeded (for example, threshold limit values[60]) than at appropriateness for research purposes. Adaptation of such data is necessary. Measurement errors arise from technical sources in addition to those for other types of exposure assessment.

Complex chemical and physical measurements have many possible sources of error, compounded by the number and complexity of technical steps necessary in all instrument calibration, sampling procedures, and measurement on the reference instrument (such as atomic absorption, spectrophotometry, microscopy, or others). It is sometimes possible to make current measurements for epidemiological study, either for prospective purposes or for extrapolating backwards in time. The latter exercise has errors proportional to the number and nature of major control measures introduced between the era of exposure and the present, and to a lesser degree to production volumes. It is also possible that the very nature of exposure will have changed, and if the chemical or physical exposures present in the workplace are no longer present no amount of statistical manipulation will help. An example was the observation that workers in one American man-made mineral fibre production factory used for the purposes of epidemiological study were found after analysis of lung tissue to have had undocumented exposure to amosite asbestos in most of the cases assessed.[61] In general, the use of current environmental measurements made to fit a specific epidemiological study design will be limited to large, well funded studies such as the Canada-France study of electric utility workers.[52]

The field of industrial hygiene is developing rapidly. Measurements which we take for granted today were not available in the past, and we must often rely on measurements taken years ago in relating past exposure to present disease. One example is provided by the study of diseases related to mineral fibres such as asbestos[13 14 16 18] or glass fibre.[26] The principal instrument available for dust air sampling in the past, the midget impinger, did not distinguish fibrous from non-fibrous particles. Although we know today that mineral fibres—of distinct dimensional classes—are the particles of real interest, we have a vast database of past exposures that relies principally on the older technology. While this does not prevent scientific study of exposure-response questions, it does lead to difficulties in the setting of standards and in calculations for risk assessment purposes. Conversion factors may be difficult to estimate, have wide confidence intervals, and may even vary between work environments.

Questionnaires

At times even job titles may be unavailable. Workers can be asked directly whether they were exposed to certain substances and if so to what quantities, but they are often unlikely to know either the specific substances present in the workplace or the degree to which these substances were present. They may be more able to describe their duties, which can then be translated into checklists of exposure for individual jobs. There is an increasing volume of information about the proper conduct and statistical considerations for the use of questionnaires in exposure assessment, although much of the information comes from other disciplines.[1] The use of standardised questionnaires such as those used in the assessment of respiratory disease would be an asset, but these are difficult to construct in a way that would make them applicable to many industries.

Instead, a number of practical and theoretical considerations must be considered in the construction or adaptation of a questionnaire for a given exposure assessment. These were well summarised by Armstrong et al.,[1] and include the choice of open or closed questions (with these authors favouring the former), the language of the questionnaire (including the level of difficulty of the language used), allowance for unforced answers, and avoidance of ambiguity including vagueness, double negatives, and obscure time reference.[1] Optimum question ordering (with questions of more interest and less threat placed early in the sequence) is also important. Subject characteristics influence questionnaire responses, the most important traits having potential effects on exposure assessment being experience and behaviour. There is little research on the effects of these variables specifically directed at the implications for exposure assessment.

Questionnaires regarding work history can be constructed as a matrix of jobs held on one axis and duties or known exposures on another. These are thus analogous and translatable to a job exposure type of data set.

In retrospective studies including case-control studies of fatal disease, questionnaires may need to be administered to proxy (such as first degree relatives) rather than workers. Issues of recall and potential bias differ for this type of study. Questionnaires may be administered either in association with interview or as a self-administered exercise.

Interviews

Many of the same issues associated with questionnaires also arise in relation to interviews of workers or proxy respondents. Interviews may be more expensive to arrange and administer but can possibly provide better information. Subjects must be properly informed before the interview and the time and place must be optimal. The content of the interview, like questionnaires, should place questions of more interest (such as those directly related to the purpose of the study) ahead of those with more threatening content (such as questions of a demographic, personal, or economic nature).[1] Interviews may be highly structured, with fixed questions and order, or open-ended, allowing more flexibility in response. The latter type of interview may extract more data, but care must be taken in its interpretation.

Interviews are subject to four principal types of error. These are errors in the content of the interview, errors in its administration, errors in recording the responses, and outright cheating by the interviewer. Content error is introduced at the design stage and for the purposes of exposure assessment can be reduced by involving experts in industrial hygiene with specific knowledge of the workplace. Errors in administration include improper asking (for all types of interview) and improper or biased probing in open-ended unstructured interviews. Most of these errors can be reduced by consistent training of interviewers. Ideally, interviewers should have some technical knowledge of the exposure assessment that they are investigating. This is particularly true for probing interviews of the open-ended variety. Demographic and educational variables of the subjects (and the interviewers) also affect the validity of interview data, as will the complexity of the exposure history that is being elicited and the time interval between interview and exposure.[11]

Biological indicators

Biological indicators of exposure have now been in use for several decades. Two types of indicator have been described in association with exposure assessment. The first include biological effect indices which are used for routine exposure monitoring purposes. This biomonitoring activity must make use of routinely available, non-invasive biological samples. These are usually urine samples for chemical exposures or their metabolites, or breath samples. Blood samples are sometimes used, although these are more common in association with actual studies of exposure rather than for surveillance. Biomonitoring methods are standardised and well described.[62] This field has become so well developed that standard biological effect indices have been established analogous to threshold limit values.[60] The American Conference of Governmental Industrial Hygienists has a list of biological effect indices which currently includes permissible levels of carbon disulphide (less than 5 mg/g urinary creatinine of 2-thiothiazolidine-4-carboxylic acid at the end of the work shift), arsenic and soluble compounds including arsine (50 μg/g urinary creatine at end of work week), and benzene (in urine and exhaled air before the next work shift). Other substances with suggested biological limits include fluorides, cadmium, carbon monoxide, lead, organic and inorganic mercury, methanol, styrene, and trichloroethylene. Biological effect indices, like threshold limit values, are subject to change with new information, and will generally be lowered as threshold limit values are lowered. For a number of exposures there are some data on potential biological effect indices but not enough to establish a limit. Malathion and polychlorinated biphenyls fall into this group, but biological measurements may nevertheless be used for exposure assessment for the purpose of epidemiological study.

The other class of biological indicators includes a wide range of tests done for evaluation of either exposure, biological effect, or disease in association with an epidemiological study. These are commonly called biologic markers or biomarkers,[4-6 63 64] and while they include some of the same measurements used in biomonitoring surveillance there is a distinction in their classification and in their use. Categories of biomarkers have been described, and are outlined in figure 15.3.

For the purposes of exposure assessment, internal dose data and biologically effective dose are the most useful concepts. Internal dose refers, as the name implies, to the dose that is deposited in and can be

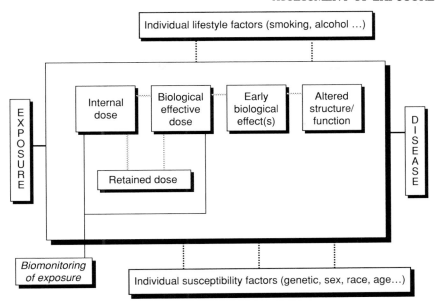

Figure 15.3   Biological indicators of exposure[75]

recovered from the organism. This is usually described in association with measurements in living subjects such as workers,[4 5] but the term is equally applicable to studies of tissues of deceased subjects or resected organs. Lung fibre analysis is one example.[18 59 61 65–71] Markers of biologically effective dose, as defined earlier, may be separated for research purposes. Both these and internal dose markers may also be or produce biological indicators that are suitable for biological monitoring of exposure as a surveillance activity. Markers of exposure that are persistent in tissue can be banked in tissue registries, and astute investigators should be aware of existing and possible collection opportunities. Unfortunately, a great deal of biologically useful material is discarded for reasons of routine maintenance and space conservation. Fixed specimens such as paraffin blocks of lung tissue should be easily conserved but are often thrown away after only a few years, and preservation of flash-frozen specimens requires both prospective design and long-term maintenance.

It is important to distinguish biomarkers of exposure from those of disease. The latter, shown in figure 15.3 as early biological effects and altered structure or function; are sometimes referred to as indicators of exposure because they may reflect, usually in a nonspecific way, the end result of exposure. These markers are not often sufficiently specific to be useful in the assessment of exposure. Many studies nevertheless attempt this. An example is a recent study of long-term shoe workers exposed to

371

benzene.[72] These workers had a 22% prevalance of a variety of chromosomal aberrations, compared with 3% in a control group. However, there was no relation between chromosomal aberrations and working period, a finding that has been confirmed in other studies of benzene exposure. The fact that non-specific chromosomal aberrations, which may or may not have biological relevance for later cancer development, are observed in working populations, does not necessarily reflect exposure in any specific or sensitive fashion. Similarly, recent attempts to develop a hybrid molecular epidemiology[63 64 73] is many years from producing information that could be useful in exposure assessment, which again should not be confused with assessment of early changes in DNA, production of DNA adducts, sister chromatid exchange, or later changes in the pathway to chronic disease.

Sources of error in the use of biomarkers are similar to those for environmental measurements. Once again, the technical aspects of measurement come into play with respect to sampling, instrumentation, and statistical manipulation. Calibration, maintenance, training, and quality control are all immensely important. Measurements range from the simple and generally reliable (for example, for benzene) to complex and unreliable except in laboratories with great experience (for example, dioxins). A huge variety of technical factors and assumptions about kinetics come into play. An example of the latter is posed by the many difficulties in the interpretation of lung fibre analysis. Although hundreds of studies have been done, inter-laboratory comparison of results is still virtually impossible,[22 71 74] and results must be interpreted with caution.[71] This is partially due to the fact that the internal dose being measured is constantly changing due to the operation of continuing exposure(s), deposition, and clearance or dissolution. At best most studies measure lung fibres that represent a lifetime of exposure with all of the above factors having dynamic effects on the end results. As a result, different fibre types have different retention. Glass fibres do not appear to be retained in the long term at all,[61] whereas tremolite asbestos fibres are retained to a much higher degree than the other fibre types which they contaminate,[18] and come to represent the bulk of lung fibre burden. This leads to difficulty in interpretation in that both the retained tremolite and the native material (for example, chrysotile asbestos or vermiculite) may be represented by the internal dose of tremolite, which is itself a biologically effective dose.[76] For this reason the term retained dose is more appropriate than internal dose in this type of study (figure 15.3).

Other types of biological indicator are also used. These include new radiological techniques that allow identification of foreign materials. Examples include identification of metals in the lung by their enhanced magnetic potential, and spectroscopy of brain lesions in vivo allowing identification of chemical make up.

372

Biological markers and routine biomonitoring data in any category can be affected by susceptibility factors such as age, sex, genetic make up, and race, as well as lifestyle factors such as alcohol intake and smoking. In addition the correlation between markers on the pathway from exposure to disease are influenced by the same factors. Some of these confounding or interactive factors can themselves be measured by biological indicators. Cotinine, a metabolite of nicotine, is a useful biological marker of exposure to cigarette smoke, whether active or passive.[77] It is virtually specific for tobacco products, and can be measured reliably in saliva, urine, and blood.[77] Urine concentration is proportional to dose, even when exposure is measured by such surrogates as numbers of smokers in the home. There are, however, as with many biological indicators, some difficulties in interpretation due to toxico-kinetic differences between individuals or groups. Non-smokers appear to clear cotinine more slowly than do smokers.

Observational surrogate measurements

At times it is not possible to measure environmental exposure or to obtain reliable information from job titles, questionnaires, or interviews. In these instances surrogates for retrospective exposure may be discovered. In the environmental epidemiology relating possible disease to electromagnetic field exposures, for example, investigators in 1979 developed a method of using wire configuration codes as a surrogate for such exposures.[78] While this study was criticised for its indirect exposure assessment at the time, further work has shown that some direct measurements may be less reliable than the wire code surrogates. This is not surprising, because wire codes may reflect past exposure tendencies, whereas direct measurements applied today may not,[53] even if they are 24-hour averages.[53 79] One Swedish study combined the characteristics of power lines with the electrical load of these lines, to produce a measure that is analogous to cumulative exposure: the dose-response correlation seen in earlier work on childhood leukaemia was supported.[80] Nevertheless, occupational studies of electromagnetic field effects should continue to use direct measurement wherever possible, and confounding or interacting exposures should be identified, if present.[52 53] The greater variation in exposure levels to be expected among electrical utility workers and others having similar exposures can be expected to clarify dose-response correlations, if the exposure measurement tools are accurate.

Variables that modify assessed exposures or their effects

Background exposure from non-occupational sources can, if sufficiently high, add to occupational exposures and should be identified. For example, recent estimates of exposure to chrysotile asbestos in the ambient air of mining and milling towns has been related as between 0·3

373

and 4 fibres/ml of air at times of greatest exposure (Camus M, personal communication). Domestic (household) exposures may have been even higher.

Interactions of exposure with other exposures or lifestyle differences are exemplified in the study of Cherry *et al.* of solvent exposures and organic brain damage. Although the main focus of the study was exposure to solvents rated for each job, information was also collected on seven sources of potential confounding or interaction, including lead, pesticides, and alcohol.[54] A principal finding was that although occupational exposure to solvents was more common in people with organic brain damage than in referents, the excess risk was concentrated among heavy drinkers. The authors postulated an interaction between alcohols and solvents, and their results support this conclusion (as opposed to a confounding effect).

Multiple routes of exposure may exist where they are not recognised, as indicated above in the discussion of total exposure assessment methodology. Chemical exposures, in particular, should always be considered by every possible site of entry including dermal absorption before the construction of an exposure index.

Persistence of materials as retained dose is a potential factor in continuing exposure. Individuals who have left the workplace but retain the toxin under study in the target organ have a complex and changing exposure which is difficult to measure accurately. Given the long latency period of some occupational diseases, this type of exposure following the end of exposure may have to be taken into account.

Lifestyle factors and individual susceptibility can be important sources of modification of exposure, including action as confounders or interaction as in the example above. Smoking is the single most important lifestyle factor to be taken into account in the proper assessment of exposure. The inhalation of cigarette smoke may act directly on another exposure, for example through the deposition of polycyclic aromatic hydrocarbons on inhaled particles. Smoking may interact with or confound exposures. This is a common problem in the correlation of occupational exposures with lung cancer. For almost every known occupational exposure that is related to lung cancer, smoking has an effect, which must be assessed.[81] Often the degree of interaction is difficult to estimate. For exposures which have not yet been shown to cause disease, smoking must be assessed if the disease has a high attributable risk for cigarette habit: lung cancer is again the best example of this. Estimation of smoking should be regarded with as much care as any other aspect of exposure assessment.

Other lifestyle factors that may need to be assessed in an individual study include drug intake (both pharmaceutical and recreational), exercise habit, and diet. Socioeconomic factors including level of education, income, and class may need to be accounted for, as all may be related to job status and therefore to exposure. Independent correlations of disease with any of these factors (for example, socioeconomic class and Hodgkin's disease[82]) may complicate exposure assessment if the same socioeconomic variable is also related to exposure. Finally, genetic make up, including race and sex, may influence biologically effective exposure through differences in metabolism or susceptibility.

Statistical considerations

Statistical theory underlying various types of exposure assessment and the potential errors introduced is beyond the scope of this chapter. Only a few basic concepts will be outlined: the reader should look to the primary statistical texts and other sources for numerical approaches.[1 3 10 11 83] All the statistical concerns relate to problems outlined above, such as the retrospective nature of exposure assessment, exposure variation over time, confounding, and interaction. To some extent statistical concerns also vary according to study design: however, most studies, particularly analytical, (case-control and cohort) have potential problems in common. These include:

- Bias in reporting of exposure.
- Exposure in referents as representative of the general population.
- Time dimensions of exposure.
- Identification of and correction for measurement error.
- Identification of and correction for confounding variables.
- Identification of and correction for interaction.

An excellent discussion of bias in the reporting of exposure was given by Schlesselman.[11] Recall bias may be defined as any systematic effect on exposure or disease status introduced by factors related to memory. These include simply forgetting the existence of past exposures, which is more likely as the time following exposure increases. Although there is a standard impression that bias may be introduced by case status, in that cases may have more of a tendency to look for past exposures that may have caused their disease, this is an area of controversy. Some have argued that people who are aware of the aetiological hypothesis of a study may be more likely to report their exposure status inaccurately.[84] However, to exclude such patients may actually bias the study by removing those with most knowledge of exposure.[85] Indeed, precisely because of a possible relationship between an exposure and a disease a person who has the disease is likely to be more adequately informed on his or her past exposure(s) than a referent. In this sense there is knowledge bias rather than recall bias, and referents may be more likely to be misclassified by exposure status than cases. This hypothesis may however hold true only when a large proportion of people do have knowledge of the aetiological hypothesis, as well as of the exposure.

In any case-referent study, referents are thought to be representative of the general population with respect to their exposure status. In addition, cases and controls must have the same theoretical opportunity to have exposure. Many factors can intervene to make this untrue.[11] For example, a condition may both cause disease, or a precursor to disease, and prevent further opportunity for exposure. Thus individuals with pre-existing lung disease are likely to avoid (or to be exluded from) dusty jobs, and those with hypertension or heart disease to avoid or be excluded from jobs involving heavy exertion. Any exposures that might cause disease of the lungs or heart could potentially be influenced. Exclusion of cases and referents who have such diseases is one possible solution. The use of proxy respondents introduces further basis for possible misclassification of exposure based on erroneous or biased recall. Relatives or fellow workers may not remember, may never have known, or may misinform the interviewer about past exposures.

Whatever the cause of an error in the assignment of exposure values to cases and referents, systematic misclassification of exposure may result. If misclassification occurs equally between cases and controls there may be a systematic reduction of the observed odds ratios, relative risk, and attributable risk.[11] If on the other hand the exposure misclassification occurs differently in cases and controls, the direction of the error cannot be predicted. It is no longer accepted that random misclassification of exposure always leads to a reduction in risk estimates: the opposite may be true in some cases.[86] [87] Adjustments for misclassification of exposure (or disease) have been suggested, but do not eliminate the possible effects.[11]

Effect of measurement error

Incorrect exposure assessment (or exposure misclassification) not only results in unreliable statistics but has an impact on the power of the study. This has been shown in studies of dietary exposure.[88] The sample size of the study appears to be inversely proportional to the square of the correlation between actual exposure and assessed exposure. Thus even a small increase in exposure misclassification may undermine assumptions about sample size made before a study begins. It is evident that accurate assessment of exposure should be a prime concern in study design, but also that the possible error in that assessment should be estimated when calculating sample size.

Validation of exposure measurements

Although the measurement of exposure is approached in a standardised manner, there has been little methodological work on the validation of past exposure measurements. Much of exposure assessment is retrospective, and as the circumstances of past exposures do not exist in many of today's industries, direct validation is not possible. Recreation of past exposure environments is likely to be impractical, expensive, or both. Despite the obvious need for continuing monitoring of exposure as input for epidemiological study, there have been few prospective studies taking advantage of contemporary measurements. It is important to note the distinction between validation and the epidemiological constructs of validity. Validation is usually an experimental or statistical exercise, which compares one measurement of exposure with another. It is often a cross-disciplinary activity, and is itself prone to errors in execution and difficulties in interpretation. A good concordance between two unrelated measures of the same exposure is more a reflection of the reliability of the two approaches in relation to each other than it is truly representative of the validity of exposure estimates.[1] In addition, if two or more methods of exposure assessment produce widely different results, it may be difficult to decide which of the measurements is more valid.

Validation of the type of exposure measurement used in a past study is possible in several ways. Exposures can be modelled using statistical techniques to account for changes in industrial practice, and the results compared with environmental exposures. The past exposure environment can be recreated. This can be done in animal experiments, but is more useful in human studies using environmental or biological measures. Measurements may be by analogy, in that they are obtained in air chambers without workers present, or more realistic, with introduction of workers into the created environment (with adequate personal protection and with personal monitoring devices to record individual exposures). In long-term or former workers, biological markers can be used to monitor the accuracy and relevance of past external environmental measurements. Finally, it is possible to use disease itself as an exposure validator. If an exposure is reliably associated with a disease in a dose-response fashion, then past exposure estimates in a study of another disease supposedly related to the same exposure may be validated by their association with the established disease.

An example combining the statistical modelling and reconstruction approaches to exposure assessment validation is offered by work on exposures to man-made mineral fibres (MMMF).[27 28] Direct measurements of exposure to MMMF were available only from 1977 onwards, and even then restricted to short-term (one to two weeks) surveys covering all jobs, and restricted to the modern technique of continuous, automated fibre production. Technological changes in the industry, including that from discontinuous batch production involving more manual handling of fibres, addition of ventilation, use of dust suppressants, and other factors could not be directly accounted for.

Cherrie et al. wished to reproduce as nearly as possible the early working conditions, as it was believed that exposures in that era were largely responsible for any excess risk presently observed.[28] They did so in a rock wool pilot plant, taking personal monitoring samples of workers both directly and indirectly involved in fibre manipulations. All technical aspects of the MMMF fiberisation process (such as melt temperature and viscosity) were monitored, as were other environmental conditions such as air exchange, temperature, and humidity. The experiment was run for one day using oil as a dust suppressant and for a second day without oil. Both total and respirable dust were measured using membrane filters and phase contrast and scanning electron microscopy: oil content of the bulk product was also measured.

Another experiment was performed using hand cutting and handling of loose wools in a small closed cabin, again with and without oil. In both experiments greater concentrations of fibre were found in air without dust suppressant oil, the ratio ranging from three to four times greater in the ventilated production environment to eight times greater in the closed cabin. In addition, fibres in the reconstructed early phase environments were thinner and longer than those in more modern facilities, and the addition of oil dust suppression had the effect of doubling the average fibre diameter, substantially reducing the respirable fraction. The authors concluded that early exposures may have been at the upper limit of that suggested previously, at least for rock wool workers. This fits well with the observation that it is in these (and slag wool) workers that a lung cancer hazard from early phase exposures has been shown most convincingly.[30-32]

An example of the use of internal dose markers was the study of chrysotile asbestos miners and millers in Quebec as compared with chrysotile textile workers in Charleston, South Carolina.[18] The major question addressed was validation of historical environmental exposure measurements, which had shown much higher levels of exposure in the chrysotile miners and millers. Lung tissue fibre concentrations were seen to be higher in this group, even though lung cancer rates were much higher in the textile workers.

An example of the use of a disease indicator for validation involves the established, dose-related association between exposure to silica dust and silicosis. The question of lung cancer and exposure to silica is less settled, because most studies are of smokers with silicosis and other possible exposures to known lung carcinogens such as asbestos, radon daughters, and others.[89] A study of silica-exposed workers in 29 metal mines and pottery factories in China found only limited support for a direct role for silica.[90] Risk was mainly in industries such as tin mines where other lung carcinogens (arsenic, polycyclic aromatic hydrocarbons, and radon gas) were highly correlated with silica exposure. As this study was based on estimates of exposure to both total dust and silica dust, it was important to know to what extent the silica estimates were accurate. One method of validation was therefore to look at the dose-response correlation between the measurements and the development of silicosis in the study groups.[91]

When this was done, a strong association between cumulative respirable silica dust exposure and silicosis was shown. The group with the strongest association between estimated silica exposure and silicosis—workers in tungsten mines—had shown no association with lung cancer.

In addition to increased use of validation procedures and more attention to the theoretical constructs of validity, continued assessment of reliability of exposure estimates is necessary. Intra- and inter-rater agreements of exposure estimation should be examined whenever possible. Reliability tests are applicable to any type of exposure estimation, from questionnaire responses to biological measurements. Inter-rater reliability was examined, for example, between the previously described JEM-derived approach of Siemiatycki et al.[78] and expert coding of exposures, and good agreement was noted.[92] On the other hand, problems have been noted in inter-laboratory comparisons of lung internal dose measurements of asbestos fibre concentration assessed by electron microscopy.[74]

Risk assessment

Quantitative risk assessment is the heart of risk analysis. It has four components:

- Hazard identification: demonstration that the substance adversely affects health.
- Dose-response: how much of the substance is needed to pose a danger?
- Exposure assessment: the subject of this chapter, but particularly the nature of existing human exposure.
- Risk characterisation: Can the threat be measured in accurate terms: do we know how much risk is posed, and with what degree of certainty?

Hazard Identification is made formally by the International Agency for Research on Cancer (for example[89]) and by government advisory bodies such as the United States Environmental Protection Agency.[93] Dose-response correlations are assessed with animal and human high-level (usually occupational) exposure data, but as with any exercise of extrapolation large errors are possible. Conservative estimators are used to allow for this, but large overestimates of risk may result. A common convention is the use of some multiple of the upper bound of the 95% confidence interval on the extrapolated risk of the substance. When this exercise produces a human risk in excess of an arbitrary standard (such as one cancer death per 1 000 000 lifetime exposed), government regulations may demand protective action. Exposure assessment in the context of quantitative risk assessment is "the process of describing, measuring, or estimating the amount of a substance that a human comes in contact with, the duration of that exposure, and the size and nature of the population exposed." [94] Hazard identification, dose-response assessment and exposure assessment together constitute the elements necessary for a quantitative risk assessment through risk characterisation. [94] The latter consists of a mathematical model or models which describe the risk in terms of its magnitude and uncertainty, which will be magnified by any doubt concerning exposure assessment. Because risk assessment is by its nature conservative, such doubt may lead to unnecessary, unrealistic, or even harmful limits on exposure.

The ultimate goal of risk assessment should be a rational limitation of exposure, both of the general population and of workers subject to higher levels. Efforts to eradicate an exposure completely for which there is evidence for a threshold will lead to threshold limit values so low they cannot be achieved or to attempts to substitute materials with unknown effects for those with quantifiable and well-understood effects. Expensive, impractical, or dangerous raw materials and products may be introduced into the workplace as a result of faulty risk assessment.

The importance of occupational exposure assessment for risk analysis is exemplified by the extrapolation of the results of epidemiological studies of radon-exposed miners to the risk of lung cancer from low-level exposure to radon daughters in houses. [95 96] The risk estimates are important because 55% of radiation exposure in the United States population consists of natural radon exposure, as compared with 18% from man-made sources. [92] The result has been an estimate of about 15 000 lung cancer deaths/year in the United States alone attributable to radon exposure, most of it at relatively low levels. This makes radon the second leading cause of lung cancer, exceeded only by cigarette smoking and having about five times the total risk of second-hand tobacco smoke exposures.

In spite of this, there remains no good direct evidence of an environmental lung cancer risk from radon. Indeed, in ecologic comparisons in the United States there appears to be an inverse correlation between lung cancer risk and radon concentration, although this may be the result of confounding by altitude, by cigarette smoking, or both. Whatever the true magnitude of the risk, the risk assessment was based on the results of studies of four occupational cohorts, with some additional assumptions. [96] Error in the original assessment of radon exposure, which is described as ". . .the inevitable systematic differences in dosimetry" in these studies might reduce the apparent risk as indicated above. [96] Conversely, one study has suggested that exposure assessment errors may have led to underestimation of the risk in ecological studies. [87] Sampling error for radon concentrations, together with failure to account for possible negative correlations between smoking rates and radon concentration, would lead to errors in effect measurement and misstate the significance of both positive and negative results of ecological analyses.

Preparation for epidemiological study: an approach to exposure assessment

The investigator who is about to launch a study into the risk of disease in relation to a specific occupation or workplace needs to take some preliminary steps. The manufacturing or other process should be studied and the materials used and produced recorded. Particularly important is a walk through the workplace—not only geographically, but also in time. If the workplace still exists there is no substitute for an actual physical walk through, preferably in the company of one or more long time workers and, if there is one, a hygienist thoroughly familiar with existing and past conditions. Present work processes should be examined in detail and possible exposures recorded. Protective equipment and control barriers should be noted, along with the date of their first installation or use. Questions should be asked about what exposures were considered by the addition of such equipment, barriers, enclosures, and so on. Changes in work processes and in raw materials used over time, as well as overall observations such as dustiness, should be elicited by questioning workers or hygienists. Workplaces no longer in existence can nevertheless be walked through using historical documents and interviews with workers and other personnel. Shipping records may be an important source of information of the types of exposure prevalent in a workplace. Workplaces where the exposures are derived from natural sources, such as mines, can be assessed by scrutiny of geological texts and documents, as well as quality control and production records. Records may not be well kept on substances that are unwanted byproducts of manufacturing or contaminants for disposal in mining and similar enterprises.

Reference to the above recommendations indicates the multidisciplinary nature of exposure assessment. Most epidemiologists do not have the necessary expertise to underake a walk through with total confidence. Experts in hygiene, at a minimum, must be consulted. Input from other professionals such as geologists, chemical engineers, and experts in control measures such as equipment or process isolation may be needed. Consultation with toxicologists and biochemists may be helpful after the investigator is familiar with the materials present in the workplace, today or in the past. While it is neither necessary nor recommended that the epidemiologist be a renaissance man when it comes to exposure assessment he or she must have sufficient working knowledge of the other disciplines to know whom to approach and what questions to ask. Failure to identify materials that are present leads to failure to identify causes of disease correctly, and failure to eliminate them. The association of a hazard with a job title is not enough: the ultimate goal must be identification of hazardous exposures at the job site, which can be removed through material replacement or control measures, or at a minimum avoided by the use of personal protective devices.

1 Armstrong BK, White E, Saracci R. *Principles of exposure measurement in epidemiology*. Oxford: Oxford University Press, 1992.
2 Ryan PB. An overview of human exposure monitoring. *Journal of Experimental Analysis of Environmental Epidemiology* 1991; 1: 453–538.
3 Checkoway H, Pearce NE, Crawford-Brown DJ. *Research Methods in occupational epidemilogy. Monographs in Epidemiology & Biostatistics #13*. New York: Oxford University Press, 1989.
4 Hulka B and Wilcosky T. Biological markers of disease. *Arch Environ Health* 1988; 43: 83–9.
5 Hulka BS, Wilcosky TC, Griffith JD. *Biological markers in epidemiology*. New York: Oxford University Press, 1990.
6 National Research Council (USA). *Environmental epidemiology volume 1: public health and hazardous wastes*. Washington: National Academy Press, 1991.
7 Siemiatycki J. Epidemiologic approaches to discovering occupational carcinogens. In: Siemiatycki J. ed. *Risk factors for cancer in the workplace*. Boca Raton: CRC Press, 1991: 17–28.
8 Siemiatycki J, Nadon L, Lakhani R, Bégin D, Gérin, M. Exposure assessment. In: Siemiatycki J, ed. *Risk factors for cancer in the workplace*. Boca Raton: CRC Press, 1991: 45–114.
9 Levy BS and Wegman DH. *Occupational health: recognising and preventing work-related disease*. 2nd edn. Boston: Little, Brown, 1988.
10 Monson RR. *Occupational epidemiology*. 2nd edn. Boca Raton: CRC Press, 1990.
11 Schlesselman JJ. *Case-control studies: design, conduct, analysis*. New York: Oxford University Press, 1982.
12 Hunter, Donald. *The diseases of occupations*. 7th ed. London: Little, Brown, 1987.
13 McDonald JC, Liddell FDK, Gibbs GW, Eyssen G, McDonald AD. Dust exposure and mortality in chrysotile mining 1910–75. *Br J Indust Med* 1993; 37: 11–24.
14 McDonald JC, Liddell FDK, Dufresne A, McDonald AD. The 1891–1920 birth cohort of Quebec chrysotile miners and millers: mortality 1976–1988. *Br J Indust Med* 1993; 50: 1073–81.
15 McDonald JC. Laboratories in epidemiology. *Public Health* 1966; 80: 212–6.
16 Dement JM, Harris RL Jr, Symons MJ, Shy C. Estimates of dose response for respiratory cancer among chrysotile asbestos textile workers. *Ann Occup Hyg* 1982; 26: 869–88.
17 Dement J and Brown DP. Lung cancer mortality among asbestos textile workers: a review and update. *Ann Occup Hyg,* 1994; 38: 525–32.
18 Sébastien P, McDonald JC, McDonald AD, Case B, Harley R. Respiratory cancer in chrysotile textile and mining industries: exposure inferences from lung analysis. *Br J Ind Med* 1989; 46: 180–7.
19 McDonald AD and McDonald JC. Epidemiology of Malignant Mesothelioma. In: Aisner J, Antmann K, eds. *Asbestos-related malignancy*. Orlando: Grune & Stratton, 1987: 31–55.
20 Peto J, Seidman H, Selikoff IJ. Mesothelioma mortality in asbestos workers: implications for models of carcinogenesis and risk assessment. *Br J Cancer* 1982; 45: 124–35.
21 Parkes RW. *Occupational lung disorders*. 2nd ed. London: Butterworth, 1982.
22 Weill HW, Abraham J, Balmes J, Case BW, Churg AM, Hughes J, Schenker M, Sébastien P. Health effects of tremolite. *Am Rev Respir Dis* 1990; 142: 1453–8.
23 Case BW. Health effects of tremolite. Now and in the future. *An N Y Acad Sci* 1991; 643: 491–504.
24 Reger R and Morgan WKC. On talc, tremolite, and tergiversation. Editorial, *Br J Ind Med* 1990; 47: 505–7.
25 Case BW. On talc, tremolite, and tergiversation. Ter-gi-ver-sate: 2: to use subterfuges. *Br J Ind Med* 1991; 48: 357–9.
26 Esmen N, Corn M, Hammad Y, Whittier D, Kotsko N. Summary of measurements of

employee exposure to airborne dust and fibre in 16 facilities producing MMMF. *Am Ind Hyg Ass J* 1979; **40**: 108–15.

27 Dodgson J, Cherrie J, Groat S. Estimates of past exposure to respirable man-made mineral fibres in the European insulation wool industry. *Ann Occup Hyg* 1987; **31**: 567–82.

28 Cherrie J, Krantz S, Schneider T, Öhberg I, Kamstrup O, Linander W. An experimental simulation of an early rock wool/slag wool production process. *Ann Occup Hyg* 1987; **31**: 583–93.

29 Öhberg I. Technological development of the mineral wool industry in Europe. *Ann Occup Hyg* 1987; **31**: 529–45.

30 Simonato L, Fletcher AC, Cherrie JW, Andersen A, Bertazzi P, Charnay N. The International Agency for Research on Cancer historical cohort study of MMMF production workers in seven European countries: extension of the follow-up. *Ann Occup Hyg* 1987; **31**: 603–23.

31 Enterline PE, Marsh GM, Esmen NA. Respiratory disease among workers exposed to man-made mineral fibers. *Am Rev Respir Dis* 1983; **128**: 1–7.

32 Doll R, Symposium on MMMF, Copenhagen, October 1986; Overview and conclusions. *Ann Occup Hyg* 1987; **31**: 805–19.

33 Statistics Canada. *Standard Industrial Classification 1980*. Ottawa: Ministry of Supply and Services Canada, #12-501E; 1980.

34 National Library of Medicine. HSDB (Hazardous Substances Data Bank). An online factual data bank focusing on the toxicology of over 4200 chemicals; including toxicity, safety, and environmental effects. Complete references; peer reviewed. Washington: NLM and Agency for Toxic Substances and Disease Registry, access by local PBX or Internet.

35 National Cancer Institute (USA). CCRIS (Chemical Carcinogenesis Information System). An online service containing scientifically evaluated data concerning carcinogenicity, tumour promotion, tumour inhibition and mutagenicity studies on over 3000 chemical substances. File built and maintained by NCI and accessed through the National Library of Medicine, Washington; access by local PBX or Internet.

36 Employment and Immigration Canada. *Canadian classification and dictionary of occupations*. 4th ed. Ottawa: Ministry of Supply and Services Canada, K1A 0S9, #MP53-8/1982E; 1982.

37 Colome S, Daisey J, Dellarco M, Pellizzari E, Quackenboss J (editors). Total exposure and assessment methodology (TEAM): An international symposium. Part I: toxic substances and Chemicals. *Journal of Experimental Analysis of Environmental Epidemiology* 1991; **1**: 1–121.

38 Pellizzari ED, Perritt K, Hartwell TD, Michael LC, Whitmore R, Handy RW *et al. Total exposure assessment methodology (TEAM) study, volume II: Elizabeth-Bayonne, New Jersey; Devil's Lake, North Dakota; and Greensboro, North Carolina*. Washington: U.S. EPA, Report #EPA600/6-87/002b, NTIS PB 88-100078, 1988.

39 Pellizzari ED, Perritt K, Hartwell TD, Michael LC, Whitmore R, Handy RW. *et al. Total exposure assessment methodology (TEAM) study, volume III: selected communities in northern and southern California*. Washington: U.S. EPA, Report #EPA600/6-87/002c, NTIS PB 88-100086, 1988.

40 Thomas KW, Pellizzari ED, Perritt RL, Nelson WC. Effect of dry-cleaned clothes on tetrachloroethylene levels in indoor air, personal air and breath for residents of several New Jersey homes. *Journal of Experimental Analysis of Environmental Epidemiology* 1991; **1**: 475–90.

41 Lioy PJ. Exposure assessment: a graduate level course. *Journal of Experimental Analysis of Environmental Epidemiology* 1991; **1**: 271–82.

42 Brain JD and Valberg PA. Aerosol deposition in the respiratory tract. *Am Rev Respir Dis* 1979; **120**: 1325–73.

43 International Commission on Radiation Protection. Models of Lung Retention based on the report of the ICRP task group. *Arch Environ Health* 1974; **28**: 1–13.

44 Kumagi S and Matsunaga I. Concentrations of urinary metabolites in workers exposed to monochlorobenzene and variation in the concentration during a workshift. *Occup Environ Med* (formerly Br J Indust Med) 1994; **51**: 120–4.

45 Ewetz L. Absorption and metabolic fate of nitrogen oxides. *Scand J Work Environ Health* 1993; **19**; Supplement 2: 21–7.

46 Brody AR, Hill LH, Adkins B, O'Conner RW. Chrysotile asbestos inhalation in rats: Deposition pattern and reaction of alveolar epithelium and pulmonary macrophages. *Am Rev Respir Dis* 1981; **123**: 670–9.

47 Pinkerton KE, Pratt PC, Brody AR, Crapo JD. Fiber localization and its relationship to lung reaction in rats after chronic inhalation of chrysotile asbestos. *Am J Pathol* 1984; **117**: 484–98.

48 Falk H, Herbert J, Crowley S, Ishak KG, Thomas LB, Popper H et al. Epidemiology of hepatic angiosarcoma in the United States: 1964–1974. *Environ Health Perspect* 1981; **41**: 107–13.

49 Green T and Hathaway DE. The chemistry and biogenesis of S-containing metabolites of vinyl chloride interactions. *Chem Biol Interact* 1977; **17**: 137–50

50 Case BW, Ip MPC, Padilla M, Kleinerman J. Asbestos effects on superoxide production: An *in vitro* study of hamster alveolar macrophages. *Environ Res* 1986; **39**: 299–306.

51 Mossman B. Mechanisms of asbestos carcinogenesis and toxicity: the amphibole hypothesis revisited. (editorial) *Br J Indust Med* 1993; **50**: 673–6.

52 Thériault G, Goldberg M, Miller AB, Armstrong B, Guénel P, Deadman J et al. Cancer risks associated with occupational exposure to magnetic fields among electric utility workers in Ontario and Quebec, Canada, and France: 1970–1989. *Am J Epidemiol* 1994; **139**: 550–72.

53 Savitz DA, Pearce N, Poole C. Update on methodological issues in the epidemiology of electromagnetic fields and cancer. *Epidemiologic Reviews* 1993; **15**: 558–66.

54 Cherry NM, Labrèche FP, McDonald JC. Organic brain damage and occupational solvent exposure. *Br J Indust Med* 1992; **49**: 776–81.

55 Hoar SK, Morrison AS, Cole P, Silverman DT. An occupation and exposure linkage system for the study of occupational carcinogenesis. *J Occup Med* 1980; **22**: 722–6.

56 Siemiatycki J, Dewer R, Richardson L. Costs and statistical power associated with five methods of collecting occupation exposure information for population-based control studies. *Am J Epidemiol* 1989; **130**: 1236–46.

57 Pannett B, Coggon D, Acheson ED. A job-exposure matrix for use in population based studies in England and Wales. *Br J Indust Med* 1985; **42**: 777–83.

58 Case BW, McCaughey WTE, Harrigan M, Sébastien P. Exposure misclassification for mesothelioma in a chrysotile mining district. *Am Rev Respir Dis* 1990; **141**; A242 (abstract).

59 Case BW, Sébastien P. Environmental and occupational exposures to chrysotile asbestos: A comparative microanalytic study. *Arch Environ Health* 1987; **42**: 185–91.

60 American Conference of Governmental Industrial Hygienists. *1993–1994 threshold limit values for chemical substances and physical agents and biological exposure indices.* Cincinatti: A.C.G.I.H., 1993.

61 McDonald JC, Case BW, Enterline PE, Henderson V, McDonald AD, Plourde M, *et al.* Lung dust analysis in the assessment of past exposure of man-made mineral fibre workers. *Ann Occup Hyg* 1990; **34**: 427–41.

62 Baselt RC. *Biological monitoring methods for industrial chemicals.* 2nd ed. Littleton, Mass: PSG Publishing and Year Book Medical Publishers, 1988.

63 National Research Council (USA). *Biologic markers in pulmonary toxicology.* Washington: National Academy Press, 1989.

64 National Research Council (USA). *Biologic markers in reproductive toxicology.* Washington: National Academy Press, 1989.

65 McDonald JC, Armstrong B, Case B, Doell D, McCaughey WTE, McDonald AD, Sebastien P. Mesothelioma and asbestos fiber type. Evidence from lung tissue analyses. *Cancer* 1990; **63**: 1544–7.

66 Case BW, Rossiter C, Saux M et al. Biological indicators and their clinical significance in persons exposed to mineral fibres: report of a workshop held in Japan: Workshop 2. *Br J Indust Med* 1993; **50**: 414–7.

67 Case BW, Sébastien P. Fibre levels in lung and correlation with air samples. in: Bignon J, Peto J, Saracci R, eds. *Non-occupational exposure to mineral fibres.* Lyon, IARC Sci. Publ., 1989: 207–218.

68 Churg A. Analysis of lung asbestos content. (editorial) *Br J Indust Med* 1991; **48**: 649–52.

69 Churg A, Wright J, Vedal S. Fiber burden and patterns of asbestos-related disease in chrysotile miners and millers. *Am Rev Respir Dis* 1993; **148**: 25–31.

70 Sebastien P, Janson X, Gaudichet A, Hirsch A, Bignon J. Asbestos retention in human respiratory tissues: Comparative measures in lung parenchyma and in parietal pleura. In: Wagner JC, ed., *Biological effects of mineral fibres*, Lyons: IARC Scientific Publ; 1980: 237–46.

71 Baker D. Limitations in drawing etiologic inferences based on measurement of asbestos fibers from lung tissue. *Ann N Y Acad Sci* 1991; **643**: 61–70.

72 Türkel B, Egeli U. Analysis of chromosomal aberrations in shoe workers exposed long term to benzene. *Occup Environ Med* (formerly Br J Indust Med) 1994; **51**: 50–53.

73 Perera FP, Weinstein IB. Molecular epidemiology and carcinogen-DNA adduct detection: New approaches to studies of human cancer causation. *J Chron Dis* 1982; **35**: 581–600.

74 Gylseth B, Churg A, Davis JMG, Johnson N, Morgan A, Mowe G et al. Analysis of asbestos fibers and asbestos bodies in tissue samples from human lung: An international laboratory trial. *Scand. J Work Environ Health* 1986; **11**: 107–10.

75 National Research Council (USA); Committee on Biological markers; modified from the figure cited in (64), National Academy Press, 1987.

76 Case BW. Biological Indicators of Chrysotile Exposure. *Ann Occup Hyg*, 1994; **38**: 503–18.

77 National Research Council (USA). *Environmental tobacco smoke: measuring exposures and assessing health effects*. Washington: National Academy Press, 1986.

78 Wertheimer N, Leeper E. Electrical wiring configurations and childhood cancer. *Am J Epidemiol* 1979; **109**: 273–84.

79 London SJ, Thomas DC, Bowman JD et al. Exposure to residential electric and magnetic fields and risk of childhood leukemia. *Am J Epidemiol* 1991; **134**: 923–37.

80 Feychting M, Ahlbom A. Magnetic fields and cancer in children residing near Swedish high-voltage power lines. *Am J Epidemiol* 1993; **138**: 467–81.

81 Samet JM, ed. *Epidemiology of lung cancer*. New York: Marcel Dekker, 1994.

82 Breslow NE and Day NE. *Statistical methods in cancer research: volume I: the analysis of case-control studies*. Davis W. ed. Lyons: IARC Scientific Publications; 1980; 32.

83 Grufferman S and Delzell E. Epidemiology of Hodgkin's disease. *Epidemiol Rev* 1984; **6**: 76–106.

84 Werler MM, Shapiro S, Mitchell AA. Periconceptional folic acid exposure and risk of occurent neural tube defects. *JAMA* 1993; **269**; 1257–61.

85 Weiss NS. Should we consider a subject's knowledge of the etiologic hypothesis in the analysis of case-control studies? *Am J Epidemiol* 1994; **139**: 247–9.

86 Dosemici M, Wacholder S, Lubin JH. Does non-differential misclassification of exposure always bias a true effect toward the null value? *Am J Epidemiol* 1990; **132**; 746–8.

87 Stidley CA and Samet JM. Assessment of ecologic regression in the study of lung cancer and indoor radon. *Am J Epidemiol* 1994; **139**: 312–22.

88 McKeown-Eyssen GE and Tibshirani R. Implications of measurement error in exposure for the sample sizes of case-control studies. *Am J Epidemiol* 1994; **139**: 415–21.

89 International Agency for Research on Cancer Monographs on the Evaluation of Carcinogenic Risks to Humans: *Silica and some silicates*. Lyons: IARC 1987; #42.

90 McLaughlin JK, Chen JQ, Dosemici M, Chen RA, Rexing SH, Wu ZE et al. A nested case-control study of lung cancer among silica-exposed workers in China. *Br J Ind Med* 1992; **49**: 167–71.

91 Dosemeci M, McLaughlin JK, Chen J-Q, Hearl F, McCawley M, Wu Z et al. Indirect validation of a retrospective exposure assessment used in a nested case-control study of lung cancer and silica exposure. *Occ Environ Med* (formerly Br J Ind Med) 1994; **51**: 136–8.

92 Goldberg MS, Siematycki J, Gérin M. Inter-rater agreement in assessing occupational exposure in a case-control study. *Br J Ind Med* 1986; **43**: 667–76.

93 United States Environmental Protection Agency (U.S. EPA). *Guidelines for carcinogen risk assessment*. Federal Register (Washington) 1986; 51(185): 33992–34003.

94 Ris CH, Preuss PW. Risk assessment and risk managment: A process. In: Cothern CR, Mehlman MA, Marcus WL, eds. *Risk assessment and risk management of industrial and environmental chemicals*. Advances in Modern Environmental Toxicology Volume XV; Princeton: Princeton Scientific Publishing; 1988; 1–22.

95 National Research Council (USA). *Health effects of exposure to low levels of ionizing radiation: BEIR V*. Washington: National Academy Press, 1990.
96 National Research Council (USA). *Health risks of radon and other internally deposited alpha-emitters: BEIR IV*. Washington: National Academy Press, 1988.

16 Measurement of outcome

PETER WESTERHOLM

Introduction

Epidemiological research is about the occurrence of health events, states, or phenomena in defined populations. The key principle is the definition of these occurrences and what to observe and to measure; (see Miettinen[1]). It is a question of identifying or designating valid and practical units of observation, which can be used for construction of such basic epidemiological measures as prevalence or incidence of disease, and criteria for selection or classification of cases for admission into case-referent studies. Classification, as was emphasised by MacMahon and Pugh in 1970,[2] is both a means and a goal of epidemiology, principles which apply also to work-related diseases or disorders.

The essence of epidemiology is the application of standard indices and criteria both for outcome variables and for exposure to possible agents. This facilitates longitudinal studies and comparison between studies carried out by different researchers. Indices designed for specific purposes may offer practical advantages in being tailored to a particular subject, but they have the drawback of being less stable and less generally understood. In this chapter I will consider outcomes and information sources commonly used in epidemiological studies of work-related disease, together with aspects of validity and reliability. For illustration, some types of outcome commonly used are reviewed in more detail but it is beyond the scope of this chapter to give a full account of the subject matter in such examples.

In measuring outcomes or occurrences the elementary step is to have a clear idea of how they relate to the objective of the study. When, for instance, we attempt to measure health we need an idea of what is meant by the term. In the following section terminology and general principles relating to validity, reliability, and other aspects of outcome measurements will therefore be outlined. These issues arise equally whether discussing laboratory findings, physical examinations, questionnaires, or other indices intended to assess health aberrations.

Validity is the ability of a measurement to reflect the underlying reality. It denotes how well the variable and measurements represent the phenomenon studied. Clearly, these measurements are limited by measurement and sampling errors. Other important concepts are precision and accuracy, or absence of systematic error. A measurement is reliable when variation as a result of error is small or negligible; inter-rater reliability refers to the results obtained by different assessors and intra-rater reliability to results by a single observer in repeated observations.

The validity of clinical observtions or laboratory measurements can often be established by comparing the observations with some accepted standard or with the results obtained from use of a method that is already well known. For other clinical measurements, such as pain and quality of life, there are no universally accepted standard criteria. As they are increasingly regarded as relevant outcome variables in studies of work-related disease other procedures have to be used in assessing their validity. Distinction has then to be made between validity based on the full content of the characteristic that is being assessed and validity based on the extent to which the results meet some criterion or gold standard representing a component part of the characteristic. Some researchers include also a predictive aspect, the capacity of the test to predict the course of disease or future health events. The validity of diagnostic tests is often assessed in terms of sensitivity, a measure of how often the disease is detected when present, and specificity, the ability of the test to register a negative result when the disease is absent. Another important quality is the positive predictive value (PPV) of a measurement or test. This is the probability of finding disease in people in whom the test is positive. The higher the PPV the better is the test at identifying disease and, conversely, the higher the negative predictive value, or NPV, the better is the test at excluding disease when the test result is negative. Sensitivity and specificity describe characteristics and validity of a particular test; predictive values measure the usefulness of the test in practice. Predictive values are determined in part by sensitivity and specificity, and in part by prevalence of the disease or phenomenon observed. In tests for low-frequency phenomena the PPV is low even if the test has a reasonably high sensitivity and specificity.

Routine statistics on mortality, cancer incidence, and congenital malformations will be discussed as a source of background information. Such data are commonly used for epidemiological purposes even if this was not intended at the time when the registers and data collection practices were established. These information sources were set up for entirely different purposes, which has an important bearing on the quality of the data collected, classified, and recorded.

Mortality statistics

Basic information on number, age, and sex of deceased people has been collected in Europe for several hundred years. The common practice throughout the western world is to register deaths and causes of death according to the procedures and rules of the International Classification of Diseases (ICD) as described by the World Health Organisation (WHO).[3] National statistics are produced from material collected from death certificates. After processing the data, these statistics are usually published by public health authorities or other governmental agencies. The WHO receives annually statistics from member countries to maintain a mortality database, beginning in 1950.

The judgement of the cause of death is usually made by a physician who completes the death certificate. Based on this certificate a single underlying cause is coded, usually following the ICD revision currently in use. There are also WHO instructions to record on the certificate other morbid conditions that are present or have contributed to death. The main value of routine mortality statistics for epidemiological studies is that they are statutory, which makes for nationwide coverage. Other positive aspects are the standard procedures for classification and coding, and usually easy access for researchers. There are, however, some aspects which have a bearing on the quality and validity of information on mortality which should be kept in mind when using it for purposes other than those originally intended.

Diagnosis

Diagnostic accuracy is a fundamentally important consideration. This will depend on a number of factors related to the medical practitioner's knowledge and experience, type of specialisation, and professional setting. It also depends on access to information about the deceased before and after death. Necropsy rates are obviously important; competently performed post mortem examinations provide more precise information and widen the range of diagnostic possibilities as compared with clinical opinion formed without use of verifying diagnostic techniques. Deaths occurring in hospital differ in this respect, sometimes considerably, from deaths occurring outside. Heasman and Lipworth in their classic report from 1966, observed substantial differences in designating cause of death between teaching hospital clinicians and pathologists.[4]

There are, however, other questions beyond the issue of diagnostic accuracy, in particular the problem of singling out one cause of death among several possible. This is a general problem of explanation theory involving, beside the ultimate and immediate causes of death, a variety of background factors affecting health. This brings in the meaning of cause, which is shared by medicine and health disciplines, and many other fields such as social and legal sciences and history research. As regards cause of death this entails consideration of a whole series of health issues and background factors, some of which may have been operating from early in life. Moreover, the increasing average age at death has resulted in chronic conditions contributing more commonly to the risk of dying.

Nomenclature and terminology

In medical statistics of mortality, the standard ICD nomenclature is commonly used, although, as emphasised by WHO, this was never intended as a standard nomenclature. The diagnostic categories reported on the death certificates are determined in practice and in degree of detail by the ICD, in specifying and coding underlying and contributing causes of death. There may also be differences between certifiers and coding personnel in recording information on the certificate and in processing it. These differences vary within and between countries, sometimes considerably. There have been comparative studies of coding and certification practices in Europe which show 10–20% differences between countries; see Kelson and Fairbrother[5] and Mackenbach et al.[6]

Other relevant issues are cultural phenomena such as tendencies among the medical community to over- or underdiagnose chronic heart disease and chronic respiratory disease. For example, it has been said that British physicians have a tendency to overdiagnose chronic respiratory disease. A cultural factor of a different kind is found in the tendency of physicians to avoid diagnoses which can be expected to be socially stigmatising for patients or their relatives. Examples of this are suicide, AIDS, sexually transmitted disease, alcohol abuse, and many others.

Geographical and social factors

An issue raised occasionally in occupational studies is the need to have appropriate denominators for the calculation of risk for some particular cause of death in a working population. Should national or regional or even local reference rates be used? And why not rates calculated for different occupational groups or socioeconomic segments of the population? The answer obviously depends on the purpose of the study and how the reference rates are to be used. In practice, however, reference rates for such subsets of the population are seldom available.

Of course, an attractive idea would be to assemble data from a seemingly homogeneous population, with regard to ethnic, socioeconomic, and life-style factors, to provide reference rates for studies of mortality or cancer incidence. The drawback lies in the smaller numbers in both numerators and denominators, leading to statistical instability. Another cause of concern is migration into and out of a specific geographical area. The possibility that such migration is selective must always be considered. Healthy persons may leave the area for career reasons and sick or elderly people may enter it, after having lived elsewhere practically all of their lives, for instance to be near their children or to stay in caring institutions. This obviously affects the mortality for that particular area. National mortality statistics are much less affected by such movements and are based on larger numbers, offering a more robust quality in expected rates of deaths or disease. Social class correction is often discussed as a means of improving precision in calculating expected numbers from reference rates. The difficulties are the poor quality of information usually available and the widely differing meanings, content, and interpretation given to the concept of social class. There are also, as has been observed in the UK, wide variations in death rates within the same social class. Social class corrections should therefore be viewed and used with caution. For further discussions of these questions, see Fox et al.,[7] [8] Kinlen,[9] McDowall,[10] and Goldblatt.[11]

Reference rates

In 1986, Gardner discussed the selection of reference rates for appropriate comparison in occupational cohort studies, emphasising that greater effort should be made to justify the use of national, local, or other types of rates in any study addressing occupational risk factors.[12] The limitations of total population mortality experience in judging the outcome of occupational cohort studies should constantly be kept in mind. For example, the general population is as a rule far from unexposed and also subject to confounding influences—social or occupational—affecting the development of the disease being studied. Another problem is the non-availability of a proportion of the population for various reasons, some connected with ill health and even early death, leading to what is often termed the healthy worker effect. This type of effect is usually ascribed to selective processes that introduce bias when comparing mortality or morbidity of employed groups with the total population. Generally, the effect is conceived as selection into employment of the more healthy, and selection out of those with poor performance or health defects. In principle, each of these mechanisms makes the unemployed seem less healthy than employed people. Obviously these mechanisms will operate with wide variation in different occupations as described by Östlin and Thorslund and Östlin.[13–15] Because of misconceptions which have sometimes arisen about the concept of the healthy worker effect, Hernberg has suggested that the term be abandoned and referred to as comparison bias, a term offering a better description of the problem.[16]

When using mortality statistics it should be remembered that this type of information is cross-sectional. The source population used to generate deaths or incident cases of disease is the one resident in the area at the time of registration; it is not a population in which all members are identified individually and then followed over a specified period of time.

Cancer incidence

In many European countries cancer registers have been organised and this trend is increasing. Usually they are geographically based, collecting information on cancer incidence within a specified region or area, or they are institution based, recording cases diagnosed and treated at a particular hospital. In many countries, for instance in Scandinavia, the UK, New Zealand, and a few others, there are national cancer registers with data based on routine reporting. Physicians who diagnose a case of cancer notify this to the registrar on a standard form. In some countries, such as Sweden where such reporting is compulsory, the information is of good quality, and often contains details of histopathology. An international review of cancer registers was made by Muir, assessing the comparability and quality of the data recorded.[17] Cancer registration in many countries includes regular analyses and publication, sometimes in the form of atlases of cancer incidence, (see Jensen et al.[18]). A cancer register is obviously as good as the information it receives. If cultural or administrative practices provide disincentives there will be underreporting from the register's catchment area. The reporting rate in Nordic countries is usually at a high level for most types of cancer, 95 percent or even higher, reflecting the high standard of diagnostic and reporting discipline, as observed by Mattsson and Wallgren.[19] Unlike statistics on causes of death, cancer registers may also receive notification of cases not yet diagnosed with certainty and these may or may not be confirmed until some time later.

Population denominators

As with cause of death statistics, the source population generating incident cancer causes is seldom defined readily in terms of number, identity, and time. Migration movements, resulting from people receiving cancer treatment within the area but living outside it or vice versa, may affect rates and cause biases. In common with mortality statistics these problems become smaller in national than in regional registers.

Record linkage

A particular use of cancer registers has been the attempt in recent years to combine register information with recorded occupation retrieved from population censuses. At least in principle, this offers the potential for comparison of cancer incidence rates in various occupational groups. In Sweden, records from the 1960 national census were linked to information collected in the Swedish cancer register for the years 1961 to 1979. Some studies were published by Malker et al. in 1985 and 1987 from the analysis of these data, with discussion of their practicality and usefulness.[20][21] There are, however, several serious problems in this approach. For example, the observed population with occupational status is usually recorded at one point in time, namely when the census was carried out. The information is thus cross-sectional, without information on employment or exposure before or after the census date and lacking information on multiple exposures and confounding factors, potential or real. As the occupational groups generally include many non-exposed persons, misclassification of occupation may easily occur. These factors tend to dilute any differences in cancer incidence between occupational groups, even if real differences exist. There is also the possibility, indeed probability, of random occurrence of extreme rates of cancer incidence leading to the statistical problem of multiple comparisons, when a large number of cancer types and locations are related to an even larger number of occupations. This inevitably results in the association of a proportion of high cancer incidence rates with occupational groups by chance alone. In Norway, efforts have been made to offset the impact of such sources of error by using data from more than one census. For example, see Tynes et al. on exposure to electromagnetic fields and cancer incidence[22] and Andersen et al. on cancer incidence in waiters.[23]

Reproductive effects

Epidemiologists have in recent years been confronted increasingly with questions concerning reproductive risks and their attribution to occupational factors or exposures to environmental pollutants in or off the work place. Public concern has been augmented by environmental accidents and disasters such as highly toxic air pollution (Bhopal, India), radioactive contamination from nuclear industries (Sellafield, UK), accidental pollution from industry (Seveso, Italy), and the nuclear plant accident in Chernobyl (former USSR). Earlier, in the 1960s, the finding that the use by pregnant women of thalidomide, caused severe congenital anomalies focused public attention on birth defects and their relation to environmental factors. In many countries surveillance systems were set up with registers of congenital malformations based on reports from hospitals and primary care units.

In any study of environmental effects on reproductive outcome two causal mechanisms must be kept in mind. These are mutagenesis, resulting from pre-conceptual effects in either or both parents causing hereditable effects, and teratogenesis, implying direct damage to developing tissues or organs in the fetus, leading to non-heritable effects. The types of outcome include infertility, extra-uterine pregnancy, spontaneous abortion, preterm birth, perinatal or neonatal mortality, congenital malformations, intra-uterine growth retardation and, in the child, mental retardation, malignant tumours and other possible long-term damage.

The methodological problems of reproductive epidemiology which address exposures at work relate primarily to the selection of endpoints or outcomes for study. Only rarely is it possible to suggest a single or specific type of outcome. It is therefore reasonable to study all conceivable types, selecting from the listing above. At the same time it is important to keep in mind that as the number of phenomena studied increases, the likelihood of one or more of these outcomes showing an excess risk as a random event is also enhanced. Also, the choice of endpoints is restricted by the availability of sources of information of reasonable quality. Once the outcomes have been selected, the investigator must deal with two main problems, case ascertainment and accuracy of information. As the concept of reproductive outcome is broad it is important to work with defined entities and to pay close attention to ascertainment procedures, with the aim of reaching a correct understanding of prevalence and incidence of specified types of outcome. Possible sources of information are birth certificates, mortality records, neonatal and other hospital records, and registers of congenital malformations; see Dolk et al. [24][25] and Källén.[26] In practise, these sources vary in quality, usually because of local differences in diagnostic methods, interpretation of clinical findings, and use of nomenclature.

Malformations

Information on congenital defects in registers depends on the quality of the data reported. Usually in such registers there is incomplete ascertainment of cases rather than the reverse. This is particularly so for minor forms of congenital defect rather than for major malformations, of which reporting is usually more complete and accurate. Also, conditions that are diagnosed some time after birth, such as hearing and mental defects, tend to be underreported in routine registers. A further problem is that the cases that are ascertained constitute a survivor group, after elimination of an unknown number of incident cases through spontaneous abortion. The proportion of affected fetuses reaching a late stage of pregnancy or birth may be influenced by both environmental factors and demographic characteristics of the population under study; see Khoury et al.[27] Kline et al.[28] and Hook and Regal.[29]

Fetal death

The use of miscarriages or miscarriage rates as an outcome variable is fraught with difficulties. The rate is most meaningful if it reflects the number of fetal deaths and premature expulsions of an embryo as a proportion of conceptions. In practice, however, this denominator is never known and instead we are forced to accept only those pregnancies that are recognised by the mother or her physician. Early abortions, occurring before the woman knows that she is pregnant, remain unknown. Evidence suggests however that these early abortions are predominantly associated with chromosomal abnormality and less often with environmental factors. In principle, advanced hormonal analyses would allow a considerable increase in the population base of known pregnancies but for many reasons, practical, economic, and other, this is seldom a real possibility in field studies.

The weak point in assessing the frequency of outcome events thus lies in ascertainment. Källén[26] has illustrated the problem with estimated survival graphs for the conceptus in four groups of women shown in Figure 16.1.[26] If group A is taken as a normal group of women, at week 28 45% of all embryos are still living and the known miscarriage rate is estimated at 10%; however, only half of these were alive when the women realised they were pregnant. Line B depicts a group of women exposed to an agent that killed some fetuses, resulting in 40% being alive at week 28 and 47% at the time of pregnancy recognition—an apparent miscarriage rate of 15%. Line C shows a group exposed to a more harmful agent, which killed the same percentage but at a still earlier age. If 45% were alive at week 28, but only 48% when pregnancy was recognised, the calculated miscarriage rate would be only 6%. Line D demonstrates the impact of a combination of early and late effects of an environmental agent during pregnancy. This example shows how misleading rates of spontaneous abortion can be when used to reflect environmental hazards, especially risk factors operating during the first few weeks of pregnancy. Induced abortion is another important factor affecting rates. If in a population there is a high rate of induced abortion early in pregnancy, this will lead to an apparent reduction in the miscarriage rate. Pregnancies which would otherwise have aborted spontaneously are interrupted by the induced abortion.

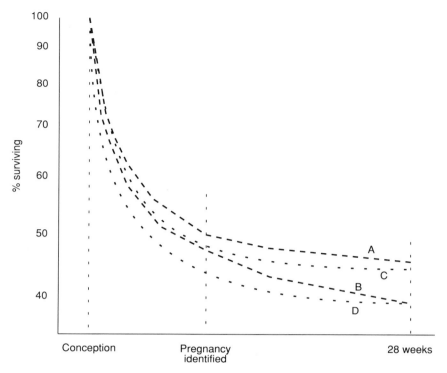

Figure 16.1 Conception survival under different assumptions (see text)

Birth weight and intrauterine growth retardation

It is common to use the birth weight of infants as an outcome variable in epidemiological studies of reproductive function. This is both under-standable and reasonable as birth weights are usually recorded with exactness and the records are well-kept and easily available. Birth weight is, however, dependent on two principal factors, growth rate of the fetus and gestational age (meaning length of pregnancy). Any factor that reduces gestational age will reduce the birth weight without implying that this necessarily reflects growth retardation. Of course, an external factor may affect both growth rate and gestational age. In principle, therefore, these two factors should be kept apart when seeking explanations in environmental factors for low mean birth weights. There are other factors also to be taken into account, such as sex, malformation, and multiple/singleton birth and, in the parents, age, height, obstetric history, smoking, alcohol and drug use, and socioeconomic background. In addition, individual factors such as maternal disease, placental dysfunc-tion, and uterine anomalies may affect growth rate and birth weight.

A recent example is an investigation by Armstrong *et al.* of preterm birth (less than 37 weeks of gestation) and low birth weight (less than 2500 g) based on a large study of work in pregnancy in Montreal.[30] Parallel analyses were carried out on birth weights with and without allowance for gestational age in a population of more than 22 000 women with singleton births. The results suggested that the association of low birth weight with specific occupations, long working hours, and fatigue was caused by a shortening of gestation. By contrast, the association with lifting heavy weights and shift work was probably caused both by fetal growth retardation and increased frequency of preterm birth.

Confounding

In this field of reproduction the problem of confounding deserves special comment. Occupation is part of the social characteristics of an individual, which include behavioural features such as smoking habits, alcohol consumption, use of drugs, and nutrition. These may or may not vary with occupation. Factors of this kind may thus confound the occupational distribution of reproductive outcomes. It is probably not possible to remove the effect of socioeconomic confounders completely, because they are largely unknown and unidentified. Still, their impact can be reduced by careful selection of groups for comparison in epidemiological studies. Equally important as potential confounders are such maternal characteristics as race, stature, and previous reproductive performance; see Källén.[26] An example of dealing with a large number of confounding variables is given by McDonald *et al.* in a study of work with visual display units (VDUs) in pregnancy.[31] In this calculation of probabilities of abortion, stillbirth, and low birth weight, the confounding variables of age, gravidity, previous miscarriage, ethnic group, educational level, smoking, and alcohol consumption were entered into a logistic regression analysis. The relative risks thus obtained did not deviate from unity, suggesting absence of an association between these outcome variables and VDU work.

A significant association between occupation and a reproductive effect may have two differing explanations—that occupation affects reproduction or that reproduction affects ability to work. If a previous pregnancy ended with the birth of a surviving child, the probability of the woman stopping work was in times past, and is still in many communities, rather high. Women who remain at work are, under such circumstances, likely to include subgroups with fertility difficulties and others who have miscarried. Both these increase the probability of reproductive wastage in a new pregnancy and lead to an increased rate of fetal death and possibly other adverse reproductive phenomena in any group of working women. This type of effect is likely to differ within and between occupations. For this reason meticulous care should be exercised in selecting groups for

397

epidemiological comparisons. Another aspect of the problem, pointed out by McDonald *et al.*, is that family size today tends to be deliberately chosen by the parents, meaning that women who have achieved the desired number of successful pregnancies do not seek a further pregnancy.[31] On the other hand, women who have had an abortion may well try to become pregnant again. This should be kept in mind when calculating observed to expected ratios for miscarriages which should therefore include information on previous pregnancies.

Musculoskeletal pain and disability

Ascertainment problems

Chronic pain and musculoskeletal disorders that affect bodily function and quality of life constitute a problem of considerable proportion throughout the western world. By and large these afflictions remain resistant to medical treatment and are difficult to measure. The pain itself is not directly observable: its measurement depends on the perception and description of the person experiencing it. It is a common ailment: between 50% and 80% of the population have had at least one episode of back pain during their lifetime (see Bergenudd *et al.*,[32] Biering-Sörensen F *et al.*,[33] Danchik *et al.*[34] and Holbrook *et al.*[35]). For extensive reviews of the scientific literature on back pain and disability the reader is referred to the recent Quebec Task Force Report[36] and to a paper by Allan and Waddell.[37] Depending on the questions asked differing information is obtained on the prevalence of back pain. For example, questions may focus on present and ongoing pain, or pain during the past or most recent few weeks, past six months or past five years. The results vary accordingly from roughly 20% to 30% in different age groups. The prevalence of neck and shoulder pain seems to be of the same or somewhat lower order of magnitude; see Takala[38] and Westerling and Johnson.[39]

McDowell and Newell published an extensive review of pain and disability in 1987 to which the reader is referred for a full discussion of concepts and techniques.[41] Pain, as many other subjective symptoms, has a time dimension. Recently experienced pain and pain in the past may, depending on the phrasing of questions, provide quite different pictures of a subject's pain experience. The concept of incidence, a basic epidemiological term for description of disease occurrence, may not easily be applied to pain symptoms, because of their episodic nature. Should a person experiencing a spell of back pain be designated as an incident case only if this is a first time event, or is it to be regarded as a recurrence of something similar, say two years ago? The validity of investigative methods for musculoskeletal pain and disability must be related to the purpose. For diagnosis and compensation, the usual objective is to distinguish between what is regarded as normal and what is abnormal, or indeed pathological. For follow-up examinations after treatment the method should discern relevant changes in disease status or time course of disease development. For descriptive epidemiological research, however, the aim is usually to detect differences in disease prevalence between defined populations. In this context, back pain of known origin, such as that caused by trauma, tumour, infection, and chronic rheumatic disease should clearly be kept apart.

A basic difficulty underlying considerations of validity in the assessment of back or shoulder pain and disability is our scant knowledge of the factors and combinations of factors that cause the pain and of the mechanisms through which these operate. In most cases of low back pain we do not even know where the pain originates or its immediate cause. Thus it is seldom possible to relate interview or examination findings to a pathological, anatomical or biochemical process. This is a substantial handicap, both in case management and aetiologic research. Another problem facing the epidemiologist is that the diagnostic entities in the WHO international classification of diseases, as applied to disorders of the musculoskeletal system, are affected by large variations in clinical and epidemiological practice. There are no generally accepted criteria for guidance and, inevitably, large variations in diagnostic competence occur.

The measurement problem

The investigator must first decide what aspects of pain are to be assessed, for example topography, severity, consequences, and timing. Pain severity can be described by the subject using a standard questionnaire or interview protocol; it can also be left to the subjects to choose their own words and terms. Pain severity is often described with its consequences or in terms of inability to carry out certain tasks. The time characteristics are obviously important, especially as to occurrence in the present or in the recent or distant past. The assessment of disability depends on what the subject can do or perform. Tests of function or capacity may include oxygen uptake or heart frequency on standard muscular work and measurements of muscular strength and endurance, joint mobility and flexibility. Such measurement techniques aim at obtaining results that are objective in the sense that the subject can influence them to a lesser extent. Nevertheless, the reliability of such methods is often highly dependent on the level of the subjects' cooperation.

Another type of measurement is based on observations of subject behaviour in standard situations or in real life. This approach can be structured as a procedure for questionnaire administration or interview. The assessment of activities of daily living (ADL) originally developed and referred to as Kant's index is one such example; see McDowell and Newell.[40] The main problem lies in the interpretation of the results, and the assessment of functional impairment. Whatever examination method is used it should be remembered that the examined subject is an active partner in the investigation. This means that the information obtained by questionnaire response or interview may be influenced by what the subject believes is possible and desirable. This category of information is thus determined by motivation, ambition, attitude, expectation, personality, culture, and other factors.

Clinical examination

In clinical practice information is usually obtained on pain location, intensity, duration and time connections, and their consequences. Such information may be recorded more or less systematically. Most often it reflects the subject's own account of the symptoms but occasionally more structured methods of assessment are applied. A pain drawing, made by the subject to locate symptoms on an anatomical diagram, as described by Randsford et al.,[41] is an example of a structured approach which has been shown by Margolis et al. to be reasonably reliable in test-retest situations.[42] The standardised Nordic set of questionnaires for analysis of musculoskeletal symptoms has become widely used; see Kuorinka et al.[43] Visual analogue scales for assessment of pain intensity and pain consequences have also been constructed and found by Million et al.[44] and McDowell and Newell[40] to have a fair degree of reliability. It is widely recognised today that chronic pain is a multidimensional phenomenon; pain intensity and persistence, pain-related disability and timing of symptoms may be important attributes of the condition. There is clear need for a global measure of pain severity for epidemiological field surveys, clinical trials, and clinical follow up. A structured approach and an instrument for such assessments has recently been put forward by Von Korff et al.[45] see also Deyo et al.[46] As to the validity of these methods, the difficulty lies in the lack of gold standard or, in simple terms, our ignorance of the truth. It is possible to compare the result of one examination technique with another and to look for correlations between them; this, however, is not validation in the proper sense; at best, it might be termed calibration.

In studies of disease and complaints deriving from musculoskeletal organs a comparison between prevalence of pain in various circumstances is usually virtually impossible to achieve, because of differences in diagnostic terminology, criteria, and methods of application. This was pointed out some years ago by Bielle et al.;[47 48] more recently, Hagberg and Wegman referred to a range of 1–100% in the prevalence of neck tension depending on study population and diagnostic criteria.[49]

Imaging techniques

Many studies have shown that changes in the lumbar spine detected in plain radiographs are associated with an increased probability of low back pain (Frymoyer et al.[50] and Biering-Sörensen et al.[51]). However, there are also studies, such as that of Witt et al., in which this an association has not been found.[52] Any comparison between them is difficult because the radiographic classification varies from one study to another.

In the cervical region both pain symptoms and degenerative radiological signs, especially the latter, increase quite steeply with age. In people over 60 years old the prevalence of radiological signs of degeneration was shown by Jung and Schumann to approach 90%.[53] The specificity of radiological signs in the older age groups was low in relation to pain symptoms and in subjects more than 60 years of age the specificity was only 9%. In younger people pain symptoms are often observed without radiological signs, implying that the sensitivity of the radiographic findings is low, although the specificity is higher. The explanation for this is partly the lower prevalence of both pain and radiographic changes in younger people and partly the relatively more common occurrence of radiographic signs of degeneration in the elderly.

Low back pain may be associated with sciatic pain, a common cause of which is a herniated lumbar intervertebral disc. With modern imaging techniques, including computed tomography and magnetic resonance imaging, the soft tissue of the spine can be better investigated. An increasing number of attempts have been made in recent years to validate these findings against nerve root and spinal cord legions found at operation. Evidence is accumulating from these studies that disc hernias and positive discography findings are common in the absence of back pain; see Bell et al.,[54] Boden et al.,[55] and Wiesel et al.[56] For a thorough review of the validity of clinical, radiological and epidemiological methods for the assessment of neck pain the reader is referred to Viikari-Juntura's doctoral dissertation[57] and surveys.[58-61] Overall, it is clear that many commonly used clinical tests for musculoskeletal disorders have unknown or doubtful reliability.

Respiratory disease

Bronchitis

From the early 1950s large differences in medical opinion on the frequency of chronic respiratory disease became widely apparent, as observed by Cochrane et al.[62] One consequence of this was an increased awareness of the need for standard methods and criteria for comparisons of prevalence and follow up studies. The British Medical Research Council took an early initiative resulting in definition of chronic bronchitis which was validated by Fletcher et al.[63] A questionnaire was developed for the standard description and classification of the disease which is still widely used, albeit in modified versions. Originally the questionnaire was intended for structured interviews; later it was developed for self-administration and found to give similar results, as described by Fairbairn et al.[64] and Samet.[65] The questionnaire and its modifications may be used to assess the prevalence of bronchitis in populations and also for case finding and screening of people with early symptoms. Its reliability in re-test trials varies from 20% to 100%, with much variation between questions. Assessments of validity by comparison of patients with bronchitic symptoms and symptom-free people usually show a sensitivity of 50–80% and a specificity of just under 80%; see Ohlson and Hogstedt.[66]

Asthma

As a separate entity this disease is attracting increasing attention with growing awareness of environmental causes and of the contribution of environmental factors to allergy and hypersensitivity. Asthma is said to be increasing both in prevalence and as a recorded cause of death although there are difficulties in defining the condition. Some 30 years ago a CIBA symposium arrived at a definition which many clinicians still regard as sound, namely "widespread narrowing of the bronchial airways which changes in severity over short periods of time either spontaneously or under treatment".[67] The comment often made, however, is that this a description and not a definition. The need for criteria which allow a person to be unequivocally classified as having or not having asthma thus remains. The episodic nature of the disorder adds to the difficulty.

These uncertainties are illustrated by results of a survey carried out by Burney et al. in the United Kingdom, which showed a high prevalence of asthma and asthma-like conditions although only 5% of people claimed to have had an attack of the disease.[67] On the other hand, a further 9% said that while working at night in the past 12 months they had experienced shortness of breath, 14% had wheeze with shortness of breath and 19% had woken in the morning with tightness in the chest. Almost any estimate of asthma prevalence is therefore possible, depending on the definition used and which of these symptoms are thought to satisfy it. If the limits are set wide, large sections of the population experience respiratory wheeze every now and then, and this results in the inclusion of mild forms of disease. If, at the other extreme, only cases undergoing treatment by asthma specialists are accepted, relatively few and more severe cases will be accepted.

The lack of an effective operational definition is a serious handicap in assessing prognosis, predictive power of examination results, and in testing for disease indicators. It is also a difficulty in assessing the validity, sensitivity, specificity, and predictive value of symptom questionnaires and interviews. To this should be added that, if earlier symptoms or disease experiences are sought retrospectively, recall bias may pose a further problem. In epidemiological studies of occupational factors this may operate as a confounder in that responses to questions on outcome may be affected by the subjects' experience of the exposure factors being studied. For additional references, see Samet,[68] Brooks,[69] Woolcock,[70] Dodge et al.,[71] and Burney and Chinn.[72]

Radiology

The sensitivity and specificity of radiological techniques for lung disease can be illustrated with the example of the correct detection of pleural plaques and other pleural changes, such as those associated with asbestos exposure. Pleural plaques are formed as circumscribed areas of connective tissue under the parietal pleura. These plaques may be situated on the chest wall, diaphragm or mediastinum and, when calcified, are easily seen on x ray films. Identification of plaques at necropsy has enabled diagnostic procedures to be validated. For example, Hillerdal and Lindgren observed plaques in 24 of 202 necropsies in people in whom plaques had previously been observed by radiography in three, a sensitivity of only 13% (3/24).[73] The corresponding specificity was 100%. With more flexible diagnostic criteria, 11 of the 24 cases were found on x ray films but the specificity decreased to 92%. Rubino and co-workers, who made a similar study, found a sensitivity of 88% for large plaques (over 100 cm^3) decreasing to 40% if all plaques were included.[74] Similarly, Hourihane et al. found a sensitivity of 14%[75] and Wain et al. of 28%.[78] In all these studies specificity approached 100%.

Pulmonary function

There are several tests of lung function that are used in epidemiological studies. The most common is spirometry, which includes measurement of vital capacity (VC), forced vital capacity (FVC), and forced expiratory volume in one second (FEV$_1$). Also, the ratio between these measures is often calculated with the FEV$_1$ expressed as a percentage of FVC. These measurements can be made with simple and reliable equipment, requiring only modest skills. However, they require cooperation from the subject and sufficient technical experience to ensure that they are made in a standard way. Several reference values have been published which take age, sex, and height into account, but with rather large differences between them. It is therefore recommended that in epidemiological studies examinations be carried out also on control groups, to avoid total dependence on standard reference values. Anyone concerned with the assessment of lung function and its association with smoking or other environmental factors is recommended to read the classic study in 1976 by Fletcher and associates of a large cohort of office employees in London, over an eight year period with repeated examinations.[77] By measuring FEV_1, these investigators were able to define the rate of decline in lung function over time and to assess the contribution of smoking habits.

Inhalation of dust containing asbestos fibres and other particles may lead to fibrotic changes in the lungs. It is therefore relevant to note three studies suggesting that such exposures may cause impaired respiratory function before any radiological changes in the lungs could be seen. Jodoin *et al.* observed a decrease in static compliance of the lungs and also a slightly lowered vital capacity and total lung capacity in workers highly exposed to asbestos whose chest radiographs were normal; the FEV_1 and diffusion capacity were not affected.[78] Weill *et al.* observed an exposure-response effect on respiratory function as assessed by measurements of vital capacity, total lung capacity, and forced expiratory volume (FEV_1) in asbestos cement industry workers.[79] Similar observations of effects on lung function in highly exposed workers in an asbestos cement industry plant were made by Ohlson *et al.*[80]

Although the reliability and validity of lung function tests are hard to assess without widely agreed reference standards, these studies illustrate that sometimes they may provide more sensitive information than radiological examinations. At least as important as this evidence of sensitivity, lung function tests have helped to establish exposure response correlations for a variety of dusts, including coal, silica, and asbestos. For references see standard texts such as that of Morgan and Seaton 1984.[81] In 1986 Järvholm *et al.* published a full review of the validity of radiological methods and lung function examinations in assessing the consequences of asbestos exposure.[82]

When considering the question of which lung function tests to choose for an epidemiological survey, the reader is referred to the recent paper by Hedenström and Malmberg.[83] In their study 32 different types of tests were made on groups of non-smokers, smokers, patients with pneumoconiosis, and others with asthma and assessments made of the different tests and combinations for their discriminatory capacity. By combining the results from different methods the discriminating capacity of the test battery was somewhat superior to the power of each test alone. Thus, the combination of transfer factor tests and dynamic spirometry increased the sensitivity from 18 to 22%, with 95% specificity, when comparing smokers with non-smokers. One should, however, beware of a simplistic view of lung function tests as it can hardly be expected that their discriminatory capacity will ever reach 100%. Lung function is a complex concept consisting of many components acting and interacting to produce what we conceive—perhaps loosely—as an overall quality. Some of these components can be observed and measured; others are still unknown to us. Thus both disease and environmental agents may affect this complex body function in many differing ways.

Neurotoxic outcomes

Neurotoxic and neurobehavioural effects of workplace exposures and their assessment have been, since historical times, one of the main challenges in occupational medicine. These effects and the agents responsible are usually grouped under three main headings: (1) organic solvents (a broad category containing roughly 20 different chemical groups), (2) metals (arsenic, lead, mercury, manganese), and (3) pesticides (organic chlorine phosphorous compounds plus a few miscellaneous chemicals). The effects of these agents are fully considered in chapter 8; here a brief overview is presented of measurement difficulties in assessing the outcome variables. Most studies have been cross-sectional or of case reports only, and few of longitudinal design. The results suggest that long term exposure to organic solvents may increase the risk of neurofunctional disorders and also possibly of chronic encephalopathy, implying organic brain damage. The symptoms described include weakening of memory, difficulties in concentration, aggressiveness, mood depression and other affective changes, together with fatigue, vertigo, decreased libido, sleeping disturbances, palpitations, and sweating. The diagnosis of neuropsychiatric dysfunction has rested mainly on the clinical evaluation of these symptoms and a history of solvent exposure.

Some of these symptoms, such as memory loss and concentration difficulties may be shown as impairment in appropriate neuropsychological tests. Such tests were developed originally to measure mild forms of brain damage and have been widely used in the diagnosis of early dementia. The neuropsychological test batteries in common use—the so-called non-hold tests—attempt to measure functions that are assumed to be sensitive to neurotoxic exposures, whereas other functions supposedly less sensitive to such exposures are thought to be identified by another group—the hold tests. The term "hold" denotes the measurement of conditions that remain relatively stable. Tests of this type are used to evaluate the pre-morbid neurobehavioural function. Their use is based on the assumption that pre-morbid level has remained unaffected. Tests currently used cover such aspects as verbal ability, cognitive non-verbal functions, psychomotor function, perceptual speed, short term memory, and simple reaction time. It is important that the results of such tests are interpreted by expert psychologists. In particular, the evaluation of the pre-morbid level in relation to the functions measured is a delicate task requiring skill and experience. In view of the numerous measurement instruments in present use the WHO has developed a test battery for the detection of group differences in working populations.[84]

The ability of neurophysiological methods to identify functional changes induced by solvent exposure has been tested in many studies. In general, the results have been discouraging. Although differences have been observed between exposed and non-exposed groups by electro-encephalography and CT scans (Örbäck et al.,[85] [86] and Mikkelsen et al.[87]), in spinal fluid proteins (Moen et al.[88]), regional cerebral blood flow (Hagstadius et al.[89]) and evoked electroencephalograph potentials (Seppäläinen et al.[90]), these are small and inter-individual variations quite large. These methods therefore have questionable validity in the assessment of individual patients or for monitoring exposed populations.

As the symptoms and disorders associated with exposure to neurotoxic agents do not easily lend themselves to operational definitions, a consensus is needed, at national or international level, on a limited number of clinical entities for use in surveys. These should be defined by normal neurological or psychiatric methods, providing standards for clinical assessment so far as possible. Appropriate guidelines were published by the American Psychiatric Association in 1987.[91] Early effects of neurotoxic agents can be studied only symptomatically as no objective correlates are likely to be found. It is important therefore to develop standard questionnaires for use in monitoring neurotoxic effects, as described by Hogstedt et al.[92] and Cherry et al.[93] A recent comprehensive review of measurements with regard to neurotoxic outcome was given by Lundberg et al.[94]

Measures of wellbeing

In recent years there has been an upsurge of interest in health assessments based on the WHO definition of health which includes physical, mental, and social aspects. As a result many instruments to measure these concepts and what is commonly known as quality of life have been constructed and put into use. Quality of life has many facets: the physical component includes daily activities, sexuality, mobility, and freedom from pain; social aspects include life with family and friends, work, and leisure time activities; the psychological functions cover cognitive and perceptual ability and capacity to cope with perceived problems. One of the first instruments of practical value was the scale of Karnowsky (1941) which emphasised physical functioning rather heavily but correlated well with indices of emotional well-being and social function. In 1963, Katz introduced a simple but robust questionnaire and accompanying scale on activities of daily living (ADL), which has proved acceptable to investigators in a wide range of disciplines. It puts emphasis on physical function in the context of daily life and, as part of an overall clinical evaluation, has come to be used extensively. For an excellent review of these and other methods and instruments in current use, see McDowell and Newell.[40] Some instruments, such as the sickness impact profile (SIP) of Gilson et al., have as points of departure a disease or therapeutic intervention.[95] Quality of life is assessed according to the SIP as a condition resulting in consequence of disease or treatment intervention. This approach has been found useful in subjects treated for various diseases such as lower back pain, cancer, hip replacement, and arthritis.

More recently, many investigators have produced their own instruments, mostly aimed at collecting data on physical and social functions, emotional or mental state, burden of symptoms, and sense of well-being. One such instrument, the quality of life index (QL) developed by Spitzer et al. in 1981,[96] comprises five equally weighted factors related to the patient's mood, perception of health, self care ability, work capability, and social interaction with family and friends. Later, Hörnquist suggested an instrument with qualitative and quantitative components within "life areas" which included biological, psychological, social, behavioural, material, and structural spheres of existence.[97] There are also others. For a more thorough review see McDowell and Newell[40] and a recent textbook on the measurement of function and well-being, edited by Stewart and Ware.[98] Spitzer has listed certain minimum criteria of validity for these instruments, which should be identified and published before their general use.[99] These include performance characteristics, panel assessments of content validity, reliability confirmed by experience and, where possible, evidence of criterion or at least construct validity.

Epilogue

In any discussion of outcome measurements in epidemiology, it is reasonable to reflect on parallel issues of diagnostic accuracy in contemporary clinical medicine. An obvious reason for this is that disease and functional impairment constitute the outcome in many studies. For the clinician, accuracy of diagnosis is essential for correct treatment. For the occupational epidemiologist a correct diagnosis offers the best prospect for an occupational hazard to be identified and its manifestations prevented. It is thus useful to remember that the training of physicians has traditionally been oriented towards pathology. The pathologist observes organs, tissues, and cells and classifies what he sees. As a rule, no causal inference is drawn from the diagnosis. Causal interpretations entail an inferential process of a type that is seldom initiated in clinical work, as was discussed by Feinstein in 1967.[100]

The clinician observes symptoms and signs and uses various additional diagnostic techniques to make inferences as to the structural or functional abnormality that can explain the observations. This implies that the appraisal of diagnostic evidence from whatever source is also an inferential process. In itself, this constitutes an important source of inter-observer variation. Depending on skills, experience, interests,

407

and proficiency, different inferences may be drawn from the same data even by competent and specialised experts. For reproducible use of diagnostic nomenclature, and of this inferential process, each disease entity must be defined using stable criteria that are understood and agreed by all concerned, a condition that seldom prevails. On the contrary, it is quite common in the health services for physicians to apply their own criteria for most clinical entities. In some fields of medicine, psychiatry for instance, the disease manifestations—outcomes for the epidemiologist—are almost wholly based on non-morphological considerations and interpretations.

Even if considerable efforts are devoted to the construction of standard nomenclature and diagnostic criteria there are hundreds of diseases, many of them quite common, for which no specific criteria exist. A group of patients designated as belonging to the same diagnostic category may therefore comprise subjects derived from many medical practitioners and may contain several sub-populations which differ significantly. To this may be added the effects of selection operating before the subject seeks medical advice and the diagnosis can be made.

It should also be kept in mind that our diagnostic skills are not infallible. Sometimes a disease or an illness cannot be identified even when the symptoms are severe, as for example with back pain. Often the underlying disease is simply not known. For the epidemiologist this means that many ailments, of widely different aetiology, can be lumped together under the simple rubric of back pain or some other name indicating how the main problem is perceived and described in easily understood terms. For some outcomes, such as sickness absence, studied epidemiologically, there is not even a common complaint, only a definable pattern of health behaviour.

The problems of setting standard criteria for complaints or health behaviour are difficult but not insurmountable. The ultimate aim of occupational epidemiology is to identify work induced disease or disturbances, thereby contributing to their prevention. Thus, in aetiological research, it is essential to identify the illness or functional disorder underlying the complaint or observed health aberration. The next problem is to find out why the observed phenomena have come about. This is aetiologically oriented thinking, in which context it is useful to consider the reflections of Miettinen and Caro on the challenges that face the epidemiologist when confronted with a complaint such as low back pain.[101] The first step in epidemiological analysis is problem description. In descriptive epidemiology it is reasonable to examine phenomena which, based on the present state of knowledge, appear related to a particular illness or disease. The challenge for the epidemiologist is then to make observations in a standard way and against explicit and distinctive criteria. Only by being rigorously faithful to this principle can the epidemiologist

contribute to aetiological research on work-related disturbances of health
and quality of life.

1 Miettinen O. *Theoretical epidemiology—principles of occurrence research in medicine.*
  Chichester: John Wiley, 1985.
2 MacMahon B, Pugh TF. *Epidemiology—principles and methods.* Boston: Little Brown,
  1970.
3 World Health Organisation. *International Classification of Diseases. Manual of the
  international statistical classification of diseases, injuries and causes of death.* Vol. 1 (9th
  revision). Geneva: WHO, 1977.
4 Heasman MA, Lipworth MB. *Accuracy of certification of cause of death. Studies on
  medical and population subjects.* No 20. London: General Registrar Office, 1966.
5 Kelson M, Fairbrother M. The effect of inaccuracies in health certification and coding
  practices in the European Economic Community (EEC) on international cancer
  mortality statistics. *Int J Epidemiol* 1987; **16**: 411–4.
6 Mackenbach JP, van Duyne WMJ, Kelson MC. Certification and coding of two
  underlying cause of death in The Netherlands and other countries of the European
  Community. *J. Epidemiol Community Health* 1987; **41**: 156–60.
7 Fox AJ, Jones DR, Goldblatt PO. Approaches to studying the effect of socioeconomic
  circumstances on geographic differences in mortality in England and Wales. *Br Med Bull*
  1984; **40**: 309–14.
8 Fox AJ, Goldblatt PO, Jones DR. Social class mortality differentials: artefact, selection
  or life circumstances. *J. Epidemiol Community Health* 1985; **39**: 1–8.
9 Kinlen L. Follow-up studies of professional and rural occupational groups. In Gardner
  MJ.: *Expected numbers in cohort studies.* Southampton: MRC Environmental
  Epidemiology Unit, 1984; Scientific report no 6: 14–20.
10 McDowall M. Reference rates from routine statistics. In Gardner MJ. *Expected numbers
  in cohort studies.* Southampton: Epidemiology Unit, MRC Environmental 1984;
  Scientific report no 6: 27–31.
11 Goldblatt P. Socioeconomic variations in mortality in England and Wales. *Finnish
  Journal of Social Medicine* 1990; **27**: 427–46.
12 Gardner MJ. Considerations in the choice of expected numbers for appropriate
  comparisons in occupational cohort studies. *Med Lav* 1986; **77**: 23–47.
13 Östlin P, Thorslund M. Problems with cross-sectional data in research on working
  environment and health. *Scand J Soc Med* 1988; **16**: 139–43.
14 Östlin P. Negative health selection into physically light occupations. *J. Epidemiol
  Community Health* 1988; **42**: 152–56.
15 Östlin P. The "health related selection effect" on occupational mortality rates. *Scand J
  Soc Med* 1989; **17**: 265–70.
16 Hernberg S. *Introduction to occupational epidemiology.* London: HK Lewis, 1992.
17 Muir C, Waterhouse. Comparability and quality of data; reliability of registration.
  Cancer incidence in five continents. Vol. 5, Muir C, Waterhouse J. eds. *Lyons, IARC
  Scientific Publication;* **88**: 45–169, 1987.
18 Jensen O, Carstensen B, Glattre E, Malker B, Pukkala E, Tulinius H. *Atlas of Cancer
  Incidence in the Nordic Countries.* Helsinki, Puna Musta, 1988.
19 Mattsson B, Wallgren A. Completeness of the Swedish cancer register. Non-notified
  cancer cases recorded on death certificates in 1978. *Acta Radiologica. Oncology* 1984; **23**:
  1–9.
20 Malker H, McLaughlin JK, Malker BK, Stone BJ, Weiner JA, Ericsson JLE, *et al.*
  Occupational risks for pleural mesothelioma in Sweden. *J Natl Cancer Inst* 1985; **74**:
  61–6.
21 Malker H, Gemne G. A register-epidemiology study on cancer among Swedish printing
  industry workers. *Arch Environ Health* 1987; **42**: 73–82.
22 Tynes T, Andersen A, Langmark F. Incidence of Cancer in Norwegian Workers
  Potentially Exposed to Electromagnetic Fields. *Am J Epidemiol* 1992; **136**: 81–8.
23 Andersen A, Bjelke E, Langmark F. Cancer in Waiters. *Br J Cancer* 1989; **60**: 112–5.

24 Dolk H, de Waals P. Congenital anomalies. In: Elliot P, Cuzick J, English D, Stern R, eds. *Geographical and environmental epidemiology: Methods for small area studies*. Oxford: World Health Organisation Regional Office for Europe, Oxford University Press, 1992.

25 Dolk H, Gojans S, Lechat MF. *EUROCAT registry description 1979–1990*, Luxembourg: Report EUR. 13615, 1991.

26 Källén B. *Epidemiology of human reproduction*. Boca Raton: CRC Press, 1988.

27 Khoury MJ, Flanders WD, James MM, Erikson JD. Human Teratogens, pre-natal mortality and selection bias. *Am J Epidemiology* 1989; **130**: 361–70.

28 Kline J, Stein Z, Susser M. From conception to birth. Oxford: Oxford University Press, 1990.

29 Hook E-B, Regal RR. Conceptus viability, malformation and suspect mutagens and teratogens in humans. *Teratology* 1991; **43**: 53–9.

30 Armstrong BG, Nolin AD, McDonald AD. Work in pregnancy and birth weight for gestational age. *Br J Ind Med* 1989; **46**: 196–9.

31 McDonald AD, McDonald JC, Armstrong B, Cherry N, Nolin AD, Robert D. Work with visual display units in pregnancy. *Br J Ind Med* 1988; **45**: 509–15.

32 Bergenudd H, Nilsson B. Back pain in middle age; Occupational workload and psychologic factors: An epidemiological survey. *Spine* 1988; **13**: 58–60.

33 Biering-Sörensen F, Hilden J. Reproductibility of the history of low back trouble. *Spine* 1984; **9**: 280–6.

34 Danchik K, Drury T. *Addressing the epidemiology of pain: pain data available from the National Center for Health Statistics*, Washington DC: NCHS, 1988.

35 Holbrook TL, Grazier K, Kelsey JL et al. *The frequency of occuurrence, impact and cost of selected musculoskeletal conditions in the United States*. Park Ridge: American Academy of Orthopaedic Surgeons, 1984: 154–156.

36 Nachemsson A, Spitzer WO et al. Scientific approach to the assessment and management of activity-related spinal disorders. A monograph for clinicians. Report of the Quebec Task Force on spinal disorders. *Spine* 1987; **12** (Supp): 1–59.

37 Allan DB, Waddell G. An historical perspective on low back pain and disability. *Acta Orthop Scand* 1989; **60**, 234 (Supp): 1–23.

38 Takala J, Sievers K, Klaukka T. Rheumatic symptoms in the middle aged population in South Western Finland. *Scand J Rheumatol* 1982; **47** (Supp): 15–29.

39 Westerling D, Johnsson BG. Pain from the neck-shoulder region and sick leave. *Scand J Soc Med* 1980; **8**: 131–6.

40 McDowell I, Newell C. *Measuring health—a guide to rating scales and questionnaires*. New York: Oxford University Press, 1987.

41 Ransford AO, Cairns D, Mooney V. The pain drawing as an aid to the psychologic evaluation of patients with low back pain. *Spine* 1976; **1**: 127–34.

42 Margolis RB, Chibnall JT, Tait RC. Test-retest reliability of the pain drawing instrument. *Pain* 1988; **33**: 49–51.

43 Kuorinka I, Jonsson B, Kilbom P, Vinterberg H, Biering, Srensen P et al. Standardised Nordic Questionnaires for the analyses of musculo-skeletal symptoms. *Applied Ergonomics* 1987; **18**: 233–7.

44 Million R, Hall W, Haavik Nilsen K, Baker RD, Jayson MIV. Assessment of the progress of the back pain patient. *Spine* 1982; **7**: 204–12.

45 Von Korff M, Ormel J, Keefe FJ, Dworkin SF. Grading the severity of chronic pain. *Pain* 1992; **50**: 133–49.

46 Deyo R, Reinvill J, Kent D. What can the history and physical exmination tell us about low back pain. *JAMA* 1992; **268**: 760–5.

47 Bielle A, Hagberg M, Mikaelsson G. Clinical and ergonomic factors in prolonged shoulder pain among industrial workers. *Scand J Work Environ Health* 1979; **5**: 205–12.

48 Bielle A, Hagberg M, Mikaelsson G. Occupational and individual factors in acute shoulder-neck disorders among industrial workers. *Br J Ind Med* 1981; **38**: 356–63.

49 Hagberg M, Wegman DH. Prevalence, rates and odds ratios of shoulder-neck diseases in different occupational groups. *Br J Ind Med* 1987; **44**: 602–10.

50 Frymoyer JW, Newberg A, Pope MH, Wilder DG, Clements J, McPherson B. Spine radiographs in patients with low back pain. *J. Bone Joint Surg* 1984; **66**: 1048–55.

51 Biering-Sörensen F, Rolsted Hansen F, Schroll M, Runeborg O. The relation of spinal

x-ray to low back pain and physical activity among 60 year old men and women. *Spine* 1985; **10**: 445–51.

52 Witt I, Westergaard A, Rosenklint A. A comparative analysis of x-ray findings of the lumbar spine in patients with and without lumbar pain. *Spine* 1984; **9**: 298–300.

53 Jung K, Schumann E. Korrelation zwischen Beschwerden im Sinne eines vertebragenen Syndroms und röntgendiagnostisch nachweisbaren Veränderungen der Halswirbelsäule. *Wien Med Wochenschr* 1975: 79–82.

54 Bell GR, Rothman RH, Booth RE. A study of computer assisted tomography: II. Comparison of metrizamide myelography and computed tomography in diagnosis of herniated lumbar disc and spinal stenosis. *Spine* 1984; **9**: 552–6.

55 Boden SD, Davis DO, Dina TS, Patronas NJ, Wiesel SW. Abnormal magnetic-resonance scans of the lumbar spine in asymptomatic subjects. A prospective investigation. *J Bone Joint Surg* 1990; **72**: 403–8.

56 Wiesel SW, Tsourmas N, Feffer HL. A study of computer assisted tomograhy: I. The incidence of positive CAT scans in an asymptomatic group of patients. *Spine* 1984; **9**: 549–51.

57 Viikari-Juntura E. *Examination of the neck—Validity of some clinical, radiological and epidemiologic methods*. Doctoral dissertation, University of Helsinki. Helsinki, 1988.

58 Viikari-Juntura E. Interexaminer reliability of observations in physical examinations of the neck. *Physical Therapy* 1987; **67**: 1526–32.

59 Viikari-Juntura E, Porras M, Laasonen EM. Validity of clinical tests in the diagnosis of root compression in cervical disc disease. *Spine* 1989; **14**: 253–57.

60 Viikari-Juntura E, Takala E-P, Alaranta H. Neck and shoulder pain and disability. Evaluation by repetitive gripping test. *Scand J Rehab Med* 1988; **20**: 167–73.

61 Viikari-Juntura E. Neck and Upper limb disorders among slaughter-house workers. An epidemiologic and clinical study. *Scand J Work Environ Health* 1983; **9**: 283–90.

62 Cochrane AL, Capman PJ, Oldham PC. Observer errors in taking medical histories. *Lancet* 1951; **2**: 1007–9.

63 Fletcher CM, Elmes PC, Fairbairn AS, Wood CH. The significance of respiratory symptoms and the diagnoses of chronic bronchitis in a working population. *BMJ* 1959; **29**: 257–66.

64 Fairbairn AS, Wood CH, Fletcher CM. Variability in answers to a questionnaire on respiratory symptoms. *British Journal of Preventive and Social Medicine* 1959; **13**: 175–93.

65 Samet JM. A historical and epidemiologic perspective on respiratory symptoms questionnaires. *Am J Epidemiol* 1978; **108**: 435–46.

66 Ohlson C-G, Hogstedt C. The MRC questionnaire on symptoms of bronchitis. A comparison with medical diagnoses and lung function. *Ann Occup Hyg* 1988; **32**: 539–43.

67 Burney PGJ. Asthma. In: Gill ERW, Trew C, eds. *Proceedings of the 7th International Congress of Life Insurance Medicine*. London: Royal Society of Medicine, 1993.

68 Samet JM. Epidemiologic approaches for the identification of asthma. *Chest* 1987; **91**: 74–8.

69 Brooks SM. The evaluation of occupational airways disease in the laboratory and workplace. *J Allerg Clin Immunol* 1982; **70**: 56–66.

70 Woolcock AJ. Epidemiological methods for measuring prevalence of asthma. *Chest* 1987; **91**: 89–92.

71 Dodge R, Clein MG, Burrows SB. Comparisons of asthma emphysema and chronic bronchitis in a general population sample. *Am Rev Resp Dis* 1986; **133**: 981–6.

72 Burney PGJ, Chinn S. Developing a new questionnaire for measuring the prevalence and distribution of asthma. *Chest* 1987; **91**: 79–83.

73 Hillerdal G, Lindgren A. Pleural plaques: correlatioon of occurrence of autopsy to radiographic findings and occupational history. *European Journal of Respiratory Diseases* 1980; **61**: 315–8.

74 Rubino GF et al. *Pleural plaques and lung asbestos bodies in the general population*. Lyons: IARC Publications, 1980; **30**: 545–51.

75 Hourihane DO'B, Lessof L, Richardson PC. Hyaline and calcified pleural plaques as an index of exposure to asbestos. A study of radiological and pathological features of 100 cases with a consideration of epidemiology. *BMJ* 1966; **1**: 1069–76.

411

76 Wain SL, Roggli VL, Foster WJ. Parietal pleural plaques, asbestos bodies and neoplacia. A clinical, pathologic and röntgenographic correlation of 25 consecutive cases. *Chest* 1984; **86**: 707–13.

77 Fletcher CM, Petro R, Tinker C, Speizer FE. *The natural history of chronic brochitis and emphysema*, Oxford: Oxford University Press, 1976.

78 Jodoin G, Gibbs GW, Machlem PT, McDonald JC, Becklake MR. Early effects of asbestos exposure on lung function. *Am Rev Respir Dis* 1971; **104**: 525–35.

79 Weill H, Ziskind M, Waggensback C, Rossiter CE. Lung function consequences of dust exposure in asbestos cement manufacturing plants. *Arch Environ Health* 1975; **30**: 88–97.

80 Ohlson CG, Bodin L, Rydman TT, Hogstedt C. Ventilatory decrements in former asbestos cement workers—a four year follow up. *Br J Ind Med* 1985; **42**; 612–6.

81 Morgan KC, Seaton A. *Occupational lung diseases*. Orlando: WB Saunders, 1984.

82 Järvholm B, Arvidsson H, Bake B, Hillerdal G, Westrin C-G. Pleural Plaques—asbestos—ill health. *European Journal of Respiratory Diseases* 1986; **68** (Supp 145): 1–59.

83 Hedenström H, Malmberg P. Optimal combinations of lung function tests in the detection of varius types of early lung disease. *European Journal of Respiratory Diseases* 1987; **71**: 273–85.

84 World Health Organisation, Office of Occupational Health. *Operational Guide for the WHO Neurobehavioural Core Test Battery*. Geneva: WHO 1986.

85 Örbäck P, Rosén I, Svensson K. Power spectrum analysis of EEG at diagnosis and follow up of patients with solvent induced chronic toxic encephalopathy. *Br J Ind Med* 1988; **45**: 409–14.

86 Örbäck P, Lindgren M, Olivecrona H, Hager-Aronsen B. Computed brain tomography and psychometric test performances in patients with solvent induced chronic toxic encephalopathy and healthy controls. *Br J Ind Med* 1987; **44**: 175–9.

87 Mikkelsen S, Jörgensen M, Braune E, Gyldensted C. Mixed solvent exposure and organic brain damage. *Acta Neurol Scand* 1988; **78** (Suppl 118): 1–143.

88 Moen B, Kyvik K, Engelsen B, Riise T. Cerebrospinal fluid proteins and free amino acids in patients with solvent induced chronic toxic encephalopathy and healthy controls. *Br J Ind Med* 1990; **47**: 277–80.

89 Hagstadius S, Örbäck P, Risberg J, Lindgren M. Regional cerebral blood flow in organic solvent induced chronic toxic encephalopathy at the time of diagnosis and following cessation of exposure. *Scand J Work Environ Health* 1989; **15**: 130–5.

90 Seppäläinen AM, Laine A, Salmi T, Riihimäki V, Verkkala E. Changes induced by short term xylene exposure in human evoked potentials. *Int Arch Occup Environ Health* 1989; **61**: 443–449.

91 American Psychiatric Association. *Diagnostic and statistical manual of mental disorders*. 3rd ed, revised (DSM-IIIR). Washington: American Psychiatric Association, 1987.

92 Hogstedt C, Andersson K, Hane M. A questionnaire approach to the monitoring of early disturbances in central nervous functions. In: Aitio A, Riihimäki V, Vainio H eds. *The Biological Monitoring of Exposure to Industrial Chemicals*. Washington: Hemisphere Publishing 1984: 275–287.

93 Cherry N, Hutchins H, Pace P, Waldron A. Neurobehavioural effects of repeated occupational exposure to toluene and paint solvents. *Br J Ind Med* 1985; **42**: 291–300.

94 Lundberg I, Hogstedt C, Lidén C, Nise G. Organic solvents. In: Rosenstock L, Cullen M eds. *Occupational Medicine*. Orlando: WB Saunders, 1994.

95 Gilson BS, Gilson JS, Bergner M *et al*. The sickness impact profile: Development of an outcome measure of health care. *Am J Public Health* 1975; **65**: 1304–10.

96 Spitzer WO, Dobson AJ, Hall J *et al*. Measuring the quality of life of cancer patients—a concise QL-index for use by physicians. *Journal of Chronic Diseases*, 1981; **34**: 585–97.

97 Hörnquist JO. Quality of life. Concept and assessment. *Scand J Soc Med* 1989; **18**: 69–79.

98 Measuring functioning and well-being—the medical outcomes study approach. Stewart AL, Ware JE, eds. London: Duke University Press, 1992.

99 Spitzer WO. State of science 1986: Quality of life and functional status as target variables for research. *Journal of Chronic Diseases* 1987; **40**: 465–71.

100 Feinstein AR. *Clinical judgement*. New York: Williams & Wilkins, 1967.

101 Miettinen O, Caro J. Medical research on a complaint: orientation and priorities. *Ann Med* 1989; **21**: 399–401.

17 Evaluation of preventive measures

NICOLA CHERRY

Introduction

Evaluation in occupational health practice, as in other fields of endeavour, necessitates making judgements. Is a policy, procedure, or intervention appropriate to the goals of the organisation? Does the procedure have the intended effect? Is this effect sufficient? Is it more effective than an alternative or cheaper strategy? Are there any adverse effects that were not intended? Answers to these questions require assessment of the nature and effect of the intervention and comparison with some alternative. In audit, the comparison is between what is done in practice and what informed opinion or consensus says should be done; it is descriptive rather than hypothesis testing. In evaluative research the questions are essentially of cause and effect; if this were done, what would be the result?

This chapter reviews the needs, methods, and practice of evaluative studies in occupational health and concludes with a brief mention of audit. It concentrates on quantitative studies of the outcome of prevention and does not consider the type of "formative" evaluation described by Menckel[1] and others in which the aim, close to that of audit, is to introduce beneficial change in occupational health services, evaluating the success by largely qualitative and subjective assessment.

The evaluative research to be discussed is either interventional or inferential. The first tests the effect of a deliberate intervention, the second generates data, often from retrospective enquiries, that permit inferences about the likely value of a future intervention. Although epidemiologists have tended to consider the two approaches separately, as evaluative and aetiological research, the issues of design and interpretation are not logically distinct and, in so far as they relate to evaluation, both are considered here.

This review concentrates on evaluative studies of the prevention of accidents and of disease which, together with promotion of well being, must be regarded as the two prime purposes of occupational health. Although control may often best be achieved by changes in the work environment by, for example, elimination of hazardous substances, enclosure of a process or improvement of ventilation, primary prevention also includes other approaches such as attempts to change attitudes and behaviour in the workforce and to reduce susceptibility by prophylaxis or selection. Measures for early detection of disease or disease markers, resulting in reduction of exposure to the hazard, are important aspects of secondary prevention at work, while attempts to reduce the consequences of disease (tertiary prevention) remain a significant part of the work of an occupational health department. Thus biological effect monitoring, treatment of accidental injuries, rehabilitation of workers, and steps to minimise emotional and practical difficulties of ill health retirement are all part of prevention.

Responsibility for these and other preventive measures lies not only with the employer and the worker, supported by occupational health services, but also with regulatory and enforcement bodies which lay down minimum standards of workplace safety, and with national and international bodies which assesses scientific evidence. Occupational health is based on scientific disciplines and it is incumbent on all who make recommendations about preventive measures, whether at an in-house safety meeting or at a prestigious international committee, to be explicit about the evidence they have used. If rational decisions are to be made about the likely outcome of a procedure or an intervention, information must be obtained from well conducted evaluative research.

Objectives

Identification of the objectives of a policy or practice may be the most difficult but critical part of the evaluation process. Any one organisation may have a huge range of objectives, both identified and implicit, for those who are involved in health and safety at work. Guidotti *et al.*, for example, list several hundred activities of an in-house occupational health service that are amenable to audit[2]; yet were an outside consultant requested to evaluate such a service he might have considerable difficulty in defining objectives in quantifiable terms. This stage of defining measurable outcomes is of the greatest importance. If over simplified, conclusions from the evaluation will not be accepted; if expressed in terms of the ultimate goal (for example, reduced mortality) the study may have neither the statistical power nor the time available to complete a useful evaluation.

Investigators have attempted to get around this in two ways, both of which have attractions as well as problems. One approach is to take the broadest possible range of objectives[3]; it is argued that any change to a system, may have effects in many directions (for example, reduced sickness absence, improved productivity, increased use of personal protection, disaffection among the control group) and use of a wide variety of outcome measures may ensure that no outcome, positive or negative, is overlooked. The difficulty here is that of multiple inference; as the number of outcomes investigated increases, so does the likelihood of some chance result. Alternatively outcomes can be arranged in a hierarchy in which, at least in theory, change at each level should be sufficient to ensure change in the next.[4] If it could be shown, for example, that increased knowledge about skin cancer leads to increased self-inspection and self-referral, resulting in early treatment and reduced mortality, it might be necessary only to show an increase in knowledge to evaluate the ultimate success of the programme in reducing mortality. Unfortunately, this would require a great leap of faith.

Such a hierarchy of objectives has a rather special role in occupational health, particularly in relation to chemical and physical hazards where exposure limits may be recommended or enforced. If an exposure level at which there is no adverse effect on health has been identified by a regulatory body, a proper objective for an industry is to maintain exposure below the level stipulated. Responsibility for establishing the link between such low exposure and reduced mortality has been taken elsewhere, informed by bodies such as the International Agency for Research on Cancer. Where no safe level can be discovered, or for new substances or new uses, health surveillance for unexpected symptoms or clusters of disease remains a prime objective of the occupational health department—as indeed it should even when a "no adverse effect level" has been established.

Evaluative research designs

Design issues in evaluative research are identical to those faced in studies of disease causation: the identification of the appropriate target population, the assessment of the exposure or intervention of interest, the definition of outcomes and methods of measuring them, and the selection of controls or an appropriate reference population. In fully controlled experimental studies problems of confounding associated with pre-existing differences between treated and comparison groups are minimised by random assignment of subjects to the arms of the experiment. In evaluative research the investigator will not be able to demand random assignment or to wait many years for the result of a prospective study. Inferences about causality are likely to be based either on observational studies of historical events (were those with lower exposure, for example, observed to have less disease?) or on short term intervention studies. In either case assumptions about the importance of pre-existing differences between groups can be examined by using one of a number of designs that have become known as quasi-experimental because treatment and comparison groups are not randomly assigned.

Bradford Hill's discussion of causality proceeds beyond the often quoted,[5] and sometimes disputed,[6] criteria of evidence to a discussion of the need to address and eliminate alternative explanations. Because science cannot prove a theory to be correct, it advances by disproving alternative hypotheses. Where practical and ethical constraints prohibit the use of strict experimental designs, the ingenuity of the investigator is of particular importance in adopting designs that, in testing and rejecting alternative hypotheses of bias and confounding, give strength to causal explanations.

The strengths and weaknesses of evaluative designs have been considered in detail by a number of authors.[4][7][8] Some of the more commonly used designs will be discussed below. It is worth noting that the cohort and case referent studies commonly used in general occupational epidemiology can be considered to be designs of the type which, in the evaluative context, are least conducive to causal inference.

Notation

Campbell introduced a system for describing designs which may be useful in attempting to understand the structure of any study, evaluative or aetiological.[9] Once the structure is clear, sources of confounding arising from the design can be systematically considered. In this system the notation X is used to designate an exposure, treatment or intervention and O a point at which observations are made. Thus if group A receives the exposure and group B does not, the design would be represented as

$$XO_A$$
$$O_B$$

The observation O, when written to the right of the X designating the intervention (or exposure), indicates that the measurement occurred after the intervention. Observations and interventions in different groups appear on different lines. In Cook and Campbell's terminology this design is a "post-test only design with non-equivalent groups."[7] The term "post-test" reflects the educational and social research settings in which this approach was first adopted, but in occupational health the O_A and O_B might be any measure of disease outcome, such as mortality from lung cancer where X represents exposure to silica in pottery workers and group B is the male population of the region where most potteries were situated.

An observation before the intervention (for example mortality before reduction of exposure) would be represented by an O to the left of the X and subscripts used to denote the number and sequence of observations. Thus a study of one group, with observations at two points before the intervention and three points after, would be represented as $O_1\ O_2\ X\ O_3\ O_4\ O_5$.

A brief review of some of the more important designs and their limitations is given below. It is based on the much more detailed discussion by Cook and Campbell, who grouped quasi-experimental designs into two classes, non-equivalent control group designs and interrupted time series designs.[7]

Non-equivalent control group designs

Cook and Campbell first described three designs which they considered do not normally permit strong tests of causal inference. These are the "one group post-test only" design (XO), "the post-test only with non-equivalent groups" (discussed above) and the "one group pretest—post-test design" (OXO). An earlier classification considered these to be pre-experimental designs, emphasising the lack of the essential feature of an experimental design, an adequate comparison group.[8]

The "one group post-test only" design provides no data against which observations in the exposed or treated group can be compared and it may be impossible to attribute the observation to the exposure or treatment. Nevertheless, knowledge about the likelihood of disease and the collection of information about the timing of the onset of symptoms may allow the generation of hypotheses about the likely cause of disease. Continued observation after removal of the suspect agent extends the design to one in which evaluation of the intervention supports, or refutes, the hypothesis.

The limitation of the second design is that it lacks information on the comparability of the two groups. The difference in post-test may result either from the intervention or from pre-existing differences between groups. The likelihood that the observation reflects group differences depends on the disease or outcome under consideration. If the exposed group develops angiosarcoma then prior group differences are unlikely to be an explanation. If, however, the exposed have a small increase in lung cancer or a small reduction in speed on cognitive tests or an increase in time-loss accidents, then pre-existing differences in smoking habit, intellectual capacity, or exposure to risk may be of considerable importance.

The third design (OXO) has limitations resulting both from the passage of time, which may bring secular changes or changes to the workforce, and, in some circumstances, from the effects of the initial observation. If the incidence of pulmonary tuberculosis decreases in the twenty years after dust controls are introduced, an observed reduction in the disease in silica workers may be the result of programmes of treatment and immunisation in the general population, rather than a result of the dust controls. The effect of a pretest also needs evaluation. If workers know that the use of protective hearing devices is being monitored before an intervention this may increase use of the device whether or not the intervening training programme, the X in the design, is effective.

Cook and Campbell list eight further non-equivalent control group designs, all of which they regard as normally interpretable. Of these the most important is the untreated control group design with pre-test and post-test—designated by

$$O_1 X \ O_2$$
$$O_1 \quad O_2$$

where measures are made of both groups before treatment and both groups after treatment. In this way, equivalence of groups before treatment, time trends, and the effects of the pre-tests can all be investigated.

An extension of this approach is the simple cross-over design in which two groups are observed in two separate time periods, one in which the intervention is given to group A, but not group B and the second with the intervention in B but not in A.

Interrupted time series

In these designs, repeated measurements are taken both before and after the intervention, either in a single group (the simple interrupted time series) designated

$$O_1 O_2 O_3 O_4 O_5 X \ O_6 O_7 O_8 O_9 O_{10}$$

or in both the treated and non-intervention group

$$O_1 O_2 O_3 O_4 O_5 X \ O_6 O_7 O_8 O_9 O_{10}$$
$$O_1 O_2 O_3 O_4 O_5 \quad O_6 O_7 O_8 O_9 O_{10}$$

Such designs are extensions of the one group pre-test and post-test design

418

(OXO) and the non-equivalent control group with pre-test and post-test

$$O_1 X \ O_2$$
$$O_1 \quad O_2$$

The advantage of the simple time series over the OXO design is that trends in the observations before the intervention can be established. If the incidence of silicosis is steadily decreasing before the introduction of dust controls the outcome of interest is a change in the slope, a faster decline, rather than simply the observation of a difference between points either side of the intervention. In a multiple time series, where the intervention occurs in one group but not the other, the possibility that the change in slope after intervention is due to extraneous causes can also be examined.

When introduction of the intervention occurs in both groups at different times (for example, the introduction of a safety awareness programme at different times at different factories) the design is known as an interrupted time series with switching replications and is designated:

$$O_1 O_2 O_3 \quad O_4 O_5 O_6 O_7 O_8 X \ O_9 O_{10} O_{11}$$
$$O_1 O_2 O_3 X \ O_4 O_5 O_6 O_7 O_8 \quad O_9 O_{10} O_{11}$$

Here each series acts as a comparison group for the other and the demonstration of effect in both groups at different times strengthens the causal inference (by replication) and gives confidence that the programme, having worked in two groups, is likely to work when used elsewhere. Increasing the number of groups, with intervention at different points in each, strengthens the design still further.

Experimental designs (with random assignment)

Finally, Cook and Campbell turned to experimental designs that might be usable in a field setting. They considered (amongst others) randomisation of individual subjects to treatment, groups to treatment and, within the same group, the random assignment of treatment to different time blocks (for example on some working days but not on others), the "equivalent time series" design. Examples of each of these can be found in evaluative studies in occupational health.

Examples of evaluative research

In the section that follows some 20 examples of evaluative studies are discussed, drawn from areas of occupational health practice. The examples are classified by type of study design rather than the nature of the outcome or intervention and are used to show the strengths and weaknesses of the formal designs as well as difficulties that may occur in interpretation. The section is not intended as a comprehensive review of all recent or influential evaluative studies but rather a demonstration of designs in practice, drawing attention to features that may be of particular importance in an occupational setting.

One group post-test only designs

X O

Such studies, in which the group is observed on one occasion only, are of "almost no scientific value" for evaluation.[8] They are, however, as has already been discussed in Chapter 14, perhaps the most productive in identifying unexpected risks in the work environment, particularly when the response is severe and of rapid onset. A group of workers with unusual signs of disease is identified, and work exposures examined to generate a hypothesis about the cause. To the extent that implicit comparisons can be made about the likely occurrence of unusual disease in the general population, an interpretation may be justified. If further information can be collected about the date of onset of symptoms it may come to resemble a comparison (OXO) of incidence before and after exposure. If incidence rates can be compared among those with and without exposure, further causal analysis becomes possible. If there are no further new cases after the removal of the suspect agent (as, for example, methyl butyl ketone[10] or dimethylaminopropionitrile[11]) the logic becomes that of an evaluative study. However, the initial design is essentially that of the observation of one group after the exposure.

Post-test only with non-equivalent groups

X O

O

The main difficulty in interpreting studies with this design is that the two groups are assumed to be similar before the intervention. Information on confounders collected after the event may be biased by either the intervention or the outcome, and may simply not be available in studies based only on records. Three evaluative studies have been chosen to illustrate different aspects of this design.

Welsh et al., investigated 1800 men from a cohort of 8047 workers employed in the Anaconda copper smelter in Montana[12] (see also chapter 2). The aim was to establish quantitative measurements of exposure to arsenic so that levels associated with excess risk of lung cancer might be identified. All highly exposed men in the original cohort (277) were taken, together with 20% of those known to have been exposed at lower levels. All men had worked for at least 12 months before 1957 and follow up was from January 1938 to December 1978. This was complete for 91% of the sample. Information on smoking habit was obtained for 82%, either from the worker or, if deceased, from a proxy.

The authors interpreted their findings as suggesting that "had men worked only in departments with low or medium arsenic exposures (for example, less than 500 $\mu g/m^3$) there would have been little excess respiratory cancer." The assumption that the incidence observed in the lower exposure groups would be found in all employees if exposure were reduced to this level depends on whether or not groups at different exposure were equivalent in terms of other risk factors. In Welsh's study cigarette smoking, the main confounder for lung cancer, was indeed shown to be similar in all exposure groups.

McDonald used information from a comprehensive survey of work and pregnancy in Montreal to evaluate benefit, in terms of fetal damage potentially prevented, of a Health and Safety Act in Quebec which permitted the reassignment or withdrawal from work of a pregnant women whose doctor certified that her work was physically dangerous for herself or the child (see Chapter 12).[13] The initial epidemiological study, of 56 000 women immediately after a live birth, still birth or spontaneous abortion, was carried out in 1982–84 and the design was essentially a cross-sectional survey with case-referent analysis. In the notation of Cook and Campbell it could be described as post-test only with nonequivalent groups. The outcomes of concern were fetal deaths, prematurity and congenital defects, and the exposures a wide range of work requirements or hazards, information on which was elicited from the women by interview.

For the evaluation of fetal damage potentially preventable by the policy of withdrawal from work, risks associated with each of 60 occupational groups were calculated from the outcome of pregnancies in the 56 000 women and these risks applied to the numbers of working women, with a child aged less than one year, in each of the 60 occupations in Quebec, as revealed by the 1986 Canadian census. In this way the number of excess deaths and preterm births potentially avoidable by removing pregnant women from high risk occupations could be estimated. It was calculated that removal of women from high risk jobs by about the tenth week of pregnancy could conceivably prevent about 6% of fetal deaths and that about 3% of preterm births might also be preventable by this intervention. The assumption underlying the conclusion was again that women in jobs with high (mainly ergonomic) work demands were similar to those in less demanding jobs for all other risk factors. The initial study, from which risks of fetal damage were estimated, permitted adjustment for a wide range of potential confounders; this is not usually the case.

The third example of this design also came from Quebec and attempted to assess the impact of legislation.[14] Eighty companies (some 70% of those eligible) agreed to take part in the study, which aimed to evaluate knowledge of the Canadian workplace hazardous materials information system

(WHMIS) following different types of (required) training of workers. All but 14 of the companies had used the services of a manufacturing sector organisation, which offered training as required under the WHMIS legislation. However, companies differed in their approach, from using the consultants to train all employees, to training selected workers who would in turn act as in-house trainers, or to adopt a less systematic approach, which meant that only a proportion of workers received any training at all. Knowledge of WHMIS was assessed by 13 multiple choice questions completed about 12 months after the training, by an average of 11 employees drawn from specified occupations within each company. The authors observed that scores on the multiple choice questions were highest when all employees had been trained by the consultants and lowest when only some of the employees had been trained by the specialists or that the training requirement had been carried out in some other way.

The requirement for training was specific to the Canadian legislation, and the availability of the specialist trade association was specific to Quebec. It is not clear how far conclusions from this study can be generalised. Equally, it is unlikely that companies choosing different training methods were equivalent in relation to risk factors for learning. In this study the 80 companies chose, from five options, the training methods perceived to be most appropriate to their needs and resources. The authors argued that in practice firms are unlikely to choose the type of inappropriate scheme that might occur with random allocation and although such an experimental approach might increase the generalisability of the results, it would be less likely to be relevant in practice. In this way, the authors attempted to make a virtue of the non-comparability of firms receiving different types of treatment; they did not, however, go beyond this to identify features of the companies that were associated with success or failure of each approach.

The one group pre-test/post-test design

OXO

In this design baseline measures are taken, the intervention put in place, and measures repeated to see if any change has occurred. The difficulty with the design is that the presence (or absence) of change may result from time related or other factors rather than the intervention. Sometimes the relation between the intervention and outcome may be so close and so specific (for example, the introduction of noise reduction measures and the reduction in noise levels[15]) that causality is a reasonable, if not always justified, presumption. In other circumstances the possibilities of bias or confounding are so great as to put in doubt any assumption of causality. The first study reviewed below is subject to some of these difficulties.

Orgel *et al.* carried out an intervention study of cashiers in a grocery store.[16] Of 34 eligible subjects, 23 agreed to take part in the initial survey of musculoskeletal symptoms and 19 completed a follow-up four months after ergnomic interventions were completed; the time taken for the implementation of the ergonomic changes (reduced reaching requirements, reduced shoulder abduction and flexion, and use of a training video) was unclear. The authors reported a significant reduction in the number of employees taking drugs for pain, 78% (18/23) at baseline but only 26% (5/19) at follow-up, and increased speed of recovery from the discomfort of working on the express checkout after it had been modified. Symptoms located in the neck, upper back or shoulders, and lower back, buttocks, or legs were reduced significantly but no change was found in the relatively low number of symptoms in the arms, forearms or wrists.

The lack of a control group in this study is a serious limitation. The interventions were designed with active participation from employees and made after a consensus conference. While this may have increased the acceptability of the changes, it also substantially increased the likelihood of bias because of knowledge of the purpose of the study. Simply being an active member of a study may improve the outcome (a phenomenon known as a Hawthorne effect[17]) and effects on motivation may be reflected in, for example, the reduced use of drugs. Other potential sources of bias or confounding include changes in the perception of workers brought about by use of a pre-test, ageing of the workforce, or increased job experience, changes in economic conditions or time of year, and regression to the mean, which would occur if those with the largest number of symptoms selected themselves for a study. While a useful example of an ergonomic intervention, the conclusions were less certain.

The investigation reported by Imbus and Suh is of the same formal design (pre-test, intervention, post-test) but support for a causal effect was much stronger.[18] In this study pulmonary function (FEV_1) was measured morning and evening for the three weeks immediately before the intervention and for three weeks immediately after; in essence a simple time series design. Subjects were workers in a cotton spinning plant where 167 (95%) of employees volunteered. Of these, 34 were eliminated from the study because of work schedule, absence or poor quality of recording of the pulmonary function tests. The intervention was unusual in that it was the effect of the removal of a protective measure—the steaming of cotton—that was to be evaluated. An FEV_1 change score was calculated for mean morning FEV_1 during steaming and mean morning FEV_1 without steaming and also for evenings before and after the intervention. Mean FEV_1 was 86 ml greater before work and 133 ml greater after work during steaming. More detailed analysis was carried out by sex and byssinosis score.

The results of this study were convincing for a number of reasons. First, the pulmonary function test results were outside the control of the subjects

423

and knowledge of the purpose of the tests and the nature of the intervention were unlikely to have affected the result. Secondly, the study took place over a matter of weeks and ageing of the population, time of year, or changes in smoking habits, for example, were unlikely to have been of great importance. The effect of practice on the pulmonary function tests could have been an issue, but would have been associated with improvement. Calibration or instrument errors remain a possibility as does the intervention of some other factor (for example, an epidemic of respiratory disease). Even in this study, the inclusion of a comparison group would have been desirable.

A third example is that of pneumoconiosis in workers exposed to crystalline silica, including a high proportion of cristobalite, in the diatomite industry.[19] A study was carried out in 1953–54 of workers in five plants in California. Among those with five years or more of exposure, 25% were found to have chest radiographs consistent with pneumoconiosis and this proportion rose to 48% in employees who had worked exclusively in processing mills. As a result of this study, greatly improved dust control measures were introduced and the evaluation study was set up to assess whether the resulting changes had been accompanied by a reduction in the prevalence of pneumoconiosis. The aim was to compare prevalence of pneumoconiosis in the 1953 study with that among workers in 1974. Radiographic classifications were made for 428 workers who had five years or more of service.

Comparison of prevalence in current workers had a number of problems, not least the possibility that those with identified changes in periodic chest radiographs, instituted since 1953, would have left the industry. Those with more than 21 years employment in 1974 had been working in part under the conditions of poor dust control and were not appropriately included in the follow up study. However recalculation of published data suggests that in the 1953 survey 142 workers had been employed for 5–10 years and of these 19 (13%) had small parenchymal opacities ($\geqslant 1/1$) or large opacities. Of the 21 employed for 10–15 years, 16 (76%) had radiographs consistent with pneumoconiosis. Amongst the 116 employees in 1974 who had been working for 10–15 years only 1 (1%) had a positive (1/1) radiograph and none of the 105 employers with exposure from 5–10 years had film classifications at this level.

This study appears to show a substantial reduction in risk following the introduction of dust controls, although the lack of information on ex-workers is a serious problem. Potential confounders that were not excluded, in the absence of a comparison group, include differences in age, race, previous occupational history of workers, changes in the use of other fibrogenic substances (for example asbestos), and differences in film quality or in readers. Earlier radiographs were not re-read and differing preconceptions about the level of pneumoconiosis were likely. Although the result of the study is consistent with expectations, the study design was not sufficiently robust to support the conclusion fully.

Other before/after cohort studies, using external standardisation, may be considered a special example of studies with referent groups and are included in the next section.

In the studies so far considered baseline and follow-up observations were of essentially the same type—repeated measurement of symptoms, of FEV_1 or of chest radiographs. This need not be the case, however. The baseline measurement may be of an underlying characteristic, genetically or environmentally determined, which may moderate the effect of the intervention. In the presence of the moderating variable the effect of exposure might be of concern, but in its absence unmeasurable. An example is of atopy and allergic response to work exposures, where the use of markers of atopy in selection has been considered as a possible preventive measure, particularly in relation to laboratory animal allergy and platinum salts.

Slovak and Hill attempted to assess the usefulness of atopy defined by family history, personal history and skin prick tests in predicting laboratory animal allergy.[20] The study is limited in that it was restricted to current employees, all 146 workers exposed to animals at two sites of a pharmaceutical company volunteering for the study; one (with occupational asthma) refused the skin prick tests. The presence of laboratory animal allergy was established by questionnaire, workers being allocated to one of three categories; asthma with rhinitis (16 workers), rhinitis but no asthma (33 workers) and no symptoms consistent with laboratory animal allergy (97 workers). When atopy was defined by skin prick tests to common allergens (a 3 mm weal in any of three tests) it was found that 80% (12/15) of asthmatics were atopic, as were 24% (8/33) of those with rhinitis without asthma, and 15% (15/97) with no symptoms. The relation between skin prick test atopy and asthma was greater than would be expected by chance and both sensitivity (80%) and specificity (82%) higher than for questionnaire based definitions of atopy, but the positive predictive value was low (34%). Slovak and Hill concluded that sensitivity and specificity of about 95% would be needed if half the cases of asthma were to be avoided by rejecting from employment those with positive skin tests to common allergens. Newill et al. discussed in more detail the implications for selection of the low predictive value of atopy in laboratory animal allergy.[21]

Untreated control group design with pre-test and post-test

$$O_1 X O_2$$
$$O_1 \quad O_2$$

In this design observations are taken at two points, in two (or more) groups and changes in the group(s) with intervention compared with those without. Studies using standardised mortality ratios in which cause specific deaths in the exposed population are compared with those expected in the general population are considered a special sub-category; use of expected figures based on era of birth and date of death take into account secular changes in cause of death (for example, decreasing mortality from stomach cancer or stroke).

An example of this approach was that of Doll *et al.* who in 1977 identified 967 men who had been employed at a nickel refinery in South Wales from the early 1900s to 1944.[22] Follow up was from 1934 to the end of 1971. Tracing was successful for 96%, of whom 689 died before 1st January 1972. The shortest period of follow up was thus 28 years. It was unclear which part of the process was hazardous, but the risk appeared greatest in the preliminary processes where major changes occurred in 1933 (see also Chapter 2).

Evaluation of the period of risk was carried out by comparing observed and expected deaths from nasal sinus or lung cancer in the cohorts starting work at 5 year intervals before 1930 and in the 15 years from 1930 to 1944. In the period to 1929 nasal sinus cancer was given as the primary cause of death in 56 cases where only 0·2 cases were expected. In workers starting employment from 1930 to 1944 no deaths from nasal sinus cancer were recorded. Similarly, 137 lung cancer deaths (with 22 expected) were found in those starting work before 1930 and only 8 (with 5·5 expected), in those 1930–44. The authors concluded that the risk continued in workers first employed up to, but not after, 1930.

In this study, while the critical feature of the improvement in the environment was unclear, dust exposures had been markedly reduced and the conclusion of an associated reduction in excess cause-specific mortality does appear warranted; both the size of the excess before 1930 and the rarity of nasal sinus cancer make it difficult to postulate a confounder of sufficient strength to explain the observation. There is, however, confounding between date of starting employment and length of follow up, with a possibility that some lung and nasal sinus cancer associated with employment in the later years has yet to arise in the group starting work 1930–44. Some 80% of workers exposed before 1930 had died by 1972, compared with 38% of the later employees. Further follow up of this younger group might be expected to show some change in cause specific mortality.

The comparison of cohorts before and after an intervention may have further problems in addition to differences in the length of follow up and the long exposure or latency required for the manifestation of chronic or malignant disease. Nurminen and Hernberg investigated cardiovascular mortality in a cohort of 343 Finnish men exposed for at least five years to carbon disulphide (CS_2) between 1942 and the start of the follow up in 1967.[23] Only men aged 25 to 64 years at the time of the examination (born between 1903 and 1942) and still alive and examined at the start of the follow up were included in the prospective cohort study. A referent cohort of 343 workers at a local paper mill without significant exposure to CS_2 was matched on age, district of birth, and type of job. Both cohorts were followed prospectively from 1967 to 1982 and deaths from cardiovascular and cerebral vascular causes noted. The outcome of particular interest appears to have been deaths from ischaemic heart disease. During the first seven years of follow up exposed workers had more deaths from this cause than the referent cohort.[24] There were 20 deaths from ischaemic heart disease among the exposed and only 9 among the unexposed. However, in the period from 8–15 years of follow up there were a further 12 deaths from ischaemic heart disease in the exposed but 15 in the referents. The authors concluded that the levelling off of risk was brought about by the measures taken to reduce CS_2 in the work environment. They also pointed out that cohort members were gradually withdrawn from exposed work, presumably in part through retirement.

Use of the same cohort to examine irreversible effects of exposure before and after intervention seems fraught with difficulties. If high exposure hastens death amongst the susceptible during the early years then reduced risk may be observed with continued follow up, regardless of exposure. Moreover, if a hazard is initially identified through a chance cluster, and this results in a reduction of exposure, the lower incidence after intervention may simply reflect a regression to the mean.

A further difficulty may arise in comparing cohorts recruited before and after an intervention, where the intervention occurs as a result of the recognition of an excess risk. If this recognition leads in turn to early detection of a disease in which a substantial proportion of patients may be successfully treated, a reduction in mortality may show the effectiveness of a screening programme rather than the successful substitution of a less hazardous material. Veys argued that in these circumstances incidence data may be preferred to mortality for detecting hazards.[25] In his study of 2090 rubber workers employed in 1946 to 1949 (that is before the removal of beta-napthylamine) the SMR for bladder cancer (to 1985) was only 112 (95% Cl 61 to 188) but the standardised incidence ratio (where expected values were obtained from registrations at the Birmingham regional cancer registry) was 174 (95% Cl 127 to 233). A difficulty in using incidence rates may arise, however, if screening of the exposed population is more thorough than of the general population. In these circumstances, the risk may appear to continue even in cohorts recruited after the intervention has taken place. Use of the untreated control group design with pre-test and post-test is well exemplified by assessing short term, often behavioural, interventions. The following examples of two such studies, of fitness programmes and training to prevent back problems, show the simplicity of the design.

In the autumn of 1971, the Los Angeles City fire department introduced a mandatory physical fitness programme for all its members, about 3250, with the aim of reducing the incidence of cardiovascular disease.[26] Although 12% did not initially meet medical criteria for inclusion in the programme, all except seven were eventually cleared to take part. The programme was of 45 minutes duration, carried out at work first thing in the morning. The effectiveness of the programme was assessed by taking a random sample of 300 periodic medical examinations and extracting data on blood pressure, cholesterol, and body weight. Analyses were presented for subjects less than 40 years, 40–49 and greater than 50 years old. The paper is not precise about procedures, but it appears that the pre- and post-tests were carried out on different people whose records appeared in the random sample of 300. Police officers formed an untreated comparison group, consisting of a random sample of 258 Los Angeles city police officers' medical records. The date of the "post-test" was around 1978.

Systolic blood pressure was unchanged, in both fire fighters and police officers, but the diastolic pressure decreased significantly between pre-test and post-test in the fire fighters but not the police. The data, presented graphically, showed a drop of at least 5 mm in each age group, and serum cholesterol was also reduced significantly amongst fire fighters in each age group, with the largest decrease (about 30 mg/dl) in men over 50. Among the policemen a non-significant drop of 0.5 mg/dl was observed. Both fire fighters and police officers gained weight slightly.

This study appeared to show a direct effect of exercise on cardiovascular fitness, but it was incompletely described. If measures were indeed on different individuals at pre- and post-test then changes could simply reflect a tendency both for the less fit to leave employment, following the introduction of the fitness programme, and for new recruits to be recruited only if they met more stringent fitness criteria.

Versloot et al. report a study to evaluate the cost-effectiveness of an intervention programme, designed to reduce absence as a result of back pain, which was carried out amongst Dutch bus drivers.[27] A postal questionnaire was completed by 82% of 41 549 drivers and random samples taken from drivers in two areas, those in the south of the country providing 200 for the intervention group and those in the north 300 as the control. The intervention group was invited to attend for a total of six hours, over three sessions, covering discussion of motivation and control over health, strength and function of the back, stress and coping mechanisms, and exercises to improve physical condition and relaxation. Nine refused to participate after the first session and 25 changed job. Only 108 attended all three sessions. Information was provided by the personnel department on numbers of days of absenteeism and length of absenteeism during three periods, the two years before the programme, the two years of the programme and the two years after the programme.

In the two years before the training programme the intervention group had a mean of 58·8 days of absence and the controls 56·9. During the two years over which the programme took place absence in the intervention group dropped to 54·6 days and rose to 63·7 days in the controls. In the final two year period, after the programme, the intervention group had 49·3 days of absence, compared with 59·9 days in the controls ($p < 0.10$). The reduction in absence in the intervention group was restricted to absences lasting between 8 and 21 days. The authors concluded that the savings arising from reduced absences easily outweighed the cost of training; however, detailed analysis of the effects on absenteeism does not suggest a clear pattern of change in the intervention group and this conclusion may be over optimistic.

An example of a simple cross-over design was presented by VanRooij *et al.*, who investigated the use of hygiene measures (washing, clean clothing, new gloves) in reducing skin absorption of polycyclic aromatic hydrocarbons (PAHs).[28] Urine was sampled before the shift on day one and at the end of the shift on day four in workers who did and did not adopt the hygiene measures. Urinary 1-hydroxypyrene was measured as an indicator of internal PAH dose. The design can be written as

$$O_1X \quad O_2 \quad O_3 \quad O_4$$
$$O_1 \quad O_2 \quad O_3X \quad O_4$$

although it would be better described in terms of change score

$$X \quad O_y \quad O_z$$
$$O_yX \quad O_z$$

where $O_y = O_2 - O_1$, and $O_z = O_4 - O_3$.

Thirteen men from two work groups took part. Half the men were first exposed during normal conditions and the other half using the special hygiene measures. The intervention was then crossed over to the other group. Analysis was of the difference in the increase in concentration of urinary metabolite between the week with and without special measures. All but 3 of the 13 workers had less increase in metabolite with the special measures and overall the increase during the week was significantly reduced.

Interrupted time series

Relatively few examples of these designs are found in the occupational health literature and the two presented here have limitations. No example was found in which the data were presented as more than two series, although the first study described might have been presented as seven time series with interventions to reduce dust being introduced at different points.

The effects of dust control and periodic medical examinations on the prevalence of silicosis were investigated in seven industrial companies in China.[29] All 26 603 workers included in the study had been exposed for at least three years and had a chest radiograph. The observation of interest was the 18 year cumulative incidence of silicosis in cohorts beginning work in four periods: before 1950, 1950–54, 1955–59 and 1960–64. Periodic medical examinations and chest radiographs were introduced in 1950–51 and then only for those working with raw materials in a glass factory or in a fire proof brick section of a steel plant. Those included in the early cohorts will have been highly selected for silica exposure as in each of these two plants silica represented at least 90% of the total dust. Dust controls and medical examinations were introduced later in the other work places, workers at lower risk forming increasing by large parts of the later cohorts.

The 18 year cumulative incidence dropped from 20.5% in those starting work before 1950 to 11·0% (1950–54) 6·4% (1955–59) and 3·3% (1960–64). No observation was made on a control group but data on dust exposure were available, showing that concentrations in the earlier years were 200–340 mg/m^3 of total dust with subsequent reduction to less than 6 mg/m^3 in all industries except for coal mines where mean exposures descreased only to 17–18 mg/m^3. The authors commented that the prevalence of silicosis in workers employed after 1960 in the coal mines was still higher than in other companies. Given the well established relation between exposure to silica and silicosis, the absence of a control group or a clear interruption to the time series is perhaps not an outstanding difficulty with this study. However, uncertainty about the composition of the successive cohorts remains.

An example of an interrupted time series together with a no treatment control time series was reported by Broadbent and Little many years ago in investigating the effect of noise reduction on error in a factory producing cine film.[30] The data were presented in a way that did not make full use of the design, but careful reading of the report provides the necessary information. Workers in the factory rotated between bays and each six weeks changed cycle of work. However, within each six week cycle the same group of men worked in bays that were, in the course of the investigation, either treated to reduce noise or left untreated. The report did not make clear how many men were involved in the study, and indeed the unit of analysis was the work produced from the treated and untreated bays during each six weeks period rather than the performance of individual workers.

Eight six week periods of work were observed, four before the intervention and four after. For each observational period data were collected both on bays which were to be (or had been) treated and on bays which were not to be treated.

The design was thus

$$O_1O_2O_3O_4X \quad O_5O_6O_7O_8$$
$$O_1O_2O_3O_4 \quad O_5O_6O_7O_8$$

Although the workers were the same for the two observations at each period, the working conditions were not identical, and in this sense the control group can be considered as non-equivalent.

The results of the study were presented by combining observations 1–4 and 5–8 in each group so that the comparison was between performance in treated bays, before and after intervention, with performance in untreated bays at the same time periods. Errors (that is broken rolls and shutdowns attributed to the operator) were greater before treatment in those bays to be treated, but the errors reduced substantially after the intervention. Some smaller reduction in errors was also observed in the bays untreated throughout but the greater reduction in the treated bays was shown to be unlikely to have arisen by chance. It was also noted that the reduction of errors in the treated bays increased with time since the intervention; the time series data were thus examined, although not fully reported.

Finally Laner and Sell, in an early study of the effectiveness of posters in increasing safe work practices (the slinging of crane hooks when not in use), included a delayed final assessment which indicated that the immediate gains of the experimental period continued to increase after the end of the main experiment.[31] The ability to evaluate the duration of an effect is an important advantage of the time series design.

Experimental designs

Randomisation of subjects

While in principal workplace experiments can be devised in which workers are randomly assigned to interventions—types of gloves, method of dealing with abrasions, distribution of rest periods—examples of truly random allocation are few. Merchant et al. constructed an exposure chamber within a cotton mill and exposed 12 men, selected for their responsiveness to cotton dust, to 33 different exposure sessions over a period of about 20 months.[32] Rather than random allocation, all men participated in each trial. For these men percentage changed in FEV_1 (before and after six hour exposure) were compared for 12 different cotton grades or treatments, together with two trials of no dust. Results showed that the steamed cotton had roughly half the biological activity (on FEV_1) as raw cotton dust. Although carried out in a cotton mill, such an experiment could well have been made in a laboratory exposure chamber, the more usual place for experiments on acute reversible responses to chemical and physical hazards.

431

Randomisation of subjects is more common in studies of the effectiveness of treatment, for example of back pain. In an early study Glover *et al.* carried out a randomised trial among 84 workers with back pain employed in a medium sized engineering works.[33] The workers were first classified by whether or not it was a first attack and, within these categories, whether or not the pain had lasted for less than seven days. Each patient was then randomly allocated to either manipulation or short wave diathermy. The outcome of interest was pain relief on a visual analogue scale from 0–100, reported by the patient immediately after treatment, three days after treatment and seven days after treatment. Patients in all groups showed a more favourable response immediately after manipulation than after diathermy, but this reached significance only in those in their first attack in whom pain had lasted less than seven days at the time of treatment. There was no other demonstrable difference between the two treatments.

A final example is taken from a randomised trial of treatment options for workers who misused alcohol.[34] Clients of an Employee Assistance Programme, who were newly identified as misusing alcohol, were randomly assigned to one of three rehabilitation regimens. During a period of 65 months, 371 employees from a work force of 10 000 were identified. Of these, 35% were ineligible according to exclusion criteria, largely because of the need for urgent medical care. Of those eligible 94% consented to participate (227 subjects) and were randomly assigned to treatment groups. The three regimens were compulsory in-patient treatment, compulsory attendance at Alcoholics Anonymous (AA) meetings, or a choice of options. Of those offered choice, 29 elected admission to hospital, 33 went to AA, three chose out-patients psychotherapy, and six opted for no organised help. The outcomes of interest were measurements of job performance and of drinking and drug use.

During a two year follow up job performance was assessed from company and study records, self reports of performance, supervisors' assessments, and hours missed from work. Measures of alcohol and drug use were largely self reported, but included referral for supplementary in-patient treatment, obtained from company records. No significant difference was found between the groups in job related outcome. On measures of drinking and drug use, the hospital group had most favourable ratings and the group assigned to AA did least well.

Randomisation of workplaces

A number of studies have been reported in which behavioural interventions have been introduced into workplaces, which were randomly assigned to intervention and control. The United Steel Workers of America, together with the University of Pittsburgh, devised a programme of education designed to increase knowledge about exposure to coke oven emissions with the aim of ensuring increased compliance with workplace safety practice.[35] Seven pairs of coke oven factories were matched on geographic location, workforce size and ethnic composition. Within each pair one was randomly assigned to receive the intervention, the other as control. In the intervention group two hour educational programmes were offered at six monthly intervals and workers could attend any or all.

The outcome of interest was knowledge of health risks and workplace practices as recorded on a questionnaire used at baseline and at one and six months following the initial programme. Less than half of those eligible to take part at the intervention plants chose to do so. Those who did not were requested to complete baseline and follow up questionnaires by telephone at the same time as the participating workers and as the workers at the control plants. The investigation showed that programme participants improved in knowledge of cancer hazards and self reported workplace practices. Non-participants at intervention factories appeared to do least well. The analysis was not made by intention to treat, that is by comparing the results for the intervention plants as a whole (both participants and non-participants) with those for the matched control plants. Even with this analysis the study would have had limited power in that, despite the several hundred employees, the number of randomised pairs of factories was only seven.

Trials of primary prevention, unrelated to work hazards, have also been carried out by random allocation of work sites to intervention. These include programmes of immunisation for influenza and other respiratory diseases and, more recently, smoking cessation and the WHO European Collaborative Group study of the prevention of coronary heart disease.[36] In this study 80 factories in Belgium, Italy, Poland and the United Kingdom were divided into 40 pairs, one of each pair being randomised to have workers receive advice about diet, smoking, weight, blood pressure, and regular exercise. Differences between the intervention and control factories were towards reductions in total coronary heart disease, fatal coronary heart disease, non-fatal myocardial infarction, and total mortality, but these differences did not reach conventional levels of significance; this was attributed largely to poor risk factor control in UK factories in which the intervention took place. With adjustment for differences in risk factors at entry, compliance (that is, reduction of risk factors) was significantly associated with decrease in fatal coronary heart disease and total mortality.[37]

Random allocation of treatments to time (the equivalent time samples design)

In this design the same individuals, or groups, are exposed, in a randomly determined sequence, to intervention or non-intervention conditions. Carry over effects of the intervention are potentially a problem with this design, and blinding the participants to the nature of the intervention may prove difficult. A recent paper by Menzies et al. provides an example[38]; it reports the result of an investigation of the effect of ventilation rate on symptoms reported by workers in four office buildings with sealed windows and mechanical ventilation systems.

Of 1838 eligible workers 1546 (84%) completed at least two symptom questionnaires. In each building observations were carried out on six occasions in three two week blocks, in each of which the ventilation system was manipulated to deliver either 20 or 50 ft^3 of outdoor air/minute/person. The order of presentation within blocks was randomly determined by the engineers and unknown to the subjects or investigators. The same ventilation level was maintained throughout the week with a symptom questionnaire being completed at mid afternoon on Wednesday or Thursday of each week.

No difference between number or type of symptoms reported was found between high and low ventilation conditions in any two week block. A tendency was noted towards reduced reporting of symptoms as the study progressed, potentially an important confounder if a balanced design had not been used.

Audit in occupational health

Medical audit has been used increasingly in recent years as an evaluative process applicable to health services in general[39] and, by extension, to those in occupational health.[40] It lies on the border between epidemiology and health service administration but because it requires an understanding of important epidemiological principles its nature and purpose deserve mention in this chapter.

The essence of the audit process is the comparison of what is done in practice with what informed opinion or consensus say should be done. If this basis has been established by credible research so much the better but, even if an arbitrary standard or code is used, comparison between the agreed standard and practice may identify areas in which improvement can be made. When lack of compliance results from legitimate differences in professional opinion, this has the advantage of identifying questions in need of properly designed evaluation.

An illustration of a systematic audit in occupational health might be to compare written procedures for preventing inhalation accidents with actions taken in practice, for example in a large chemical manufacturing plant. The first requirement for audit would be the collection of information in standard format on all such accidents and dangerous occurrences over a defined period, whether or not any injury resulted.

This would require effort and ingenuity, with care to manage sources of bias in assessment, not all which will be obvious. The data once assembled would then have to be recorded for analysis in a standard manner, with sufficient detail of what happened and was done but without identifying information on personal and mitigating facts. A review panel, working independently, would then be asked to assess the case histories for degree of compliance, or otherwise, with the company code of practice. Membership of the panel would require careful thought to ensure that the views of employees, supervisors, responsible professionals and, perhaps, outsiders were recorded. Properly conducted, such an audit would be informative, lead to improvements in practice, and quite possibly identify important questions in need of research.

A possible threat to the objectivity of this approach lies in the fact that the case histories, albeit unidentified, will be familiar to the panel and seen as personal events rather than as examples on which to build future policy. An alternative method used successfully in assessing the appropriateness of a specific surgical procedure—coronary artery bypass grafting—reduced this problem.[41] In this example, the audit process had four components. First, a comprehensive, classified conspectus was prepared by experts of all possible circumstances in which such an operation might be justified. Secondly, details were extracted in standard format about a representative sample of the operations selected for audit. Thirdly, these case summaries were allocated to one of the categories in the conspectus by a technically competent group—a fairly easy task. Finally, the review panel, working individually, scored each of the selected conspectus categories (not the case summaries) for appropriateness on a 10 point scale. This method has great strengths; it focuses the evaluation on well defined but abstract categories, rather than on personal case histories and it allows unlimited flexibility in panel membership and case series for assessment.

A similar approach could be taken with the rather simpler problem of inhalation accidents. A detailed conspectus would be prepared on the prevention and management of these accidents in all possible circumstances. Many other examples in which this method would or might be helpful are given by Guidotti et al. who list, under 17 headings and some 400 sub-headings, important aspects of occupational health practice which in any plant might require audit.[2] For each of the 17, or for the list in toto, some aspect of the conspectus method might prove useful.

Conclusions

This chapter has considered the design of evaluative studies, both observational and interventional, and the examples found have been adequate. This is not to suggest that evaluative studies are frequently included amongst reports of occupational research nor, indeed, that those studies that have been carried out are readily accessible in occupational health journals. In a recent review of intervention studies only 33 reports were found from 1988–93; of these only half were published in occupational health or hygiene journals.[3]

It seems likely that a relatively high proportion of evaluative studies remain unpublished. There are several reasons for this. First, evaluation within an organisation may be undertaken to address problems that are seen as of purely local concern; even if an intervention is successful this may not be felt to be of interest to a wider community. Secondly, studies in this field may be particularly susceptible to political or administrative events that lead to a curtailment of the investigation. Thirdly, even if the study is completed and publication is desired, this may not be easy. Reviewers may be unfamiliar with evaluative designs and fail to recognise the strength of even a well designed study. Finally, there is a high proportion of largely negative studies among those that have been published; if a promising intervention is shown to have little or no effect it may be suspected that either the design or conduct of the study was deficient and editors will be reluctant to publish.

The most compelling reasons for the paucity of published studies, however, are the lack of commitment or interest by those responsible for interventions to evaluate whether or not the intervention is successful[42] and the indifference of a scientific community, trained in the virtues of evaluation by randomised clinical trials, which fails to recognise that valid data can be obtained by any other approach.

Because of these difficulties, rather than despite them, the arguments for more evaluative studies seem overwhelming. Immense amounts of money are being spent on policies and procedures (inspecting work sites, taking chest radiographs, eliminating suspected carcinogens) for which the evidence of effectiveness is either wholly missing or highly suspect. The larger the infrastructure and the more entrenched the practice, the more difficult it may be to put the evaluation in place. However it can and should be done. Secondly, much evaluation is based on inference from observational data; if action is taken based on these inferences, the intervention requires evaluation. Thirdly, intervention studies, particularly those in which the design cannot fully control bias or confounding, need to be replicated under circumstances where these can be minimised; a second study with the same bias and the same result does not advance knowledge but a replication that avoids the recognised weaknesses of the first one does. Fourthly, more studies are needed to show the effectiveness of simple behavioural changes, such as safer work practices and increased personal hygiene.[28] Exhortation to adopt such measures may be much less effective than demonstration of effect within the target workforce (although this assertion could usefully be evaluated).

Fifthly, the nature of industry, with multiple but similar workforces, lends itself to use of the powerful interrupted time series design with multiple replications. A prerequisite is the ongoing recording of outcomes and working conditions so that the change, if any, attributed to an intervention can be evaluated against knowledge of preceding and subsequent events. Increasing emphasis on audit in occupational health may serve to improve records of changes over time. Finally, use of biological markers of exposure and disease, particularly where the outcome of concern is associated with a long exposure or latency, may permit prospective interventions rather than inferential studies of the effects of exposure. Such a molecular epidemiological approach to evaluation will depend critically on success in determining and validating markers of early stages of disease.[43]

Wegman has argued persuasively that occupational epidemiology is of little value unless results of research are applied to prevention and that the academic discipline of epidemiology is in danger of becoming divorced from applications in the workplace.[42] Understanding of evaluative research is critical if decisions are to be based on evidence, but at present the more competent intervention studies are being carried out by behavioural scientists who understand the designs but seldom have training in epidemiology or managerial responsibility for decision making in occupational health. Given that preventive measures may entail considerable expense and effort, and that their introduction implies that a hazard has been recognised, the occupational health service has at least a responsibility to conduct both audit, to ensure that procedures agreed are indeed being carried out, and surveillance, to ensure that the outcome to be prevented does indeed not occur. From either of these activities unexpected problems may be found, providing hypotheses for aetiological research and suggesting further interventions in which formal evaluation may finally form part of the plan.

1 Menckel E. *Evaluating and promoting change in occupational health services.* Stockholm: Swedish Work Environment Fund, 1993.
2 Guidotti TL, Cowell JWF, Jamieson GG. *Occupational health services: a practical approach.* Chicago: American Medical Association, 1989.
3 Goldenhar LM, Schulte PA. Intervention research in occupational health and safety. *J Occup Med* 1994; 36: 763–75.
4 Suchman EA. *Evaluation research.* New York: Russell Sage Foundation, 1967.
5 Hill AB. The environment and disease: association or causation? *Proc R Soc Med* 1965; 58: 295–300.
6 Rothman KJ. *Modern epidemiology.* Boston: Little, Brown, 1986.
7 Cook TD, Campbell DT. *Quasi-experimentation.* Chicago: Rand McNally, 1979.
8 Campbell DT, Stanley JC. *Experimental and quasi-experimental designs for research.* Chicago: Rand McNally, 1967.
9 Campbell DT. Factors relevant to the validity of experiments in social settings. *Psychol Bull* 1957; 54: 297–312.
10 Allen N, Mendell JR, Billmaier DJ, Fontaine RE, O'Neill J. Toxic polyneuropathy due to methyl n-butyl ketone. *Arch Neurol* 1975; 32: 209–18.

11 Kreiss K, Wegman DH, Niles CA, Siroky MB, Krane RJ, Feldman RG. Neurological dysfunction of the bladder in workers exposed to dimethylaminopropionitrile. *JAMA* 1980; 243: 741–5.

12 Welch K, Higgins I, Oh M, Burchfiel C. Arsenic exposure, smoking and respiratory cancer in copper smelter workers. *Arch Environ Health* 1982; 37: 325–35.

13 McDonald AD. The 'retrait préventif': an evaluation. *Can J Public Health* 1994; 85: 136–9.

14 Saari J, Bédard S, Dufort V, Hryniewiecki J, Thériault G. Successful training strategies to implement a workplace hazardous materials information system. *J Occup Med* 1994; 36: 569–74.

15 Fairfax RE. Noise abatement techniques in southern pine sawmills and planer mills. *Am Ind Hyg Assoc J* 1989; 50: 634–8.

16 Orgel DL, Milliron MJ, Frederick LJ. Musculoskeletal discomfort in grocery express checkstand workers: an ergonomic intervention study. *J Occup Med* 1992; 34: 815–8.

17 Last JM (ed). *A dictionary of epidemiology*. New York: Oxford University Press, 1988.

18 Imbus HR, Suh MW. Steaming of cotton to prevent byssinosis—a plant study. *Br J Ind Med* 1974; 31: 209–19.

19 Cooper WC, Jacobson G. A 21-year radiographic follow-up of workers in the diatomite industry. *J Occup Med* 1977; 19: 563–6.

20 Slovak AKM, Hill RN. Does atopy have any predictive value for laboratory animal allergy? A comparison of different concepts of atopy. *Br J Ind Med* 1987; 44: 129–32.

21 Newill CA, Evans R, Khoury M. Pre-employment screening for allergy to laboratory animals: epidemiologic evaluation of its potential usefulness. *J Occup Med* 1986; 28: 1158–64.

22 Doll R, Matthews JD, Morgan LG. Cancers of the lung and nasal sinuses in nickel workers: a reassessment of the period of risk. *Br J Ind Med* 1977; 34: 102–5.

23 Nurminen M, Hernberg S. Effects of intervention on the cardiovascular mortality of workers exposed to carbon disulphide: a 15 year follow-up. *Br J Ind Med* 1985; 42: 32–5.

24 Nurminen M. Reappraisal of an epidemiological study in *Epidemiology of occupational health*. Karvonen K, Mikheev MI, eds. Copenhagen: World Health Organisation Regional Office of Europe, 1986.

25 Veys CA. Bladder tumours among UK rubber workers—reply. *Ann Occup Hyg* 1994; 38: 105–6.

26 Barnard RJ, Anthony DF. Effect of health maintenance programs on Los Angeles City firefighters. *J Occup Med* 1980; 22: 667–9.

27 Versloot JM, Rozeman A, van Son AM, van Akkerveeken PF. The cost-effectiveness of a back school program in industry. *Spine* 1992; 17: 22–7.

28 vanRooij JGM, Bodelier-Bade MM, Hopmans PMJ, Jongeneelen FJ. Reduction of urinary 1-hydroxypyrene excretion in coke-oven workers exposed to polycyclic aromatic hydrocarbons due to improved hygiene skin protective measures. *Ann Occup Hyg* 1994; 38: 247–56.

29 Lou J, Zhou C. The prevention of silicosis and prediction of its future prevalence in China. *Am J Public Health* 1989; 79: 1613–16.

30 Broadbent DE, Little EAJ. Effects of noise reduction in a work situation. *Occup Psychol* 1960; 34: 133–40.

31 Laner S, Sell RG. An experiment on the effect of specially designed safety posters. *Occup Psychol* 1960; 34: 153–69.

32 Merchant JA, Lumsden JC, Kilburn KH, Germino VH, Hamilton JD, Lynn WS, et al. Preprocessing cotton to prevent byssinosis. *Br J Ind Med* 1973; 30: 237–47.

33 Glover JR, Morris JG, Khosla T. Back pain: a randomised clinical trial of rotational manipulation of the trunk. *Br J Ind Med 1974;* 31: 59–64.

34 Walsh DC, Hingson RW, Merrigan DM, Levenson SM, Cupples LA, Heeren T, et al. A randomised trial of treatment options for alcohol-abusing workers. *N Engl J Med* 1991; 325: 775–82.

35 Parkinson DK, Bromet EJ, Dew MA, Dunn LO, Barkman M, Wright M. Effectiveness of the United Steel Workers of America coke oven intervention program. *J Occup Med* 1989; 31: 464–72.

36 World Health Organisation European Collaborative Group. European collaborative trial

of multifactorial prevention of coronary heart disease: final report on the 6-year results. *Lancet* 1986; **i**: 869–72.

37 Rose G. European collaborative trial of multifactorial prevention of coronary heart disease. *Lancet,* 1987; **i**: 685.

38 Menzies R, Tamblyn R, Farant J-P, Hanley J, Nunes F, Tamblyn R. The effect of varying levels of outdoor-air supply on the symptoms of sick building syndrome. *N Engl J Med* 1993; **328**: 821–7.

39 Royal College of Physicians. *Medical audit. A first report. What, why and how.* London: The Royal College of Physicians of London, 1989.

40 Agius RM, Lee RJ, Murdoch RM, Symington IS, Riddle HFV, Seaton A. Occupational physicians and their work: prospects for audit. *Occup Med* 1993; **43**: 159–63.

41 Gray D, Hampton JR, Berstein SJ, Kosecoff J, Brook RH. Audit of coronary angiography and bypass surgery. *Lancet* 1990; **335**: 1317–20.

42 Wegman DH. The potential impact of epidemiology on the prevention of occupational disease. *Am J Public Health* 1992; **82**: 944–54.

43 Schulte PA, Perera FP (eds). *Molecular epidemiology.* San Diego: Academic Press, 1993.

18 Analysis and interpretation

GEOFFREY BERRY

Introduction

There are many texts on statistical methods applied to the analysis of data in medical research, and it is not intended to go over the basic theory, which can more conveniently be referred to there.[1-3] Rather the emphasis will be on methods that are particularly appropriate to the types of data that arise in occupational health. In chapter 14 the types of study design used in occupational health are described. The methods of analysis to be discussed will focus on these types of study design using mainly examples included in the earlier chapters. The main emphasis will be on the use of linear models and the chapter concludes with a short section on statistical aspects of meta-analysis.

Basic considerations of statistical modelling

Before particular problems are considered some basic points of statistical analysis aimed at detecting an association between a health effect or outcome, and a study or exposure variable are discussed. In its simplest form the question of interest is "Is exposure associated with the outcome?" or symbolically

$$E \rightarrow D$$

where E represents exposure and D the outcome, and the symbol $\rightarrow$ denotes "causes," "influences" or "is associated with" according to the circumstances. This question can be assessed statistically by basic methods; for example if exposure consists of two categories, exposed and non-exposed, and the outcome is a continuous variable approximately normally distributed, such as forced expiratory volume (FEV), then the significance of the effect of exposure can be calculated using the two-sample t test, and the size of the effect and its precision, the 95% confidence interval, can be estimated using the same methodology. Frequently, the problem becomes multivariate because of the presence of possible confounders, or effect modifiers, the effects of which must be eliminated from the assessment of the effect of exposure. In the above example, we would wish to be assured that the effects on FEV of age, height, and smoking were properly taken into account. Thus the relationship is now:

$$E, C_1, C_2, C_3 \rightarrow D$$

where C_1, C_2, and C_3 represent age, height, and smoking considered as potential confounders. The method to be used would then be multiple regression.

If the outcome variable is not a continuous variable but a dichotomous variable, such as presence or absence of a condition, then methods appropriate to that type of variable must be used and this leads to the method of logistic regression. In another case the outcome variable might be the number of cases of a condition occurring in a population followed over time and would be characterised by a count of cases occurring over a known number of person-years of follow up. The outcome is then a Poisson variable and the method of Poisson regression, or the log-linear model, would be appropriate. In studies of survival the outcome is the length of survival before an event such as death, death resulting from a particular cause, or the onset of a disease or condition. Typically in such studies there will be individual subjects, possibly the majority, in whom the event has not occurred up to the time of the latest observation. Although the survival to the event is unknown for such a subject, there is some information on its value as it must exceed the known survival time; such an observation is termed a *censored* value. Methods of survival analysis often incorporate regression methods.

While the details of the various methods differ, it is important to note that conceptually they have many similarities.

In general terms the relationship may be expressed as

$$x_1 \, x_2 \ldots x_p \rightarrow y.$$

While this is convenient it is important never to lose sight of the fact that one of these variables is the exposure (of course in some cases there might be several variables representing exposure) and the others are potential confounders or effect modifiers whose effects may be of little direct interest.

Classical multiple regression is given by the relationship

$$y = \alpha + \beta_1 x_1 + \beta_2 x_2 + \ldots + \beta_p x_p + \varepsilon$$

where ε is the error term which is independently normally distributed, α is the *intercept*, and β_i is the *partial regression coefficient* of y on x_i. This is the amount by which y changes on average when x_i changes by one unit and the other xs remain constant. The outcome variable, y, is sometimes referred to as the dependent variable, and the explanatory or predictor variables, x_is, are sometimes called the independent variables.

There are no assumptions on the form of the variables on the right hand side and forms often used include:

- continuous (for example, $x_1 = $ age);
- transformed (for example, $x_2 = $ age^2);
- categorical with two levels (for example, exposed or unexposed to an occupational substance, represented by the dummy or indicator variable $x_3 = 0$ for unexposed and 1 for exposed);
- categorical with more than two levels (for example, smoker, ex-smoker, or non-smoker, represented by two indicator variables: $x_4 = 1$ for a current smoker and zero otherwise, and $x_5 = 1$ for an ex-smoker and zero otherwise);
- product term [for example, if $x_1 = $ age, $x_2 = $ smoking (1 for a smoker, 0 otherwise), $x_3 = x_1 \times x_2$].

This last type of variable arises in the assessment of whether a variable is acting as a confounder or as an effect modifier. Then the regression equation is

$$\begin{aligned} \text{FEV} &= \alpha + \beta_1 x_1 + \beta_2 x_2 + \beta_3 x_3 \\ &= \alpha + \beta_1 \, \text{age} && \text{for non-smokers} \\ \text{and} &= (\alpha + \beta_2) + (\beta_1 + \beta_3) \, \text{age} && \text{for smokers} \end{aligned}$$

Thus, β_3 is the difference between the slopes on age for smokers and non-smokers—it represents interaction or effect modification; that is, the effect of smoking is modified by age. If $\beta_3 = 0$ then

$$\begin{aligned} \text{FEV} &= \alpha + \beta_1 x_1 + \beta_2 x_2 \\ &= \alpha + \beta_1 \, \text{age} && \text{for non-smokers} \\ \text{and} &= \alpha + \beta_1 \, \text{age} + \beta_2 && \text{for smokers} \end{aligned}$$

This is the analysis of covariance model with age as the covariate, and β_2 is the smoking effect after allowing for age; the effect of smoking is uninfluenced by age.

These two models are illustrated in figure 18.1. In figure 18.1(a) the relationship between FEV and age is given by two non-parallel lines for

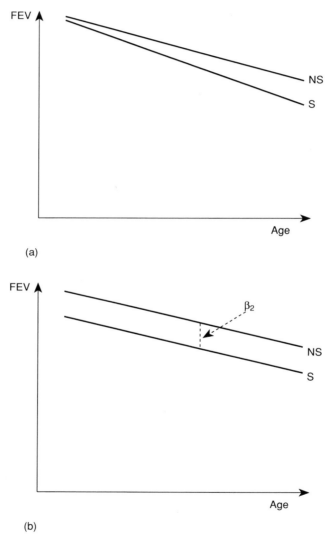

(a)

(b)

Figure 18.1 Connection between FEV and age for smokers and non-smokers. In (a) age is an effect modifier as the effect of smoking increases with age. In (b) the effect of smoking is constant over the age range.

smokers and non-smokers; the effect of smoking is larger at older than at younger ages, or the effect of smoking is modified by age. In figure 18.1(b) the lines are parallel and the vertical displacement between them represents the effect of smoking independent of age. The phenomenon here, of statistical interaction, has been described as effect modification. Effect modification is dependent on the scale in which the variables are measured. To take a well-known example, the relative risk of contracting lung cancer in terms of smoking and exposure to asbestos is approximately multiplicative. Relative to non-smoking unexposed subjects, those who smoke but are unexposed to asbestos experience the smoking risk, and non-smokers exposed to asbestos experience the asbestos risk. For smokers who are exposed to asbestos the relative risk due to the combination of risks is the product of the separate risks of smoking and asbestos exposure. This may be described as an interaction, or effect modification, on the scale of relative risk. But if the risk is transformed to its logarithm the effects are additive and there is no interaction or effect modification. Whether there is biological interaction, synergism, or antagonism, depends on the biological mechanism which may be unknown and cannot necessarily be concluded from the presence of effect modification.

Model fitting strategy

In any analysis the question arises of how the terms to be included in the final model are chosen. There are three types of variables to be considered:

- the exposure factor, E;
- potential confounders, C_i;
- terms representing effect modification (that is, product terms between the exposure variable and potential confounders, $E \times C_i$).

The first principle is that the exposure factor must be retained in all models irrespective of its statistical significance or the size of its effect. The determination of association between the outcome and the exposure factor is the purpose of the study and, therefore, of the analysis and this can only be achieved by retaining this factor.

Another principle is that if a conceptual factor is represented by a set of two or more indicator variables then inclusion or exclusion of the set of indicator variables must be as a whole; exclusion of some but not all of the indicator variables would not necessarily make sense. While there may be occasions in which the number of indicator variables is reduced by amalgamating categories with similar effects, this should be done only after careful assessment of the results and the epidemiological rationale, and not through a sequence decided only on statistical criteria.

The third principle is the hierarchical principle, which states that if an interaction term is included then all lower order terms that contribute to that interaction must also be included. Thus if an effect modification variable, $E \times C_i$, is included then so also must the variable C_i (E is always included). Contravention of this principle, by omitting C_i but retaining $E \times C_i$, involves the arbitrary specification that the effect of C_i is zero when E is zero, and leads to results that are dependent on the way a variable is coded (0,1 or 1,2). From the hierarchical principle it follows that a variable must be considered for effect modification before it is considered as a confounder.

These principles lead to systematic ways of arriving at a final model. The discussion will be in terms of a number of models:

- Baseline model containing the exposure term and all the potential confounders;
- Full model containing the exposure term, all the potential confounders, and all the effect modification terms.

The first step is to eliminate as many effect modification terms as possible. Two approaches can be followed. In the backward-elimination approach one would start with the full model and delete interaction terms one set at a time starting with the least significant and continuing until all the remaining interaction sets are significant. The forward-selection approach is to start with the baseline model and to add the most significant interaction term, and continue to add interaction terms until none of those excluded are significant. Except when there are only a few potential confounders the forward approach is the more feasible.

Retention or exclusion of interaction terms is usually based on statistical significance. Unless there are *a priori* reasons to suggest that effect modification is likely, a stringent significance level such as 0.01, may be set to take account of the multiple testing of several effect modifier sets. The end result of this stage of the analysis is to arrive at a model intermediate between the baseline and full models, usually nearer the former, and in many cases there will be no effect modification and the baseline model will be used.

The next step is to try to simplify the model by excluding potential confounders. The only candidate variables for exclusion will be those already shown not to be effect modifiers. The backward method is the most appropriate here but the criteria for removal should not solely be statistical significance. The degree of confounding that a variable exerts may be measured by the absolute or relative change in the value of the regression coefficient on the exposure factor when the variable is excluded from the analysis. If there is an appreciable change then the variable should not be omitted even if its effect is insignificant. What constitutes an appreciable change is a matter of judgement but values such as 5% or 10% may be used for risk factors.[4] Thus if exclusion of a potential confounder changes the risk ratio of the exposure variable by less than 5% then that potential confounder may be removed on this criterion.

Another criterion is that of precision of the regression coefficient of the exposure variable. A potential confounder should not be removed if to do so reduces the precision of the exposure effect to a material extent. When the outcome variable is a continuous variable removal of a potential confounder may well increase the standard deviation, and hence the standard error of the exposure regression coefficient. With a dichotomous outcome this will not occur, so this criterion will not be critical. Finally a variable that has itself a significant effect may be retained on the grounds of giving a complete model of the data, but this is not essential for a valid assessment of the exposure variable's effect provided that the other two criteria have been satisfied.

For a discussion on strategy in fitting multivariate models see Kleinbaum *et al.*[5] (chapter 21) and Greenland.[4]

Generalised linear models

We now consider the models appropriate to different types of outcome variable. These were unified by the concept of a generalised linear model by Nelder and Wedderburn[6] and an overall account is given by McCullagh and Nelder.[7] A generalised linear model consists of two components:

- y is distributed with mean (or expectation) Y according to a certain error distribution.
- there is a transformation of Y, $g(Y)$, such that a linear model holds, that is

$$g(Y) = \alpha + \beta_1 x_1 + \beta_2 x_2 + \ldots + \beta_p x_p.$$

Classic regression

Classic linear regression is a particular case of this more general form, for which the error distribution is the normal distribution, and no transformation is necessary for a linear regression model on the explanatory variables, that is $g(Y) = Y$ the null transformation. Classic multiple regression is a well-known method and further details are available in many texts.[1 2 8 9]

The adequacy of a regression model should be checked and methods of doing this are available with statistical software. Many methods involve the examination of residual plots to detect non-linearity in the relationship, a non-normal distribution, or a non-constant variability (heteroscedasticity).

More formal regression diagnostic methods are available, which are sensitive in identifying points that are either discrepant from the regression through the remaining points (outliers), have a disproportionate influence on the fitted regression equation, or both. A point is regarded as influential if it exerts more than its fair share in determining the values of the regression coefficients. A standardised measure of influence is Cook's distance.

When outliers or influential points are identified the problem arises of whether it is legitimate to exclude them. Points should not be excluded simply because they appear discrepant from the remainder of the data, but the data corresponding to such points should be checked carefully in case there has been an error at some stage. When this is not the case it is important to recognise such discrepant data and assess how they influence the interpretations.

Another source of difficulty arises if some of the explanatory variables are highly correlated; this is termed collinearity or multicollinearity. In general terms collinearity arises if there is a near linear relationship between some of the explanatory variables in the regression. When this occurs changes in one explanatory variable can be compensated for by changes in other variables, so that different sets of regression coefficients fit the data almost equally well. This leads to estimated regression coefficients with large standard errors and possibly quite implausible values. Collinearity is a feature of the explanatory variables and is unrelated to the values of the outcome variable. Often collinearity can be detected by examination of the correlation matrix of the explanatory variables. If two variables are highly correlated then this implies collinearity between those two variables; an example is given on page 451. It is possible for collinearity to occur between a set of three or more variables without any of the correlations between pairs of these variables being clearly large enough to indicate a problem, so it is useful to have a more formal check in the regression calculations. A measure of the influence of collinearity involving x_i is the variance inflation factor (VIF), which indicates the degree of inflation of the variance of the regression coefficient due to collinearity.

A fuller description of regression diagnostic methods is given in Kleinbaum et al.[9] (chapter 12) and Armitage and Berry[2].

Logistic regression

Where y is a dichotomous or binomial variable with probability of P from a sample of n, then the mean is nP. As P is between 0 and 1, a transformation is required to convert this to an unlimited range. The most appropriate transformation in epidemiology is the logit transformation

$$\text{logit}(P) = \ln\left(\frac{P}{1-P}\right)$$

where ln = natural or Naperian logarithms. This leads to the logistic

448

regression model

$$\ln\left(\frac{P}{1-P}\right) = \alpha + \beta_1 x_1 + \beta_2 x_2 + \ldots + \beta_p x_p$$

with a binomial error distribution.

A reason for the value of the logit transformation in epidemiology follows from the relationship

$$\text{logit}(P) = \log(\text{odds}).$$

As the odds ratio can be estimated in a case-control study it follows that logistic regression can be used to analyse the data from such studies, as well as from other designs.

The regression coefficients require back-transformation for a meaningful interpretation. β_i is the increase in logit (P), or the log (odds), for an increase of one unit in x_i, with all the other xs constant. Hence $\exp(\beta_i)$ is the odds ratio corresponding to an increase of one unit in x_i, with all the other xs constant. The confidence limits of the odds ratio are calculated as the exponential transformation of the limits of β_i.

Poisson regression

This type of model arises when y is a Poisson count, such as the number of cases in P person-years at risk. If the incidence of disease $= \lambda$, then the mean value is λP.

The log transformation is used to give

$$\ln(\text{incidence}) = \alpha + \beta_1 x_1 + \beta_2 x_2 + \ldots + \beta_p x_p$$
$$\ln(Y/P) = \alpha + \beta_1 x_1 + \beta_2 x_2 + \ldots + \beta_p x_p$$
$$\ln(Y) = \ln(P) + \alpha + \beta_1 x_1 + \beta_2 x_2 + \ldots + \beta_p x_p.$$

This is a generalised linear model with a Poisson error distribution, and an extra term $\ln(P)$ forced into the model.

The interpretation of β_i is obtained after transforming back, $\exp(\beta_i) = $ risk ratio corresponding to an increase of one unit in x_i, with all the other xs constant.

Survival analysis, proportional-hazards model

Strictly speaking this is not a generalised linear model but, in conceptual terms, it shares many characteristics with the models discussed earlier. The data consist of the times of death or of some other end-point. Such studies usually include subjects who have not reached the end-point, so the time is unknown for these—but it is known that the time to the end-point exceeds the current survival time (censored value).

449

The analysis is in terms of the hazard (death rate). The proportional-hazards model of Cox,[10] is

$$\lambda(t) = \lambda_0(t) \exp(\beta_1 x_1 + \beta_2 x_2 + \ldots + \beta_p x_p)$$

where $\lambda(t)$ is the death rate at time t, and $\lambda_0(t)$ is the time-dependent part of the hazard. This model may be written

$$\ln[\lambda(t)] = \ln[\lambda_0(t)] + \beta_1 x_1 + \beta_2 x_2 + \ldots + \beta_p x_p.$$

The interpretation of β_i is again obtained after transformation, $\exp(\beta_i)$ is the relative death rate corresponding to an increase of one unit in x_i, with all the other xs constant.

Mortality analyses have been used a lot in occupational epidemiology and a further account of some of the methods is deferred until p 452.

Fitting models

All of the above models may be fitted to data to give tests of statistical significance of effects, estimates of effects, and their standard errors, which may be used in statistical inference. For classic regression the method of least squares is used. Essentially this method consists of finding the regression that fits the data points best. This method is a particular case of the more general method of maximum likelihood which is used to fit generalised linear models. Fortunately the details need not concern us, as the availability of statistical software, such as SAS,[11] SPSS,[12] BMDP,[13] and GLIM,[14] allows the complex calculations to be performed quickly and accurately. Indeed it is only the availability of such software that makes these models feasible and that has led to their increasing use over the past 15 years or so.

Other texts covering generalised linear models are Dobson;[15] Cox and Snell,[16] Hosmer and Lemeshow,[17] Kleinbaum,[18] and Breslow and Day[19] for logistic regression; and Cox and Oakes[20] for survival analysis.

Examples of generalised linear models

In this section examples are presented that illustrate the methods discussed above.

Logistic regression

Yiming et al. carried out a cross-sectional study to investigate the effect of industrial noise on hypertension in a group of 1101 female textile workers.[21] The presence of hypertension was defined in terms of standard criteria on the blood pressure or the current use of hypertensive drugs. This binomial variable was used as the outcome variable in a logistic regression analysis. The study factor was sound pressure level (SPL) represented by a continuous variable in units of dB(A). Possible confounders considered were age, years worked, use of salt (low, normal, high; represented by two indicator variables), and a history of hypertension in either parent (present or absent).

The possibility of interaction effects on hypertension between the five explanatory factors was investigated and none was found. Therefore, a logistic regression with all these five factors, that is six variables, was fitted. Highly significant effects were found for the use of salt and a family history of hypertension. When included together neither age nor years worked was significant but this was because of the high correlation between these two variables ($r = 0.97$). This resulted in the problem of near collinearity and after excluding years worked the regression on age was significant. This illustrates that reduction of a regression model by eliminating variables must be done one variable at a time; it may be invalid to eliminate all non-significant variables in one step. Following the approach discussed at the bottom of p 446 it was possible to eliminate the use of salt and a family history of hypertension because, although these two variables were statistically significant, they had little confounding effect on the value of the regression coefficient on SPL. The value of the regression coefficient on SPL for a logistic regression that also included age ranged between 0·028 and 0·030, according to the inclusion of some or all of the variables representing salt use, family history, and years worked. It was essential to retain age in the regression since its exclusion changed the coefficient on SPL to 0·052. The final model, therefore, included age and SPL.

Another step in the analysis is to check the adequacy of the final model in terms of its fit to the data. Yiming *et al.* checked this by forming 12 groups classified by three age-groups and four groups for SPL, and comparing the observed numbers with and without hypertension with the numbers predicted from the logistic equation. This gave a chi-square variable of 27·3 with 20 degrees of freedom, a value that could easily occur by chance ($P = 0·13$). This indicated that the regression coefficient on SPL, 0·030, is a valid estimate of the effect of a change of 1 dB(A) in SPL on the logarithm of the odds of hypertension. An increase of 30 dB(A) increases the odds by $\exp(30 \times 0·030)$, that is by a factor of 2·5, for constant values of age, use of salt, and family history. The overall prevalence of hypertension was 7% and this factor corresponded to an approximate doubling of the prevalence. Although the effect of noise could be assessed after allowing only for the confounding effect of age, when predicting the prevalence of hypertension for individuals or groups it was necessary to use the full model containing the effects of use of salt and family history.

This example illustrates all the steps of a logistic regression analysis: checking for effect modification, reduction of number of potential confounders, and checking the adequacy of the final model. The way that the model was checked in this example involved dividing the explanatory variables into groups, and this approach is not always possible; for example, if more explanatory variables had been included there could be too many groups with small counts to give a valid test. An alternative general test, introduced by Lemeshow and Hosmer, involves forming groups in terms of the predicted probabilities and comparing observed and expected numbers within these groups.[22]

Poisson regression

McDonald et al. reported a study of preterm births in almost 23 000 single live births in relation to maternal employment.[23] A number of non-occupational risk factors, which could possibly be confounders, such as age, gravidity, educational level, smoking, and alcohol consumption, had to be taken into account. The analysis was conducted in two stages. In the first a multivariate logistic regression was carried out on the non-occupational confounders. From this logistic regression the probability of a premature delivery for each woman was calculated. In the second stage of the analysis the observed numbers of premature deliveries were compared with the expected numbers, obtained by adding up the probabilities calculated using the logistic regression.

In the second stage, various occupational factors were considered in analysis using Poisson regression; the occupational factors included sector of employment, adverse working requirements such as lifting heavy weights, standing, working long hours, and adverse environmental conditions such as noise and vibration. The only factors consistently associated with preterm delivery were lifting heavy weights (relative risk 1·25) and working long hours (relative risk 1·35). These estimates of risk were adjusted for sector of employment and were unaffected after taking account of the other occupational variables.

Poisson regression may also be used in mortality studies and an example is discussed in the next section.

Mortality analysis

A common study design in occupational epidemiology is the *cohort study*, in which a group, classified by exposure to some feature of the environment, is followed over time and the vital status of each member determined up to the time at which the analysis is carried out. Often it is possible to use existing records to establish exposure in the past, and this gives the historical prospective cohort study. Such studies often cover periods of 20 or 30 years or longer. A review of cohort study design and application was given by Liddell.[24] The aim is to compare the mortality experience of subgroups, such as high exposure with low exposure, to establish whether exposure might be contributing to mortality, either from all causes or from specific causes.

As such studies cover a long period of time, individuals are ageing through the follow up period and their mortality risk is changing. In addition there may be period effects on mortality. Both the age and period effects need to be taken into account in the analysis. Individuals are at risk over different periods of time and may change their exposure classification over this period; for example, if exposure is classified by cumulative exposure, then so long as a subject is accumulating exposure there will be changes from one category to the next. Of course the outcome can only occur in the final category of exposure, but it is important to distribute the risk over all the exposure categories relevant to that subject's past experience.

A common method of taking account of age when comparing death rates is to use standardised death rates. Standardisation for age and period simultaneously is a straightforward extension of the method used when standardising for age alone; in what follows only age is specially mentioned for simplicity of expression, but age and period should be understood. Two methods of standardisation are in common use. Both involve dividing the age range into categories, usually five years wide. In the direct method of standardisation the age-specific death rates in the population under study are applied to a standard population. This gives the number of deaths that would have occurred in the study population, if that population had the same age structure as the standard population. If this number is divided by the actual number of deaths in the standard population then the ratio, which is termed the comparative mortality figure (CMF), is the relative death rate. In the indirect method, the number of deaths that occurred in the study population is compared with the number that would be expected if the study population had experienced the age-specific death rates of the standard population. The ratio of observed to expected deaths is the standardised mortality ratio (SMR).

Both standardised rates may be regarded as weighted means, over the separate age groups, of the ratios of the age-specific death rates in the study population to the age-specific deaths rates in the standard population. In the direct method the weights are determined solely by the standard population and hence the method will give comparable standardised rates when applied to different subgroups. In contrast the weights used in the indirect method depend on the age distribution of the study population. This means that SMRs calculated for different subgroups are not strictly comparable.[25] The lack of comparability is because of confounding by age and will therefore be a problem only if the age distributions of the subgroups are appreciably different and if the relative deaths rates are associated with age.[26]

When the ratio of the death rates in the study and standard populations is independent of age, the SMRs are comparable. Equally if the age distributions of the groups under comparison are similar the SMRs are comparable. An advantage of the indirect method is that it provides a more precise result than the direct method, that is confidence intervals are narrower and comparisons sharper. This is because in the direct method the observed deaths in the study subgroups are used and some of these may be unstable because they contain few deaths.[26] SMRs may be non-comparable when exposure categories that are defined in terms of duration of exposure are compared; workers with more than 20 years' exposure are likely to be older than those with less than 10 years' exposure and this opens up the possibility of confounding by age.

Subject-years method (indirect standardisation)

The indirect method of standardisation is the basis of the subject-years method or modified life-table approach. Since this method was used by Doll,[27] it has been commonly applied in occupational mortality studies. In this approach the expected number of deaths in an exposed group, or in subgroups, is calculated by applying the age- and period-specific death rates of a standard population to the subject-years at risk in each of the age-period intervals. The standard population is usually a national or regional population for which published death rates are available. Thus the observed number of deaths is compared with the number expected if the individuals had experienced the same death rates as the population of which the group is a part. The ratio of observed to expected is the usual measure of effect and, by analogy with indirect standardisation, is often referred to as an SMR.

The method has usually been applied to single groups or descriptively to a few subgroups without much formal comparison of subgroups. The method is easily extended to compare mortality between subgroups, or more generally to take account of other variables recorded for the subjects in the study. The extension involves expressing the SMR as a proportional-hazards regression model of the variables.[28] An example, in which mortality from lung cancer in men with asbestosis was studied in terms of three levels of severity of asbestosis, three intervals of length of follow up since diagnosis, and two cities in which the diagnosis was confirmed, showed that city of diagnosis and severity of asbestosis had significant influences on the lung cancer risk.[28] There was also an interaction between these two variables. The risk did not depend on length of follow up and none of the other interactions was important.

Internal standardisation

A disadvantage of the subject-years approach is the assumption that the death rates in the study population and the external reference population are in a constant proportion in all the age-period strata, that is, that the reference death rates apply to the study population at least to a constant of proportionality. The approach may be modified by working entirely within the data set and avoiding reference to an external population. The expected deaths are then calculated using the death rates observed in the whole study for each cell of the array of age groups by period of time (see top of p 454[26]). With more than two subgroups, comparison of these internal SMRs still depends on proportional hazards of the subgroups across the age-period strata. This approach is conservative and may be improved by a Mantel-Haenszel approach.[26 29]

Standardised rate ratios (direct standardisation)

The use of directly standardised rates eliminates the possibility of confounding by age that can occur in the comparison of indirectly adjusted rates. When an external reference population is used as standard the CMF is obtained. The CMF may be unstable if the study population contains age groups with few deaths and so its advantage in eliminating confounding may be overcome by an increase in its sampling variability.

When an internal reference group is used as standard the CMF is referred to as the standardised rate ratio (SRR)[30 31] (see also p 456). If a study contains an unexposed group then an appropriate choice for the internal reference would be that group. All exposed subgroups are standardised with respect to the unexposed group and the standardised rates are comparable because of the direct method of standardisation. As with the CMF, some of the SRRs may be unstable. This can be avoided by using a Mantel-Haenszel method of combining the age groups; this reintroduces the possibility of confounding by age, but the amount of any confounding is less than in an SMR analysis.

Poisson modelling

The methods discussed above involve stratification for all the variables to be taken into account. When there are more than a few such variables to be considered simultaneously, then methods based on stratification will produce many cells with small numbers and the comparisons become imprecise. Also, when a variable is measured on a continuous scale it may be inappropriate or wasteful to transform the values into a set of categories.

The most general approach is Poisson modelling. For a subgroup i and age-period stratum j, if n_{ij} is the number of subject-years and γ_{ij} the death rate then the expected number of deaths, μ_{ij}, is given by

$$\ln \mu_{ij} = \ln n_{ij} + \ln \gamma_{ij}.$$

If γ_{ij} is modelled in terms of the age-period stratum and a set of covariates by

$$\ln \gamma_{ij} = \alpha_j + \beta_1 x_{ij1} + \beta_2 x_{ij2} + \ldots + \beta_p x_{ijp}$$

then

$$\ln \mu_{ij} = \ln n_{ij} + \alpha_j + \beta_1 x_{ij1} + \beta_2 x_{ij2} + \ldots + \beta_p x_{ijp}.$$

This is a generalised linear model of a Poisson variable (p 449) with the addition of the term $\ln n_{ij}$. Breslow and Day (chapter 4) give fuller details of the method and worked examples.[26]

In the above the index i is used for subgroups but could equally refer to individuals. The covariates $x_{ij1}, x_{ij2}, \ldots, x_{ijp}$ are referred to with suffix j as some may change value as an individual passes through the age-period strata, for example transfer from low to high exposure. Some of the covariates may, of course, be constant throughout.

Some examples

Energy research workers

Checkoway et al. presented the results of an historical cohort study of workers at an energy research laboratory.[32] The mortality of the whole group was compared with that expected if the national (US) or state (Tennessee) death rates had applied to the group using indirect standardisation. There were 194 deaths from cancer of all types compared with an expectation from US rates of 250. Thus the SMR was estimated as 0·78 (95% CI 0·67 to 0·89).

It was necessary to assess whether mortality was related to various features of the working environment. In one analysis the cumulative dose of radiation was the exposure variable of interest. This was defined in categorical form as 0, 0·001–0·999 rems, 1·000–4·999 rems, and 5 or more rems. It was necessary to assess this after a ten year latency. The first 10 years of employment were excluded from the analysis, and thereafter each person contributed person-years at risk to the exposure category reached ten years previously. Age and calendar period were classified in five-year groups. The unexposed group (0 rem) was taken as the standard for the calculation of the SRRs for the three exposed groups. The results are summarised in table 18.1 (p 457).

The combination of the external and internal comparisons led to the conclusion that the workers experienced a lower cancer mortality than the general US population, and that there was no association of cancer mortality with the dose of radiation to which workers were exposed.

Workers in the diatomaceous earth industry

Checkoway et al. conducted a cohort mortality study of workers employed in the mining and processing of diatomaceous earth.[33] The

Table 18.1   Standardised rate ratios (SRRs) for deaths due to cancer according to radiation dose category with a 10 year latency for workers at an energy research laboratory (from Checkoway et al.[32])

Dose category (rems)	Observed	SRR
0 (reference category)	34	1·00
0·001–0·999	73	1·06
1·000–4·999	36	0·97
≥5	11	0·90

methods of analysis included comparison with US national death rates using the SMR and internal analyses using Poisson regression. The SMR for lung cancer relative to US rates was 1·43 (95% CI 1·09 to 1·84) based on 59 observed deaths and 41·4 expected. Poisson modelling was used to analyse this excess according to duration of employment in dust-exposed jobs, and adjusting for age, calendar year, duration of follow-up, and ethnicity. The results are given in table 18.2 for a latency of 10 years.

There was an increasing trend in the relative risk of lung cancer with increasing duration of work in dust-exposed jobs. This was tested formally by fitting a trend parameter and was significant (p = 0·003; proportional increase in risk per year 0·044 with standard error 0·015).

The combination of methods led to the conclusion that there was an excess of lung cancer in the workforce and that this excess was associated with duration of employment in dust-exposed jobs.

General remarks

The choices of methods of analysing mortality data might appear to give a confusion of possibilities. One distinction between the methods is whether there is reference to an external standard. It is usually useful to have an overall assessment of how the mortality in the study population compares with that of the larger population from which the working group was selected. Any differences are not necessarily related to those features of the working environment that might have been of most concern.

There is often a reduced mortality in a working group because of the so called healthy worker effect, but it is perhaps salutary to be reminded that

Table 18.2   Trend of lung cancer mortality with latency of 10 years by duration of employment in dust-exposed jobs, adjusting for age, calendar year, duration of follow-up and ethnicity (from Checkoway et al.[33])

Duration (years)	No of deaths	Relative risk (95% CI)
<5 (reference)	28	1·00
5–9	10	1·56 (0·75 to 3·25)
10–19	12	1·67 (0·83 to 3·35)
≥20	9	2·58 (1·17 to 5·66)

there may be aspects of the working environment that are beneficial to health. The usual method of external standardisation is through the calculation of the SMR. Although comparison of SMRs is potentially confounded by age or calendar period, this possibility does not usually have serious consequences. The only conditions in which there is a problem is when groups are compared, which differ in their age distribution and for which their relative deaths are dependent on age.

Once the mortality experience of the whole group and main subgroups have been compared with an external reference, the features of the working environment that may be associated with the mortality are most appropriately analysed using internal methods. The choices are an SRR analysis, a Mantel-Haenszel analysis, or Poisson modelling. The last of these becomes the most feasible option when the number of variables to be considered is such that stratification becomes unwieldy. For simpler problems a stratified analysis is feasible. Breslow and Day in their section 3.6 consider the Mantel-Haenszel method the most appropriate type of stratified analysis.[26] A feature of this method is that as well as combining age and period groups to give a summary risk, a test of heterogeneity is available to test the assumption of proportional risks over the age groups that are being combined. If there is no evidence of heterogeneity then this provides reassurance that there is no serious confounding by age so that it is unnecessary to carry out an SRR analysis. If heterogeneity is found it is prudent to investigate this more closely rather than produce a combined rate based on heterogeneous contributions.

Meta-analysis

It is common to find that in many areas of research into occupational health a number of studies have been carried out that provide information on the same type of association. A summary analysis of the set of studies is then useful. Examples are given by Berry et al. who combined the results of six studies that examined the combined effects of smoking and asbestos exposure on lung cancer,[34] by Coleman and Beral who combined nine studies on the incidence of acute myeloid leukaemia in electrical workers,[35] and by Parazzini et al. who combined the results of eight case-control studies on spontaneous abortion in women working with video display terminals during pregnancy.[36]

There are likely to be differences in the way that the studies were conducted, for example, because of variations in the way the exposure was classified, but nevertheless the measures of association between exposure and outcome may be expected to be similar. It is often useful to combine the results of the different studies to give an overall estimate of effect, which will have the precision of the total amount of data. Such

Table 18.3   Meta-analysis combining studies on acute myeloid leukaemia in men in electrical occupations (data from Coleman and Beral[35])

Study	Observed	Expected	Relative risk (95% CI)	w	w*
1	60	36·7	1·63 (1·25 to 2·10)	25·2	4·9
2	22	10·6	2·07 (1·30 to 3·14)	7·3	3·3
3	36	14·5	2·48 (1·73 to 3·44)	10·0	3·8
4	31	29·8	1·04 (0·71 to 1·48)	20·5	4·7
5	33	26·8	1·23 (0·85 to 1·73)	18·4	4·6
6	4	3·4	1·19 (0·32 to 3·04)	2·3	1·7
7	41	36·2	1·13 (0·81 to 1·54)	24·9	4·9
8	2	0·9	2·33 (0·26 to 8·40)	0·6	0·6
9	6	2·6	2·33 (0·85 to 5·06)	1·8	1·4
Totals	235	161·5	1·46 (1·27 to 1·64) (fixed-effects estimate) 1·57 (1·21 to 1·93) (random-effects estimate)	111·0	29·8

combinations are referred to as meta-analyses or overviews. The full methodology includes consideration of ways of compiling the studies to be included to reduce selection bias and publication bias, and an assessment of the quality of the different studies in terms of other possible biases. These issues will not be pursued here but attention is given to the statistical methods of combining the results from the separate studies. As illustration the data used by Coleman and Beral will be considered.[35] The data are given in table 18.3.

The most natural way of combining the studies is to add the observed and expected numbers of cases and work with the totals. This is equivalent to treating the combination of nine studies as one large study and gives the overall estimate in the row of totals in table 18.3. Another way of looking at this is that the overall relative risk is a weighted average of the separate estimates of relative risk, each study being weighted by the inverse of its variance; that is by the expected number of cases divided by the overall estimate of relative risk. This approach provides a more general framework that can be used for different measures of risk. The method proceeds as follows:

E_i = the estimate of effect from the ith study;
v_i = the variance of E_i;
$w_i = 1/v_i$ (the weight).

Then the overall estimate of the effect and its standard error are given by

$$E = \Sigma w_i E_i / \Sigma w_i$$
$$SE(E) = 1/\sqrt{\Sigma w_i},$$

where the summation is over all the studies being combined.

Another question is whether the studies give heterogeneous estimates of risk. The test statistic for this is

$$X^2 = \Sigma w_i E_i{}^2 - (\Sigma w_i E_i)^2 / \Sigma w_i$$

which is approximately distributed as a chi-square with $k-1$ degrees of freedom where k is the number of studies.

For the analysis of Coleman and Beral the test of heterogeneity is 23·02 with 8 degrees of freedom which provides strong evidence of heterogeneity $(P=0·003).$[35] Two approaches are now possible. The first is to report the heterogeneity but to regard the combined estimate and its standard error as appropriate to the set of studies being combined; this is the fixed-effects approach. The second approach is to regard the heterogeneity as representing another form of random variation and to incorporate this extra random variation into the estimation process; this is the random-effects approach, which can also be regarded as an empirical Bayes method. The method was given by DerSimonian and Laird[37] and is described in Berlin et al.[38] The method consists of estimating the extra variability and adding this to the variability of each estimate. The extra variability is represented by a variance of τ^2 which is estimated by

$$\tau^2 = \max\left(0, \frac{X^2 - (k-1)}{\sum w_i - \left(\sum w_i{}^2 \Big/ \sum w_i\right)}\right).$$

A revised weight $w_i{}^\star$ is defined for each study as $1/(v_i + \tau^2)$ and the calculations repeated using this weight.

These approaches have been applied to the data summarised by Coleman and Beral, using relative risk as the measure of effect.[35] The variability between studies (τ^2) is estimated as 0·164; that is the standard deviation between the separate estimates of relative risk is 0·4 in addition to the sampling error within each study. The weights, w and $w^\star$, are shown in table 18.3, together with the combined estimates of relative risk using the fixed-effects and random-effects approaches. The estimates of relative risk are similar but the confidence interval with the random-effects model is about twice the width of that with the fixed-effects approach because of the extra variability taken into account.

The random-effects approach involves giving more weight to the smaller studies and less to the larger studies than the fixed-effects approach; with the latter the range of relative weights is over 40-fold, but only 8-fold with the former.

Often combinations of studies are carried out after logarithmic transformation of the relative risk, and for the above meta-analysis this gives similar conclusions; 1·39 (95% CI 1·23 to 1·58) with fixed-effects and 1·48 (95% CI 1·18 to 1·84) with random effects.

ANALYSIS AND INTERPRETATION

1 Altman DG. *Practical statistics for medical research.* London: Chapman and Hall, 1991.
2 Armitage P, Berry G. *Statistical methods in medical research,* 3rd ed. Oxford: Blackwells, 1994.
3 Bland M. *An introduction to medical statistics.* Oxford: Oxford University Press, 1987.
4 Greenland S. Modelling and variable selection in epidemiologic analysis. *Am J Public Health* 1989; 79: 340–9.
5 Kleinbaum DG, Kupper LL, Morgenstern H. *Epidemiologic research—principles and quantitative methods.* Belmont, California: Lifetime Learning Publications, 1982.
6 Nelder JA, Wedderburn RWM. Generalized linear models. *Journal of the Royal Statistical Society A* 1972; 135: 370–84.
7 McCullagh P, Nelder JA. *Generalized linear models,* 2nd ed. London: Chapman and Hall, 1989.
8 Draper NR, Smith H. *Applied regression analysis,* 2nd ed. New York: Wiley, 1981.
9 Kleinbaum DG, Kupper LL, Muller KE. *Applied regression analysis and other multivariable methods,* 2nd ed. Boston: PWS-Kent, 1988.
10 Cox DR. Regression models and life-tables (with Discussion). *Journal of the Royal Statistical Society B* 1972; 34: 187–220.
11 SAS Institute Inc. *SAS/STAT user's guide,* version 6, 4th ed., Volumes 1 and 2. Cary, North Carolina: SAS Institute Inc, 1989.
12 SPSS Inc. *SPSS reference guide.* Chicago: SPSS, 1990.
13 Dixon WJ (chief ed.). *BMDP statistical software manual,* Volumes 1 and 2. Los Angeles: University of California Press, 1990.
14 Francis B, Green M, Payne C (eds). *The GLIM system: release 4 manual.* Oxford: Oxford University Press, 1993.
15 Dobson AJ. *An introduction to generalized linear models.* London: Chapman and Hall, 1990.
16 Cox DR, Snell EJ. *Analysis of binary data,* 2nd ed. London: Chapman and Hall, 1989.
17 Hosmer DW, Lemeshow S. *Applied logistic regression.* New York: Wiley, 1989.
18 Kleinbaum DG. *Logistic regression—a self-learning text.* New York: Springer-Verlag, 1994.
19 Breslow NE, Day NE. *Statistical methods in cancer research, volume 1—the analysis of case-control studies.* Lyons: International Agency for Research on Cancer Scientific Publications No 32, 1980.
20 Cox DR, Oakes D. *Analysis of survival data.* London: Chapman and Hall, 1984.
21 Yiming Z, Shuzheng Z, Selvin S, Spear RC. A dose response relation for noise induced hypertension. *Br J Ind Med* 1991; 48: 179–84.
22 Lemeshow S, Hosmer DW. A review of goodness of fit statistics for use in the development of logistic regression models. *Am J Epidemiol* 1982; 115: 92–106.
23 McDonald AD, McDonald JC, Armstrong B, Cherry NM, Nolin AD, Robert D. Prematurity and work in pregnancy. *Br J Ind Med* 1988; 45: 56–62.
24 Liddell FDK. The development of cohort studies in epidemiology: a review. *J Clin Epidemiol* 1988; 41: 1217–37.
25 Yule GU. On some points relating to vital statistics, more especially statistics of occupational mortality. *Journal of the Royal Statistical Society A* 1934; 97: 1–84.
26 Breslow NE, Day NE. *Statistical methods in cancer research, volume 2—the design and analysis of cohort studies.* Lyons: International Agency for Research on Cancer Scientific Publications No. 82, 1987.
27 Doll R. The causes of death among gas-workers with special reference to cancer of the lung. *Br J Ind Med* 1952; 9: 180–5.
28 Berry G. The analysis of mortality by the subject-years method. *Biometrics* 1983; 39: 173–84.
29 Breslow NE. Elementary methods of cohort analysis. *Int J Epidemiol* 1984: 13: 112–5.
30 Miettinen OS. Standardization of risk ratios. *Am J Epidemiol* 1972; 96: 383–8.
31 Checkoway H, Pearce N, Crawford-Brown DJ. *Research methods in occupational epidemiology.* New York: Oxford University Press, 1989.
32 Checkoway H, Mathew RM, Shy CM, Watson JE, Tankersley WG, Wolf SH, *et al.* Radiation, work experience, and cause specific mortality among workers at an energy research laboratory. *Br J Ind Med* 1985; 42: 525–33.

33 Checkoway H, Heyer NJ, Demers PA, Breslow NE. Mortality among workers in the diatomaceous earth industry. *Br J Ind Med* 1993; **50**: 586–97.
34 Berry G, Newhouse ML, Antonis P. Combined effect of asbestos and smoking on mortality from lung cancer and mesothelioma in factory workers. *Br J Ind Med* 1985; **42**: 12–18.
35 Coleman M, Beral V. A review of epidemiological studies of the health effects of living near or working with electricity generation and transmission equipment. *Int J Epidemiol* 1988; **17**: 1–13.
36 Parazzini F, Luchini L, La Vecchia C, Crosignani PG. Video display terminal use during pregnancy and reproductive outcome—a meta-analysis. *J Epidemiol Commun Health* 1993; **47**: 265–8.
37 DerSimonian R, Laird N. Meta-analysis in clinical trials. *Controlled Clin Trials* 1986; **7**: 177–88.
38 Berlin JA, Laird NM, Sacks HS, Chalmers TC. A comparison of statistical methods for combining event rates from clinical trials. *Stat Med* 1989; **8**: 141–51.

COMMENTARY

19 Epidemiology and occupational medical practice

H A WALDRON

Whereso'er I turn my view,
All is strange, yet nothing new;
Endless labour all along,
Endless labour to be wrong.

Samuel Johnson

The mathematician, GH Hardy, wrote in his memoirs that "It is a melancholy experience for a professional mathematician to find himself writing about mathematics" [1]; the same might be said of an epidemiologist writing about epidemiology. However, if nothing else, it does provide an opportunity to make some observations that one might not be able to do in any other context.

The question that I have been asked to consider is, does occupational epidemiology have an impact upon the practice of occupational medicine? And I suppose that the answer, like the answer to so much else in medicine, is no—and yes.

Occupational epidemiology has a long history. Studies of printers, workers in the rag trade, textile workers, miners, and lead workers were reported, mostly in the American literature in the early 1900s, and Cushing recognised in 1920 that recording the occupation of patients in hospital

. . ."though amusing, . . . is of no great interest [unless we] know

463

what ailments these various people presented [and] whether their tasks, or absence of tasks, had any possible bearing on these disorders. . ."[2]

However that may be, I doubt whether the practice of individual occupational physicians was altered one whit then, nor is it altered now, by the constant outpouring of papers into the medical literature by the epidemiologists. It is one thing to know that lead workers, or some solvent workers may have a relative risk greater than unity of having slowed motor nerve conduction velocities, or that workers in the radiation industry seem to be at greater risk of contracting leukaemia, but when dealing with an individual patient, this information is of little value to the clinician. When dealing with individual workers as patients, occupational physicians are concerned to know whether or not the signs or symptoms with which they present are actually caused by work. Does the work bring them into contact with the putative toxic agent and if so, to what degree, and is there any evidence of over-exposure? Finally, are the symptoms of which the patient complains, and the signs that may be elicited compatible with the work experience, or is there some more likely explanation?

If they are competent, occupational physicians ought to be good at making this decision because this is what marks them out as specialists. In the normal doctor–patient contact the abstract concept of relative risk has no place. The cause of belly ache in a lead worker is discovered on grounds other than the fact that epidemiologists have shown that lead workers have a high relative risk for this condition; neurological symptoms in a solvent worker are much more likely to be from causes other than solvent exposure despite studies showing a relative risk of neuropsychiatric disorders, and so on.

Monson described the role of the occupational physican, vis-à-vis that of the epidemiologist rather well in the preface of the first edition of his *Occupational epidemiology*. "Occupational physicians over the years have dealt primarily with acute diseases resulting from short-term exposures to physical and chemical agents," he wrote. ". . . a practising physician has little opportunity to assess whether 20 years of working with benzene leads to leukaemia. The exposure may have produced no intolerable symptoms; the disease may not have developed until 10 years after the exposure has stopped."[3]

Where the findings of epidemiological studies do impinge upon the work of the occupational physicians is in what one might call their advisory—one might even say defensive—role. Occupational physicians are often required to submit reports to management outlining current thinking about levels of exposure, often in response to media coverage of a *cause célèbre*, or the clamourings of a pressure group, or as part of the evidence submitted in response to a governmental consultative document, which might have some effect upon the workings of industry. The most usual course here is to take a broad view of the literature and produce a conclusion on the basis of published work. And for this reason, occupational physicians need to be aware of some of the pitfalls that can be encountered during such an exercise. Some of these will be considered in what follows; I am aware that there may be others that I have not come across.

It is as true in occupational epidemiology as in any other field of research that those who undertake it do so for many different reasons, but it is probably only in occupational (and environmental) medicine that papers are published or criticised for purely political or social reasons. There are two extremes; on the one hand there may be a member of a university department who has the conviction that workers in some area are being exploited and that his duty is to do all that he can to correct this wrong; on the other hand there is the company medical officer who has been instructed to counter the bad press that his company's product has been receiving. In either case they may falsify results in papers to journals, or they may try to destroy results that are already in press by criticising papers or by denigrating the credentials of the authors of these papers. I do not suppose that the number of such people in either category is large, but neither do I suppose that most readers of this book will not know one or more people to whom these descriptions would apply. Some readers will have had the experience of being castigated by one side or the other and will know what an uncomfortable business it is.

There is no means of knowing what prompts people to undertake research and publish in the area of occupational health although personal knowledge of those who work in the field may provide some clues; once a paper is in the press, however, whether it is good or bad, it is there to lend weight to a point of view that is being put forward and I will say more about this later.

Many people carry out research because they have a genuine curiosity about the world and its inhabitants, but there is increasingly a tendency to carry out research solely to provide departmental or institutional funds. This is not necessarily a bad reason and any good head of department nowadays has perforce to be as much a fund raiser or business manager as a thinker, so that his staff do not swell the ranks of the unemployed. But this trend has led, in my view, to some unfortunate outcomes for occupational epidemiology.

The methods used in epidemiological research are not unique to any field of interest. Rather as a spanner can be used for many different purposes, so epidemiological methods can be used to investigate many problems. Occupational groups are relatively well defined and easy to get at and so they present attractive targets for epidemiologists who want to extend the range of their studies and the extent of their fund gathering activities (even though the scope for the latter may not be great). It is no

465

surprise then to find that most occupational epidemiology (in the UK at least) is being pursued by those whose principal training and experience is not in the field of occupational health.

In occupational epidemiology one is trying to relate outcomes with exposures but whereas the outcomes can readily be understood by anyone with some medical knowledge, the exposures cannot. There are three components of exposure, which need to be known in advance of any study of occupational epidemiology. These are the nature of the process, the likelihood of workers at difference stages of the process being exposed and the degree to which this will occur, and finally, the likely consequences of exposure. It is reasonable to expect that those trained in occupational health will have this knowledge and that those not so trained will not.

Of course everyone knows that the measurement of exposure, especially in an historical cohort study, is the most difficult part of the study, and for this reason it is generally glossed over—if it is mentioned at all—in text books and seldom referred to in papers. Even with expert input, assessments are often no better than educated guesses, but at least these are better than uneducated guesses. It is often impossible to categorise the exposure of workers with any precision and no one should be fooled into thinking that classification schemes or job exposures matrices are anything more than guesswork with an added air of sophistication. The end result is that there is a general tendency to underestimate the effects of exposures and in the absence of reliable biological or environmental monitoring data, dose response or dose effect correlations should be treated with a good deal of circumspection.

Measurement of exposure is undoubtedly liable to serious error if investigators are not familiar with methods of work but this error can be further compounded by another, that of misinterpretation of the meaning of results, if they are not conversant with the toxicology of the material to which exposure is presumed to occur. And being conversant requires a more serious knowledge than can be gained from a computerised literature search.

With the amount of statistical analysis now almost routinely undertaken in any study, it is likely that "significant" results will be found; the task is to separate those that are biologically relevant from those that are merely statistically significant. Or, when do we know that we are dealing with real phenomena and not confounders? Davey Smith has explored this in two interesting papers and I will not comment further but refer those who wish to follow it up to his work.[4][5]

When confronted with an apparently anomalous outcome, it is not difficult to construct an explanation. Backache more common in nurses who smoke? Well obviously the vessels arising from the spinal artery are constricted in smokers, hence the pain. Carcinoma of the vagina in female solvent workers? Explained by the fact that cells of the vaginal epithelium can metabolise organic compounds. There is no limit to the ingenuity displayed and probably almost no result which cannot be attributed to some more or less plausible cause, however toxicologically bizarre. Authors all too often forget (if they had ever known) Bradford Hill's strictures about the necessity to use common sense in the interpretation of data. As he said, ". . . far too much emphasis is placed upon the use of statistical tests without a full and thoughtful consideration of the actual results." And ". . . the more anxious we are to prove that a difference between groups is the result of some particular action that we have taken or observed, then the more exhaustive should be our search for an alternative and equally reasonable explanation of how that difference has arisen."[6]

Probably the most celebrated explanation of an unusual result in terms of a plausible cause in recent years has been the so-called Gardner hypothesis which sought to explain the cluster of cases of childhood leukaemia in Seascale (a small town close to the Sellafield nuclear reprocessing plant) in terms of paternal exposure to radiation. The results of Gardner's investigation were published in the *British Medical Journal* in 1987 and the hypothesis gained wide acceptance and support even though the doses of radiation received by the men at the plant were far less than those recognised to double the spontaneous gene mutation rate in humans.[7] In their careful review of the evidence, Doll and his colleagues have recently concluded that the hypothesis "does not accord with what is known of radiation genetics or the hereditability of childhood leukaemia."[8]

Gardner's suggestion attracted a great deal of attention because its ramifications were potentially of great importance to the nuclear industry and those working within it and it was taken up especially vociferously by the antinuclear lobby. Doll's analysis leaves no room to suppose that the cause of the Seascale cases was what Gardner suggested, however, and that is what most toxicologists think. Other less important, or emotive issues, however, will not receive anything like the same degree of attention and the scientific literature is in my view likely to become increasingly cluttered up with reports of unlikely associations accompanied by plausible mechanisms, all more likely to reward the lawyer than the doctor.

I said earlier that from time to time, individuals or organisations have a vested interest in undermining the credentials of workers whose results they wish to repudiate or discredit. One way to do this is to impugn the research because of the origin of its funding. The stance one sees most often is that any study paid for by industry, or reported by industry, is necessarily biased in favour of that industry. A study that fails to find an effect between lead exposure and behaviour in children is only to be expected if it was funded by the lead industry—isn't it? And of course, research funded by the asbestos industry will find that there are levels of exposure at which men may work with no apparent ill effects on their health. By contrast, studies supported by apparently neutral organisations are always to be supposed free of such bias or misinterpretation.

This places those who wish to pursue occupational epidemiology in something of a dilemma since, as Hans Weill has remarked, it has never been easy to obtain funding for occupational epidemiological studies and there are relatively few sources of funding outside industry.[9] In this country the Medical Research Council does not see occupational health within its purview and the Health and Safety Executive, which has limited resources, seems intent on funding only goal-directed research from which nothing of importance has been known to arise.

Industry itself remains the principal source of research funds and, understandably, companies will not be overly anxious to publicise their own research if it is thought to reflect badly on them or give a supposed advantage to a competitor, or to allow investigators into the worst of their factories.

To this extent, occupational epidemiology in the UK is considerably constrained financially. In some other countries—Sweden and Finland are examples of which I have personal knowledge—funds for research into occupational health are substantial and raised by a levy on employers. This seems an attractive proposition, rather on the lines of the "polluter pays" principle relating to cleaning up the environment, but in the present political climate in this country, any scheme to tax employers so as to provide funds for research into occupational health has not the slightest chance of coming to fruition, nor is there much prospect of change in the foreseeable future as occupational health research does not seem to have a high priority in any political manifesto.

The absence of a substantial, independent research fund must act to the detriment of the health of those at work as it is accompanied by lack of information on which to base sound and sensible health and safety policies.

There are many potential forms of bias in an epidemiological study, selection, observation, information, and confounding, and much of the effort in a well run investigation goes into trying to reduce the effect of these biases on the outcome. I do not propose to discuss these any further here as they are covered in detail elsewhere, but I do wish to mention some forms of bias that exist outside the study, but which can also have an important effect on the apparent connection between exposure and outcome. I refer to these as biases in the press.

The publication of a paper, whatever its intrinsic merits, does give the data and conclusions it contains a gravitas that they could never have otherwise. Once "in the literature" an author's opinions, however flawed, are never able to be ignored, if only because they will be trawled by an on-line search and be cited by those who add references to their own papers to illustrate their own profound knowledge rather than the point they are trying to make. The decision to publish a paper, however, is subject to as

468

many whims and vagaries as any other human activity and there are biases in the press of which readers should be aware, and I will mention just a few as they have an important bearing on the advisory role of occupational health professionals.

I suppose all authors will know that it is easier to have a paper published if it contains positive rather than negative results. Most scientists would subscribe to the view that advances in knowledge depend upon new facts being discovered and editors, who wish their journal to be at the front of their field, naturally imagine that positive results are progressive and negative ones retrogressive, or at best neutral. And where competition for space in journals is great, progressive papers are the more attractive. This is a somewhat limited view of progress, however, and there are many examples of important advances being made by the failure to corroborate a current theory. In the area of occupational health it is important to be able to show a lack of effect at some level of exposure as this helps to define safe working limits.

Be that as it may, pressure is undoubtedly put upon authors to produce positive results if they wish to see their work in print and fortunately, statistical analyses, if carried out for sufficiently long can almost always be relied upon to produce a positive result, which can be seized upon to form the main discussion point of a paper, or, preferably, the basis for the next grant proposal.

Publication bias will tend to skew associations between exposure and outcome towards a positive effect and this may be reflected in the kind of "weighing" procedure which is undertaken in some literature reviews. By this I mean that the number of positive results is put on one side, the number of negative on the other and the outcome determined simply by the ratio of the two.

It is difficult to see what can be done to counter this bias in the press. It might be possible for a reviewer or a statistician considering a meta-analysis to find out from grant giving bodies what studies they have funded in the area of interest and write to all the grant holders to ask for both published and unpublished results; it might also be possible to write to all those who have appeared in print to ask if they have unpublished results which they would be willing to make available. Neither possibility seems entirely feasible and even were they to be attempted, there is no guarantee that complete coverage would ever be attained, nor that all authors would collaborate.

Fraud in science seems fortunately to be rare, or is rarely discovered, and when perpetrated it is usually in the furtherance of the perpetrator's career.[10] As the scientific community seems unable or unwilling adequately to detect or control fraud, however, its true extent is unknown. There have been some famous cases of scientific fraud in recent years, none in the field of occupational health. When fraud is

469

committed in occupational health—and I suggested earlier that some instances of this may be known to readers—then it is most likely to be in the form of the introduction of spurious data to protect a particular vested interest rather than to promote the career of the author.

I think that we can agree that outright fraud in occupational epidemiology is rare, but there are some sharp practices which undoubtedly are indulged in and of which readers of research journals should be aware. The most significant is duplicate publication.

Duplicate publication is an example of sharp practice against which readers of journals should be on guard; it is common. I became aware of it first when I was interested in the neurological effects of lead exposure. Specifically, I wished to find out if there was good evidence to show that motor nerve conduction velocity was slowed at low blood lead levels and if so, if it was possible to construct any kind of dose-effect correlation. Having conducted the literature review which did indeed show that most papers were in favour of an association, but it became apparent that some authors were describing the same group of subjects on more than one occasion, or reporting a second study of, say, 20 workers, of whom 18 had been the subject of an earlier paper.

A similar exercise some time later of the neuropsychological effects of solvent exposure also showed the magnitude of the extent to which the same results appeared more than once in the press.

My next experience of duplicate publication was as editor of the *British Journal of Industrial Medicine* when a reviewer reported to me on two separate occasions that she had been sent a paper from me that was identical with one sent to her by the editor of another journal. It was this that prompted me to investigate the extent of duplicate publication in my own journal and the results were not encouraging.[11] I extracted the details of all the papers published by authors who had contributed main articles to the journal between 1988 and 1990 and where the abstract of a paper was similar to one in the journal I obtained the full paper and compared this with the paper in the *British Journal of Industrial Medicine*. Of the 110 main articles published in 1988, 6 (6%) had been published elsewhere; in 1989 the proportion was 10 of 128 (8%) and in 1990, it was 15 of 126 (12%). Few of the papers had been published in an exactly similar form on the two occasions, but in most of them there had been only slight modifications. It was common for the authors to be listed according to the specialty of the journal. For example, in the *British Journal of Industrial Medicine* the first author was likely to be an occupational health professional, but if the results were then published in a journal of chest diseases, then the first author would be the chest physician on the team, and so on.

Duplicate publication can be justified under some circumstances. Few editors would object to considering a paper that had first been published in a minority language, or if a paper which they had already published were to be published in one, although they would expect mention to be given to the prior publication. Some authors make special pleading by suggesting that as the subject of their research covers two disparate fields—epidemiology and radiology, for example—then the results should be published in two specialist journals, emphasising the epidemiological or the radiological features as appropriate. Sometimes this is reasonable, again so long as the other publication is acknowledged and it is made plain that the same study is being reported, not two separate studies. Conference proceedings notoriously breed duplicate publications but mercifully these are usually difficult to obtain and rarely cited and so they can generally be ignored.

Journals are now trying to take steps to curb duplicate publication, although probably not for altruistic reasons, but simply because they do not want to be the second journal to publish a paper. Almost all require authors submitting papers to sign a declaration that the work has not been sent elsewhere which does not, of course, deter any duplicate publisher. Reviewers may sometimes pick up duplicate submissions, especially in a small field, and some journals now routinely run literature searches on authors whose papers they are considering to see first how many papers they have published recently and secondly, if any of these have titles bearing on the paper in hand. Journals with small budgets and a small staff are not able to go to those lengths, however, and the onus must be on the reader to be vigilant and read carefully.

The structured abstract is a great boon to the duplicate publisher as it is designed, as I understand it, to stand alone and readers need do no more than scan the abstract to gain the salient points of the paper. Given that most of us do not read the scientific press for pleasure, this saves time and possibly a great deal of tedium, but as there are no references to previous work in the abstract, it is easy for the duplicate publisher to conceal the fact that the abstract is based on data that have appeared elsewhere. Incidentally, the structured abstract does nothing to increase the pleasure of reading and is a poor substitute for the summary still required by the better journals.

I cannot see the time when bias, methodological, editorial, and authorial, will be totally eliminated from the papers in our scientific journals and so readers and reviewers must try to ensure that they are able to distinguish the evidence that can be relied upon from that which cannot, and that, like medicine, is a "craft so long to lerne."

The nature of research into occupational health has changed substantially in the last few decades. When I was preparing a piece to mark the 50th volume of the *British Journal of Industrial Medicine*, I examined the content of the first five volumes and the last five. The first five were characterised by a greater proportion of clinical than epidemiological papers, whereas in the last five, the position was

471

completely reversed and the great majority of papers published were concerned with epidemiology (the proportions were 22% for clinical papers and 18% for epidemiology in the first five years and 9% and 63%, respectively for the second five). Nowadays, research into occupational health is inconceivable without the application of epidemiological methods, especially as we look for decreasingly small effects of decreasingly small exposures.

Nevertheless, I doubt whether the day-to-day practice of occupational physicians is influenced by these research findings although I acknowledge their importance when trying to arrive at a consensus view for briefing, advising, or educating others. Some of the biases likely to be encountered in carrying out the studies have been discussed elsewhere in this book; some of those resulting from their publications I have dealt with here.

There are some serious issues that depend on the results of epidemiological studies, the most significant of which are the setting of standards and regulations (discussed in the next chapter) and I would like to think that the studies and opinion on which they rely were soundly based, but regrettably, impartiality like generosity is not a common commodity and as Francis Bacon reminds us ". . . what a man would like to be true, that he more readily believes." [12]

1 Hardy GH. *A mathematician's apology*. Cambridge: Cambridge University Press, 1940: 1.
2 Cushing H. *Sixth annual report of the Peter Bent Brigham Hospital for the year 1919*, Cambridge: Cambridge University Press, 1920: 74.
3 Monson RR. *Occupational epidemiology*. Baton Rouge: CRC Press, 1980.
4 Smith GD, Phillips AN. Confounding in epidemiological studies: why "independent" results may not be all that they seem. *BMJ* 1992; 305: 757-9.
5 Smith GD, Philips AN, Neaton JD. Smoking as an "independent" risk factor for suicide: illustration of an artifact from observational epidemiology? *Lancet* 1992; 340: 709-12.
6 Hill AB, Hill ID. *Principles of medical statistics*, 12th ed, London: Edward Arnold, 1991: 277-8.
7 Gardner MJ, Hall AJ, Downes S, Terrell JD. Follow up study of children born elsewhere but attending schools in Seascale, West Cumbria (schools cohort), *BMJ* 1987; 295: 819-22; Follow up study of children born to mothers resident in Seascale, West Cumbria (birth cohort), *ibid*: 822-7.
8 Doll R, Evans HJ, Darby SC. Paternal exposure not to blame. *Nature* 1994; 367: 678-98.
9 Weill H. Future of research into occupational lung disease. *Br J Ind Med* 1993; 50: 481-3.
10 Anon. What to do about scientific misconduct. *Nature* 1994; 369: 261-2.
11 Waldron T. Is duplicate publishing on the increase? *BMJ* 1992; 304: 1029.
12 Bacon F. *Novum Organum*, book 1, aphorism 49.

20 Occupational epidemiology and public policy

HANS WEILL

The *raison d'être* for the development of policy options which deal with the diseases due in whole or in part to workplace exposures is their prevention. The underlying scientific basis by which this is done may come from various sources, ranging from the fundamental biologist to the physician-scientist, and includes industrial hygienists, statisticians, engineers, and chemists, as well as others. All these disciplines can, however, inform the research conducted by the epidemiologist, who is engaged in the assessment of exposure and dose, and the measurement of disease outcomes, the relationships between them, and how other factors influence these relationships. Ultimately, the epidemiologist (along with his or her interdisciplinary team) presents the findings to policy-makers, and because the quantitative data come from human populations, these results are more likely to gain the regulators' acceptance and, indeed, also that of the general population.

Studies in the animal model, particularly when not accompanied by positive human evidence, while relied on by government and international agencies (for example, the United States Environmental Protection Agency and the International Agency for Research on Cancer) fail to convince many of the primary players in protecting worker health: industry management, the workers themselves, and the general public from which often comes the lament "not another rat carcinogen". As it turns out, however, most environmental and occupational health policy decisions are made in the absence of epidemiologic studies, with reliance of necessity on animal studies.

Even when human population studies are available, they are often inadequate or too few, and may be conflicting in their results or show marginally "positive" associations which may or may not be causal in nature. It is also useful to note that "negative" studies are far less likely to be published, making the totality of the published epidemiologic database in this field often unbalanced. Of course, when the science is readily summarised, and correlations are found consistently and are robust, consequent policy decisions should emerge quite easily. Regrettably, this is not common.

It is my intention to provide several examples of which I have personal knowledge of how the results of occupational epidemiology can play either a useful or detrimental role in regulatory policy or judicial decisions, including instances in which the results of sound epidemiologic research have been ignored by the policy-makers, usually at the behest of vested interests.

One would be hard pressed to find more common examples of interfacing between occupational disease and public policy than for the asbestos-related diseases, in which epidemiology has had both successes and failures. Appropriate use of epidemiological data on asbestos health effects has often been thwarted by advocacy and, at times, those who have identified themselves as the guardians of worker health have successfully pushed policy positions which have undoubtedly resulted in more exposure-related disease and death. More about this later.

As the amount of asbestos used in the industrialised world declined (in the late 1970s and early 1980s) increasing concern was being expressed in the United States that airborne asbestos fibres could be released from asbestos-containing materials in buildings, mainly in and above acoustic ceilings, and consequently result in exposure-related health effects in occupants. Schools were an early focus of this concern, a focus which sometimes led to emotional public testimony by scientists and erratic advice from the US Environmental Protection Agency (EPA). This, in turn, resulted in understandable fear among parents of schoolchildren, widespread removal of asbestos-containing materials (most often in good repair) in schools and other buildings, and massive filings of lawsuits against the manufacturers of the products to recover the removal costs.

Science ultimately contributed to the resolution of this issue in two important ways, although the litigation continues. First, extensive measurements of airborne fibres resulted in objective exposure assessment.[1][2] Secondly, quantitative risk assessment was performed using the epidemiological database provided by studies of occupationally asbestos-exposed populations, in which cumulative exposure estimates for individual members of the cohorts were possible and correlated with health outcome.[3] Models were widely agreed to, calculated risks were extrapolated to the exposure levels found in buildings, and the risks estimated. These risks could be readily compared with a host of well known risks that were accepted daily by the general public. The issue was largely diffused in the media, and the EPA reversed its earlier implicit position, now expressing publicly that asbestos-containing material should be left in place until time for demolition or renovation. Putting the calculated negligible risks to occupants in perspective was made possible by the epidemiological studies which provided the data necessary for quantitative risk analysis.

Asbestos provides another kind of example. Scientific studies from many parts of the world did not induce United States regulators to take the different types of asbestos fibres into account in the asbestos regulatory process. The data that showed that amphibole asbestos (the commercial varieties of which are crocidolite and amosite) is far more potent than chrysotile in relation to mesothelioma risk grew steadily stronger for at least the past two decades.[4] A similar fibre type-related gradient in risk for lung cancer and asbestosis is also likely to exist, although the evidence is more limited[5-7] (see also Chapter 5).

Most countries accepted this evidence and regulated amphiboles more stringently, either by lower workplace standards for permissible exposure limits, or by banning their use and/or importation altogether. Why have the United States officials not accepted the same compelling evidence? The answer certainly lies in the political pressure from sections of the scientific and legal communities, which have convinced the government agencies that to regulate amphiboles more stringently is to accept exposure to chrysotile more readily. This is, of course, nonsense—chrysotile exposures must be controlled in accord with the scientific data regarding exposure-related risks of that fibre. One wonders how much lethal disease might have been prevented had the United States taken firm action on the amphiboles, as did other countries, when the evidence was certainly sufficient in the 1970s and even earlier?

Epidemiologic studies on fibres have not been limited to asbestos; man-made mineral fibres have also been the subject of much study since the early 1980s. Large multi-company mortality studies have been published from both Europe and the United States[8 9] (see also Chapter 5). In general, workers engaged in the manufacture of glass and rock wool have not shown an excess risk of lung cancer. Those exposed to slag wool, contaminated with arsenic and perhaps other carcinogens, have shown an excess risk, but whether this has been related to past fibre exposure is quite uncertain. No risk of mesothelioma has thus far been demonstrated in any of these worker groups.

A recent follow-up morbidity study of workers engaged in the manufacture of fibrous glass and mineral (rock and slag) wool has not

475

detected evidence of exposure-related non-malignant respiratory disease.[10] The mortality studies are of large populations, but the generally low exposures (in comparison with asbestos fibre concentrations in past working populations) have suggested to some commentators that there is inadequate sensitivity to detect what could be a substantial risk.

When rats were used in large inhalation studies using glass fibres, no tumours were found,[11] but it was contended that this animal model was not sensitive enough to show the risk.[12] On the other hand, rats seem to be particularly sensitive in regard to the development of lung cancer in response to a variety of inhaled particles (for example, crystalline silica), perhaps because of their susceptibility to dust overload leading to nonspecific inflammation, cell proliferation, and tumours. The results of these epidemiological and animal inhalation studies on glass and rock wool fibres should have been reassuring especially when the animal and human research agreed, which is not always the case. At present the policy issue involved is the classification of glass, rock, and slag wool; regulators (National Toxicology Program in the US) have chosen to list all of these materials as carcinogenic.

In addition to the prevention or mitigation of occupational health risks, epidemiology also has a role in policies that govern the compensation of workers who have been injured as the result of their workplace exposures. In seeking to answer the question, "When is lung cancer attributable to a worker's asbestos exposure?," my colleague, Janet Hughes, and I made a prospective mortality study in workers in asbestos products manufacturing. We found that a substantial excess risk (four-fold) was seen in those members of the cohort who had radiographic evidence consistent with asbestosis, but no excess risk if such evidence was absent, even when pleural effects alone were present.[13] Other, but possibly not all, studies are consistent with these findings.[14-16] As virtually all instances of lung cancer in asbestos-exposed populations are in workers who have smoked (all of those with lung cancer in our study were smokers), it is reasonable to maintain that, in the presence of fibrosis and cigarette smoking, asbestos should be considered a causal factor. This evidence has been largely accepted by those who make decisions regarding workplace-induced diseases for which compensation can be claimed as a fair way of dealing with a difficult problem.

Almost all the epidemiological evidence that links crystalline silica exposure to lung cancer risk comes from workers compensated for silicosis.[17] Only limited evidence can be brought to bear on the question: "Does crystalline silica exposure *per se* result in excess lung cancer risk?" The fact that people with asbestosis and silicosis have elevated lung cancer risks should be added to the finding that subjects with lung fibrosis not of occupational origin may also have a greater risk of lung cancer than the general population lending plausibility to the hypothesis that there may very well be linkage between inflammation, fibrosis, and lung cancer.[18] Does this give support to the common practice of providing compensation for lung cancer only if the mineral dust exposure has also resulted in fibrosis? It surely must, at least until there is convincing epidemiologic evidence to the contrary.

The last decade has brought considerable focus to the question of crystalline silica as a potential human carcinogen. As indicated above, excess lung cancers have been observed primarily in subjects with silicosis, and the issue of a selection bias has been raised.[17] Risks in compensated workers should not be compared with general population statistics (see Chapter 5). Cohort studies of silica-exposed populations have not been able to relate quantitative estimates of past crystalline silica exposure to lung cancer risk. In one study, however, dose-dependency of an excess lung cancer risk was shown when exposure (to cristobalite), was assessed using an ordinal approach.[19] For silicosis, the risk in occupationally exposed populations appears not only to be dose-related, but also with a threshold ("no-effect") level.[20] If one accepts that excess lung cancer had to date been adequately shown only in those with silicosis, the prevention of lung fibrosis can be expected to protect from the cancer risk. Does it then appear to be a reasonable use of public funds to protect the public from cancer at levels of general environmental exposure far below that at which silicosis occurs? The epidemiologic studies to date clearly do not support this policy, although that is currently the direction being taken by some governmental agencies in the United States.

That acute airways constriction occurs in relation to the working shift in the cotton textile industry has been recognised for many years. Richard Schilling first showed that this occupational disorder, called byssinosis, was related to the airborne concentrations of cotton dust in textile mills[21] and the United States Occupational Safety and Health Administration workplace textile dust standard is based on a cross-sectional study of this disease.[22] The long-term course of respiratory health in mill workers was less clear, and a five-year longitudinal multi-plant study was undertaken, the results of which have been published.[23] Our investigations of textile workers showed a correlation between cotton dust exposure and annual decline in function, and between this annual decline and the acute post-shift drop in lung function. Additional analyses have shown that excess annual decline in function (a predictor of chronic airways obstruction) was limited to workers engaged in yarn manufacturing (early textile production) who were also smokers. The current permissible exposure limit in the United States of 200 μg/m^3 of elutriated dust did not adequately protect workers in yarn production who were also smokers, leading to our recommendation that smokers be excluded from working in this section of the industry, and that the dust exposure limit be lowered to 100 μg/m^3.[23] These findings raise the important policy issue of mandating

477

shared responsibility for worker health—in this instance, by modifying personal behaviour or limiting employment to non-smokers and workplace exposure levels. In the past, there has been essentially total reliance on the latter, and considerable resistance to the former. Whether this continues to be the case remains to be seen.

The enormous burden of litigation in the United States dealing with asbestos-related disease in exposed workers has been complicated by defendants found liable in tort claims having to institute additional litigation, to obtain insurance coverage which they thought they had, to compensate workers claiming to have been injured by their exposure to asbestos. Such coverage has been contested by insurers for a variety of reasons, and the courts have ruled inconsistently concerning the time period when the "trigger" of coverage occurs. For example, some courts have held that coverage is triggered when the exposures began, and continues through the time of diagnosis of an asbestos-related disease, or beyond; others have maintained that coverage begins at the time of diagnosis. Obviously, it is in the insured's interests to maximise the coverage to include the longest possible time. In a Boston court, the trigger of coverage was defined as the date on which the diagnosis was made. The Appellate Court, however, sent the case back to the trial judge and asked her to decide instead "when the disease could reasonably have been capable of being diagnosed." My colleagues and I were asked if we had a data set that could be analysed in order to answer the question. We did indeed!

We had for some time been following a population of workers engaged in the manufacture of asbestos-containing building products and had recently collected the data for a ten year longitudinal study of the determinants of progression of asbestos-related disease. Our population of 244 workers was first studied while they were actively employed. Most had four examinations over the next 10 years (at about three-year intervals). There were 855 films available for independent classification by three readers experienced in the use of the ILO classification of chest radiographs; the films were read independently and in random order without regard to others in that set of films.

Sixty-three of the 244 workers had a positive film; 37 had at least one negative previous film. Survival analysis provided probabilities of the diagnosis having been made at varying times previously. From the exponential model, which provided a good fit to the data, 50% of the diagnoses could have been made at least 6·14 years before the actual diagnosis (confidence interval was 4·4 to 10·3 years), or there was a 51% probability of a positive film six years before a current positive. The Court accepted what became known as a "rollback" of six years, meaning that the company had six more years of insurance coverage to apply to awards or settlements made to plaintiffs. The rollback lengthened as the number of small opacities on the last film increased. In accepting this study and its results in resolving a dispute with substantial economic implications for compensating individuals with asbestos-related disease, the judge could not resist mentioning in her opinion that this, like other epidemiological studies, was not perfect. The decision was challenged by the insurance companies, but was upheld by the Appellate Court.

The tools of occupational epidemiology are likely to become more sensitive and specific in the future with the increased use of biological markers of exposure, the adverse pre-clinical effects of that exposure, and host susceptibility to any such effects (see Chapter 15). The biomarkers will increasingly measure dose, not just exposure, and genetic predisposition will be increasingly identified by the molecular techniques even now available. With regard to biological effects, there will, however, be greater difficulty in understanding and communicating, for example, the impact of subtle biochemical or immunological alterations (even if shown to be dose-dependent) in terms of their long-term impact on health. When the health implications of such changes are sorted out, more precise dose-response information will result, risk assessment will be improved, and resulting policy more readily defended in the public arena.

I have tried to provide illustrations of the potential use of occupational epidemiology in the policy decision-making which impacts on occupational and environmental health—both prevention of disease and equitable recompense of disease produced by workplace exposures. It will be apparent that the results have been mixed. The "gold standard," a term aptly applied to the results of studies on human populations, has at times provided answers that were resisted for non-scientific reasons. Epidemiologists must be more persuasive in marketing their product in the public arena. They must also take steps to assure that population studies of workers can continue to be done, at a time when the future of this type of research is uncertain for a number of reasons which I have reviewed elsewhere.[24] Both workers and their employers are showing less and less enthusiasm for participation in these studies. Workers do not trust investigators to detect, or make public, hazards in the workplace. Management is scared off by overzealous researchers who confuse scientific objectivity with social objectives. These conflicts are exacerbated by lawyers on both sides whose primary interest is all too clear. The historical dependence on occupational epidemiological research of regulators and other policy-makers should be the primary selling point.

1 Health Effects Institute. *Asbestos in public and commercial buildings: a literature review and synthesis of current knowledge.* Cambridge, Massachusetts: Health Effects Institute-Asbestos Research, 1991.

2 Health Effects Institute. *Asbestos in public and commercial buildings: supplementary analyses of selected data previously considered by the Literature Review Panel.* Cambridge, Massachusetts: Health Effects Institute-Asbestos Research, 1992.

3 Hughes JM, Weill H. Asbestos exposure—quantitative assessment of risk. *Am Rev Respir Dis* 1986; **133**: 5–13.
4 Weill H, Hughes JM. Asbestos health effects: resolving the scientific uncertainties. *Postgrad Med J* 1988; **64** (suppl 4): 48–55.
5 Weill H, Rossiter CE, Waggenspack C, Jones RN, Ziskind MM. Differences in lung effects resulting from chrysotile and crocidolite exposure. In: Walton WH, ed, *Inhaled Particles IV*. Oxford and New York: Pergamon Press, 1977; 789–98.
6 Jones RN, Diem JE, Hughes JM, Hammad YY, Glindmeyer H, Weill H. Progression of asbestos effects: a prospective longitudinal study of chest radiographs and lung function. *Br J Ind Med* 1989; **46**: 97–105.
7 Hughes JM, Weill H. Asbestos and man-made fibres. In: Samet JM, ed, *Epidemiology of lung cancer*. New York: Marcel Dekker, 1994; 185–205.
8 Marsh GM, Enterline PE, Stone RA, Henderson VL. Mortality among a cohort of U.S. Man-made mineral fibre workers: 1985 follow-up. *J Occup Med* 1990; **32**: 594–604.
9 Simonato L, Fletcher AC, Cherrie J, Andersen A, Bertazzi P, Charnay N, *et al*. The man-made mineral fibres (MMMF) European historical cohort study: extension of the follow-up. *Ann Occup Hyg* 1987; **31**: 603–23.
10 Hughes JM, Jones RN, Glindmeyer HW, Hammad YY, Weill H. Follow-up study of workers exposed to man-made mineral fibres. *Br J Ind Med* 1993; **50**: 658–67.
11 Hesterberg TW, Miller WC, McConnell EE, Chevalier J, Hadley JG, Bernstein DM, *et al*. Chronic inhalation toxicity of size-separated glass fibres in Fischer 344 rats. *Fundam Appl Toxicol* 1993; **20**: 464–76.
12 Pott F, Roller M. *The carcinogenic effect of fibres with special regard to inhalation experiments*. Dortmund: Federal Institute for Industrial Safety, 1993.
13 Hughes JM, Weill H. Asbestosis as a precursor of asbestos related lung cancer: results of a prospective mortality study. *Br J Ind Med* 1991; **48**: 229–33.
14 Sluis-Cremer GK, Bezuidenhout BN. Relation between asbestosis and bronchial cancer in amphibole asbestos miners. *Br J Ind Med* 1989; **46**: 537–40.
15 Sluis-Cremer GK, Bezuidenhout BN. Response to letter to the Editor. *Br J Ind Med* 1990; **47**: 215–6.
16 Kipen HM, Lilis R, Suzuki Y, Valciukas JA, Selikoff IJ. Pulmonary fibrosis in asbestos insulation workers with lung cancer: a radiological and histopathological evaluation. *Br J Ind Med* 1987; **44**: 96–100.
17 Weill H, McDonald JC. Crystalline silica exposure and lung cancer risk: the epidemiologic evidence. *Thorax* 1995, in press.
18 Turner-Warwick M, Lebowitz M, Burrows B, Johnson A. Cryptogenic fibrosing alveolitis and lung cancer. *Thorax* 1980; **35**: 496–9.
19 Checkoway H, Heyer NJ, Demers PA, Breslow NE. Mortality among workers in the diatomaceous earth industry. *Br J Ind Med* 1993; **50**: 586–97.
20 Muir DCF, Julian JA, Shannon HS, Verma DK, Sebestyen A, Bernholz CD. Silica exposure and silicosis among Ontario hardrock miners: III. Analysis and risk estimates. *Am J Ind Med* 1989; **16**: 29–43.
21 Roach SA, Schilling RSF. A clinical and environmental study of byssinosis in the Lancashire cotton industry. *Br J Ind Med* 1960; **17**: 1.
22 Merchant JA, Lumsden JC, Kilburn KH, O'Fallon WM, Ujda JR, Germino VH, *et al*. Dose response studies in cotton textile workers. *J Occup Med* 1973; **15**: 222–30.
23 Glindmeyer HW, Lefante JJ, Jones RN, Rando RJ, Weill H. Cotton dust and across-shift change in FEV^1 as predictors of annual change in FEV^1. *American Journal of Respiratory and Critical Care Medicine* 1994; **149**: 584–90.
24 Weill H. Future of research into occupational lung disease (editorial). *Br J Ind Med* 1993; **50**: 481–3.

Index

Epidemiology books from the BMJ Publishing Group

CHILDHOOD CANCER AND NUCLEAR INSTALLATIONS

Edited by Valerie Beral, Eve Roman, Martin Bobrow

This collection of papers outlines the controversy over childhood cancers at the site of nuclear installations – from the television programme on Windscale in 1983, through Martin Gardner's remarkable statistical studies to the present day.

ISBN 0 7279 0815 4   496 pages

NEW PERSPECTIVES IN LUNG CANCER

Edited by N Thatcher and S Spiro

Recently advances in lung cancer have been limited to specific areas. This book addresses the issues that are most controversial and brings the reader up to date with the latest knowledge. Leading experts discuss quality of life for the patient; how far to investigate; the role of tobacco; as well as the newest therapeutic and scientific advances.

"Offers the reader an excellent and balanced overview of many aspects of lung cancer."
Annals of Oncology

ISBN 0 7279 0786 7   203 pages

MOTHERS, BABIES, AND DISEASE IN LATER LIFE

D J P Barker

Following the internationally successful publication of *Fetal and Infant Origins of Adult Disease*, David Barker has now written a book for the non-specialist. He describes the scientific basis for the argument that improving the diet and health of young women will prevent coronary heart disease, stroke, and diabetes in the next generation; reviews the link between early infection and adult diseases; and presents strategies for preventing disease in the future.

ISBN 0 7279 0835 9   192 pages

FETAL AND INFANT ORIGINS OF ADULT DISEASE

Edited by D J P Barker

This collection of papers from the MRC Environmental Research Unit at Southampton University sets out the evidence that some adult diseases originate in impaired development during fetal life and infancy.

"This exciting book covers the ages of man, history, social change and diet, and thus impinges on many branches of medicine. It is of wide interest and is highly recommended." *Hospital Update*

ISBN 0 7279 0743 3   368 pages

For further details of these books and our full range of titles write to:

Marketing Department
BMJ Publishing Group
BMA House
Tavistock Square
London
WC1H 9JR

Or telephone Diana Chapple on 0171 383 6541